INTRAPARTUM
OBSTETRICS

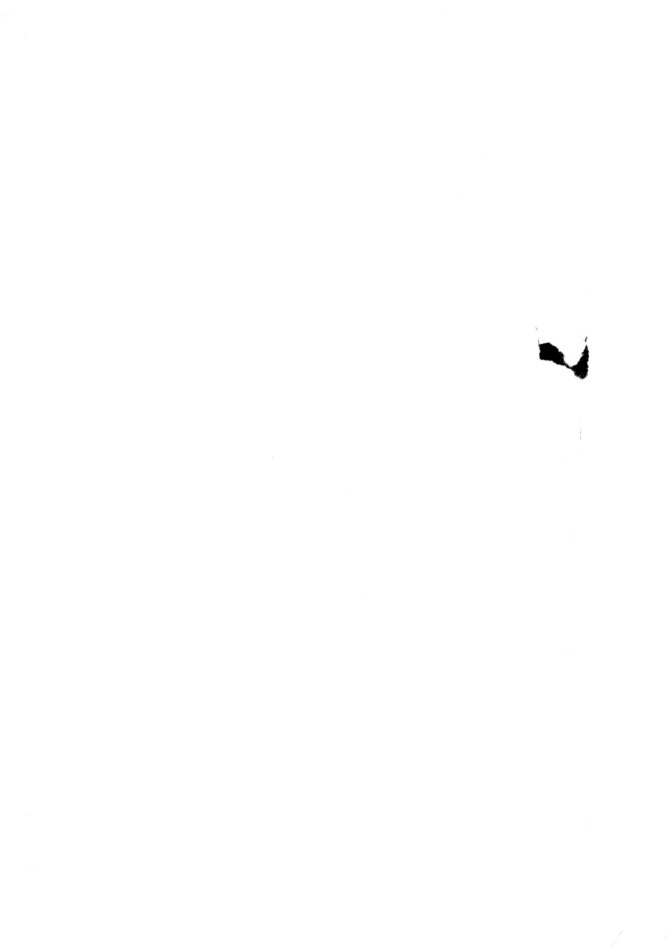

INTRAPARTUM OBSTETRICS

Edited by

JOHN T. REPKE, M.D.

Associate Professor
of Obstetrics, Gynecology,
and Reproductive Biology
Harvard Medical School
Director
Center for Labor and Birth
Department of Obstetrics
and Gynecology
Brigham and Women's Hospital
Boston, Massachusetts

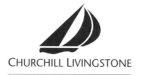

CHURCHILL LIVINGSTONE

New York, Edinburgh, London, Melbourne, San Francisco, Tokyo

Library of Congress Cataloging-in-Publication Data

Distributed in the United Kingdom by Churchill Livingstone, Robert Stevenson House, 1–3 Baxter's Place, Leith Walk, Edinburgh EH1 3AF,and by associated companies, branches, and representatives throughout the world.

Accurate indications, adverse reactions, and dosage schedules for drugs are provided in this book, but it is possible that they may change. The reader is urged to review the package information data of the manufacturers of the medications mentioned.

The Publishers have made every effort to trace the copyright holders for borrowed material. If they have inadvertently overlooked any, they will be pleased to make the necessary arrangements at the first opportunity.

Acquisitions Editor: *Jennifer Mitchell*
Production Editor: *Dorothy J. Birch*
Production Supervisor: *Sharon Tuder*
Cover Design: *Jeannette Jacobs*

Printed in the United States of America

First published in 1996   7 6 5 4 3 2 1

I would like to dedicate this book to more people than I can possibly name: to my parents, Jack and Rose, who provided me with the emotional and financial security to grow and develop; to Jaque, my wife, who has always been there when I needed her; to the late Richard J. Weber, Ph.D., who helped me to appreciate the beauty of science and medicine, and finally, to the OB/GYN residents of the Johns Hopkins Hospital and the Brigham and Women's Hospital, whose dedication and intellectual curiosity has always served to stimulate my own pursuit of excellence.

Contributors

Richard E. Besinger, M.D.
Associate Professor, Division of Maternal-Fetal Medicine, Department of Obstetrics and Gynecology, Loyola University of Chicago Stritch School of Medicine, Maywood, Illinois

Ronald T. Burkman, M.D.
Professor, Department of Obstetrics and Gynecology, Tufts University School of Medicine, Boston, Massachusetts; Chairman, Department of Obstetrics and Gynecology, Baystate Medical Center, Springfield, Massachusetts

Samuel Charache, M.D.
Professor, Departments of Medicine and Pathology, Johns Hopkins University School of Medicine; Director, Hematology Laboratory, Department of Pathology, Johns Hopkins Hospital, Baltimore, Maryland

Mary E. D'Alton, M.D.
Associate Professor, Department of Obstetrics and Gynecology, Tufts University School of Medicine; Chief, Division of Maternal Fetal Medicine, Department of Obstetrics and Gynecology, New England Medical Center Hospitals, Boston, Massachusetts

Sanjay Datta, M.D.
Professor of Anaesthesia, Harvard Medical School; Director, Obstetric Anesthesiology, Brigham and Women's Hospital, Boston, Massachusetts

Lawrence D. Devoe, M.D.
Director, Section of Maternal-Fetal Medicine, and Professor, Department of Obstetrics and Gynecology, Medical College of Georgia School of Medicine, Augusta, Georgia

John P. Elliott, M.D.
Professor, Department of Obstetrics and Gynecology, University of Arizona College of Medicine, Tucson, Arizona; Co-Director, Division of Maternal-Fetal Medicine, Department of Obstetrics and Gynecology, Good Samaritan Hospital, Phoenix, Arizona

Sebastian Faro, M.D., Ph.D.
Professor and Chairman, Department of Obstetrics and Gynecology, University of Kansas School of Medicine; Chairman, Department of Obstetrics and Gynecology, University of Kansas Medical Center, Kansas City, Kansas

Terry I. Feng, M.D., M.P.H.
Assistant Professor, Division of Maternal-Fetal Medicine, Department of Gynecology-Obstetrics, Emory University School of Medicine; Chief, Department of Obstetrics, Crawford W. Long Memorial Hospital, Atlanta, Georgia

James E. Ferguson II, M.D.
Director, Division of Maternal Fetal Medicine, Mamie A. Jessup Associate Professor, Department of Obstetrics and Gynecology, and Associate Professor, Department of Radiology, University of Virginia School of Medicine, Charlottesville, Virginia

Katherine S. Foley, M.D.

Fellow, Division of Maternal Fetal Medicine, Department of Obstetrics and Gynecology, Madigan Army Medical Center, Tacoma, Washington

Frederic D. Frigoletto, Jr., M.D.

Charles Montraville Green and Robert Montraville Green Professor of Obstetrics, Gynecology, and Reproductive Biology, Harvard Medical School; Chief, Vincent Memorial Obstetrics Division, Department of Obstetrics and Gynecology, Massachusetts General Hospital, Boston, Massachusetts

Bernard Gonik, M.D.

Professor and Associate Chairman, Department of Obstetrics and Gynecology, Wayne State University School of Medicine; Chief, Department of Obstetrics and Gynecology, Grace Hospital, Detroit, Michigan

Michael F. Greene, M.D.

Associate Professor of Obstetrics, Gynecology, and Reproductive Biology, Harvard Medical School; Director, Maternal-Fetal Medicine, Department of Obstetrics and Gynecology, Mass-achusetts General Hospital, Boston, Massachusetts

Janet B. Hardy, M.D., C.M.

Professor Emeritus, Department of Pediatrics, Johns Hopkins University School of Medicine; Past Director, Adolescent Pregnancy Programs, Johns Hopkins Hospital, Baltimore, Maryland

Stephen K. Hunter, M.D., Ph.D.

Fellow Associate, Department of Obstetrics and Gynecology, University of Iowa College of Medicine, Iowa City, Iowa

John W. C. Johnson, M.D.

Professor, Division of Maternal-Fetal Medicine, Department of Obstetrics and Gynecology, University of Florida College of Medicine, Gainesville, Florida

Timothy R. B. Johnson, M.D.

Chair and Bates Professor of Diseases of Women and Children, Department of Obstetrics and Gynecology, Research Scientist, Center for Human Growth and Development, University of Michigan Medical School, Ann Arbor, Michigan

Linda J. Kobokovich, R.N.C., M.Sc.N.

Clinical Specialist, Birthing Pavilion, Dartmouth-Hitchcock Medical Center, Lebanon, New Hampshire

Jerome N. Kopleman, M.D.

Assistant Professor, Department of Obstetrics and Gynecology, Uniformed Services University of the Health Sciences F. Edward Hébert School of Medicine, Bethesda, Maryland; Assistant Professor, Department of Obstetrics and Gynecology, University of Washington School of Medicine, Seattle, Washington; Chief and Fellowship Director, Division of Maternal Fetal Medicine, Department of Obstetrics and Gynecology, Madigan Army Medical Center, Tacoma, Washington

Mabel Koshy, M.D.

Professor, Department of Medicine, University of Illinois College of Medicine, Chicago, Illinois

E. Y. Kwawukuma, M.B, Ch.B., F.W.A.C.S.

Lecturer, Department of Obstetrics and Gynecology, University of Ghana Medical School; Consultant, Obstetrician, and Gynecologist, Department of Obstetrics and Gynecology, Korle Bu Teaching Hospital, Accra, Ghana

Ellice Lieberman, M.D.

Assistant Professor of Obstetrics, Gynecology, and Reproductive Biology, Harvard Medical School; Assistant Professor, Department of Maternal and Child Health, Harvard School of Public Health; Chief, Obstetric and Perinatal Epidemio-logy, Department of Obstetrics and Gynecology, Brigham and Women's Hospital, Boston, Massachusetts

Diane Lorant, M.D.

Assistant Professor, Department of Pediatrics, University of Utah School of Medicine, Salt Lake City, Utah

William C. Mabie, M.D.

Associate Professor, Division of Maternal-Fetal Medicine, Department of Obstetrics and Gynecology, University of Tennessee, Memphis, College of Medicine; Director, Obstetric Intensive Care Unit, Regional Medical Center at Memphis, Memphis, Tennessee

Glenn R. Markenson, M.D.

Assistant Chief, Division of Maternal Fetal Medicine, Department of Obstetrics and Gynecology, Tripler Army Medical Center, Honolulu, Hawaii

Arthur S. Maslow, D. O.

Chief, Antepartum Diagnostic Center, Division of Maternal Fetal Medicine, Department of Obstetrics and Gynecology, Madigan Army Medical Center, Tacoma, Washington

Richard Molteni, M.D.

Associate Professor, Department of Pediatrics, University of Utah School of Medicine; Director, Medical Services, Division of Neonatology, Department of Pediatrics, Primary Children's Medical Center, Salt Lake City, Utah

Peter E. Nielsen, M.D.

Clinical Instructor and Fellow, Division of Maternal-Fetal Medicine, Department of Obstetrics, Gynecology, and Reproductive Sciences, University of Texas Medical School at Houston, Houston, Texas

Lisa L. Paine, C.N.M., Dr.P.H.

Associate Professor, Department of Obstetrics and Gynecology, Boston University School of Medicine; Director, Nurse-Midwifery Education and Maternal and Child Health Programs, Boston University School of Public Health, Boston, Massachusetts

Thomas C. C. Peng, M.D.

Associate Professor, Division of Maternal-Fetal Medicine, Department of Obstetrics-Gynecology, Virginia Commonwealth University, Medical College of Virginia School of Medicine, Richmond, Virginia

Jeffrey P. Phelan, M.D.

Co-Director, Division of Maternal-Fetal Medicine, Department of Obstetrics and Gynecology, Pomona Valley Hospital Medical Center, Pomona, California; Co-Director, Division of Maternal-Fetal Medicine, Department of Obstetrics and Gynecology, San Antonio Community Hospital, Upland, California

Eva Pressman, M.D.

Assistant Professor, Department of Gynecology-Obstetrics, Johns Hopkins University School of Medicine; Director, Obstetrics Clinics, Department of Gynecology and Obstetrics, Johns Hopkins Hospital, Baltimore, Maryland

William F. Rayburn, M.D.

John W. Records Chair, Professor, and Chief, Section of Maternal/Fetal Medicine, Department of Obstetrics and Gynecology, University of Oklahoma College of Medicine, Oklahoma City, Oklahoma

Jaque R. Repke, R.N.C., M.S.

Clinical Director, Perinatal/GYN Nursing, New England Medical Center, Boston, Massachusetts

John T. Repke, M.D.

Associate Professor of Obstetrics, Gynecology, and Reproductive Biology, Harvard Medical School; Director, Center for Labor and Birth, Department of Obstetrics and Gynecology, Brigham and Women's Hospital, Boston, Massachusetts

Jo-Anna L. Rorie, C.N.M., M.S.N., M.P.H.

Assistant Professor, Nurse-Midwifery Education and Maternal and Child Health Programs, Boston University School of Public Health, Boston, Massachusetts; Senior Nurse-Midwife, Dimock Community Health Center, Roxbury, Massachusetts

Kenneth J. Ryan, M.D.

Kate Macy Ladd Distinguished Professor of Obstetrics, Gynecology, and Reproductive Biology, Harvard Medical School; Chairman, Ethics Committee, Brigham and Women's Hospital, Boston, Massachusetts

Leonard E. Safon, M.D.

Associate Clinical Professor of Obstetrics, Gynecology, and Reproductive Biology, Harvard Medical School; Attending Obstetrician-Gynecologist, Department of Obstetrics and Gynecology, Brigham and Women's Hospital, Boston, Massachusetts.

Philip Samuels, M.D.

Director, Maternal-Fetal Medicine Fellowship Training, Associate Director, Obstetrics and Gynecology Residency Program, Associate Professor, Division of Maternal-Fetal Medicine, Department of Obstetrics and Gynecology, Ohio State University College of Medicine, Columbus, Ohio

Thomas D. Shipp, M.D.

Instructor of Obstetrics, Gynecology, and Reproductive Biology, Harvard Medical School; Assistant, Vincent Memorial Obstetrics and Gynecology Service, Massachusetts General Hospital, Boston, Massachusetts

Lynn L. Simpson, M.D.

Fellow, Division of Maternal Fetal Medicine, Department of Obstetrics and Gynecology, Tufts University School of Medicine; Instructor, Division of Maternal Fetal Medicine, Department of Obstetrics and Gynecology, New England Center Hospitals, Boston, Massachusetts

Thomas H. Strong, Jr., M.D.

Associate Professor, Department of Obstetrics and Gynecology, University of Arizona College of Medicine, Tucson, Arizona; Associate Director, Phoenix Perinatal Associates, Phoenix, Arizona

John M. Thorp, Jr., M.D.

Assistant Professor, Division of Maternal and Fetal Medicine, Department of Obstetrics-Gynecology, University of North Carolina at Chapel Hill School of Medicine; Attending Physician, Department of Obstetrics and Gynecology, University of North Carolina Hospitals, Chapel Hill, North Carolina

Michael Trautman, M.D.

Associate Professor, Department of Pediatrics, University of Utah School of Medicine; Director, Neonatal Life Flight, Division of Neonatology, Department of Pediatrics, Primary Children's Medical Center, Salt Lake City, Utah

Carl P. Weiner, M.D.

Director, Division of Maternal-Fetal Medicine, and Professor, Departments of Obstetrics and Gynecology, University of Iowa College of Medicine, Iowa City, Iowa

Bruce A. Work, M.D.

Professor, Section of Maternal-Fetal Medicine, Department of Obstetrics and Gynecology, Medical College of Georgia School of Medicine, Augusta, Georgia

Carolyn M. Zelop, M.D.

Instructor of Obstetrics, Gynecology, and Reproductive Biology, Harvard Medical School, Boston, Massachusetts

Preface

The term *intrapartum obstetrics* can have different meanings for different individuals. My original concept for this book was not simply management of labor and delivery, but integrated management of patient care in labor and delivery units as they are utilized today. Those of us actively engaged in clinical obstetrics and perinatology know well that the labor and delivery unit has become much more than a place simply for management of labor and delivery. It has become a center for screening health and disease, for counseling of bereaved families who have lost a newborn, for critical care management of patients with medical complications that even two decades ago would have precluded delivery of a viable infant, for management of antepartum medical complications of pregnancy, and yes, a center for the management of uncomplicated labor and delivery.

With that in mind, I embarked on a project that has culminated with the production of this book, *Intrapartum Obstetrics,* which can be useful to clinical practitioners who work in labor and delivery units in the management of patients who fit any and all of the above categories. In putting this work together, I have tried to make it sufficiently encyclopedic to serve as a resource for factual information pertaining to management decision making as well as a practical guide to obstetric management. Both goals could only have been accomplished with the participation of the group of experts who agreed to donate their knowledge and time to the completion of this book. It is my hope that the readers of this book will appreciate the complexity of the decision-making process in high risk obstetrics and how opinions may differ from individual to individual, and institution to institution.

I have tried to solicit contributions from those experts recognized as leaders in the field of obstetrics and perinatology, nursing, and midwifery. For their part, they have all unselfishly given of themselves, their knowledge, and their clinical opinions to help in the completion of this book.

In addition to the unending gratitude I offer to my co-professionals who have helped in completing a valuable contribution to the obstetric literature, I would like to take this opportunity to thank the publishers and production editors at Churchill Livingstone, specifically Jennifer Mitchell, Jennifer Hardy, Bridgett Dickinson, and Dorothy J. Birch, whose support and patience were instrumental in the development and completion of this book. Additionally, I would like to thank the secretarial and professional staff of the Brigham and Women's Hospital for providing me with an environment conducive to the completion of such a monumental task. I would also like to thank Mikki Senkarik for her excellent illustrations, for her suggestions, and for her occasional "faxed cartoons" that were a frequent source of amusement during the sometimes stressful process of editing.

This is what I hope will be the first of many editions of *Intrapartum Obstetrics.* I hope its readers will find that it does fulfill its mission and serves their needs well and that our patients are the ultimate beneficiaries.

John T. Repke, M.D.

Contents

Chapter 1

A Brief History of Modern Obstetrics

John T. Repke

The evolution of modern obstetrics is indeed an interesting one. Obstetricians, or midwives as they were called in earlier times, occupied a particularly mysterious place within the realm of medicine. Two thousand years ago, the major role of the midwife was not to assist women in difficult childbirth, but to comfort them until they died.[1] A review of medical history is striking in terms of how the practice of obstetrics has changed and how the human relationships within it have been altered. In the succeeding pages, experts in the field have provided an outline of how modern obstetrics is practiced and how medically complicated pregnancies are managed.

CONDUCT OF NORMAL LABOR AND DELIVERY

"The cardinal rule for good midwifery is to be scrupulously clean," wrote Baas in 1889.[2] Asepsis remains an important part of modern obstetric practice. In past times, however, most deliveries did not occur in hospitals. This becomes apparent as one peruses older obstetrics textbooks and finds separate chapters devoted to the contents of the obstetrics kit. A review of the suggested "kit" at the Rotunda Hospital in the mid-19th century reveals a lengthy list of equipment. It is noteworthy that Tweedy and Wrench, addressing obstetricians in 1908, asserted that "the first business to which you have to attend when a pregnant woman asks you to conduct her

childbirth is to get a nurse."[2] Perhaps some things have not changed that much after all.

MANAGEMENT OF LABOR

It is interesting that in our current era of high technology, in which interventions abound, a look back at history shows that the most important function of the obstetrician was to do nothing. Hirst[3] states that:

> Everyone in possession of a medical diploma is popularly supposed to possess the ability to manage a labor case, and everyone who essays the practice of medicine would have his ability put to the proof before his medical career has run a very long course. To a beginner in obstetric practice there is much that is trying and embarrassing. . . . Some consolation however, can always be found in the reflection that labor is a natural and a comparatively easy process in the large majority of cases; that a physician's duty is one mainly of inaction and non-interference and that most probably the labor will terminate fortunately for mother and child in spite of his inexperience.

Another perspective is offered by Parvin,[4] who states that:

> In cases of labor for time advancing favorably, sudden accidents imperilling the life of mother or of

1

Contents of the Obstetrics Kit of the Rotunda Hospital, Dublin (1908)

Bonds forceps with Neville's axis-traction

Martin's needle holder

Large and small curved needles for perineum and cervix

Large and small Bozemann's catheters

Rheinstadter's flushing spoon curette

Bullet forceps

A pair of stout sharp point scissors

Small scissors

Plucking forceps

Two glass vaginal nozzles

Two needles for infusion under the breast

A metal female catheter

A No. 12 or 14 gum elastic male catheter

Carton's mucus catheter

Baby's silver catheter

A pocket lancet

A small trocar and cannula

Rotunda douche

Rubber gloves

Nail brushes

Infusion apparatus

Sterile cat gut

Chloroform

Opium tabloids

Sodium chloride soloids for infusion

Biniodide of mercury tabloids

Squibb's ergot

Creolin

Lysol

Duhrssen's tins of iodoform gauze

Sterile wadding

A hypodermic kit with morphia, strychnine, ergotinine, digitalin, cocaine, and atropine

A small bottle of brandy for hypodermic injections

A small bottle of ether for hypodermic injections

Stout binder pins

A batist apron

Soap

(From Tweedy and Wrench[2] with permission)

---

child may arise, and professional knowledge and skill be needed to meet them; while the common role of the obstetrician is to observe, to control, to alleviate, and to protect, emergencies may come which demand his promptest action and greatest ability, though it is only in a small minority of births, not more than 5 per cent, [that] any other interference is required."

One is also struck by the manner in which obstetricians from a bygone era emphasized the importance of anatomy and clinical judgement, and the responsibility of the obstetrician to the mother and also, although clearly secondarily, to the fetus. To appreciate the evolution of obstetrics, one need only re-

view the brief monograph by Landis.[5] Intended for use as a review book for medical students and physicians, the monograph makes some things readily apparent, such as the emphasis on anatomy and physiology that persists today, yet in other ways illustrates how far the practice of obstetrics has come. Examples of some of Landis's questions are presented in the boxed list below. What becomes more apparent at the dawn of the 20th century is the ability of medicine to begin to deal with the medical complications of pregnancy, previously largely ignored because the frequent result was the death of the mother or fetus, or both. A review of the table of contents of the first edition of Williams's textbook of obstetrics,[6] published in 1904, shows that nearly all of the book is

---

Selected Review Questions of Landis (1887)

1. What is obstetrics? The science and art of affording aid to women in labor.
2. What is meant by science and art? The science of obstetrics embraces the definite rules of procedure founded upon a correct knowledge of the nature of labor and its complications; the art consists in a skillful carrying out of these rules. The science may be taught in books and lectures; the art must be acquired by practice at the bedside.
3. What are the ordinary duties of the physician in a case of labor?
   a. To examine the woman and ascertain the exact state of affairs.
   b. To watch the progress of the case.
   c. During the first stage to encourage the woman, see that the bed is properly prepared, that due provision is made for the infant when born, and to keep others from meddling.
4. What is the fetal mortality in the breech presentation? From 30 to 50 percent.
5. How should transverse presentation be managed? We should not await any of the spontaneous methods, but turn the child to a vertex or breech presentation. If this is impossible, we would have to perforate the chest and reduce the size of the child (see embryotomy).
6. What are the dangers in placenta previa? Death of the mother from hemorrhage and of the child from asphyxia. The maternal mortality is one in four; fetal mortality one in two to three.
7. When a version fails in a transverse presentation, what alternative operation have we? Embryotomy.
8. What is embryotomy? The operation by which the size of the child is reduced by cutting and mutilation. It is now restricted to mutilation of the body; when applied to the head it is called craniotomy.
9. What are the indications for the cesarian section?
   a. A pelvis contracted by two inches in the conjugate, or obstructed by tumors, or other insurmountable obstacles to delivery by the natural way.
   b. For the rapid delivery of a supposed living child after the death of the mother. Children have been saved when the mother had been dead for more than one hour.

(From Landis,[5] with permission.)

---

devoted to anatomy and physiology, a substantial portion to pathology of labor, and only a relatively small portion to medical complications of pregnancy. At that time, those complications centered almost entirely on obstetric trauma, infection, and toxemia.

The following pages take the reader through the best knowledge that is available in modern obstetric medicine. By comparison with the textbooks of yesterday, the emphasis on technology is extraordinary. The changes in human relations and in the provider/patient relationship, and the relatively new emphasis on the fetus, have all worked to make obstetrics a markedly different specialty than the one practiced by our predecessors. Nonetheless, the importance of disseminating knowledge in obstetrics cannot be overstated. As one studies the past, writes about it, or engages in modern scientific and clinical research, one clearly sees the extraordinary responsibility of the obstetrician, still perhaps best summarized more than a century and a half ago by Burns[7] in *Principles of Midwifery:*

Should this work fall, only, into the hands of those competent to judge in their profession, it would, if faulty or deficient, do little harm; but, as it has been circulated extensively, it must, like other systems and elements, have an influence on the opinions, and future practice of the student of midwifery; and would prove useful or injurious to society, according to the correctness of the principles it contains.

REFERENCES

1. Baas JH: Outlines of the History of Medicine and the Medical Profession. (Handerson HE, Trans.) J.H. Vail, New York, 1889
2. Tweedy EH, Wrench GT: Rotunda Practical Midwifery. Oxford University Press, London, 1908
3. Hirst BC: A Textbook of Obstetrics. 2nd Ed. WB Saunders, Philadelphia, 1899
4. Parvin T: The Science and Art of Obstetrics. 2nd Ed. Lea Brothers, Philadelphia, 1890
5. Landis HG: A Compend of Obstetrics. 3rd Ed. P. Blakiston Son, Philadelphia, 1887
6. Williams JW: Obstetrics: A Textbook for the Use of Students and Practitioners. D. Appleton, New York, 1904
7. Burns J: The Principles of Midwifery; Including the Diseases of Women and Children. 10th Ed. Longman, Brown, Green, and Longmans, London, 1843

Chapter 2

Prenatal Care: Preparation for a Safe Childbirth

Janet B. Hardy

In this chapter, a public health or preventive approach is taken in the discussion of prenatal care. Such an approach is important, since good health both before and during pregnancy provides the foundation for a successful outcome. Additionally, prenatal care can provide an unparalleled opportunity for promoting good health practices which, while important to the outcome of the immediate and subsequent pregnancies, can continue beyond termination to the benefit of the mother and her family. The obstetric components of prenatal management are sketched only briefly, since excellent sources for this information exist elsewhere.[1-3] The major sources for this chapter are three publications and many years of research and programmatic experience with adolescent pregnancy, low-birth-weight (LBW) infants, and infant mortality. The publications include the following:

1. "Caring for Our Future, The Content of Prenatal Care," a report of the U.S. Public Health Service Select Panel on the Content of Prenatal Care.[1] Members of the Panel, prior to making recommendations, examined current practice in terms of the scientific evidence supporting each prenatal care activity and its relevance for the care of all pregnant women or only for some.
2. *New Perspectives in Prenatal Care*, published in 1990 and edited by Merkatz and Thompson.[4]

3. The 1985 report of the U.S. National Institute of Medicine's Committee on Preventing Low Birth Weight.[5]

Together, these three publications provide broad and detailed information about the objectives and content of prenatal care. An earlier U.S. Public Health Service report, "Promotion of Child Health: A National Strategy"[6] points out that "people are the assets of a society" and that "healthy newborns are a singularly important societal resource while those unable to function normally represent harm to society and, through loss of human capital, to the individual." Prenatal maternal care is recognized as an important pathway to a safe delivery and birth of a healthy infant. Others have been less emphatic in endorsing such care and have questioned its cost effectiveness, especially for healthy women.[5,7,8] Without detracting from the importance of good prenatal care, it has become increasingly clear that the ecologic context of a pregnancy is also an important determinant of both immediate and longer range outcome. Because comprehensive prenatal care can in part offset the adverse effects of poverty and social disadvantage, it is particularly important to poor women. From these and other sources, it is clear that

1. A strong consensus exists for the efficacy of good prenatal care in terms of improving the health

of the mother and fetus and reducing the risk of maternal and infant mortality and low neonatal birth weight.

2. Little scientific evaluation has been done on the effectiveness of the various components of prenatal care to guide the development of cost-effective programs by emphasizing effective components and discarding ineffective ones.

3. It seems likely that no one pattern of prenatal care will be cost effective in meeting the needs of all women.

4. Obstetrics, like other disciplines within the health care system, has reached a watershed. The system is changing in response to the lack of balance between highly specialized and highly expensive technologic medicine, which can often produce life-saving results for patients with major obstetric problems, and low-cost preventive strategies that could be applied to many more women, preventing many of those conditions that call for much of the expensive tertiary care required today.

The need for change in the United States in the content of prenatal care or access to such care, or both, is obvious from the 1989 ranking of the United States as 22nd in infant mortality and 31st in risk of LBW among westernized countries,[9] despite its being among the most affluent of all nations. More recent reports show continued but minimal improvement in the infant mortality rate[10] and an increase, particularly among black women, in the frequency of LBW infants.[11] The frequency of LBW in 1991 was 7.1 percent, the highest observed since 1978, with a 5.8 percent rate for white and 13.6 percent rate for black infants. While 7 percent of all infants are LBW, 60 percent of all infant deaths occur among LBW babies. Furthermore, among those LBW infants who survive the risk of short-term morbidity, long-term disability is two to three times that of infants of normal birth weight.[5] The frequencies of LBW and infant mortality vary widely among ethnic and socioeconomic groups in the United States. Rates for black women and those who are poor are much higher than the national average, and are comparable to those found in some less developed countries.[9]

Poverty in the United States has been increasing in recent years. Of the 4-million babies born each year, approximately 25 percent are born into families living below the federal poverty level.[9] Poor women are the least likely to be adequately nourished, to live under favorable environmental conditions, or to have the information required to protect their own health, and the most likely to engage in risk-taking behavior and to have inadequate prenatal care. Poor women of all ethnic groups are at a higher risk of complications of pregnancy, labor, and delivery.[4,5] The increased need for additional services for these women comes at a time of decreasing resources for intervention at federal, state, and local levels. A compelling reason for changes in the health-care system is the need to provide adequate maternal and infant care for all women and children.

HISTORICAL NOTE

Because the history of obstetrics both reinforces the perceived value of prenatal care and provides useful insights for the current status of such care a much abbreviated review of this history helpful. Throughout recorded history, pregnancy has been surrounded by cultural traditions, taboos, and myths. Traditionally, women giving birth were attended by other women, but before this century, information about their prenatal care was generally unavailable. Lacking understanding about reproduction and contraceptive methods, many women had large numbers of closely spaced children. Maternal, fetal, and infant mortality rates were extremely high. Eclampsia, dystocia, hemorrhage, and puerperal infection were major causes of maternal death. These conditions still prevail in some developing countries where family planning is not yet readily available and large family size is valued.

In westernized countries, the advent of scientific methods of medical care in the latter part of the 19th century, and their application to obstetrics, produced information about reproductive pathophysiology, diagnosis and treatment of disease, aseptic techniques, and anesthesia, which laid the foundation for modern obstetrics. Concomitant with the development of scientific medicine was a gradual change in the birthing process from a "natural" event assisted by midwives to a "medical" event controlled by physicians. During the latter half of the 20th century, the growth of scientific knowledge and technology has accelerated, and maternal mortality in the United States is now a rare event. In 1991, a year in which 4,110,907 births were recorded, only 323 maternal deaths were attributed to complications of pregnancy, the birth process, or the puerperium, for a rate of 7.9 deaths per 100,000 live births.[10] In less developed countries where professional obstetric care is generally not available, many women still die from complications of childbirth.

A forerunner of modern prenatal clinics was the clinic established in Dublin in 1858. Poor women who wanted hospital delivery were required to register some months before the expected delivery date to secure a bed. At registration, they were examined by a physician, and those with evidence of preeclampsia were admitted and treated with rest, fresh air, and good food. The frequency of eclampsia was much reduced among these women.[12] Similarly, poor women admitted during pregnancy to the Preston Retreat, which opened in Philadelphia in 1866, had more favorable outcomes than women who delivered in other Philadelphia hospitals.[13] It should be noted that Dr. William Goodall, organizer of the Preston Retreat, was the first physician in the United States to use antiseptic and aseptic techniques in obstetric practice.

Organized prenatal care in the United States was begun early in the 20th century by nurses and other women who saw the need for social reform and were concerned about the high rates of infant mortality among the poor.[4] As medical knowledge advanced, obstetricians and public-health physicians soon assumed control of such care. Initially the emphasis was on preventing maternal death. An early landmark in this evolution was a study reported in 1914 by Dr. J. Whitridge Williams[14] of 705 fetal deaths among 10,000 consecutive deliveries at the Johns Hopkins Hospital. The results suggested that organized prenatal care could reduce the frequency of fetal deaths by 40 percent. Williams postulated that competent obstetric evaluation coupled with health education during pregnancy would substantially reduce the hazards of toxemia, dystocia, and prematurity. Dr. Nicholson J. Eastman, William's successor at Johns Hopkins, credited the development of organized prenatal care "with having done more to save mother's lives than any other single factor."[15]

When the emphasis on preventing maternal mortality began to be successful, a shift to preventing infant mortality began. In 1918, the New York Maternity Center Association was established to oversee the development of maternity centers for all of Manhattan. A 1921 study of the 8,743 women who had received prenatal and postnatal care through the Centers showed a 30 percent reduction in neonatal deaths and a 21.5 percent reduction in maternal mortality.[4] The work of the public-health nurses was viewed as an essential ingredient in the success of these centers. These nurses had responsibility for finding pregnant women, gaining their confidence, and imparting to them an understanding about the value of medical care. In 1922, Dr. Lobenstine described the components necessary for good prenatal care.[16] Included were an examination by a physician as early as possible in pregnancy; a visit with a social worker for poor women; regular home visits by a public-health nurse throughout pregnancy; hospital admission for intercurrent illness or complications; and hospital delivery for all abnormal pregnancies. The Metropolitan Life Insurance Company found home visits to pregnant and postpartum women to be cost effective, and this practice continued from 1909 to 1952.[17]

In 1909, the U.S. Government became involved in improving outcomes for poor women and children. The first White House Conference on Dependent Children was convened. An important outcome of this conference was the establishment of a federal Children's Bureau. Among the first initiatives of the new bureau were studies to determine the causes of infant mortality. Two findings from these studies are noteworthy. One linked infant mortality with poverty. The other demonstrated that prenatal care enhanced infant survival.[18] The first publication by the Children's Bureau was titled "Prenatal Care"; it appeared in 1925 and became a classic, promulgating standards for the medical and educational components of prenatal visits. Dr. Lobenstine was among the physicians whose advice the Bureau sought in defining standards for prenatal care.[19] Standards proposed in the 1980s differ relatively little from those the Bureau published in 1925. During the Second World War, the services of the Children's Bureau were extended by the development of the Emergency Maternity and Infant Care Program (EMIC), which provided free, high-quality care for the wives and children of military servicemen in the lowest four pay grades.

Other important federal initiatives included the Sheppard-Towner Maternity and Infant Protection Act of 1921,[20] which strengthened the public health role by providing federal and state funding for instruction about nutrition and hygiene in pregnancy, child health clinics, and public-health nurse visits to pregnant women and children. Unfortunately, for poor women, it was terminated after 7 years, largely as the result of intensive lobbying by the American Medical Association, as physicians apparently felt threatened by the Act's emphasis on public-health services.[4] Even though the funds were withdrawn, the interest generated by this program continued and helped in the passage of the Social Security Act of 1935, which led to the development of Title V. This important law, which continues to exist, provides joint federal/state funding to promote maternal and child health and provide services for crippled children. Notwithstanding these government initiatives, poor women and children in the United States have not generally had the unrestricted access to the preventive pregnancy, and infant care available to all women in most westernized countries. In recent years, access to such care has become even more difficult for American women, and the proportion without prenatal care has increased.[9] Because of escalating malpractice costs, inadequate Medicaid reimbursement, and burdensome paperwork, some obstetricians have withdrawn from providing services to poor women. In 1987, 17 percent of all births were subsidized by Medicaid.[4] Recent efforts to improve reimbursement and access by adjusting eligibility have been helpful, but much more is needed.

In the period since the Second World War, major changes have occurred in obstetrics, including continuing emphasis on research and technical advances, with implications for acute obstetric and intensive perinatal care and preventive efforts to improve maternal health and pregnancy outcome. During this period, however, the roles of the public-health nurse and nonprofessional home visitor have declined. Recent studies by Olds[21] and others[22] indicate the preventive value of home visits to poor families during pregnancy and infancy, and nationally supported special programs such as Healthy Start

have reintroduced this useful practice as a part of prenatal care.

In 1983, the American College of Obstetricians and Gynecologists (ACOG) collaborated with the Academy of Pediatrics in producing *Guidelines for Perinatal Care.*[2] This volume and its subsequent editions are based on the concept of a coordinated, multidisciplinary approach to perinatal care within a regionalized system of care. This approach is based on the provision of the level of care, whether primary, secondary, or tertiary, required for the management of each woman's pregnancy and delivery.

Levels of Prenatal Care

Level I, *primary care:* Appropriate for the normal, healthy, low-risk woman who can be expected to have a normal pregnancy.

Level II, *secondary care:* Appropriate for women considered to be at moderate risk of pregnancy complications that can be managed at the community level when adequate care is available

Level III, *tertiary care:* Desirable for women and fetuses considered to be at high obstetric risk, and requires highly sophisticated care by trained personnel

---

This regional system has worked well in terms of the provision of better care for pregnant women and infants through the establishment of facilities and expertise in the management of high-risk pregnancies and neonates. Maternal and infant mortality have been reduced. The system has also facilitated research relating to maternal, fetal, and neonatal medicine and the postgraduate education of physicians, nurses, and public-health and allied health personnel. However, change in the system appears to be necessary in response to the changing patterns in the provision of medical services and the increasing development of health maintenance organizations (HMOs) and similar systems that stress continuity of primary care and cost containment. While primary preventive care for all pregnant women should be a major goal, the maintenance of a system of high-risk perinatal care is essential for the optimal management of high-risk pregnancies and for the training of the highly specialized personnel on whom optimal care and research depend.

The success of the regional system has depended on (1) initial and periodic patient evaluation, with maternal and fetal risk assessment throughout pregnancy, so that potential problems can be identified early and patients transferred to facilities with the capability to deal with the individual's level of risk; (2) an understanding of different regional systems and coordination between levels of care so that patient transfer can be facilitated; (3) a regional system of emergency transport for high-risk women and their fetus before delivery (preferably before labor), and of sick or tiny newborn infants at high risk of mortality. The major emphasis has become fetal survival. Although an essential goal of the regional system is to optimize outcome for high-risk infants (and reduce disability among survivors), emphasis on the primary prevention of conditions leading to maternal and fetal complications should be of even greater importance.

PROVIDERS OF PRENATAL CARE

Obstetricians/Gynecologists

A woman's socioeconomic status and the area of the country in which she lives largely determine the type of reproductive health and pregnancy care she receives. A major component of this is the providers of prenatal care. Specially trained and certified obstetrician/gynecologists provide pregnancy and delivery care for most American women, particularly those above the poverty level. The setting in which prenatal care is provided (i.e., the organizational structure whether private practice, HMO, public-health clinic, hospital clinic) and the availability of obstetric and other medical specialists help to determine the services that family physicians, certified nurse midwives (CNMs), nurses, and other personnel provide. As stated above, adequate services are essential for patients perceived to be at obstetric risk.

Certified Nurse Midwives

Since the 1950s, CNMs have begun to play an increasingly important role in obstetric care in hospital and prenatal care settings. In recent years, free-standing birthing facilities staffed by CNMs, backed up by certified obstetricians, have begun to provide prenatal and delivery services for women with normal, low-risk pregnancies who prefer to deliver in a more "natural," home-like environment. These deliveries make up only a small fraction of all deliveries. Pregnancy and the birthing process in the United States are largely controlled by obstetricians and other physicians, but it seems clear that CNMs can and will play increasingly important roles in these areas, in part because women appreciate the added time spent with them and the breadth of midwife services, and in part as a response to the increasing emphasis on the preventive and social aspects of medical services, service areas in which CNMs are very effective. However, in view of the increased time that midwives generally spend with pregnant women and of recent, justified increases in nursing salaries, it is unlikely that prenatal care by midwives will be significantly less expensive than that provided by physicians.

Family Physicians

Approximately 50 percent of general and family physicians provide obstetric services for their patients and receive approximately 20 percent of visits for pre- and postnatal care.[4] These services are a logical extension of these physicians' continuing care for all family members. Their services are particularly important in rural areas and areas with large proportions of patients from lower socioeconomic backgrounds; their effectiveness depends on referral of high-risk patients for specialized obstetric care.

Ancillary Services

During the second half of the 20th century, increasing sophistication in pregnancy planning and in controlling the birth of undesired, ill-timed, or potentially defective children through contraception, abortion, and female and male sterilization have contributed in a major although unquantifiable way to reductions in both maternal and infant mortality.

DETERMINANTS OF PREGNANCY OUTCOME

A variety of factors influence pregnancy outcome. Pregnancy and childbirth are special times for women in which many experience joy, happy expectation and a sense of accomplishment. For others, however, pregnancy and childbirth are times of depression and even despair. For all women, whether the pregnancy was planned and was wanted or not, these events represent major changes in the course of their lives, requiring personal, physiologic, and emotional, as well as family, adjustments. Although they are "natural" events, their successful conclusion depends on many factors, both intrinsic and extrinsic to the pregnant woman. An understanding of these factors is the foundation on which optimal care is based. Because women's characteristics and backgrounds vary widely, as do those factors that determine pregnancy risk, care during preg-

nancy must be both flexible and broadly based to meet individual needs. The goal of prenatal care should be primarily preventive and directed at identifying problems that may jeopardize maternal or fetal health (or both), through health promotion and the earliest possible identification of risk factors so that they may be eliminated or their potentially adverse effects mitigated.

Determinants of pregnancy outcome are shown in Figure 2-1 and detailed in Table 2-1. Characteristics in the areas indicated have been shown in many studies to be associated with pregnancy outcome, including stillbirth, neonatal death, preterm delivery, and LBW.[5,23,26] It should be noted that risk factors associ-

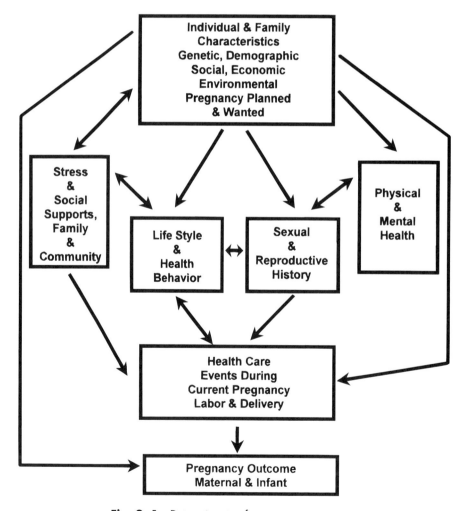

Fig. 2–1. Determinants of pregnancy outcome.

Table 2-1. Theoretical Construct for the Examination of Factors that Determine Maternal and Infant Outcomes, Proximal and Ultimate[a]

Maternal Factors	Obstetrical Factors	Placental Function	Factors Influencing Initiation of Labor and Delivery	Infant Outcome
Culture—SES	Prenatal Care	Blood flow	At term 37+ wk.	Proximal
Age	Time of registration	Size/weight	Premature <37 wk.	Preterm
Education	Type of care	Implantation	Very premature	delivery, low
Marital status	Number of visits	site	delivery <32 wk.	birthweight,
Medical	Special programs	Pathology		intrauterine
assistance	Nutrition	Previa		growth
Source of care	WIC, food stamps	Abruption		retardation
Income	Weight gain	Infection		Congenital
Physical	Obstetric risk factors	Infarction		malformation
characteristics	History of spontaneous	Membranes		Immaturity
Height	abortion	Infection		Injury
Prepregnant	History of prior LBW infant			Sick
weight	History of stillbirth, neonatal			Ultimate Outcome
General health	death			Neonatal death
Weight gain	Parity (high)			Intrauterine
Behavior	Incompetent cervix			infant death
Smoking	Genital malformation			Neurologic
Alcohol	Bleeding			deficit
Eating habits	Blood volume (hypovolemia)			Cognitive
Exercise	Premature rupture of			deficit
Drugs	membranes			Unimpaired
Stress and social	Other medical conditions			
support	Hypertension			
Environmental	Sexually transmitted disease,			
Toxins (e.g.,	vaginitis			
lead)	Heart disease			
Trauma	Diabetes			
Family violence	Endocrine problems			
Sexual abuse	Anemia (type)			
	Viral infections			
	Antenatal hospital admission			

[a] The effect of maternal characteristics on outcome is mediated through obstetrical factors, placental function, and those that determine the initiation of labor.

ated with adverse pregnancy outcome may be directly and independently related to specific outcomes, as in the case of cigarette smoking and LBW, or may, through their association with some other, independently related variable, be "markers" for risk. For example, our studies have shown low maternal age (<18 years) to have no direct relationship with LBW.[27] However, LBW is strongly and independently related to socioeconomic status. Because most adolescents (<18 years at delivery) are poor, maternal age is a useful marker of social risk. However, the mechanisms responsible for the relationships between poverty and pregnancy outcome have not been clearly defined.

Working in collaboration with James McCarthy, Ph.D. and John T. Repke, M.D., we have developed material relating to individual risk factors for LBW and infant mortality. Material was derived from a study population of 14,509 women and their infants, identified by Certificate of Live Birth, who were resident in Baltimore City, and who delivered a single, live-born infant of known gestational age on the obstetric service of the Johns Hopkins Hospital between 1979 and the end of 1986. Of these women,

12,266 were black and 2,243 were white; 8 percent of the black and 54 percent of the white women were private patients. The remainder were from the surrounding, socially disadvantaged community, and most were eligible for Medicaid coverage of obstetric care. Black women in the study had similar risks of LBW and infant mortality to those in Baltimore City as a whole, but the white women had considerably higher rates of infant mortality than all white residents of the city, partly reflecting the referral of high-risk obstetric-patients for tertiary care and partly reflecting the low socioeconomic status of white women from the community.

The data were drawn from matched birth and infant-death records; computerized obstetric and neonatal summaries; and maternal and infant hospital records. Contextual variables from the 1980 census provided the characteristics of the census tract of the mother's residence. Statistical methods used in the study employed descriptive and multivariate techniques, particularly multiple-regression analysis, with emphasis on the prediction of LBW and infant mortality from maternal characteristics. The study has been described elsewhere.[28] Because of the overriding effect of fetal gestational age and birth weight on mortality, and the effect of obstetrical complications on preterm delivery (PTD) and LBW, a number of multivariate equations were designed to examine the effect of maternal characteristics on outcome in four domains: sociodemographic, behavioral, physical, and obstetric. The results are summarized in Tables 2-2 through 2-4.

Table 2-2 shows the distributions and simple associations between selected maternal demographic, physical, and behavioral characteristics and infant death rates per 1,000 live births for each ethnic group separately. Table 2-3 shows similarly arranged data for selected obstetric characteristics. The bivariate analyses reflected in Tables 2-3 and 2-4 suggest that, with the exception of the analysis pertaining to young maternal age, most of the variables shown are related to infant mortality (and, in data not shown, to LBW). For example, women whose height was 60 in. or less, or whose prepregnant weight was less than 100 pounds, were at greater risk of adverse outcome than women with other heights or weights. Cigarette smoking was also associated with increased risk and, in this inner-city population, just over half the women smoked. Alcohol use, which was reported by

21 percent was not associated with increased risk. Delayed (third trimester) or no prenatal care, found in 16 percent of the population, increased the risk of infant mortality more than twofold.

Among obstetric characteristics, a history of spontaneous (but not induced) abortion was strongly associated with infant mortality in black women, but less so among white women. A history of delivery of a prior LBW infant was also associated with risk, as was a history of prior and existing medical conditions, including endocrine problems, heart disease, and asthma. Sexually transmitted diseases (STDs) and hypertension had no significant association with infant mortality. An amalgam of obstetric conditions that suggested a high obstetric risk (see the footnote in Table 2-3) was also significantly associated with infant mortality.

When the conditions were entered into logistic-regression models for sociodemographic, physical, behavioral, and obstetric risk factors as described above, somewhat similar findings remained. It is noteworthy that low maternal age (i.e., <18 years) was not a risk factor for infant mortality.

For some variables, substantial proportions of data were missing. When the frequency of missing data reached 8 percent or more, dummy variables to indicate missing information were entered into the multivariate equations. These missing values were found to be important indicators of risk, and show the need for caution in the statistical handling of missing information if bias is to be avoided.

Space does not permit a detailed description of the results for factors affecting infant mortality but two points must be made. One is that these results and those for similar analyses of LBW were generally in accord with the findings of other studies mentioned elsewhere in the text. The second is that the results emphasize the possibilities for prevention and the need for life-long preparation for optimal childbearing, at both the personal and societal levels.

Analyses such as those described above are in accord with the literature, and indicate areas in which pregnancy care can be effective. It should be noted that some of these factors (i.e., enduring poverty[29]) may well have antedated the onset of pregnancy, indicating the desirability of offsetting their effects before the onset of pregnancy.

Table 2-2. Infant Deaths in Relation to Selected Maternal Characteristics by Race[a]

Maternal Characteristic, Demographic	Black				White			
	Group		Infant Deaths		Group		Infant Deaths	
	n	%	n	Rate[b]	n	%	n	Rate[b]
Age (years)								
≤17	2,339	19.1	34	14.5	196	8.7	1	5.1
18–34	9,570	78.0	132	13.9	1,792	79.9	29	16.1
≥35	259	2.1	1	3.9	230	10.3	1	4.3
N.S.	98	0.8	1	10.2	25	1.1	0	0.0
Parity								
0	5,607	45.7	66	11.8	1,081	48.2	15	13.9
1	3,516	28.7	54	15.4	705	31.4	9	12.8
2+	3,143	25.6	48	15.3	457	20.4	7	15.3
Age/parity risk[c]								
Low	11,609	94.6	155	13.3	2,152	95.9	29	13.4
High	657	5.4	13	19.8	91	4.1	2	22.0
Marital status								
Married	1,908	15.6	17	8.9	1,452	64.7	23	15.9
Single	10,358	84.4	151	14.6	791	35.3	8	10.1
Education (yr)								
<12	5,616	45.8	86	15.3	711	31.7	9	12.6
≥12	5,623	45.8	59	10.4	1,342	59.8	16	12.0
Not stated	1,027	8.4	23	22.4	190	8.5	190	31.6
Prenatal care status								
Private	934	7.6	7	7.5	1,219	54.4	10	8.2
Clinic	10,772	87.9	134	12.5	977	43.6	19	19.4
None	533	4.6	27	48.2	47	2.1	2	42.0
Height (in.)								
≤60	630	5.1	10	15.9	89	4.0	1	11.2
60–68	10,767	87.8	135	12.6	1,985	88.6	23	10.2
≥69	389	3.2	2	5.1	94	4.2	2	21.2
N.S.	459	3.9	21	43.8	75	3.3	5	66.7
Prepregnant weight (lb)								
<100	654	5.3	10	15.3	92	4.1	1	10.9
100–119	2,920	23.9	34	11.6	591	26.4	6	10.2
120–179	5,056	41.2	60	11.9	1,048	46.7	10	9.5
≥180	875	7.1	13	14.9	127	5.7	1	7.9
Not stated	2,752	22.0	51	18.6	385	17.2	13	33.8
Used cigarettes								
No	5,983	48.8	69	11.5	1,293	57.7	14	10.8
Yes	6,283	51.2	99	15.7	950	42.3	17	17.9
Used alcohol								
No	9,639	78.6	132	13.7	1,496	66.7	21	14.0
Yes	2,627	21.4	36	13.7	747	33.3	10	13.4
Late/no prenatal care								
No	10,313	84.1	122	11.8	2,029	90.5	26	12.8
Yes	1,953	15.9	46	23.6	214	9.5	5	23.4
Total	12,266	100	168	13.7	2,243	100	31	13.8

[a] Single live births of known gestational age, n = 14,509.

[b] Numbers expressing rates per 1,000 live births have been rounded.

[c] High age/parity risk for all births to adolescents <16 years of age; multiparous births to 16- and 17-year-old patients; ≥3 births to 18- and 19-year-old patients; ≥4 births to women ≥20 years of age.

Table 2-3. Infant Deaths in Relation to Selected Obstetrical Characteristics by Race[a]

	Black				White			
	Group		Infant Deaths		Group		Infant Deaths	
Obstetrical Characteristics	n	%	n	Rate[b]	n	%	n	Rate[b]
History of spontaneous abortion								
No	10,466	85.3	134	12.8	1,834	81.8	24	13.6
Yes	1,800	14.7	34	18.9	409	18.2	6	14.6
History of prior low birthweight infant								
No	11,184	91.2	141	12.6	2,114	94.3	29	13.7
Yes	1,082	8.8	27	15.0	129	5.8	2	15.5
Hypertension								
No	11,111	90.6	158	14.3	2,068	92.2	27	13.1
Yes	1,155	9.4	10	8.7	175	7.8	4	13.8
Other medical conditions								
No	10,381	84.6	135	13.0	1,957	87.6	25	12.8
Yes	1,885	15.4	33	17.5	283	12.8	6	21.0
Significant bleeding before labor								
No	12,010	97.9	147	11.0	1,203	98.2	28	12.7
Yes	256	2.1	21	82	40	1.8	3	75.0
PROM >12 hours								
No	11,673	95.2	150	12.8	2,159	96.3	28	12.9
Yes	593	4.8	18	30.3	84	3.7	3	35.7
High obstetric risk[c]								
No	8,473	69.1	82	9.7	1,698	75.7	17	10.1
Yes	3,790	30.9	86	22.7	548	24.3	14	25.7

PROM, premature rupture of membranes.
[a] Single live births of known gestational age n = 14,509.
[b] Numbers expressing rates per 1,000 live births have been rounded.
[c] High risk, high age/parity risk, prior spontaneous abortion, prior low birthweight prepregnant weight <100, hypertension, other medical conditions.

PRECONCEPTION CARE

A major recommendation of the Expert Panel on the Content of Prenatal Care[1] is that women should be encouraged to make a preconceptual medical visit or seek such care as part of their ongoing primary health care. Because the purpose of the visit is to ensure that women begin their pregnancy in optimal health, its content is directed toward risk assessment and the reduction of risk.

Sites for Preconception Care

Several venues in addition to the offices of obstetrician/gynecologists and CNMs exist for achieving these objectives. Ideally, because health and well-being from birth to adulthood have a major impact on a woman's ability to have a healthy pregnancy, primary care-givers, such as pediatricians, internists, and family practitioners, have key roles in this objective. Family planning and STD clinics, as well as other health services for women and girls, are alternative medical-care sites. Educational and health services in schools and colleges also have the potential to help young women prepare for healthy pregnancies. Routine medical contacts with nonpregnant adolescents and adult women should include an inquiry into plans for childbearing. As pointed out by Summers and Price,[30] family-planning clinics facilitate reaching adolescents and low-income women. Places providing pregnancy-testing services usually offer counseling and make appropriate referrals for

Table 2-4. Determinants of Infant Mortality: Results of Logistic Regression Analysis

Maternal/Obstetric Characteristics	Relative Risk	Confidence Interval
Age (yr)		
≤17	0.74	0.88–1.74
≥18	1.00	
Parity		
0	1.04	0.70–1.55
1	1.11	0.76–1.61
2+	1.00	
Marital status		
Single	1.18	0.79–1.76
Married	1.00	
Education (yr)		
0–9	0.97	0.53–1.76
10–12	1.05	0.65–1.72
13+	1.00	
Unknown	1.81	1.01–3.25
Race		
Black	1.00	
White	0.79	0.51–1.22
Late/no prenatal care	1.52	1.07–1.91
Height (in.)		
≤60	1.19	0.64–2.21
60–68	1.00	
≤69	1.68	1.08–2.59
Prepregnant weight (lb)		
<100	1.2	0.8–2.6
100–179	1.00	
180+	1.15	0.66–2.02
Unknown	1.65	1.13–2.39
Used cigarettes	1.42	1.05–1.91
Used alcohol	.89	0.62–1.24
History of spontaneous abortion	1.36	0.94–1.95
History of prior low birthweight	1.73	1.13–2.64
Hypertension	.78	0.45–1.36
Other medical conditions	1.45	1.02–2.08

patients with positive tests. Those who test negatively should also be counseled about appropriate contraception or preconception care. As shown by Zabin,[31] adolescents with a "pregnancy scare" are at risk of a subsequent unintended pregnancy. Health services offered in industries employing large numbers of women and occupational health centers are also sites where preconception care or referral for such care could be provided as part of health-promotion activities.

Content of Preconceptual Care

Preconceptual screening procedures for all women cover risk factors for adverse pregnancy outcome, and are similar to those recommended by ACOG[3] and the Select Panel on the Content of Prenatal Care.[1] Screening procedures should include (1) a historical review of each woman's background in terms of demographic, economic, psychosocial, and life-style characteristics; and (2) a medical and reproductive assessment by history and physical examination, including pelvic and breast examinations and certain laboratory tests. For women with high-risk life styles or potential genetic or environmental risks, additional tests may be indicated. These include screening for illicit drugs; syphilis, gonorrhea, and other infections that may be sexually transmitted (chlamydia, herpes simplex, hepatitis B, human immunodeficiency virus, [HIV], cytomegalovirus [CMV]); tuberculosis; and toxoplasmosis; tests for hemoglobinopathies; and tests for potential genetic problems as indicated by history. The screening results should be discussed with the woman and plans made for any remediation that may be indicated.

Another important component of the visit is education and counseling to promote a healthy life-style by practicing good nutrition, reasonable exercise, and "safer" sex, and by avoiding cigarettes, alcohol, and drugs. Risks attendant on family violence and sexual abuse should also be considered, and appropriate referrals made.

In summary, preconception care should ideally be a part of ongoing primary care, but as many women do not receive preconception care and counseling in the course of their routine health care or in other contacts with health-care providers, a preconception visit is advised to ensure that a woman enters pregnancy in optimal condition for childbearing.

As recommended by the Select Panel, the male partner should be included in the preconceptual planning, particularly in its educational and counseling components to promote both his own health and that of his partner. His participation will also help to enhance compliance by his partner.

PREGNANCY OPTION COUNSELING

Because many pregnancies are unintended, mistimed, result from physical abuse, or are simply unwanted,[32–34] and because undesired fetuses and children may be at risk of unfavorable outcomes, it is important, once the diagnosis of pregnancy is made, to ascertain the woman's feelings about it and to let her know of her rights with respect to deciding whether to continue the pregnancy, terminate it, or place the child for adoption. Such planning will often include the partner or, in the case of the unmarried adolescent, the parent. Planning and referral for appropriate services should be done promptly. A decision to continue the pregnancy should be followed by prompt referral for prenatal care.

The First Prenatal Visit

The objective of the first prenatal visit, like that for a preconceptual visit, is to help the pregnant woman along the path to a healthy pregnancy and thus prevent or minimize maternal and fetal problems during the prenatal period.

The First Prenatal Visit

1. If not already done, establish that the woman is pregnant, determine the duration of the pregnancy, and estimate an expected date of confinement (EDC)
2. Pregnancy option counseling, if not already provided
3. Assessing the woman's current health status, including nutrition, by means of medical and obstetric history, physical examination, and appropriate laboratory tests; provision should be made for the diagnosis and treatment of any adverse conditions
4. Perform risk assessment, an important function of the visit; both maternal and fetal risks must be considered; as indicated, identified risk factors may include medical and obstetric conditions, and behavioral, socioeconomic, and environmental factors

---

Risk Assessment

Several standard risk-assessment instruments have had wide use during the past 25 years. Because both their specificity and sensitivity are relatively low,

some controversy exists about their value.[4] However, systematic assessment is a useful approach to both preventive and acute care for individual patients. The primary focus is on identifying risks related to maternal characteristics, pregnancy complications associated with PTD and LBW, and genetic risks for fetal anomalies of structure or function. While many risk factors for these problems have been well documented since at least the 1950s, the mechanisms mediating the effect of many such factors are not clearly understood. As a society, the United States has had considerable success in the management of genetic, general medical, and obstetric risk, with the result that maternal and infant mortality and morbidity have been significantly reduced. Some success, although imperfect, has been achieved in reducing such behavioral risks as cigarette smoking and alcohol intake, particularly among better educated and more affluent women. However, these problems continue to be associated with substantial infant mortality and morbidity. Recent years have seen little progress in reducing the risks that stem from poverty and social disadvantage. Despite nutritional programs for poor and disadvantaged women and infants, such as WIC (supplemental nutrition for Women, Infants, and Children) and food stamps, poverty remains a serious risk factor for PTD, LBW, and infant mortality for women and infants of all ethnic groups. For reasons not well understood, black women and their infants have higher rates of PTD, LBW, and infant mortality than white women regardless of their socioeconomic background.[35,36] Furthermore, women eligible for maternal and infant benefit programs sometimes fail to understand the importance of nutrition and avoiding risky behavior, and fail to receive instruction or needed referral for these services from busy practitioners.

Several specific behavioral risks may be more amenable to intervention than is structural poverty.

Behavioral Risks

Behavioral risks related to PTD, LBW, and infant mortality include failure to have adequate prenatal care even when access is available. Poor and uneducated women are particularly likely to have delayed or no prenatal care. Table 2-2 shows that substantial numbers of women fail to receive such care. Other life-style-related risk factors include single mother-hood and failure to practice "safer" sex.

Sexually Transmitted and HIV Infections

Women who initiate sexual activity as young adolescents, who have multiple sex partners, and who fail to use condoms or other barrier methods of contraception are at increased risk of STDs, including hepatitis B and HIV infection. Their fetuses are at risk of STD acquired during pregnancy or delivery. Specifically, HIV infection is a serious risk for women and their infants in high-risk areas such as poor inner-city neighborhoods where alcohol and drug abuse are prevalent.[4] In some large city hospitals, infection rates among pregnant women may reach 5 to 8 percent. Whitley and Goldenberg[37] report that 50 percent of the neonates of HIV-infected women will have congenitally acquired HIV infections, and that most of these infants will develop symptoms of acquired immunodeficiency syndrome (AIDS).

Illicit Drug Use

A survey in 18 metropolitan hospitals found that the frequency of drug-exposed neonates in recent years has increased three to fourfold in 15 of them. One in six neonates exposed had withdrawal symptoms. No source of treatment had been available to the mothers prenatally in two-thirds of the hospitals. Maternal deaths during labor from cocaine use have been reported in Los Angeles and Washington, DC. Eight of the hospitals in the survey reported growing numbers of "border" babies (i.e., infants abandoned by their drug-addicted mothers). This is a substantial problem, as 15 percent of American women aged 15 to 44, or a total of 8 million women, use illicit drugs. Drug education and treatment facilities are urgently needed for pregnant drug users. Illicit drug use and its maternal and fetal consequences are well reviewed by Jones and Lopez.[38]

Other Substance Use

The adverse effects of cigarettes and alcohol during pregnancy have been well recognized for many years, yet many women still smoke and drink alcoholic beverages during pregnancy. Cigarette smoking is associated with increased risks of LBW and infant mortality, and with certain maternal complications associated with placental bleeding.[39] The frequency of smoking during pregnancy is higher among young and poor women, corresponding to the association of poverty with high-risk behavior.

Alcohol use, even in early pregnancy and in small amounts, may have adverse fetal effects. Fetal alcohol syndrome, characterized by facial anomalies and mental subnormality, is a serious problem best prevented by education before the onset of pregnancy. The frequency of heavy drinkers varies with the population studied (3–9 percent).[4,p.177]

Physical Abuse During Pregnancy

During the past several years, increasing attention has been directed toward the role of physical abuse during pregnancy on adverse outcome in terms of maternal complications, premature delivery, LBW, and fetal or neonatal death. The reported frequency of abuse during pregnancy varies from 3 percent to 29 percent, depending on the population studied. Additionally, the proportion of women reporting abuse depends on the way in which the data are collected. McFarlane and colleagues,[40] using a simple three question, self-administered questionnaire, among a sample of 691 black, hispanic, and white women surveyed during prenatal care in Houston and Baltimore, reported a frequency of 17 percent. However, when the questions were asked face-to-face by the health care provider, 29 percent of the women reported abuse, versus only 8 percent on a standard medical-history intake form. Abuse was found to be more frequent and more severe among white than among black or hispanic women. The potential for being victims of homicide was also found to be greater for white women.[41] Others have reported an association between alcohol and illicit drug use and the risk of physical abuse.[42] While it seems likely that physical abuse is related to high levels of family stress and poverty, the problem has been recognized in all educational and socioeconomic levels of society. It should be noted that physical abuse is accompanied by a heavy burden of emotional abuse, anxiety, and depression. Efforts should be made to identify abused women and provide them with prompt, appropriate referral, education, and counseling.

Prepregnant Weight, Height, and Weight Gain in Pregnancy

Prepregnant weight and height and weight gain during pregnancy have a strong association with pregnancy outcome. While height and weight are to some extent genetically determined, health and nutrition during infancy, childhood, and adolescence are also important. Infant birth weight is associated with both prepregnant weight and height, as seen in Tables 2-2 and 2-4. Adequate health care and nutrition during childhood and adolescence can help prepare a woman for a healthy pregnancy, and attention to nutrition during pregnancy can reduce the frequency of LBW and associated infant mortality. Weight gain in pregnancy bears an important association with birth weight. Data from the Collaborative Perinatal Study[23-25] indicated 20 years ago that a 30-pound weight gain was optimal during pregnancy, rather than the 15 to 20 pound gain that was in vogue when the study began. Because of its strong relationship to gestational age at delivery, weight gain is a difficult variable to use in research, and must be controlled for gestational age. The WIC program and the food stamp program, through which nutritional supplements have been made available to poor and near-poor families, have made an important and effective contribution to the health of American women and children. It is fair to say that if these programs are seriously curtailed, both the rates and the associated costs of LBW and infant mortality will increase.

Effectiveness of Risk Assessment

Regardless of their assigned risk category, not all women within such a category experience the same degree of pregnancy risk. Large proportions of high-risk women have normal pregnancies, while some ostensibly low risk women develop serious and unexpected complications. An excellent review by Selwyn of the effectiveness of risk-assessment instruments in predicting LBW and PTD is included in the text by Merkatz and Thompson.[4]

Ultrasound Screening

The use of ultrasound to visualize uterine contents has had a marked impact on obstetric care. Its routine use has been adopted by several European countries and recommended by others.[43] A consensus conference held in 1984 by the National Institutes of Health (NIH)[44] produced a list of 28 clinical circumstances in which ultrasonography was of potential value in clinical management, but found no evidence that routine screening leads to reductions in perinatal mortality or morbidity. Recommendations from the NIH conference were that ultrasonography be performed only on the basis of a specific obstetric indication, and that randomized clinical trials of its use be conducted to assess its value in the United States. The report of a recent, large (n = 15,151) clinical trial, the RADIUS study,[45] involving low-risk pregnant women showed no improvement in perinatal outcome with routine ultrasonography as compared with its selective use on the basis of clinical judgment. The results of this study are generally supported by a meta-analysis of four previous studies.[46] However, perinatal mortality was lower in the screened group because of an increased frequency of induced abortion to terminate pregnancies in which the fetus was malformed. More fetal malformations than commonly reported were also detected in the RADIUS study but this had no effect on perinatal outcome.

It would seem that we are left without a clear-cut answer. From the population viewpoint, routine ultrasonography is probably unjustified. Screening should be done on medical indication. From the individual's viewpoint, those women who are anxious about the possibility of carrying a malformed fetus (which, if identified, would be aborted) should be screened if they so desire.

Return Visits

The first return visit for prenatal care is often scheduled 1 to 2 weeks after the first visit. Its purpose is to discuss with the woman plans for her continuing care based on the findings at the initial visit and any laboratory or other tests performed at that time.

Subsequent follow-up visits for the normal, low-risk patient are usually scheduled at monthly intervals until the 28th week, after which they are scheduled every two weeks through the 36th week, and thereafter usually at weekly intervals until the onset of labor.

The purpose of the return visits includes continued obstetric screening; education on the course of pregnancy and fetal development; reinforcement of the importance of good nutrition and avoiding smoking, alcohol, and other substances that may undermine maternal and fetal health; encouragement of appropriate exercise; and preparation for labor and delivery. The content of the visits is spelled out in *Guideline for Perinatal Care*.[2] Many pregnant women are depressed and anxious. Encouragement, information about what to expect, and clear directions about what to do in case of emergency and where to go at the onset of labor can be of great help in allaying their fear and in obtaining their compliance, thereby changing a potentially stressful time into a positive experience. Seriously depressed women require referral for appropriate mental health services.

COMPREHENSIVE PRENATAL CARE: DOES IT WORK?

Comprehensive care is designed to provide an array of preventive and crisis-oriented services to optimize pregnancy outcomes for all women, particularly those deemed to be at high risk.[2] A useful example of an effective comprehensive care program was initiated in the 1970s for pregnant adolescents by King at the Johns Hopkins Hospital.[33] This program was designed to improve the pregnancy experience and outcome of inner-city adolescents, many as young as 10 to 13 years of age. Between 300 and 350 adolescents, younger than 18 years of age who wished to continue their pregnancies were enrolled annually. Over 90 percent were eligible for Medicaid assistance. Over 80 percent were from families begun by a adolescent birth, 51 percent by birth to an adolescent under age 18. Most of the families were headed by a single parent and most were welfare-supported. Needs-assessment studies indicated that the adolescents and their mothers had little accurate information about reproduction, contraception, nutrition, and parenting. Only 12 percent of adolescents reported that their pregnancy was intended. The frequency of sexually transmitted infection and other health problems was high. All the adolescents were at high risk of complications on the basis of their medical, behavioral, social, economic, and environmental background. The average gestation at registration was 17 weeks and the average number of prenatal visits was nine.

Table 2-5 documents the comparability of the background characteristics of patients receiving comprehensive care at the Hopkins Adolescent Clinic (HAC) and those receiving care in other, traditional Johns Hopkins clinic programs. Table 2-6 compares the obstetric courses of the two groups. Those receiving comprehensive care gained significantly more weight and had fewer instances of anemia and pre-eclampsia. They made an average of 9.2 visits and kept 80 percent of the appointments, as compared with 50 percent for control patients. While there was no difference between the two groups in mean gestational age at delivery (Table 2-7), they did show substantial differences in the frequency of LBW and very-low-birth-weight (VLBW), infants. The frequency of LBW was below 10 percent for HAC mothers, compared with 16.4 percent for the control mothers and the frequency of VLBW was 1.9 percent versus 3.9 percent, respectively. The frequencies of both LBW and VLBW were lower among the HAC clinic patients than among adult patients in the regular obstetric clinic. Neonatal deaths among control infants (1.2 percent) were three times more common than among the infants of HAC patients (0.4 percent). Evaluation suggested that the added program costs were offset by savings from averted expenditures for hospital costs associated with LBW and pregnancy complications in the comprehensive HAC program.

Because the medical care received by both groups of patients was of the same high standard, we conclude that the additional services that rendered the HAC program comprehensive were what improved outcome, that is, (1) the team approach with case management providing continuity of care; (2) the social service component with its psychosocial support and ability to access a range of needed community services and nutritional supplements; (3) the educational program providing the information and motivation needed for responsible self-care and the management of anxiety; and (4) the caring and supportive program environment. Similar programs for poor, socially disadvantaged women of all ages would be likely to enjoy similar success were resources available to support them. Medicaid does not currently provide reimbursement for social services, beyond crisis management, and provides none at all for health- and parenting-education services.

SUMMARY AND RECOMMENDATIONS

The question is not whether prenatal care works, given the ample historical and more recent evidence for its effectiveness, but rather how can it be made

A Summary of the Comprehensive John Hopkins Adolescent Clinic Program

This program, designed to provide services for a high-risk group, is described briefly below in terms of its guiding principles and ingredients, both of which can be adapted to other sites and risk groups.

1. It was postulated that a *caring,* multidisciplinary staff, led by a senior obstetrician, was needed to provide service, and that staff members should understand
   a. the exigencies and limitations inherent in poverty and social disadvantage
   b. adolescent development, with younger adolescents requiring more services because of being less physically and emotionally mature than older adolescents
   c. the importance of establishing trust in relationships between clients and staff
2. A *team approach* was needed to provide continuity of care in a teaching institution in which obstetric care was provided by house officers under the supervision of senior faculty members; Nurses, social workers, health educators, and supporting staff all provided important elements of continuity
3. An effective team approach required an *individual case management system.* Each new patient's history was reviewed and plans for care were made at weekly staff meetings: Patients already in the system were discussed as problems arose or appointments were missed. Plans for care were formulated by the staff working in concert, and decisions were made with respect to implementation
4. High-quality obstetric care was available with an ongoing albeit informal process of obstetric *risk assessment,* which was part of the standard prenatal care. Because adolescents need continuing reassurance and educational reinforcement, routine prenatal visits were scheduled every 3 weeks rather than every 4 weeks initially, then every 2 weeks from 26 weeks' until 38 weeks' gestation, and then weekly

5. Each adolescent was required to participate in the clinic's *educational program,* which was offered at each visit. This program consisted of semistructured, small-group discussions led by an educator, obstetric nurse and/or social worker, or midwife. Individual sessions were arranged as indicated with the clinic health educator, nurses, or social worker. Topics covered included reproductive physiology, fetal development, nutrition, exercise, work, substance abuse (i.e., drug, alcohol, and smoking cessation), family planning, parenting and child care, and preparation for labor and delivery. These sessions also involved preparation of a significant other (mother, boyfriend) who would support the adolescent during labor
6. Each adolescent was required to meet with the clinic *social worker* for assessment of socioeconomic and family resources and support, and of possible physical and sexual abuse. The adolescent and her family were linked with a network of community agencies for any needed support and continued schooling. The social worker involved the adolescent's mother and/or husband or boyfriend in the planning process. Additional social work visits for counseling about family relationships, schooling, and financial support were scheduled as needed. The social worker often became involved in issues of compliance with visits or special medical or nutritional regimes, failure to keep appointments, and other problem areas. Home visits were made by a paraprofessional to all pregnant adolescents below age 16 and to others when indicated. The need for continuing education was stressed. Issues related to pregnancy option counseling, such as abortion, adoption, sexual abuse, and so forth were referred to the social worker

(Continued)

7. A postpartum visit was scheduled for each adolescent 4 weeks after delivery to
   a. ensure her return to health after pregnancy, labor, and delivery
   b. reinforce good health habits learned
   c. provide family planning education and supplies
   d. review plans for continued health care for the mother and child
8. The *obstetric nurses* were central to the program's success. They personally knew each adolescent, including the details of her history and plans for her care. They interviewed her at the end of each visit to be sure that she understood what had occurred and why. They provided substantial individual support, counseling, and education in an informal way as part of their patient contacts, and were leaders or co-leaders of educational sessions. They were available every day by telephone or in the clinic to provide advice, support, or emergency service. They provided linkage with the labor and delivery suite, the hospital floors, and outside medical services as needed. They visited adolescents admitted to the hospital. They became the adolescent's friends and mentors
9. Well-documented *medical records*, including flow sheets to document care during each visit, were an integral part of the system, providing continuity of medical care. Records were available on the labor and delivery suite, providing prenatal information needed for optimal obstetric and pediatric care.
10. An ongoing *evaluation of process and patient outcome* was built into the program. The process evaluation was informal and revealed areas for improvement. The outcome evaluation was more formal and was designed to measure program effectiveness in meeting its goals of improved health for mother and infant. Two major evaluation efforts were facilitated by the availability of control groups composed of adolescents of similar backgrounds, with infants delivered in the same facilities and by the same staff, but differing in the site of prenatal care. The results of the evaluations are presented in Tables 2-5 to 2-7 and discussed further in the text.

Table 2-5. Comparison of Adolescents Enrolled in the Comprehensive Program and Traditional Johns Hopkins Prenatal Programs

Characteristics	Comprehensive Care (n = 744)		Traditional Care (n = 744)	
	Mean	%	Mean	%
Education, highest grade completed	8.3		8.4	
History of				
Prior abortion		11.6		11.4
Prior birth		7.3		10.3
Duration of pregnancy at registration	17.3		17.0	
Age at delivery (mean)	16.1		16.0	

(Adapted from Hardy and Zabin,[33] with permission)

more effective and less costly. Few research findings exist as bases for judging the cost effectiveness of various components of such care, but ample information about important risk factors for poor outcome is available to guide effective strategies for prenatal care.

Revisions of the generally accepted standards for prenatal care are needed to improve pregnancy outcome for all mothers and infants, and for society as well. These revisions are needed to provide documented, cost-effective care within the overall health care system, and to make such care acceptable to this generation of childbearing women. To accomplish the latter, the revised care programs need to involve the mother's partner and to emphasize a caring, humane, broad-based preventive approach rather than one that emphasizes the purely scientific and technical aspects of care. It is necessary to overcome the

Table 2-6. Obstetric Course and Outcome: Comparison of Adolescents Receiving Comprehensive versus Traditional Prenatal Care

Maternal Characteristics	Comprehensive Care (n = 744)		Traditional Care (n = 744)		P Value[a]
	Mean	%	Mean	%	
Prenatal					
Prepregnant weight	121.8		120.7		
Weight gain		28.9		23.5	0.0001
Anemia (hematocrit level <30 mm)		10.9		15.6	0.002
Pre-eclampsia		3.5		5.9	0.02
Gonorrhea		7.9		5.4	
Gestation at delivery (completed weeks)	38.5		38.4		
% ≤36 weeks		18.7		21.5	
PROM >12 hours		3.5		5.5	0.03
Cervical laceration		2.8		4.2	0.05
Cesarean section ≤14 years		17.1		19.5	

PROM, premature rupture of membranes.
[a] P values that are not significant are not indicated.
(Adapted from Hardy and Zabin,[33] with permission.)

sometimes rather chauvinistic management of pregnant women manifested by some obstetricians who have tried to control rather than guide the course of pregnancy, labor, and delivery. The revisions should not be limited to issues that affect only an existing pregnancy, but should also include provision for education in child care and early parenting. The de-

Table 2-7. Fetal Outcome Following Comprehensive (HAC) Prenatal Care Compared with Traditional Care

Fetal Outcome	Comprehensive Care (n = 744)		Traditional Care (n = 744)		P Value[a]
	Mean	%	Mean	%	
Birth weight	3,083		3,038		
<2,500 g		9.9		16.4	0.006
<1,500 g		1.9		3.9	0.02
Apgar ≤6 at min		4.0		6.7	0.02
Mortality					
Stillbirth		1.2		1.0	
Neonatal deaths		0.4		1.2	0.08
Hospital days (mean)	4.9		6.0		

[a] P values that are not significant are not indicated.
(Adapted from Hardy and Zabin[33] with permission.)

sirability of breast feeding, because of its many benefits to mother and child, should not be overlooked.[47]

To meet these goals, those responsible for the health of female infants, children, adolescents, and women must bear in mind that pregnancy and motherhood are expected life-course events. Preparation for these events in terms of optimal health, nutrition, and education in the self-determined, behavioral aspects of health, family planning, and parenting are essential for an optimal outcome. Clearly, personnel in many disciplines are involved in the health care and education of future parents. All women should have access to continuing primary care and family planning services, and a preconception visit to assure a healthy, successful pregnancy.

In addition to providing good obstetric care, prenatal care should assure optimal health during pregnancy by

1. Monitoring risk, both individual and population group
2. Risk reduction through
   a. referral, if necessary, for medical, nutritional, and obstetric problems
   b. behavioral change of risk factors such as smoking, illicit drug use, or lack of compliance with pregnancy care

c. provision of social services for crisis situations, financial support, and other social needs
3. Health education through group discussions or individual sessions with respect to reproductive physiology, nutritional needs in pregnancy, fetal development, substance abuse, family planning, preparation for labor and delivery, and infant parenting
4. Providing such emotional support and confidence building as the woman may require to understand her pregnancy, allay her anxieties, and derive comfort and pleasure from her experience
5. Ensuring that ongoing primary care is arranged for both the mother and infant when the pregnancy is over

The manner in which these goals are met will depend on the structure in which prenatal care is provided and the available staff. While a reduced number of prenatal visits may be sufficient for the obstetric monitoring of healthy women, it would be insufficient to provide the breadth of continuing care needed for even low-risk women. The additional routine contact needed by women in this group may be provided by nurses working individually or with small groups, or at home visits or by scheduled telephone calls. These contacts can provide excellent opportunities for psychosocial support, education, and counseling. Clinical trials are needed to determine the effectiveness and cost of such a system.

Women at risk need closer supervision, and socially disadvantaged women, because of their educational and socioeconomic deprivation, will have the most favorable outcome from comprehensive prenatal care with referral for nutritional and social services, such as that described earlier for adolescents. This kind of care is demonstrably cost-effective in high-risk groups when the averted costs of more frequent prenatal hospital admissions, longer hospital stays after delivery, and the costs of LBW are considered.[33]

REFERENCES

1. Public Health Service Expert Committee on the Content of Prenatal Care: Caring for Our Future: The Content of Prenatal Care. U.S. Department of Health and Human Service, Public Health Service, Washington, DC, 1989
2. Guidelines for Perinatal Care. 3rd Ed. American Academy of Pediatrics, Amercan College of Obstetricians and Gynecologists, Washington, DC, 1992
3. Standards for Obstetric and Gynecologic Services. 7th Ed. American College of Obstetricians and Gynecologists, Washington, DC, 1989
4. Merkatz IR, Thompson JE (eds): New Perspectives in Prenatal Care. Elsevier, New York, 1990
5. Institute of Medicine's Committee to Study the Prevention of Low Birthweight: Preventing Low Birthweight. National Academy Press, Washington, DC, 1985
6. Promoting Health/Preventing Disease: Objectives for the Nation. U.S. Public Health Service, Washington, DC, 1980
7. Hall M, MacIntyre S, Porter M: Antenatal Care Assessed. The University Press, Aberdeen, 1985
8. Rush CB, Entman SS: Antenatal care and intrapartum management. Gen Obstet 5(5):647, 1993
9. Troubling Trends Persist: Shortchanging America's Next Generation. National Commission to Prevent Infant Mortality, Washington, DC, 1992
10. National Center for Health Statistics: Advance report of final mortality statistics 1991: Monthly Vital Statistics Report Suppl 8/31/93 42:2, 1993
11. National Center for Health Statistics: Advance report of final natality statistics 1991: Monthly Vital Statistics Report Suppl 9/93 42:3, 1993
12. Sinclair EB, Johnson G: Practice of midwifery in Dublin 1858. Cited by Taussig FJ: The story of prenatal care. Obstet Gynecol 34:731, 1937
13. Penman WP: William Goodall and the Preston Retreat. Trans Stud Coll Physicians Phila 37:124, 1969
14. Williams JW: The limitations and possibilities of prenatal care. JAMA 44:95, 1915
15. Eastman NJ: Our Obstetrical Heritage: The Story of Safe Childbirth. Cited by Thomas H. Shoe String Press, Hamden, CT, 1960
16. Lobenstine RW: Practical means of reducing maternal mortality. Am J Publ Health 12:39, 1922
17. Hamilton DB: The Metropolitan Life Insurance Company Visiting Nurse Service: 1900–1953. University of Virginia Press, Charlottesville, VA, 1987
18. Bradbury DE: Five Decades of Action for Children: A History of the Children's Bureau. Children's Bureau, Washington, DC, 1962
19. Children's Bureau: Standards of Prenatal Care: An Outline for the Use of Physicians. U.S. Government Printing Office, Washington, DC, 1925
20. Klerman LV: The need for a new perspective on prena-

tal care. p. 3. In Merkatz IR, Thompson JE (eds): New Perspectives in Prenatal Care, Elsever, New York, 1990

21. Olds DL, Henderson CR, Tatelbaum R, Chamberlin R: Improving the delivery of prenatal care and outcomes of pregnancy: A randomized trial of nurse house visitation. Pediatrics 77:16, 1986

22. Hardy JB, Streett R: Family support and parenting education in the home: an effective extension of clinic-based preventive health care services for poor children. J Pediatr 115:927, 1989

23. Niswander K, Gordon M: The Women and Their Pregnancies: A Report from the Collaborative Perinatal Study. WB Saunders, Philadelphia, 1972

24. Hardy JB, Drage SS, Jackson E (eds): The First Year of Life. The Johns Hopkins Press, Baltimore, 1979

25. Weiss W, Jackson E: Results of a multivariate analysis of factors associated with low birthweight in the collaborative perinatal study. p. 31. In Hardy J, Drage F, Jackson E (eds): The First Year of Life. The Johns Hopkins Press, Baltimore, 1979

26. Kramer M: The etiology and prevention of low birthweight. In Berendes, Kessell, Yaffee (eds): Current Knowledge and Pirorites for Future Research in the Prevention of Low Birthweight, an International Symposium. National Center for Education in Maternal and Child Health, Washington, DC, 1991

27. McCarthy J, Hardy JB: Age at first birth and birth outcomes. J Res Adolesc 3(4):373, 1993

28. Hardy JB, McCarthy J, Repke J: Low Birthweight and Perinatal and Infant Mortality. Final Report to NICHD on Grant No. HD24127, July 1992

29. Starfield BH, Shapiro S, Weiss J, et al: Race, family income and low birthweight. Am J Epidemiol 134:1167, 1992

30. Summers L, Price RA: Preconception care: an opportunity to maximize health in pregnancy. J Nurse-Midwifery 38:188, 1993

31. Zabin LS, Hirsch MB, Boscia JA: Differential characteristics of adolescent pregnancy test patients: abortion, childbearing and negative test groups. J Adolesc Health Care 11:107, 1990

32. Zelnik M, Kantner JF, Ford K: Sex and Pregnancy in Adolescence. Sage Library of Social Science, Beverly Hills, CA, 1981

33. Hardy JB, Zabin LS: Adolescent Pregnancy in an Urban Environment. The Urban Institute, Washington, DC, 1991

34. Reitman C (ed): Abortion and the Unwanted Child. Springer, New York, 1971

35. Kleinman JC, Kessel SS: Racial differences in low birthweight: Trends and risk factors. N Engl J Med 317:749, 1987

36. Wise PH: Confronting racial disparities in infant mortality: reconciling science and politics. Am J Prev Med 9:7, 1993

37. Whitley RJ, Goldenberg RL: Infectious disease in the pre-natal period and recommendations for screening. p. 363. In Merkatz IR, Thompson JE (eds): New Perspectives in Prenatal Care. Elsevier, New York, 1990

38. Jones CL, Lopez RE: Drug abuse and pregnancy. p. 273. In Merkatz IR, Thompson JE (eds): New Perspectives in Prenatal Care. Elsevier, New York, 1990

39. Meyer MB: Effects of maternal smoking and attitude on birthweight and gestation. p. 81. In Reed DM, Stanley FJ (eds): The Epidemiology of Prematurity. Urban Schwarzanberg, Baltimore, 1977

40. McFarlane J, Parker B, Soeken K, Bullock L: Assessing for abuse during pregnancy: severity and frequency and associated entry into prenatal care. JAMA 267:3176, 1992

41. Berenson AB, Stiglich NJ, Wilkinson GS, Anderson GD: Drug abuse and other risk factors for physical abuse in pregnancy among white non-hispanic, black and hispanic women. Am J Obstet Gynecol 164:1491, 1991

42. Amaro H, Fried LE, Cabral H, Zuckerman B: Violence during pregnancy and substance use. Am J Public Health 80:575, 1990

43. Berkowitz RL: Should every pregnant women undergo ultrasonography? N Engl J Med 329:874, 1993

44. National Institutes of Health, Office of Medical Applications of Research: The use of diagnostic ultrasound imaging during pregnancy. JAMA 252:669, 1984

45. Ewigman BC, Crane JP, Frigoletto FD, et al: Effect of prenatal ultrasound screening on perinatal outcome. N Engl J Med 329:821, 1993

46. Bucher HC, Schmidt JG: Does routine ultrasound scanning improve pregnancy outcome? meta-analysis of various outcome measures. BMJ 307:13, 1993

47. Oski, F: A warm chain for breastfeeding. Lancet 344:1239, 1994

Chapter 3

Nursing in the LDR(P) Era

Linda J. Kobokovich and Jaque R. Repke

The primary purview of the intrapartum nurse is the management of the patient and her family's response to the patient's labor and delivery situation. The nursing goal is to provide a safe and satisfying labor and delivery experience within the context of each patient's specific clinical situation. While this remains its central focus, the past several decades have seen evolution in the practice of intrapartum nursing. Influenced by patient-driven, epidemiologic, and economic forces, both the scope of intrapartum nursing practice and the physical setting of the intrapartum period have been redefined.

Reflecting a shift from practitioner- to patient-driven practice, labor, delivery, and recovery, (LDR) units emerged as patients expressed the desire to undergo all three processes in a single setting, with an emphasis on family-oriented care. Taking the concept one step further, labor, delivery, recovery and postpartum (LDRP) units incorporate the entire postpartum course within a single room dedicated to maternity care, creating the need for postpartum and nursery competencies for intrapartum nurses. These approaches have been found to be not only economic in terms of decreased transfer and paperwork, but also successful in facilitating continuity by nursing-care providers, thus strengthening the practice of primary nursing.

From an epidemiologic standpoint, women who were previously incapable of or advised against childbearing now have the possibility of a successful outcome of pregnancy as a result of improvements in the practice and technology of obstetrics and neonatal care. These patients have also prompted the adaptation of personnel and the care environment to their needs. Knowledge and competency in intrapartum critical care have thus become new requirements for the nurses who care for these patients. This chapter discusses the current use and design options of both LDRs and LDRPs, and the impact of new competency requirements on intrapartum nursing practice. It also explores future opportunities for nursing roles in the intrapartum setting.

LDR/LDRP ERA

The past decade has seen dramatic change in the design of obstetric services, owing in great part to forces dictated by the consumer public. As health-care organizations continue to improve their systems and strive toward a family-centered approach to such care, the collaborative efforts of physicians, nurses, and administrators are essential to the success of such efforts.

Interestingly, the concept of a family-centered approach to intrapartum care began with a LDR room that was first implemented in 1969 at a South African hospital by physician Morris Notelowitz.[1] This design was intended for use by women with both low- and high-risk pregnancies, with the goal of having the mother remain in the same room for labor, birth, and recovery before moving to a postpartum room. Ten years passed before a similar concept appeared in the American medical literature. In 1979, Dr. Loel Fenwick expanded the concept when he described single-room maternity care (SRMC), which included labor, delivery, recovery, and postpartum care in a single room (called the LDRP room).[1] By that time however, the major maternal-and-infant care organizations in the United States had published "Joint Statement of Family Centered Maternity Care." American families had begun a revolutionary effort in the mid-1970s to put the family back into the experience of birth.[2] Fenwick's proposals acknowledged this societal revolution.

While advocating SRMC, Fenwick suggested that the traditional multiroom system of providing obstetric care was actually detrimental to the quality of such care. He believed that the traditional system was not as safe as it should be, was expensive to run, and was difficult to staff. In 1980, Ross Planning Associates[3] described an LDR system. Both concepts represented an attempt to move from the traditional multiroom delivery system to a more home-like atmosphere that encouraged family participation but maintained a sense of safety in terms of managing medical complications. Even though the SRMC design was the first to be discussed in the United States, the LDR design became the more popular. Only recently have more health-care organizations moved to the complete SRMC design.

Appeal of Family-Centered Maternity Care

Those health-care providers who embrace family-centered maternity care endorse a particular philosophic approach to obstetric care. The driving force behind the movement toward family-centered care and the use of LDR and SRMC facilities is convenience and comfort for the mother. The change to these alternative designs has clearly been driven by consumer forces.[4]

Labor, Delivery, Recovery System

In modern health-care organizations, family-centered designs take the form of an LDR room or an SRMC room (LDRP room). The LDR room was the

---

Philosophy of Family-Centered Care

The belief that

1. Childbirth is an emotional, dynamic, and highly individualized time in a family's life
2. The collaborative efforts of the childbearing family, the nurse, and the physician are necessary to provide optimal care
3. Health-care providers should be flexible
4. The mother and infant should be cared for as a single unit, with the infant spending most if not all of its time with its mother
5. Active participation and support by the mother's husband, friends, and support personnel enhance the birthing process[1]

---

first such design to be embraced and is the design most frequently used today.

The LDR room began as a *birthing room.* This was usually a private room that was tastefully redecorated. However, such rooms initially received little use because of the restrictive requirements for their use, which included a commitment from both the patient and the physician that the birth would be completed without anesthesia. In general, these first attempts at alternate delivery options were unsuccessful because they were not supported by the medical staff.[3,5] However, the birthing room did serve one purpose in demonstrating that standards for safety could be met in an alternate design. The continuing success of the LDR room is largely due to the minimal risk entailed in 80 percent of births.[3]

Subsequent LDR rooms were sized to comfortably accommodate up to eight persons during the birth process, and were equipped to provide care for all noncesarean births. Even though LDR rooms were initially intended for use by low-risk mothers, they are now used to accommodate all vaginal births. In addition, health-care facilities that have LDR units now exist throughout the United States.[3]

When designing a unit that incorporates the concept of the LDR room, several considerations are necessary. These are based on an estimated length of stay (LOS) in the LDR room of 12 hours. The first consideration is the number of LDR rooms needed. This is determined by using a formula that includes the number of projected births per year, the average LOS (ALOS), and the occupancy rate, as follows[3,6]:

$$\text{Number of rooms needed} = \frac{\text{number of births} \times \text{ALOS}}{365 \times \text{occupancy rate}}$$

A second consideration when using the LDR room concept is that of the additional space needed to support the concept. The LDR room entails reliance on a traditional postpartum space. Once the recovery period is completed, the family is transferred to the postpartum setting. Designated space is also needed for an early labor lounge, an operating room for cesarean births, an anesthesia storage space, a clean supply and equipment storage area, a clean-up area, locker rooms, and on-call rooms. It is also recommended that a conference room be planned into the design of the unit.[3] Most LDR rooms are completely equipped for delivery, and the turnover for each room is fairly rapid.

The LDR design has distinct advantages. It often requires less space than a traditional system, and offers an increased measure of flexibility for movement between a more progressive and more traditional system, as needed. Because only one room must be cleaned, the LDR design also saves money in both material and human resources. Currently, a unit designed to include LDR rooms is a powerful marketing tool for the public, in being conducive to family-centered care. The atmosphere is home-like and the family makes only a single move from the delivery to the postpartum unit.[3] Disadvantages of the design are its greater equipment costs and the extra space and nursing resources necessary for the postpartum unit.[3]

Schmidt,[5] in evaluating the LDR design in a Level-III perinatal center performing over 5,000 births annually, found that the LDR design could accommodate virtually every type of delivery, including a wide range of intrapartum complications affecting mothers and their infants. In addition, parents were unanimous in their enthusiasm for both the continuity of care and the comfort and convenience of the room.[5] In a more current evaluation of the LDR design,

Williams and Mervis[7] found that in their urban tertiary-care hospital, all but 3.8 percent of vaginal deliveries were performed in the LDR room. Transfers to a operative delivery room were most often for ominous fetal heart-rate (FHR) tracings and patients with twin gestations for vaginal delivery. Mortality statistics were essentially unchanged over those in the previous year when a traditional multiroom system was used.[7] These two studies confirm both the success and safety of the LDR design.

Single-Room Maternity Care

Even though the LDR room was the pioneering design for family-centered care, the SRMC concept has recently become increasingly popular. In the SRMC design, labor, delivery, recovery, and postpartum care occur in the same room. This avoids disruptive moves at inappropriate times and allows the family to remain together.[8]

The mother and infant stay in the SRMC room for 12 hours to 2.5 days after parturition. Women having vaginal deliveries are usually discharged at 12 to 36 hours, depending on their condition and that of their infant, as well as on the ALOS for the geographic region. Women experiencing cesarean births are discharged 2.5 to 4 days after parturition. Because of the longer lengths of stay in the SRMC system, a health-care facility would need more SRMC rooms than LDR rooms. The number of SRMC rooms needed is also based on ALOS, number of births, and the planned occupancy rate.[6] Generally, an SRMC room will accommodate 100 patients annually.

$$\text{SRMC rooms} = \frac{\text{number of annual births} \times \text{ALOS}}{365 \times \text{planned occupancy rate}}$$

The SRMC room can be slightly smaller than the LDR room. Because there are more rooms in the SRMC design than in the LDR design, equipment for delivery is shared between SRMC rooms. Consequently, equipment in the SRMC system is stored in a central location rather than in each room. This consideration can also be cost-saving in terms of equipment dollars.

The benefits of the SRMC design are many. First and foremost is the provision of family-centered care in a safe environment. As previously noted for the LDR design, all but a few selected births can be accomplished safely within the SRMC system. The design maximizes the use of space and personnel, provides for greater flexibility in the provision of nursing care, prevents disruptive moves, decreases time and cost in cleaning, and allows the newborn infant to remain with its family. Because the infant spends most of its time with the family, a traditional nursery is not required. In contrast to a traditional nursery design, all that is needed is a smaller holding area adjacent to the central nurses' area. This decreases the cost for nursery space and nursery personnel, and also facilitates infection control.[3] Whereas a single nurse might circulate among several babies in a traditional nursery, and potentially spread infection among them, the SRMC design enables the mother or family to provide much of the care for the infant, and the nurse cares only for one particular infant for a particular period. The nurse then goes to another room to provide further care, increasing the likelihood of good hand washing and infection-control techniques. Finally, airborne infection cannot simultaneously affect several infants when each is located in a different room. The greatest adjustment for units adopting the SRMC concept is the provision of maternal-plus-infant care.

Comparison of LDR and SRMC Designs

In planning for the future, many health-care organizations weigh the options of both the LDR design and the SRMC design. Some of the items considered are the number of rooms needed, room size, equipment, cesarean deliveries, anesthesia considerations, antepartum and postpartum care, nursery needs, and staffing patterns. Table 3-1 provides a comparison of these eight factors for the LDR and SRMC designs.

Table 3-1. Comparison of LDR and SRMC Designs

	LDR	SRMC
Number of rooms needed	Requires fewer rooms but requires a traditional postpartum space	Total number of square feet needed to provide maternity service is less; requires more individual SRMC rooms.[5,6]
Room size (subject to some state regulations that are usually more limited than the recommendations given here)	350 sq ft per room; 2,800 sq ft for service of eight rooms	300 sq ft per room (less space required as equipment is stored centrally)[5,6]
Equipment cost and storage	Greater equipment cost as each room is permanently equipped for birth	Equipment cost is less as equipment is shared between rooms; requires space for equipment storage.
Cesarean deliveries (number of operating rooms dependent on volume of deliveries)	Requires operating room space (number required will reflect type of populations served and number of deliveries)	Requires operating room space; (number required will reflect type of populations served and number of deliveries.)
Anesthesia equipment (requirements vary more by institution than by design)	May be permanently placed in each room	Usually found only in the operative area.
Antepartum and postpartum care	Usually takes place on separate unit; requires additional space and staffing costs	Incorporated into SRMC design; women strongly prefer the privacy afforded by the SRMC design[6]
Nursery	Most often maintains a traditional nursery space; mother/infant care can be accomplished in this setting	Incorporates mother/infant care with 24-hour rooming in; requires only downsized "holding areas"[5,6]
Staffing	Nurses often maintain traditional activities of each unit, with expertise found in one area; staffing costs increase	Requires cross-training of staff; initial financial outlay, but payoff is tremendously increased staffing flexibility, which translates into financial savings[6]

Cross-Training

The SRMC concept requires that nurses be reoriented from their specialty in perinatal nursing, whether labor and delivery or postpartum, antepartum, or nursery care, to being able to care for women and their infants through all stages of the hospital stay and birth. This reorientation process has been called cross-training, and is the single greatest adjustment for the staff when moving to SRMC and maternal-plus-infant care. It is important that this cross-training process be carefully planned and communicated to the nursing staff. The staff must know how the process will be accomplished and what is expected of them. This sensitivity to the staff is critical in fostering a positive attitude with regard to the change.[1]

Because of increasing emphasis on competencies in nursing practice, the optimum cross-training program would include a preceptor-based program consisting of didactic and experiential learning components, as well as establishing clearly defined competencies and showing how they can be achieved. The process of orienting a nurse to maternal-plus-infant care takes from 3 to 6 months, while orientation to intrapartum care takes approximately 1 year.[1,8] The concern and effort put into this process are critical, since a positive attitude about the change to maternal-plus-infant care is essential for success in making the transition. Even though cross-training is costly and lengthy, the extra time spent in the effort translates into job satisfaction, increased productivity, increased flexibility in the daily provision of care, and greater cost efficiency.[1,5,6]

Besides keeping the nursing staff informed about changes and progress related to cross-training, it is critical that communication also occur with the medical staff. In order for the transition to progress smoothly, collaboration between the nursing and medical staff is essential.

Consideration of an Alternative Design

The LDR and SRMC designs have proved to be safe and satisfying for both the consumer and health-care provider.[5,7] The transition to one of these designs is a process that must be collaborative and carefully thought out. Some health-care organizations are converting either to an LDR design or an SRMC design. Others are combining these two concepts into a single unit with some LDR rooms and some SRMC rooms. As noted earlier, the inherent disadvantage in the LDR design is the reliance on a traditional postpartum unit. This continues to fragment nursing resources and often creates tension between nursing units. The need for transfer between units creates inherent problems and dissatisfaction for consumer and provider alike. The SRMC design, now recognized as cost-effective, can be efficiently accommodated by almost any size health-care facility.[3] This design is being expanded to accommodate obstetric services with volumes of as many as 3,000 to 5,000 deliveries annually and comprising 40 to 60-bed units.[1,6] Another important advantage of the SRMC design is continuity of nursing care. With all aspects of birth occurring in the same location and with the same staff, a particular nurse can participate in the birth and then follow-through with the family in the postpartum period. This atmosphere promotes primary nursing and LOS accountability for the nursing staff, and translates into patient satisfaction.

Most health-care facilities moving to the SRMC design do so because of market competition. Women are becoming increasingly insistent in making known their desires for family-centered care. When planning their childbearing experiences, expectant mothers are "shopping around" for health-care facilities that are less technologically oriented and more family centered.[9] Facilities that want to remain competitive are redesigning the ways in which they provide maternity care. However, the support of the physician and the nursing staff is, as noted earlier, critical to the success of the redesigning process. The current trend toward a decreasing postpartum length of stay favors the SRMC design. Currently, the ALOS for vaginal birth is 1.5 days, and for most hospitals, approximately 80 percent of births are vaginal.[10] This rapid turnover is well suited to the efficiency of the SRMC unit. Additionally, the ALOS for cesarean birth is just over 3 days,[1,3,10] a short period that can also be easily accommodated within the SRMC design. Currently, most obstetric beds in the United States remain traditional postpartum beds. However, LDR designs now account for 16 percent of obstetric beds, and their proportion of LDR beds grew by 11 percent from 1988 to 1992. SRMC designs account for 8.3 percent of obstetric beds, and grew by 4 percent over the same period.[10] Most SRMC designs are currently found in smaller hospitals, although this trend seems to be changing.[1,3,10]

When considering a change to one of the alternative designs, it is important to consider the following points:

> The planning must be collaborative, with representation by the facility administration, nursing providers, physician providers, and consumers
>
> The criteria and needs of the particular healthcare facility and of the parties involved in the planning must be carefully considered.
>
> Modifications in care by both physician and nursing staffs should be made before structural changes begin
>
> The desires of all parties should be kept in mind
>
> A positive attitude should be continually fostered by reassuring nursing and physician staffs that they are doing excellent work

Awareness of these points will help create success in the transition to a more family-centered approach to childbirth. It is important to remember, however, that childbirth will become steadily demedicalized. As we move into the 21st century, the American childbirth experience will be increasingly located in free-standing birth centers, with the majority of low-risk care provided by certified nurse midwives and nurse practitioners. The driving force behind these changes will be pressures to contain health-care costs. High cost, high-technology care will be directed only at those women who experience high-risk pregnancies and a need for greater intervention.[11] American obstetricians have seen a tremendous shift in women's childbirth demands over only the past 20 years. The daughters of women who were thankful for the "natural childbirth" techniques of Lamaze and Bradley are now thankful for improved epidural and intrathecal narcotic techniques.[2] The key to success in the future health-care environment is putting oneself and one's health-care institution into a position of flexibility with the capacity to accommodate change.

CHANGING NURSING ENVIRONMENTS

The expectations, requirements, and opportunities for nurses in intrapartum settings have changed drastically in the past decade. This change has been prompted by consumer demand, which has led to a greater emphasis on improvement in the quality of care and an increasingly litigious society. These changes have created opportunities for greater autonomy in the scope of nursing practice, and to the renegotiation of procedural boundaries for nurses, accompanied by increasing accountability and liability for their actions. The opportunities for and responsibilities of nurses in maternal-and-infant health care arena will continue to change and evolve drastically. Critical components to consider in relation to these changes are nursing competencies and expanded nursing roles.

Nursing Competencies

The requirements for demonstrated nursing competency has become foremost in the nursing-practice arena. In discussing this trend it is important to begin by defining the concept of competency. An important distinction in this regard is that of competency as opposed to proficiency. Although the two are often interchanged, it is important to understand the difference between them. Competency refers to a minimum standard that protects society, whereas proficiency implies expertise.[12]

The concept of nursing competency became more prominent as nursing education was influenced by the movement of competency-based education in the field of teacher education.[12] Initially, competency concepts in nursing were simply equated with behavioral objectives. Current perspectives on nursing competency, however, are derived from evaluations of actual practice. The current working definition of competency involves an integration of performance objectives that reflect cognitive awareness, psychomotor skills, and attitudes.[12]

The movement toward demonstrating competency in nursing is in keeping with current trends toward ensuring quality standards of care. The 1991 Joint Commission on Accreditation of Healthcare Organizations (JCAHO) Nursing Care Standards speaks directly to the evaluation of competence in Standard 2. This standard states that all members of an institution's nursing staff must be competent to fulfill their assigned responsibilities.[13] Accreditation agencies are increasingly requiring that nurses be "credentialed" in clinical procedures that involve a high level of risk or are highly technical. The particular skills in question are described as a competency, with a definition of the specific knowledge and psychomotor skills needed to achieve the competency. Organizations such as the Association of Women's Health, Obstetrical, and Neonatal Nurses (AWOHNN) assist nurses in meeting this requirement by publication of specialty standards.[14] The benefits of this compentency demonstration include quality care and documented clinical competence that can be presented in the nurse's and institution's defense if malpractice accusations are made.[15]

The concept of competency is becoming increasingly evident in intrapartum nursing, with competency-based orientation and evaluation becoming the norm. Evaluation based on competency is derived from principles of criterion-referenced measures, with the nurse's performance in caring for childbearing families being measured against existing criteria rather than against the performance of other nurses. The existing criteria reflect the ability, skill, judgment, attitude, and values that the nurse needs to function in a particular position.[16] The emphasis on competency is an attempt to ensure that nurses provide quality patient care to each consumer.

Accrediting organizations' emphasis on competency has also increased the sense of each institution's and each nurse's liability in the provision of care. Long past are the days when a nurse could state that "the doctor told me to do it." The American legal system now holds that each nurse must be competent and accountable for decisions made when providing care. It is also expected that each health-care organization will make every effort to ensure that nurses working within their purview are competent and capable. These pressures often lead to tension in interactions between nurse providers and physician providers. This is especially true in the field of intrapartum care, in which the liability of providers is particularly high. For this reason it has become increasingly important for physician and nurse care-givers to collaborate and cooperate when planning and providing care for individual patients.

Expanded Nursing Roles

The role of intrapartum nurses has changed steadily through the 20th century. This trend will continue into the next century as the demands made on intrapartum and maternal/infant-care nurses evolve with the progressively decreasing length of stay and the inevitable changes in the provision of health care. American society is mandating humanistic and available care for all citizens, the delivery of which will effect profound changes in the health-care system. Ernst,[17] in writing about health-care reform, predicts that methods for decreasing the cost of health care will include significant change in the providers of prenatal and intrapartum care. Institutions that now employ medical residents to staff their prenatal clinics will turn to nurse midwives as being more economical and able to provide primary care to women of childbearing age. This trend will also work toward bringing the skill and expertise of the provider in line with the patient's needs. Eventually the ratio of obstetricians to nurse midwives must reflect the ratio of women who have perinatal and intrapartum complications to those who have uncomplicated births.[17] Roles more specific to the intrapartum experience are also emerging. McGee[18] has described the role of the perinatal nurse practitioner as including expertise in advanced physical and psychosocial assessment, history taking, and technologic skills in procedures such as basic ultrasonography, biophysical profiling, the insertion of internal monitoring devices, hemodynamic monitoring, and providing first assistance for obstetric surgical cases. Not only does this role meet the need of health-care facilities, it is also widely accepted by patients. Other nursing curricula across the United States are being altered to incorporate the growing demand for nurses skilled in primary, ambulatory, and home care.[2]

As health-care choices and technology become more complex, nurses will become increasingly important to consumers. They will serve as consultants and buffers in a fast-paced and highly technologic system,[2] as well as sources of support during uncomplicated births. More frequently, the nurses will become the manager of the care planned by a physician-nurse team. Fortunately, intrapartum nurses, and nurse midwives in particular, have a long history of collaboration during the process of birth. This collaboration has affected the quality of care provided to childbearing families. The needs of future consumers and of the health-care system demand the comprehensive and complex services that can be successfully provided through the continued partnership and collaboration of intrapartum nurses and physicians.

CHANGE AGENTS IN MATERNITY CARE

As patient needs change, so must the practice and practitioner. As health care providers, we must be able to reflect on our practice in an organized manner. This allows us to make improvements and to enhance those aspects that are good now but that could be better. These improvements should always emanate from a patient-centered, quality-oriented philosophy, and require a collaborative approach. Overriding the forces shaping our practice are the economic realities of health-care today. Interdisciplinary quality assessment and improvement programs are the vehicles that should be used to determine the changes required in obstetric care without sacrificing quality. The intrapartum setting will continue to change as a result of putting the patient at the center of our practice. Collaboration with our physician and nurse-midwife colleagues is the key to success in these ventures. Only together can we improve on and shape intrapartum health care for our patients.

REFERENCES

1. National Association of Women's Health Professionals: Focus. Hill Rom, Evanston, IL, 1988
2. Covington C, Collins J: Back to the future of women's health and perinatal nursing in the 21st century. J Obstet Gynecol Neonatal Nurs 23:183, 1994
3. Ross Planning Associates: Perspectives in Perinatal and Pediatric Design. Ross Laboratories, Columbus, OH, 1988
4. Koska M: One-stop LDRP units redefine obstetrics care. Hospitals 62:60, 1988
5. Schmidt R: Labor-delivery-recovery room: planning the delivery suite for current need. Clin Perinatol 10: 49, 1983
6. Doodan J: LDR v LDRP: Contemporary Obstetrical Design Trends. Frontline Planning Vol. 2. Ross Planning Associates; Columbus, OH, 1989
7. Williams J, Mervis M: Use of the labor-delivery-recovery room in an urban tertiary care hospital. Am J Obstet Gynecol 162:23, 1990
8. Reed G, Schmid M: Nursing implementation of single room maternity care. J Obstet Gynecol Neonatal Nurs 15:386, 1985
9. Klerman L: Perinatal health care policy: how will it affect the family in the 21st century. J Obstet Gynecol Neonatal Nurs 23:124, 1994
10. American Hospital Association: Survey of Obstetric Services: Executive Summary—1992. Section for Maternal and Child Health, American Hospital Association, Chicago, 1993
11. Freda M: Childbearing, reproductive control, aging women, and health care: the projected ethical debates. J Obstet Gynecol Neonatal Nurs 23:144, 1994
12. Feeney J, Benson-Landau M: Competency-based evaluation: not just for new nurses. Dimens Crit Care Nurs 6:368, 1987
13. Kelly K: Nursing Staff Development: Current Competence, Future Focus. JB Lippincott, Philadelphia, 1992
14. AWHONN's Didactic Content and Clinical Skills Verification for Professional Nurse Providers of Basic, High Risk, and Critical Care Intrapartum Nursing. Association of Women's Health, Obstetrical, and Neonatal Nurses, Washington, DC, 1993
15. Lohrman J, Kinkade S: Competency-Based Orientation for Critical Care Nursing. CV Mosby, St. Louis, 1992
16. Wagner P, Kenney M, Martz J: Competency based evaluation. p. 216 In Pinkerton S, Schroeder P (eds): Commitment to Excellence. Aspen Publications, Rockville, MD, 1988
17. Ernst E: Health care reform as an ongoing process. J Obstet Gynecol Neonatal Nurs 23:129, 1994
18. McGee D: The perinatal nurse practitioner: an innovative model of advance practice. J Obstet Gynecol Neonatal Nurs (in press)

Chapter 4

Evolution of Modern Pain Management

Sanjay Datta

HISTORICAL ASPECTS

Benjamin Rush[1] had a vision that a medicine would one day be available that "should suspend sensibility altogether and leave irritability or the powers of motion unimpaired and, thereby, destroy labor pains altogether." Unfortunately, more than a century later, the ideal agent for the relief of pain in childbirth remains unavailable. Long before the era of modern anesthesia, attempts were made to relieve labor pain. The very first effort for this even met significant opposition. Eufame MacAlyane of Edinburgh was a victim of this opposition, and was buried alive on Castle Hill in that city while seeking assistance from Agnes Sampson for her labor pain.[2]

Sir James Y. Simpson must be credited with the introduction of modern anesthesia in obstetric practice. He first used ether in childbirth on January 19, 1847, and reported his results before the obstetric society of Edinburgh on February 10 of that year. At the same time, Simpson began experimenting with a few colleagues in an attempt to find a better anesthetic agent. On November 8, 1847, he first used chloroform in an obstetric case, and presented a paper on the new agent at the first winter meeting of the Edinburgh Medico-Chirurgical Society.[3] Chloroform was made popular by John Snow when he used it during the birth of Prince Leopold, eighth child of Queen Victoria.[4] Interestingly, although surgical anesthesia was first used in the United States, a long time passed before anesthesia was used for obstetric practice. The first case report of the use of ether for the relief of labor pain in the United States was published as a letter in the *Boston Medical and Surgical Journal* on April 14, 1847, by Nathan Colley Keep. Walter Channing, Professor of Obstetrics at the Harvard Medical School, used ether extensively in obstetric procedures, and wrote his famous *A Treatise on Etherization in Childbirth. Illustrated by Five Hundred Eighty-one Cases.*[5] Augustus Kinsley Gardner of New York City was the first in the United States to use chloroform in obstetrics, on February 2, 1848. In 1849, during the American Medical Association's Second Annual Meeting, the report of the committee on obstetrics was presented by the acting chairman, C.R. Gilman of New York. The main part of the report was related to the application of anesthetics in obstetric practice. It stated that the use of these agents "was not only justifiable for the purpose of alleviating the pain of labor, but also that, in all difficult and instrumental labors, their application could not be rightfully withheld." For the next 35 years, ether and chloroform were used extensively, until nitrous oxide and oxygen for obstetric analgesia were popularized by J. Clarence Webster of Chicago in 1909. With the acceptance of anesthesia to relieve pain for the second stage agents to produce amnesia during the first stage became popular. Combinations of large doses of scopolamine and morphine were used for so-called twilight sleep. A high incidence of depressed and asphyxiated babies from this technique made it unpopular. Barbiturates given either orally or intravenously were also tried from 1928, but never became popular. Another interesting anesthetic "cocktail," which was used by Gwathmey, and called "synergistic analgesia," consisted of hypodermically administered morphine and magnesium sulfate with the rectal installation of ether. Although these different methods helped parturients with their labor pain, they were associated with high incidences of nausea and vomiting, as well as sedation of mothers. Hence, local infiltration block as well as caudal epidural and spinal anesthesia with local anesthetics began to become popular.

On January 12, 1931, Eugen Bogdan Aburel presented a paper titled "L'anesthésie locale continue (prolongée) en obstetrique" at a meeting of the Obstetric and Gynecologic Society of Paris.[6] Most probably this is the first paper to describe the technique of continuous epidural (caudal) and lumboaortic plexus block for the relief of pain in childbirth. Other names important in the development of continuous caudal anesthesia were Hingson and Edwards.[7] Cosgrove was responsible for demonstrating the safety of spinal anesthesia,[8] whereas the saddle block technique for delivery was popularized by Adriani and Parmely[9] in 1946.[10] Today, the epidural block is one of the most popular techniques for the relief of labor pain, during both the first and second stages. Epidural block was first achieved unintentionally by Corning in 1884,[11] but did not gain acceptance until Graffagnino and Seyler[12] reported the results of its use in obstetrics in 1935. Flowers, Hellman, and Hingson[13] first used vinyl tubing for continuous epidural block in obstetric patients, and this made the epidural technique the most popular method for obstetric anesthesia. Apgar, Marx, Bonica, Bromage, and Shnider were responsible for popularizing modern anesthesia practice in obstetrics.

CURRENT TRENDS

Regional analgesia and anesthesia for obstetric patients are undergoing revolutionary changes that will ultimately benefit both parturients and neonates. These changes have taken place in the arena of techniques and equipment, as well as in medications.

VAGINAL DELIVERY

Pain of labor is carried by different peripheral nerves, depending on the stage. The first stage of labor is mediated through the afferent nerve supply of the uterus via the sympathetic nerve, ultimately to the T10–L1 segments. Pain of the second stage of labor is carried by the S2, S3, and S4 spinal segments (pudendal nerve).

Different Nerve Block Techniques for First and Second Stages of Labor

First Stage
  Epidural analgesia
  Caudal analgesia or anesthesia
  Spinal analgesia or anesthesia
  Bilateral sympathetic block
  Paracervical block

Second Stage
  Epidural analgesia
  Caudal analgesia or anesthesia
  Spinal analgesia or anesthesia
  Pudendal nerve block

Of the different nerve-block techniques, epidural analgesia has become the most popular for both the first and second stages of labor. Spinal analgesia and anesthesia have recently been tried for this purpose with some success. Caudal analgesia or anesthesia is seldom used at present for labor.

Epidural Analgesia

Epidural analgesia has become the most popular method for the relief of labor and delivery pain in the parturient. It can be achieved in two ways: (1) the segmental-block technique with intermittent injections, and (2) the complete block technique with intermittent injections or continuous infusion.[14]

Epidural Analgesia Techniques

1. *Segmental block technique:* can be used during the first stage of labor by limiting the sensory analgesia to segments T10–L1. As labor progresses to the second stage, analgesia can be extended to block the sacral innervation. The main disadvantage of this regimen is the possibility of failure to provide perineal analgesia if the timing of the top-up is not perfect, this is not uncommon in a busy hospital
2. *Complete block technique:* can provide sensory analgesia from T10–S5 from the very first dose. With the advent of continuous infusion technique, this method has become popular

---

Whatever the final procedure, the use of small concentrations of local anesthetic for labor and delivery has become the accepted technique. As suggested by Bromage,[15] an ideal local anesthetic for labor and delivery should be associated with maximum sensory analgesia with minimal motor block (Fig. 4-1). At present, 0.125 percent bupivacaine fulfills the motor-anesthetic requirement to a certain extent, although sensory analgesia may not be adequate in a significant number of patients.

Combination of Opiates and Local Anesthetic Agents

The combination of opioids and local anesthetic agents in recent years has dramatically changed the management of labor and delivery pain. The site and mechanism of action of opioids and local anesthetics are different. Presynaptic and postsynaptic receptors in the substantia gelatinosa of the dorsal horn of the spinal cord have been suggested as the major sites of action of spinal opiates,[16] whereas blockade of the axonal membrane of the spinal nerve roots, as well as the anterior and posterior horn cells, is the mechanism of action for local anesthetics. One of the major advantages of spinal opiates is the capability to produce selective blockade of pain without blocking the sympathetic nervous system, thus maintaining a stable cardiovascular system. There are different types of opiate receptors (e.g., μ, δ, κ, and ϵ), and these bind specific opioid

agonists. Mixtures of epidural opiate and local anesthetic are associated with several advantages. First, They are efficacy during both the first and second stages of labor. Second, A reduction in the doses of both the local anesthetic and the narcotic, and a consequent minimizing of their side effects. Use of low concentrations of local anesthetic will be associated with minimum motor blockade, which is suitable for parturients. Finally, there is a possible synergistic effect. Different opioids, such as fentanyl, sufentanil, alfentanil, and butorphanol, had been used mixed with bupivacaine, either in an intermittent or a continuous infusion technique. At present, the bupivacaine and fentanyl mixture has become the combination of choice in most hospitals in the United States. A combination of 0.125 percent or 0.0625 percent bupivacaine with 2 μg/ml of fentanyl at an infusion rate of 8 to 10 ml/hr is most commonly used.

Continuous Epidural Infusion

Although continuous infusion for epidural analgesia in obstetrics was first described as early as 1963, it never became popular because of a lack of availability of the proper instruments as well as of local anesthetic. With the advent of long-acting local anesthetics like bupivacaine, as well as better mechanical infusion pumps, continuous infusion has become the technique of choice for vaginal delivery.

Main Advantages of Continuous Epidural Analgesia Infusion

1. A more stable depth of analgesia, which becomes an important part of patient satisfaction
2. The possibility of lower blood concentrations of local anesthetic
3. A reduced risk of total spinal block in the presence of an inadvertent injection of local anesthetic into the subarachnoid space
4. Lower blood concentrations of local anesthetic if the catheter is accidentally placed in the vein
5. A lower incidence of hypotension due to the possibility of decreased sympathetic blockade

---

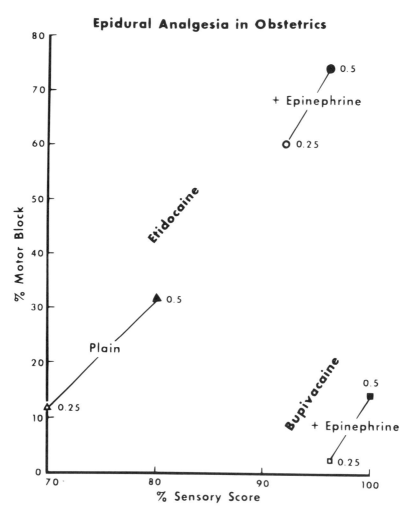

Fig. 4-1. Sensory-motor dissociation. (From Bromage,[38] with permission.)

A loading dose of the local anesthetic is given before the start of the infusion in order to establish an adequate sensory block as well as to confirm correct placement of the epidural catheter. From 10 to 12 ml of 0.25 percent bupivacaine has been the most popular agent for this purpose. While this method provides adequate analgesia for the first stage of labor, there might be a possibility of inadequate perineal analgesia with the use of continuous infusion. This problem can be counteracted to a certain extent if the mother is gradually eased from the horizontal into the reclining position with the progress of labor.

Subarachnoid Block

Subarachnoid block with local anesthetic delivery never became popular because of its short duration and also because of the motor block it produces. However, with the advent of the microcatheter, several investigators used the intermittent spinal anesthetic technique for labor and delivery.[17] From 0.5 to 1 percent isobaric lidocaine solution was used for pain during labor, whereas 1 percent hyperbaric solution was used for perineal anesthesia during delivery. Unfortunately, the U.S. Food and Drug Administration (FDA) has withdrawn the microcatheters used in the technique from the market. It is hoped that in the future, microcatheters will again be used, and an ideal local anesthetic-narcotic mixture will be found for use in this technique.

Subarachnoid morphine at a dose of 0.5 to 1 mg was associated with adequate pain relief, mainly for the first stage of labor, and to a certain extent also for the second stage.[18] However, it had several disadvantages, including a slower onset (45 to 60 minutes) of pain relief, as well as side effects such as nausea, vomiting, pruritus, and the possibility of delayed respiratory depression. A dose of 0.25 morphine mixed with 25 µg fentanyl was used to hasten the onset of anesthesia, but side effects remain a major problem.[19] Intrathecal opiates might be beneficial in situations in which an absolutely stable cardiovascular system is essential (e.g., patients with severe Eisenmenger syndrome or the tetralogy of Fallot).

Meperidine for Labor and Delivery

Meperidine, a phenylpiperidine opioid, has been observed to have local anesthetic activity. A 10 mg dose of hyperbaric meperidine (5 percent dextrose) was associated with 2 to 3 hours of pain relief during labor. One must, however, remember that intrathecal meperidine may be associated with hypotension, most probably related to sympathetic block and also to motor blockade.[20]

Combined Spinal-Epidural Technique

The combined spinal-epidural technique is a novel approach in which the advantages of subarachnoid as well as epidural technique are sought to provide optimal pain relief for labor and delivery. A 4.5-in, 17-gauge epidural needle is inserted into the epidural space through the loss-of-resistance technique. A 4 11/16-in, 25-gauge Whitacre spinal needle is then passed via the epidural needle into the subarachnoid space until clear cerebrospinal fluid is observed. Intrathecal opioid is injected at this time. The spinal needle is withdrawn at this stage, and an epidural catheter (2 cm) is inserted in the epidural space. The catheter can be used either for the intermittent or continuous epidural infusion technique or to provide adequate perineal analgesia with local anesthetic. Sufentanil in doses of 10 µg has been used successfully in our institution.[21] The addition of 15 µg epinephrine did not prolong the duration of analgesia, but 2.5 mg bupivacaine extended the labor analgesia. A mixture of sufentanil and 2.5 mg bupivacaine may be extremely useful in patients who request pain relief in the latter part of their labor. The absence of motor blockade and hypotension in the presence of excellent sensory analgesia may make this technique useful for the initiation of epidural analgesia during labor.

Why should a small concentration of local anesthetic and opioid mixture be used? The combination of these two agents will provide parturients with a minimal degree of motor block, which may be associated with a reduced incidence of both instrumental delivery and surgical intervention.[22]

Future Prospects

New Local Anesthetic Agents

Ropivacaine is a new amide local anesthetic agent structurally related to bupivacaine and mepivacaine. Unlike these two agents, it is prepared as an isomer(s). This agent has a few extremely beneficial properties as compared with bupivacaine, which remains the most popular local anesthetic for obstetric patients. These advantages include less cardiovascular toxicity and wider differences in sensory versus motor effects. Animal and human studies have shown that ropivacaine produces an equivalent degree of sensory anesthesia to bupivacaine, but a lesser degree of motor blockade.[23] This obviously will be beneficial for laboring patients. Combining opioids with ropivacaine may permit a reduction in the concentration of local anesthetic to the point of reaching Bromage's goal of 100 percent sensory analgesia with 0 percent motor block.[15]

Other Medications

Clonidine, an α_2-adrenergic-receptor agonist, can decrease the sympathetic outflow and can modulate pain sensation. Different trials are being undertaken to define the advantages of combining this agent with other opioids in different applications of pain control. Studies in the obstetric population will ultimately ascertain the usefulness of the α_2-adrenergic-receptor agonists in relieving labor as well as pain following cesarean section. Nonsteroidal anti-inflammatory drugs (NSAIDs), such as intravenous ketorolac, may also play a part in this.

Inhalation Analgesia

Although inhalation analgesia in combination with oxygen has been used in the United Kingdom and a few centers in the United States,[24] this technique has never been used in our institution because of the possibility of vomiting and aspiration of acid stomach contents.

CESAREAN SECTION

Spinal Anesthesia

Spinal anesthesia is becoming popular for elective cesarean section throughout the world because of the advent of the new pencil-point needles, which have virtually abolished the incidence of headache.

Advantages and Disadvantages of Spinal Anesthesia for Cesarean Section

Advantages
  Simplicity
  Speed of onset
  Reliability because of the definite end point (cerebrospinal fluid)
  Minimal fetal exposure because of the use of small amounts of local anesthetic
  Awake patient, hence less chance of gastric aspiration
  Less incidence of maternal shivering[25]

Disadvantages
  Greater risk of hypotension
  Intraoperative nausea or nausea and vomiting
  The possibility of postdural puncture headache
  Limited duration of action (unless continuous spinal technique is used)

Several studies have been performed to counteract or minimize the side effects of this technique to make it more attractive.

Hypotension

Maternal hypotension may be defined as a decrease in systolic blood pressure to below 100 mm Hg or by more than 30 mm Hg from preanesthetic values.

The higher the segmental sympathetic blockade, especially above T4, the greater the risk of hypotension. Because of its rapidity of action, hemodynamic alterations (hypotension) are significantly greater in spinal than in epidural anesthesia. Arterial hypotension may be exacerbated when sympathetic blockade from spinal anesthesia coincides with the assumption of the supine position, since the gravid uterus will further impair venous return. Without preventative measures, maternal hypotension develops in 82 to 92 percent of cases.

Prevention and Treatment

Prehydration (acute volume expansion) is one of the most effective means of decreasing the magnitude and rapidity of a decrease in blood pressure during obstetric anesthesia. From 1,500 to 2,000 ml of lactated Ringer's solution is usually recommended. Dextrose-containing solutions should not be used unless indicated because of the possibility of neonatal hyperglycemia and hyperinsulinemia, which will produce neonatal hypoglycemia following delivery.

Choice of Vasopressors

Ephedrine is the vasopressor of choice for obstetric patients because it will increase the blood pressure by increasing the force as well as the rate of cardiac contraction without causing uterine vasoconstriction. Infusion of small boluses of ephedrine should be used to maintain the baseline blood pressure. In the presence of maternal ischemic cardiac disease, valvular stenosis, fetal tachyarrhythmia, or maternal tachycardia, ephedrine may be contraindicated. In such cases small bolus doses of phenylephrine may be indicated.

Prevention of Nausea and Vomiting

Peripartum emetic symptoms during induction of spinal anesthesia can be prevented by avoiding maternal hypotension. Traction of the uterus or peritoneum during surgery may also be a significant source of intraoperative nausea and vomiting. An adequate amount of local anesthetic as well as the addition of an opioid with a local anesthetic will reduce the afferent discharges from the peritoneum and abdominal viscera, and can therefore reduce the incidence of these annoying side effects. Use of metoclopramide (10 mg IV) 30 minutes before the surgery has also been shown to be effective in reducing the incidence of nausea and vomiting.

Local Anesthetics

The introduction of hyperbaric bupivacaine for spinal anesthesia for cesarean section has made a significant contribution to patient satisfaction. Hyperbaric bupivacaine is associated with good sensory anesthesia, and the coincidental regression of sensory and motor block is also helpful for the patient. Use of 0.2 mg epinephrine is associated with better sensory anesthesia. Recent studies have observed the lack of correlation between patient height and the total dose of local anesthetic. A dose of 1.6 ml of 0.75 percent hyperbaric bupivacaine has been suggested as the dose of choice for the average patient (148 to 178 cm height).[26]

Intrathecal Opioids

The use of opioids with a local anesthetic during the induction of spinal anesthesia will improve the intensity of sensory anesthesia. This will be associated with better intraoperative, as well as postoperative, pain relief. Fentanyl, sufentanil, meperidine, and morphine have been used for this purpose[27] (Table 4-1). Intrathecal preservative-free morphine sulfate in a dose of 0.1 to 0.5 mg has been shown to provide postoperative pain relief for 17 to 27 hours. However, pruritus, nausea, vomiting, and delayed respiratory depression may be side effects of this regimen.

Role of Meperidine as the Sole Agent for Spinal Anesthesia in Cesarean Section

Interestingly, meperidine has been noted to have local anesthetic properties. Lower extremity and perineal as well as urologic procedures have been performed under subarachnoid block achieved with meperidine alone. A group from France originally used intrathecal meperidine for elective cesarean delivery. At the Brigham and Women's Hospital, cesarean section was done on a patient allergic to both classes of local anesthetics, under spinal anesthesia using preservative-free meperidine alone.[28] A 1 mg/kg dose of 5 percent hyperbaric meperidine was used for the induction of spinal anesthesia following proper hydration. Within 5 minutes a sensory level to four thoracic dermatomes was achieved with a significant degree of motor block. Hypotension was corrected with intravenous ephedrine. However, I believe that intrathecal meperidine should currently be used only in special circumstances.

Postdural Puncture Headache

Postdural puncture headache (PDPH) used to be one of the major problems with spinal anesthesia for cesarean section. Different measures were undertaken to reduce the incidence of this problem. A smaller needle size was associated with a lower incidence of PDPH. The incidence of PDPH with a 26-gauge spinal needle is approximately 5 percent, and with a 27-gauge needle is 2.7 percent, whereas 29 to 30-gauge needles are associated with an incidence of PDPH of less than 1 percent. The incidence of headache has also been decreased by inserting the cutting needle parallel to the dural fibers. Finally, the availability of pencil-point spinal needles such as the Whitacre and Sprotte needles has also helped to reduce the incidence of PDPH. With 25 gauge Whitacre pencil-point needles, the incidence of headache in our institution remains only 0.8 percent.

Limitation of Surgical Time

A fixed anesthesia time has always been a limitation for spinal anesthesia because of the use of a fixed amount of local anesthetic at one time. The continuous catheter technique was not popular because of the high incidence of PDPH associated with the use of larger gauge needles. The advent of microcatheters showed considerable promise in this regard, but as noted earlier, the FDA has banned the use of microcatheters for continuous spinal anesthesia. It is hoped that, in the future, problems encountered with the use of the microcatheters can be solved with

Table 4-1. Intrathecal Opioids for Cesarean Delivery and Postoperative Analgesia

Opioid	Dose	Onset (min)	Duration (hr)
Morphine	0.2–0.3 mg	30–40	12–27
Meperidine	1 mg/kg	2–3	1 (anesthesia) 6 (analgesia)
Fentanyl	6.25–15 μg	5	3–5
Sufentanil	10–20 μg	5	3–5

(From Lussos and Datta,[27] with permission.)

the use of better techniques in the hands of skilled anesthesiologists.

Spinal anesthesia for cesarean section is becoming popular throughout North America and also in Europe. The introduction of new local anesthetics, opioids, spinal needles, and catheters will make this technique ideal for cesarean delivery.

Epidural Anesthesia

Epidural anesthesia remains a popular technique, especially in Europe.

Advantages and Disadvantages of Epidural Anesthesia for Cesarean Section

Advantages
  Lower frequency and severity of maternal hypotension
  Absence of time limitation because of use of continuous technique
  Awake patient, hence, less chance of gastric aspiration
Disadvantages
  Slower onset of surgical anesthesia
  Higher failure rate
  Need for larger amounts of local anesthetic
  Greater incidence of shivering

Cardiovascular Effects of Anesthesia

The gradual onset of sympathetic blockade with incremental dosing causes only minor alterations in maternal hemodynamics. The compensatory sympathetic response also remains intact for a longer time.

Local anesthetic agents with epinephrine (1:200,000) contain 5 μg of epinephrine/ml. When gradually absorbed, 100 to 125 μg epinephrine used with a local anesthetic for cesarean section will have a predominantly β-mimetic effect. Heart rate and stroke volume may increase in association with a decrease in total peripheral resistance and mean arterial pressure. However, accidental intravascular injection of epinephrine will be associated with maternal tachycardia and hypertension.

Choice of Local Anesthetic Agent

Lidocaine 2 percent with epinephrine remains the drug of choice in the United States for elective cesarean section. Its rapid onset and relatively long duration of action, associated with good sensory anesthesia, make it popular for elective cesarean section in patients without cardiovascular problems. Bupivacaine 0.5 percent has a slower onset of action and may therefore be used in situations in which cardiovascular stability is important, such as in the presence of pregnancy-induced hypertension. 2-Chloroprocaine should be the drug of choice in the presence of fetal distress, especially with acidosis. Its rapid onset of action, short half-life (in both mother and neonates), and good sensory and motor anesthesia make it suitable for this purpose. However, because of its quick offset of action, reinforcement doses should be administered every 30 minutes. In the early 1980s, a few cases of chronic adhesive arachnoiditis were reported when a large volume of 2-chloroprocaine was used in the presence of inadvertent dural puncture. 2-chloroprocaine was formerly supplied with 0.2 percent bisulfite with low pH, posing the risk of generating sulfurous acid, which may act as a neurotoxic agent. The 2-chloroprocaine now in use contains no methylparaben, and the antioxidant sodium bisulfite has been replaced by ethylenediaminetetraaceticacid (EDTA).

Mixture of Local Anesthetics

A recent study in the United Kingdom reported that the combination of 0.5 percent bupivacaine and 2 percent lidocaine with epinephrine (50:50 mixture) provided excellent anesthesia for cesarean section, and was superior to 2 percent lidocaine with epinephrine.[29] The authors also suggested that the reduction of the bupivacaine dose may reduce the risk of cardiotoxicity.

Addition of Bicarbonate to Local Anesthetics

Use of bicarbonate with local anesthetic agents has become very popular in recent years. The combination produces a more rapid onset of local anesthetic block. Addition of bicarbonate to local anesthetic will increase the pH of these solutions and, ultimately, the percentage of the uncharged form of the anesthetic agent, which is important for diffusion through the nerve membrane. The quality of block has also been observed to improve.

Epidural Opioids for Intraoperative and Postoperative Pain Relief

Different opioids have been tried epidurally for improved intraoperative pain relief, as well as for postoperative analgesia. Fentanyl at a dose of 50 to 100 µg was associated with intense sensory anesthesia when mixed with 2 percent lidocaine with epinephrine or 0.5 percent bupivacaine.[30–32] Sufentanil was also found to be effective when used with 2 percent lidocaine with epinephrine.[33] A fourfold reduction in visceral pain was observed when epidural sufentanil was used in varying doses. However, neonates whose mothers received 50 µg or more exhibited depressed primary reflexes. One problem of sufentanil in the epidural space is its lack of potency. It has been observed that sufentanil is only 2 to 3 times more potent than fentanyl when used epidurally, whereas it is 5 to 10 times more potent when used systemically. Thus, accidental intravascular injection of 30 to 50 µg of epidural sufentanil may cause acute respiratory depression and possible chest-wall rigidity. To have an optimal effect, the opioids have to be injected with at least 10 to 15 ml of preservative-free normal saline. Epidural morphine at 3 to 5 mg, hydromorphone at 1 mg, and butorphanol at 1 to 4 mg also have been used for this purpose. The duration of analgesia with different opioids following cesarean section is shown in Table 4-2.[27]

Although morphine has been found to be very effective for postoperative pain relief, it produces delayed respiratory depression. The incidence of life-threatening respiratory depression is 0.1 percent. The side effects of epidural morphine can be counteracted by infusion of naloxone or oral naltrexone (6 mg).

Monitoring the Patient Following Spinal Opiates

Different investigators have suggested various devices for monitoring delayed respiratory depression. These include pulse oximetry, end-tidal carbon dioxide pressure monitoring, and impedance plethysmography. However, most investigators agree that good nursing care and vigilance remain the most effective methods in caring for postoperatively patients having spinal opiate anesthesia.

Combined Spinal–Epidural Block

In 1988, Rawal and colleagues[34] suggested the use of combined spinal and epidural block for cesarean section. The authors observed that (1) surgical anesthesia and muscular relaxation following block for cesarean section were superior, as shown by a lesser need for supplementary analgesics; (2) the dose of 0.5 percent bupivacaine used epidurally to obtain a T4 block following the use of 1.5 to 2 ml of 0.5 percent hyperbaric spinal bupivacaine was about three times smaller (this was also reflected in total maternal and fetal blood bupivacaine concentrations); (3) the incidence of hypotension was lower (4) in the duration of the procedure was more flexible because of the presence of the epidural catheter. This technique has been used in Europe, but has not yet become popular in the United States.

Future Local Anesthetic Agents

The new long-acting amide local anesthetic ropivacaine is undergoing extensive clinical trials. Ropivacaine is associated with less cardiovascular toxicity than bupivacaine. It also produces a greater degree of differential blockade (sensory > motor) than bupivacaine. Hence, ropivacaine may be ideal for parturients undergoing cesarean section since this patient population prefers to be mobile soon after the surgery. With adequate sensory anesthesia this will be associated with better maternal and neonatal bonding.

New Postoperative Medications

Different α-adrenergic-receptor agonists are being tried for the management of postoperative pain. The future will reveal the practical applications of this

Table 4-2. Epidural Opioids for Cesarean Delivery Postoperative Analgesia

Opioid	Dose	Onset (min)	Duration (hr)
Morphine	3.0–5.0 mg	30–60	12–27
Methadone	5.0 mg	15–20	6–8
Meperidine	20–50 mg	10–15	3–4
Fentanyl	50–100 µg	5–10	2–4
Sufentanil	20–30 µg	5–10	2–4
Butorphanol	1–4 mg	10–15	2–8

(From Lussos and Datta,[27] with permission.)

Advantages and Disadvantages of General Anesthesia for Cesarean Section

Advantages
  Speed of induction
  Reliability
  Reproducibility
  Controllability
  Avoidance of hypotension
Disadvantages
  Possibility of maternal aspiration
  Problems of airway management
  Narcotization of the newborn
  Maternal awareness during light general anesthesia

Induction Agents Used for General Anesthesia

Thiopental (3 to 4 mg/kg)
  Advantages: safe, reliable, standard agent at present
  Disadvantages: cardiovascular depression
Ketamine (1. to 1.5 mg/kg)
  Advantages: anesthetic and analgesic, increased heart rate and blood pressure
  Disadvantages: increased heart rate and blood pressure; should not be used in hypertensive patients.
Methohexital (1 mg/kg)
  Advantages: recovery is more rapid
  Disadvantages: may be contraindicated in epileptic patients
Etomidate (0.3 mg/kg)
  Advantages: minimal alteration in cardiorespiratory state, recovery is faster
  Disadvantages: pain on injection, myoclonus, adrenal suppression
Propofol (1 to 1.5 mg/kg)
  Advantages: recovery is more rapid
  Disadvantages: higher incidence of hypotension

---

group of drugs for cesarean delivery. Ketorolac, a new nonsteroidal anti-inflammatory agent given intravenously, is undergoing trials for postoperative pain relief. This agent, on its own or in combination with smaller doses of opioids, may be ideal for pain relief following cesarean section.

In summary, the future of regional analgesia and anesthesia for obstetric patients is encouraging and bright. New agents, instruments, and techniques will make this technique safer for both mothers and babies.

General Anesthesia

The use of general anesthesia for cesarean section has decreased dramatically in recent years. At our institution, only 5 percent of all cesarean sections are now done under general anesthesia. The indications for such anesthesia usually include acute severe fetal distress and cases in which regional anesthesia is contraindicated. Routine use of nonparticulate antacid and metoclopramide intravenously unless contraindicated are absolutely essential.

Airway Management

Parturients experience a more rapid decrease in arterial oxygen saturation than do nonpregnant patients. This is related to an increased oxygen demand and decreased functional residual capacity. Difficulty or inability to intubate are the main prob-

lems in using general anesthesia. Hence, a drill procedure for difficult intubation[35] should be planned by every anesthesiology team involved in obstetric anesthesia. The feasibility of this might be discussed with the relevant obstetricians.

Anesthesia should be maintained by 50 percent oxygen and 50 percent nitrous oxide, with a small amount of volatile anesthetic to prevent maternal recall.[36] After delivery, narcotics and tranquilizers can be used instead of volatile anesthetics. The mother should be extubated when fully conscious.

Effect of Induction-to-Delivery Interval and Uterine Incision-to-Delivery Interval

Several investigators observed a better neonatal status when the induction-to-delivery (I–D) interval was less than 10 minutes in the case of general anesthesia. However, in the case of regional anesthesia, if hypotension was prevented, there was no correlation of a prolonged I–D interval and neonatal depression. However, the uterine incision-to-delivery (UI–D) interval is important both for general as well as regional anesthesia. A UI–D interval of more than 180 seconds was associated with low Apgar scores as well as neonatal acidosis.[37]

CONCLUSION

Understanding of the physiology, pharmacology, and clinical management of anesthesia for cesarean section has advanced significantly in recent years. If one routinely follows the criteria meticulously, one should expect an excellent maternal and fetal outcome with either general or regional anesthesia in normal parturients. However, we prefer regional anesthesia for cesarean section unless contraindicated.

REFERENCES

1. Rush B: Medical Inquiries and Observations. p. 221. 4th ed. Vol. 4. Ayer, Philadelphia, 1972
2. Ellis E: Ancient Anodynes—Primitive Anaesthesia and Allied Conditions. Heinemann, London, 1946
3. Priestly W, Storer H (eds): The Obstetric Memoirs and Contributions of James Y. Simpson. 2 Philadelphia, 1856
4. Claye A: The Evolution of Obstetric Analgesia. Oxford University Press, London, 1939
5. Heaton C: The history of anesthesia and analgesia in obstetrics. J Hist Med 1:567, 1946
6. Curelaru SL: Eugen Bogdan Aburel (1899–1975). Anaesthesia 37:663, 1982
7. Hingson R, Edwards W: Comprehensive review of continuous caudal anesthesia during labor and delivery. Curr Res Anesth 4:181, 1943
8. Cosgrove S, Hall P, Gleson W: Spinal anesthesia with particular reference to its use in obstetrics. Curr Res Anesth Analg 16:234, 1937
9. Adriani J, Roman-Vega D: Saddle block anesthesia. Am J Surg 71:12, 1946
10. Parmley R, Adriani J: Saddle block anesthesia with Nupercaine in obstetrics. Am J Obstet Gynocol 52:636, 1946
11. Corning J: Spinal anaesthesia and local medication of the cord. NY State J Med 42:483, 1985
12. Graffagnino P, Seyler W: Epidural anesthesia in obstetrics. Am J Obstet Gynecol 35:597, 1938
13. Flowers CE, Hellman L, Hingson R: Continuous peridural anesthesia/analgesia for labor, delivery and cesarean section. Curr Res Anesth Analg 28:181, 1949
14. Datta S: Relief of labor pain by regional analgesia/anesthesia. In Datta S (ed): The Obstetric Anesthesia Handbook. Mosby-Year Book, St. Louis, 1992
15. Bromage P, Datta S, Dunford L: Etidocaine: an evaluation in epidural analgesia for obstetrics. Can Anaesth Soc J 21:535, 1974
16. Cousins M, Mather L: Intrathecal and epidural administration of opioids. Anesthesiology 61:276, 1984
17. Huckaby T, Skerman J, Hurley R et al: Sensory analgesia for vaginal deliveries: A preliminary report of continuous spinal anesthesia with a 32-gauge catheter. Reg Anesth 16:150, 1991
18. Abboud T, Shnider S, Dailey P et al: Intrathecal administration of hyperbaric morphine for the relief of labor pain in labor. Br J Anaesth 56:1351, 1984
19. Leighton B, Simone CD, Norris M: Intrathecal narcotics for labor revisited: the combination of fentanyl and morphine intrathecally provides rapid onset of profound, prolonged analgesia. Anesth Analg 69:122, 1989
20. Johnson M, Hurley R, Datta S: Continuous microcatheter spinal anesthesia with subarachnoid meperidine for labor and delivery. Anesth Analg 70:658, 1990
21. Camann W, Denney R, Holby E, Datta S: A comparison of intrathecal, epidural and intravenous sufentanil for labor analgesia. Anesthesiology 77:884, 1992
22. Naulty J, Smith R, Ross R: The effect of changes in labor analgesic practice on labor outcome. Anesthesiology 69:A76, 1988
23. Bader A, Datta S, Flanagan H, Covino B: Comparison of bupivacaine- and ropivacaine-induced conduction blockade in the isolated rabbit vagus nerve. Anesth Analg 68:724, 1989
24. Cohen S: Inhalation analgesia and anesthesia for vaginal delivery. In Schnider SM, Lennson G (eds): Anesthesia for Obstetrics. 3rd Ed. Williams & Wilkins, Baltimore, 1993
25. Helbo-Hansen S, Bang U, Garcia R et al: Subarachnoid versus epidural bupivacaine 0.5% for cesarean section. Acta Anaesthesiol Scand 32:473, 1988
26. Norris M: Height, weight, and the spread of subarachnoid hyperbaric bupivacaine in the term parturient. Anesth Analg 67:555, 1988
27. Lussos S, Datta S: Anesthesia for cesarean delivery. Part II. Epidural anesthesia, intrathecal and epidural opioids, venous air embolism. Int J Obstet Anaesth 1: 183, 1992
28. Camann W, Bader A: Spinal anesthesia for cesarean

delivery with meperidine as the sole agent. Int J Obstet Anesth 1:156, 1992

29. Howell P, Davies W, Wrigley M et al: Comparison of four local extradural anesthetic solutions for elective caesarean section. Br J Anaesth 65:648, 1990

30. Naulty J, Datta S, Ostheimer G, et al: Epidural fentanyl for post-cesarean delivery pain management. Anesthesiology 63:694, 1985

31. Gaffud M, Bansal P, Lawton C et al: Surgical analgesia for cesarean delivery with epidural bupivacaine and fentanyl. Anesthesiology 65:331, 1986

32. Preston P, Rosen M, Hughes S et al: Epidural anesthesia with fentanyl and lidocaine for cesarean section: maternal effects and neonatal outcome. Anesthesiology 68:938, 1988

33. Courtney M, Bader A, Hartwell B et al: Perioperative analgesia with subarachnoid sufentanil administration. Reg Anesth 17:292, 1992

34. Rawal N, Schollin J, Wesstrom G: Epidural versus combined spinal epidural block for caesarean section. Acta Anaesthesiol Scand 32:61, 1988

35. Lussos S, Datta S: Anesthesia for cesarean section. Part III. Int J Obstet Anesth 2:208, 1992

36. Warren T, Datta S, Ostheimer G et al: Comparison of the maternal and neonatal effects of halothane, enflurane, and isoflurane for cesarean delivery. Anesth Analg 62:516, 1983

37. Datta S, Ostheimer G, Weiss J et al: Neonatal effects of prolonged anesthetic induction for cesarean section. Obstet Gynecol 58:331, 1981

38. Bromage PR: Epidural Analgesia. p. 50. WB Saunders, Philadelphia

Chapter 5

Expanding Role of Nurse-Midwifery

Lisa L. Paine and Jo-Anna L. Rorie

The heart of nurse-midwifery care for women and newborns lies more in the nature of that care than in its specific components. Nurse-midwifery practice has a firm foundation in the critical thought process and is focused on the prevention of disease and the promotion of health, taking the best from the disciplines of midwifery, nursing, public health and medicine to provide safe, holistic care. Nurse-midwives are partners with women in the provision of health care, engaging in a dynamic re-evaluation of each woman's health needs and providing continuous attendance for women during birth. Nurse-midwives would rather nurture a woman's progress with hands-on care than diagnose her problems from afar, rather listen than lecture, rather teach a health principle than treat an illness, rather empower a woman to join in decision-making than decide for her, rather urge her to speak for herself than be her advocate, rather support natural processes than employ technological interventions, rather instill in a woman a trust for her body than demonstrate the nurse-midwife's technical proficiency, although nurse-midwives will do all these things when necessary. Nurse-midwifery is a profession born of a woman's vision, nurtured in an understanding of women's developmental phases, and committed to assuring women in all populations that it is their birthright to be part of this unique model of care.[1]

For more than 50 years, nurse-midwives have been leaders in the family-centered maternity care move-

ment in the United States.[2-4] Although nurse-midwives are well-known as alternative health-care providers for the lowest-risk women, their lengthy and significant history in providing care for the most vulnerable childbearing families is now being broadly recognized.[5-7] Using support, education, counseling, and high-quality clinical care, nurse-midwives have consistently demonstrated that the care they provide in all settings of practice is comprehensive, safe, acceptable, affordable, and accessible.

Numerous reports have shown that care by nurse-midwives results in high levels of satisfaction, excellent pregnancy outcomes, and very reasonable health-care costs.[8-18] In the past decade, reports such as these have led to consistent recommendations by policy makers about the expanded role of the nurse-midwife as a means of improving access to care, improving the quality and outcomes of care, and decreasing health-care costs.[7,19-21]

More recently, physicians and health-care administrators have joined policy makers in recognizing the benefits of collaborative obstetric practices that include nurse-midwives. Nurse-midwives are being called on with increasing frequency to complement the range of obstetric care services to more adequately meet the needs and desires of today's childbearing families.[22-24]

This chapter describes the expanding role of the nurse-midwife in obstetric practice, and explores the future role of the nurse-midwife in education, research, and administration. Specific aspects of midwifery practice and philosophy are explored in sufficient detail to provide the reader with a better understanding of the ways in which nurse-midwives adhere to practice philosophies while making sound clinical-practice decisions, especially regarding consultation with physicians and the use of technology. Nurse-midwife-attended births in various practice settings are also explored, including examples of innovative collaborative practice models both in and out of the hospital.

EVOLUTION OF NURSE-MIDWIFERY IN THE 20th CENTURY

Nurse-midwifery in the United States has its roots in rural Kentucky, where the first nurse-midwifery service was started in 1925.[25] Public-health nurses who were dually educated in midwifery and nursing provided comprehensive care to the most vulnerable women and infants in this remote area of the country. Dramatic improvements in access to health care for mothers and their families, and improvements in perinatal outcomes such as maternal and infant mortality, were documented.[26]

Numerous other examples of the impact made by nurse-midwives in an array of underserved and remote areas have been documented throughout this century,[27,28] including the less-known work of Maude Callen in rural South Carolina[29] and of Agnes Reinders of the Catholic Maternity Institute in New Mexico,[30] and the more widely reported examples of nurse-midwifery in urban and inner-city areas,[31–35] remote and rural locations,[8,9,36,37] and alternative birth settings.[38–42]

Results of a recent nationwide study[5–7] of nurse-midwives in clinical practice indicate that certified nurse-midwives (CNMs) continue to make a substantial contribution to the care of women of all backgrounds, particularly to that of women from underserved and vulnerable groups, such as the poor, adolescents, minority ethnic groups, women of immigrant status, and women living in medically underserved areas. Fifty-six percent of women who visit CNMs annually live in inner-city or rural locales. Over 40 percent of all women who visit CNMs annually have health-care coverage from Medicaid or Medicare, and over 25 percent are covered by pri-

vate insurance or are enrolled in managed-care programs. The study also showed that while most of the care provided by CNMs is related to pregnancy and birth, as many as 20 percent of all visits to nurse-midwives are made by women seeking care "outside the maternity cycle."[7] Ambulatory care is provided by nurse-midwives in a variety of health-care settings, including hospital clinics (43 percent), private offices (42 percent), public clinics (36 percent), health-maintenance organizations (HMOs) (10 percent), and birth centers (9 percent)[5]

Although there are over 5,000 CNMs in the United States today,[43] an increase from a mere 300 in the mid-1960s,[44,45] the number is low compared to the nearly 70,000 obstetrician/gynecologists.[46] In the past decade, the growth in the number of nurse-midwives and in the number of nurse-midwifery education programs has been rapid. This growth is largely due to consumer demand,[47,48] increased emphasis at the policy level on the role of the nurse-midwife in today's health-care system,[19–21] government policies that remove artificial barriers and mandate reimbursement for care,[49,50] and the initiatives of the American College of Nurse-Midwives (ACNM) to achieve broader support for nurse-midwifery education.[51]

Through the rigorous ACNM accreditation process approved by the U.S. Department of Education,[52] close to 40 American colleges and universities house nationally accredited programs that prepare graduates to take the national certifying examination for nurse-midwifery.[53] After passing the national examination, the nurse-midwife may use the title certified nurse-midwife. Nurse-midwifery education programs offered in conjunction with a master's degree vary in their emphasis on graduate work in such areas as public health, nursing, research, administration, and health policy. Programs that offer certificates rather than academic degrees use the same core midwifery curriculum,[54] but often focus on excellence in clinical care for certain vulnerable populations, such as low-income inner-city immigrants,[17] or care in specific settings, such as the free-standing birth center.[55]

Individual states determine licensing, practice statutes, and other regulations related to nurse-midwifery practice, including prescriptive authority, scope of clinical practice, and reimbursement for clinical services rendered.[56–59] A great deal of vari-

Table 5-1. Live Births by Physicians and Midwives, 1992

Birth Attendant Place of Birth	All Births	Physicians	CNMs	Other Midwife	Other
Total	4,065,014	3,834,502	185,005	14,190	31,317
In-hospital	4,021,608	3,824,176	176,117	2,420	18,895
Out-of-hospital	43,017	10,214	8,878	11,767	12,158

(From Centers for Disease Control and Prevention/National Center for Health Statistics.[62])

ance in these regulations occurs from one state to another, and ultimately determines both the number of practicing CNMs[50] and the volume of clinical care provided.[7,60] Further credentialing for intrapartum practice occurs within the hospital or birth center in which the nurse-midwife practices.[59,61]

NURSE-MIDWIFE-ATTENDED BIRTHS

The steady increase in the number of practicing CNMs is reflected in national birth data that indicate increasing numbers of CNM-attended births. From 1975 to 1992 there was a sevenfold increase in the number of nurse-midwife-attended births in the United States.[62] By 1992, the most recent year that data are available, nurse-midwives attended nearly 5 percent of all births nationwide[62] (Table 5-1). Con-

trary to assumptions that nurse-midwifery intrapartum practice occurs primarily outside the hospital, the hospital is by far the most common site of birth. In 1992, 95 percent of all CNM-attended births occurred in hospitals, with 4 percent in free-standing birth centers and less than 1 percent in the home. Although the hospital is the most common site of CNM-attended births, a recent study[5] indicates that 12 percent of all practicing CNMs use the birth center and 8 percent use the home as a birth site. The researchers attribute these findings to the fact that some CNMs use more than one birth site, and that the higher volume multimember practices are located in hospitals.[5]

Table 5-1 also allows for comparisons about births attended by physicians, CNMs, and other midwives in 1992. Figure 5-1 shows the proportion of 1992

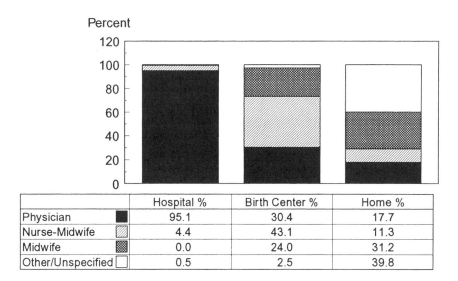

Fig. 5-1. Attendants at U.S. births in three settings: hospital, birth center, and home, 1992.

births in each of three settings—the hospital, the free-standing birth center, and the home—that were attended by physicians, nurse-midwives, and other midwives. Nurse-midwives attend 4 percent of all hospital births, 43 percent of all births in free-standing birth centers, and 11 percent of all home births. Most out-of-hospital births attended by nurse-midwives occur in free-standing birth centers, whereas out-of-hospital births by other midwives occur most often in the home.[62]

INTRAPARTUM PRACTICE OF NURSE-MIDWIFERY

Philosophy of Care

Nurse-midwifery philosophy[63] is based on the premise that health care should be safe and satisfying. Emphasis is placed on self-determination for women in their birth process and a woman's right to full information about her health care. Respect for human dignity and cultural variations are also essential philosophical components of the care rendered by nurse-midwives. Since the 1950s, prominent physicians[64–69] have noted that the strong practice philosophy of nurse-midwives "sets them apart"[64] from other obstetric-care providers.

Examples of Intrapartum Midwifery Management

Encourage whenever safe and possible
  Involvement of women's family in all aspects of care
  Natural onset of labor
  Frequent ambulation and position change
  Tub bath or shower
  Oral hydration
  Auscultation of the fetal heart rate
  Nonpharmacologic pain relief
  Varied labor and birth position
  Nonpharmacologic labor stimulation
  Gentle maternal second-stage pushing effort
  Early and consistent family interaction
  Early breast-feeding
  Early postpartum discharge

Use only as needed
  Intravenous fluids
  Electronic fetal monitoring
  Vaginal examination
  Pharmacologic pain relief
  Pharmacologic labor stimulation
  Amniotomy
  Episiotomy
  Regional anesthesia

Key Components of Nurse-Midwifery Philosophy

Every Individual has the right to
  Safe, satisfying health care
  Respect for human dignity and cultural variation
  Self-determination
  Complete information
  Active participation in health care

Normal pregnancy is enhanced by
  Education
  Health care
  Supportive intervention

(From American College of Nurse-Midwives, with permission.[63])

These same conclusions about philosophic distinctions have been made by researchers attempting to explain variations in the use of obstetric interventions and differences in perinatal outcomes between physicians and midwives.[17,70,71] Nurse-midwifery philosophy includes the appropriate use of technology in childbirth and supportive interventions in the natural process when needed and when the benefits of such technology outweigh the risks. Clinical-practice statements of the ACNM further describe the ways in which this philosophy is translated into intrapartum practice.[72]

Standards of Practice

The quality of nurse-midwifery practice is addressed by the ACNM through its *Standards for the Practice of Nurse-Midwifery*.[73] These standards specify that the

CNM maintain policies that provide a safe and reliable mechanism for obtaining medical consultation, collaboration, and referral when needed. A national Continuing Competency Assessment program is available as a means for nurse-midwives to meet the ACNM quality-assurance standards.[74] In all settings, nurse-midwives engage in some form of quality assurance or peer review.[75] Because of the similarities in medical liability from attending births,[76] nurse-midwives are frequently enrolled in obstetric risk-management programs along with their medical colleagues.[43] Concerns are sometimes voiced about the CNM meeting obstetric/gynecologic standards, but data from a recent study exploring the extent to which obstetrician/gynecologists, family physicians, and CNMs met certain standards of the American College of Obstetricians and Gynecologists (ACOG) do not support these concerns. The results indicated that CNMs adhere to the standards even more closely than their physician counterparts.[86]

Nurse-Midwifery Clinical Management

Midwives are expert in clinical management of the normal labor process.[77] This expertise is particularly valued in hospital-based situations, in which the

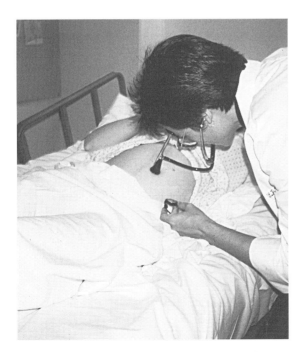

Fig. 5-2. Fetoscope auscultation in early labor.

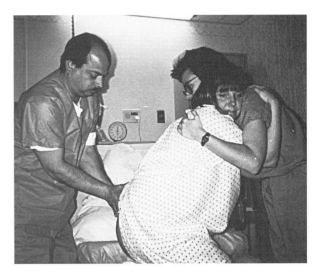

Fig. 5-3. Labor support by midwife and father.

presence of a midwife on the labor and delivery unit brings a level of knowledge, both learned and intuitive, that is highly respected by the unit staff. The nurse-midwife's educational preparation and commitment to the philosophy of midwifery care set the stage for a birth with maximum safety and satisfaction and minimal intervention.

The midwife's presence, patience, and communication with the laboring woman, and the ability to forge a synergistic relationship with her, are undoubtedly the features of midwife-attended birth that onlookers often find difficult to understand. The midwife's knowledge that "something is not quite right" or that "everything is progressing smoothly" often consists of 90 percent data and 10 percent intuition. Using the eyes, the ears, the hands, and the heart, the midwife formulates and implements the scientific process that lies behind every management decision. This is both the art and the science of midwifery practice, as shown in Figures 5-2 to 5-5.

The midwife practices safely while using low-technology methods by implementing a methodical process of careful and rational decision-making known as the "nurse-midwifery management process." The steps of the process, as enumerated in Varney's classic American nurse-midwifery textbook,[25] are to gather necessary information for a complete clinical evaluation, identify problems or diagnoses after cor-

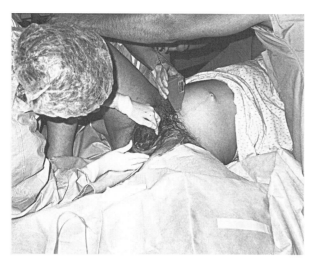

Fig. 5-4. Doptone auscultation in late second-stage fetal heart rate monitoring.

rect interpretation of the data, anticipate potential problems or diagnoses, evaluate the need for immediate midwifery intervention or physician consultation/collaboration, develop a comprehensive plan of care supported by a valid rationale, direct or implement the plan of care efficiently and safely, and evaluate the effectiveness of the care and repeat the process when care is ineffective.

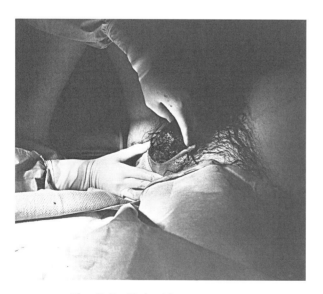

Fig. 5-5. Birth without episiotomy.

Using the management process, the midwife approaches the labor and delivery experience with the premise that *nothing* is routine. Because each woman's labor requires an individualized approach, each management plan differs according to her unique needs. The challenge for every midwife is to know when and why each management decision or intervention is needed, how it will affect the woman's experience of birth and the birth outcome, and when and how to prepare the woman when intervention is needed to achieve an ultimate safe outcome, without implying any failure of the natural process.

Selective Use of Technology in Midwifery Practice

Several examples of intrapartum nurse-midwifery management in the boxed list titled, *Examples of Intrapartum Midwifery Management.* Included in the list of procedures to be used only as needed are electronic fetal monitoring and episiotomy. Both procedures have been studied extensively and rigorously in recent years by clinicians and scientists,[78,79] and despite the substantial scientific support for the use of selective episiotomy and against routine electronic fetal monitoring, they continue to be routine in many settings. One explanation for this is that both auscultation of the fetal heart rate with a fetoscope and delivery over an intact perineum require a great deal of manual skill that has in recent years often been overshadowed by technology. Fortunately, in many contemporary birth settings, this trend is changing as physicians and nurses call on nurse-midwives to help them regain the use of these methods.

Recently a number of low-technology procedures and noninterventive practices were evaluated for clinical-trial evidence of their effectiveness.[80,81] Table 5-2 lists several procedures used frequently by nurse-midwives that have been shown to improve pregnancy outcomes. Using the same rigorous evaluative methods, the researchers further identified a number of "routine" medical procedures, long rejected by midwives that should be abandoned immediately in the light of scientific evidence.

Support During Labor and Birth

The benefits of support during labor and birth are well-documented.[77,80] During labor the midwife assures the woman giving birth that she is strong and

Table 5-2. Effects of Selected Interventions on Pregnancy and Childbirth Outcomes

Intervention	Effect
Enhanced social and psychological support from caregivers	Reduced Poor communication with staff Dissatisfaction with care Not feeling "in control" Worries and unhappiness Feeding problems with baby Feeling physically unwell 6 weeks postpartum
Social and psychological support during labor	Reduced Augmentation of labor Caesarean section
Upright versus recumbent position during first stage of labor	Reduced Use of narcotics/epidural anesthesia
Upright versus recumbent position during second stage of labor	Reduced Abnormal fetal heart rate patterns Severe pain Low umbilical artery pH (<7.25)
Lateral tilt versus dorsal position during second stage of labor	Reduced Mean umbilical arterial pH
Exhalatory versus sustained bearing down during second stage of labor	Reduced Abnormal fetal heart-rate patterns Low Apgar scores
Restricted versus liberal use of episiotomy at delivery	Reduced Overall trauma Perineal trauma
Unrestricted mother-infant contact following delivery	Reduced Breast-feeding failure
Unrestricted breast-feeding	Reduced Breast-feeding failure
Social support and information for breast-feeding mothers	Reduced Breast-feeding failure

(From Enkin et al,[81] with permission.)

capable, and that with the midwife's knowledge, experience, and support, and the natural forces of her own body, she can gather the courage to safely give birth to her baby. The midwife's protective stance allows the woman ample opportunity to trust herself and others around her, to "let go" and allow the baby to be born, and to feel pleased about her accomplishments, even if her own powers must be augmented with intervention to result in a safe birth. In situations in which consultation and intervention become necessary, continued support, encouragement, and advocacy are essential for a safe birth environment.

Fear is always present for the laboring woman, and it is imperative that the midwife create a birth environment in which the woman feels safe. To minimize fear and facilitate the woman's mastery over it, the midwife often encourages the woman to develop a labor and birth plan. Such plans can foster education or counseling, especially when begun during the antepartum period when expectations are unrealistic. As a means of individualizing care, the birth plan fosters communication between the woman and her care-giver, which has been shown to minimize malpractice exposure and claims.[82] The midwife uses the birth plan as a means of building trust and further developing communication with the woman about her goals and desires for a safe and satisfying birth experience. The birth plan is not viewed as a mandate, but rather as a useful tool of advocacy for

---

Forms of Intrapartum Care That Should Be Abandoned

Failing to involve women in decisions about their care

Failing to provide continuity of care during pregnancy and childbirth

Leaving women unattended during labor

Involving doctors in the care of all women during pregnancy

Involving obstetricians in the care of all women during pregnancy

Insisting on universal institutional confinement

Shaving the perineum routinely prior to delivery

Administering enemas or suppositories routinely during labor

Limiting duration of second stage of labor arbitrarily

Restricting maternal position during labor and delivery

Directing maternal pushing during second stage of labor

Performing episiotomy routinely

Separating healthy mothers and babies routinely

Scheduling the timing and duration of breast-feedings routinely

Failing to take account of women's social circumstances postpartum

(From Enkin et al,[81] with permission.)

---

women when they are in the most active phases of labor. When birth plans have not been documented before birth, the midwife uses the time available during labor to accomplish as much trust-building and mutual decision-making as possible.

Participation in the decision-making process, information about her labor progress, and the constant assurance that she is strong and capable are but a few of the needs of the laboring woman that the midwife must be equipped to address. The classic work of Lesser and Keane[83] describes the needs of a laboring woman as (1) bodily or physical care, (2) a sustaining human presence, (3) relief from pain, (4) acceptance of her attitudes and behaviors, and (5) information about and reassurance of a safe outcome for herself and her baby. Toward this end, Varney[25] enumerates the midwife's "armamentarium" of support measures as a means to address these needs, including positioning, relaxation exercises, breathing exercises, prevention of exhaustion and provision for rest, assurance of privacy and prevention of exposure, explanation of the process and progress of labor, explanation of procedures and imposed limitations, attention to basic hygiene, support during vaginal examinations, alleviation of leg cramps, use of physical touch, and involvement of significant others. Because of the intensity of the task of providing supportive care for the laboring woman, the midwife often shares this role with family members, nurses, and other hospital staff members in order to meet these very important needs.

Consultation, Collaboration, or Referral for Complications

The need for both prevention-oriented and treatment-oriented care in all perinatal-care settings allows ample room for physicians and nurse-midwives to work both cooperatively and collaboratively. Interdependence in providing care to women with higher-risk pregnancies also allows for a collaborative relationship, with the physician focusing on high-risk medical care and the midwife concentrating on the normal aspects of pregnancy and the associated needs of the childbearing family. This interdependent practice relationship between obstetrician/gynecologists and CNMs has been defined since 1971 in a joint statement by the ACOG and ACNM, with revisions made in 1975 and 1982.[84]

During labor and birth, the nurse-midwife consults with a specialist in obstetric or surgical intervention when that individual's expertise is necessary for timely and appropriate intervention. The physician contact may be a consultation only, or may result in referral for care or collaboration between the two providers.[85] Collaborative management involves two key components: knowledge on the part of the midwife about the appropriate timing for collaboration, and a well-developed relationship with the physician(s) in which there is a mutual respect for one another and for the differences in practice philosophy that may exist. The timing of consultation depends on a variety of factors, including the relationship between the midwife and the physician consultant; the urgency of the circumstances surrounding the consultation; the specifics of the written guidelines or protocols; and the characteristics of the population and practice setting.

Although there is substantial overlap in the clinical roles of the physician and the CNM, and of the CNM and the nurse in the intrapartum setting, laboring women can benefit from a team approach that allows for their full range of needs and desires to be met. The type of care offered by midwives can be beneficial irrespective of the woman's risk status. Laboring women with complicated pregnancies often need medical care, midwifery care, and nursing care. In the case of obstetric emergencies, when time is of the essence, the midwife can be invaluable in providing emergency clinical and surgical care, intensive supportive care for the woman and her family, and support to all other members of the obstetric and surgical team. Collaborative teams of physicians, midwives, and nurses maximize the possibilities for comprehensive, family-centered care for all women.

NURSE-MIDWIFE-ATTENDED LABOR AND BIRTH IN TWO SETTINGS

The following case studies illustrate the similarities and differences in nurse-midwife-attended births in two sites that are becoming frequent locations for birth: the in-hospital birth unit and the free-standing birth center. The scenarios characterize the experience of two women who are typical of the women in a nurse-midwife intrapartum caseload: a 16-year-old, unmarried, low-income, inner-city adolescent receiving clinic-based midwifery services; and a 27-year-old, married, middle-income woman from a small community receiving midwifery care at a birth center. These scenarios serve to demonstrate how the standard of midwifery care is rendered in two very different settings to two women from very different backgrounds.

The In-Hospital Birth Unit

Keisha is a 16-year-old single, primapara who registered at 16 weeks' gestation for prenatal care with the local clinic midwives. The prenatal visit took place at a neighborhood health center located in a high-infant-mortality area. A well-documented barrier to prenatal care in this area had been problems with access to care.[87] Since nurse-midwives have a long and successful history of working with disenfranchised populations, the statewide response to the problem of access was to develop midwifery services in health centers, with the midwife as the primary care provider for childbearing women.[88] This enabled women such as Keisha to seek and obtain prenatal care in the community in which they lived.

Keisha's prenatal course was uneventful, and 2 days after her due date she began having mild contractions. At 2:00 AM she telephoned the midwife on call and explained that the contractions were coming every 15 to 20 minutes and lasting approximately 30 seconds. She was able to talk through the contractions, but worried about timing her trip to the hospital. The midwife explained to Keisha that she was in very early labor, and encouraged her to try and get some sleep.

At 5:00 AM Keisha telephoned the midwife and stated that the contractions were coming closer and beginning to bother her. The midwife asked about the baby's level of activity and questioned Keisha about the presence of bloody show. Keisha confirmed that the baby was active and denied the appearance of bloody show. She was still able to talk through her contractions and was advised to remain home as long as she was comfortable doing so, and to telephone the midwife within 1 hour. At 7:00 AM Keisha reported a change in her labor pattern and was no longer able to speak through her contractions. The CNM spoke with Keisha's mother and advised her to bring Keisha to the hospital.

Keisha was met by the CNM in the hospital's labor and delivery unit. The external fetal monitor was briefly applied as per hospital protocol. Within a short time the fetus was reactive, and the CNM planned to continue using intermittent auscultation unless otherwise indicated. Keisha was examined and found to be 5 cm dilated, with a bulging bag. Shortly after the pelvic examination her bag of waters broke, the labor intensified, and things began to move very quickly. Keisha was no longer able to focus and became very tense and upset. Keisha's mother helped her to focus and concentrate on dilating, while the CNM worked with Keisha to find a more comfortable position and began a back massage. After the massage, Keisha was encouraged to walk. Although Keisha had planned for natural childbirth and had expressly requested not to be medicated, she began asking about the possibility of receiving medication. Thirty minutes later, Keisha returned to bed and insisted on being medicated.

Keisha was offered oxymorphone hydrochloride (Numorphane), a semisynthetic narcotic. This slowed her labor, allowing her time to rest between contractions, and enabled her to gain the strength needed for pushing. An hour and a half later her contractions were coming every 2 minutes. Keisha's behavior had changed; she was inwardly focused and made a slight grunting sound with each contraction. There was also an increase in the bloody show. On examination, the CNM saw that Keisha was fully dilated and ready to push. The nurse and the CNM prepared the room for delivery.

Keisha's mother remained at the head of the bed, giving her support and encouragement. Keisha was instructed to push slowly, allowing the perineum to stretch out for the baby's head, and minimizing the need for an episiotomy. In a calm and directed manner, the CNM asked Keisha to look to her for directions during the contractions. The nurse positioned a mirror to enable Keisha to see. Warm compresses and a mineral oil massage were applied to the perineum. After a 35-minute second stage the baby was crowning. The CNM supported the perineum and gently guided the infant's emerging head, shoulders, back, and feet. Keisha's new daughter was placed on her abdomen. The infant was dried and her nose suctioned. Keisha looked at her daughter in amazement and disbelief, and stated, "Oh my God! I can't believe I did this." There was a palpable air of reverence in the delivery room for what this young woman had accomplished.

The Free-Standing Birth Center

Patty and David made the decision to have their second child in a birthing center with a group of four nurse-midwives. The birth center was located ap-proximately six miles from the hospital, and Patty and David were interested in birthing in a more relaxed, home-like setting. Nurse-midwives who deliver in this type of setting have developed protocols for careful screening of potentially high-risk women, and Patty had been screened for any complications associated with her previous delivery that would prohibit her from delivering at the birth center. The backup physician was available if consultation was needed. If a complication occurred, transfer to the hospital would take place within 15 minutes and physician backup within 20 minutes.

Patty began labor 2 days after her due date, at 2:30 PM. She telephoned the midwife on call and reported that her contractions were stronger at this point in the labor than she remembered them being for her first baby. She also told the midwife that she noticed a small amount of bloody show. Patty had been 3 cm dilated for over 2 weeks, and the midwife advised her to come in for checking and monitoring.

When Patty arrived at the birth center she was found to be 3 cm dilated, with the infant's head at zero station and a bulging bag of forewaters. An intravenous infusion was not started because Patty was well hydrated and had no history of anemia or heavy bleeding. The CNM suggested the use of a warm bath to facilitate the labor, as well as to aid Patty in relaxation and help alleviate pain. Patty remained in the warm bath for approximately 90 minutes, with the CNM monitoring the fetal heart tone with an intermittent Doppler ultrasonograph. Patty's labor continued, with her contractions coming every 2 to 3 minutes. After 3 hours her cervical examination remained unchanged.

The use of pitocin augmentation of her labor was discussed, and Patty was told that she would need to be transported to the hospital for further monitoring. With the use of pitocin, contractions are of greater intensity, are specifically timed, and do not evolve gradually, leaving no time to prepare for them. The CNM consulted with her physician colleague, who agreed that based on the clinical data pitocin augmentation was an appropriate option. The CNM explained to Patty that the use of pitocin is not a benign procedure, and although the written protocols and procedures at the birth center stated that the CNM could institute pitocin augmentation, it must be administered in the hospital.

Patty wanted to wait another hour before agreeing

to the pitocin augmentation. The fetus was reactive and Patty returned for continued warm-water therapy with the understanding that she was approaching a time at which a decision would have to be made. Patty and David trusted the CNM to make a decision based on the best interests of Patty and her unborn fetus. Approximately 45 minutes later Patty reported pressure on her rectal area. On examination the CNM found that Patty was 8 cm dilated.

Patty and David returned to the birthing room. The room was pleasantly decorated, and Patty remarked that it "felt like home." Her membranes soon ruptured and she was found to be fully dilated. Because she wanted to push while lying on her side, David helped to support her legs while the CNM massaged the perineum in preparation for delivery. The delivery was uneventful; afterward the baby went immediately to Patty's abdomen and breast-feeding was begun.

After the delivery of the placenta Patty continued to have very heavy bleeding. The CNM examined the placenta while the nurse massaged the uterus. Although the placenta appeared to be intact, the CNM was concerned about the color and nature of the bleeding. She started an intravenous infusion and asked the nurse to call for the physician consultant. The CNM reassured Patty and David by explaining that this was one of the situations they had discussed prenatally that could require timely intervention and physician consultation. On closer vaginal and cervical inspection the CNM discovered trailing membranes, which were promptly removed with ring forceps.

By the time the physician arrived, the bleeding had abated and the uterus was firm. Patty and David had met with the physician consultant on two occasions during the prenatal period, and felt very pleased that she arrived quickly. They were also pleased that no additional intervention was needed and that their plans for an early return to their home were not changed.

Follow-up Care

Despite the differences in their backgrounds and the settings in which they received care, both Keisha and Patty had the benefit of excellent midwifery care and access to high-quality medical and nursing care. Both women had minimal intervention at birth, and

both experienced no postpartum complications. Both were discharged from their settings within 24 hours of giving birth, feeling good about themselves and their experience. Both women were satisfied with their care and their providers. Both successfully breast-fed their babies, both received a follow-up phone call from their midwife, and both returned for follow-up visits. After spending time at home with their babies, Keisha returned to school and Patty returned to work. Keisha and Patty's experiences and outcomes were ideal, and represent those that can be expected when nurse-midwives provide care in a comprehensive, family-centered maternity care setting.

INTRAPARTUM PRACTICE MODELS: IN-HOSPITAL AND OUT-OF-HOSPITAL

Several reports have described model practices in which CNMs working in collaboration with other members of the obstetric team offer high-quality care that results in improved access, outcomes, and satisfaction with intrapartum care.[89-97] The following discussion of intrapartum practice models provides the foundation needed to explore the multitude of collaborative practice innovations used in the settings in which nurse-midwives practice. No attempt has been made to represent all types of practice, but rather to provide enough information to stimulate new ideas about the role of the nurse-midwife in modern obstetric practice.

Characteristics of the Women Served Across Birth Sites

The contribution of nurse-midwives to the care of vulnerable populations is discussed earlier. Table 5-3 shows several interesting comparisons of the percentages of CNMs who serve vulnerable women in various birth settings. CNMs in practices that include home births serve more rural women and fewer inner-city women than do CNMs in practices that attend births in birth centers or hospitals. CNMs who attend births in hospitals are more likely to serve inner-city women and other vulnerable groups than are CNMs using other birth sites; the lowest percentage of CNMs serving adolescent, black American, Asian, Hispanic, and immigrant women are those with home-birth practices. Women whose

Table 5-3. Location of Residence, Population Characteristics and Care Payment Source for Recipients of Nurse-Midwifery Care in Three Birth Settings, 1991

Variable	Hospital (%) (n = 1,494)	Birth Center (%) (n = 191)	Home Birth (%) (n = 132)	Total (%) (n = 1,879)
Location of residence				
Inner City	36	22	14	34
Urban	18	26	17	19
Surburban	25	32	29	25
Rural	21	20	39	22
Vulnerable population groups[a]				
Adolescents	96	92	77	95
African Americans	89	87	76	89
Native American	36	40	40	36
Asian/Pacific islander	59	59	40	57
Hispanic	80	81	63	79
Poor	89	84	86	89
Immigrant	53	39	35	51
Uninsured	78	82	93	79
Source of payment for care				
Self paying	8	19	35	11
Health Maintenance Organization	15	18	0	15
Insurance	19	32	33	19
Medicaid	42	26	19	40
Military	6	0	0	5
Indian health	2	0	1	2
Free/other	7	13	13	8

[a] Respondents could select all that applied.
(Adapted from Schupholme et al,[5] with permission.)

care is reimbursed by Medicaid are more commonly cared for by CNMs in hospital settings and least commonly by CNMs in home-birth settings; the reverse is true for women who pay for their own care. Insurance is the most common source of reimbursement for CNMs whose practice includes births in birth centers and hospitals.[5]

In-Hospital Birth Models

A wide range of hospital birth models have flourished in recent years, as have reports about their success in offering collaborative-practice opportunities for physicians, midwives, and nurses. In the past, some reports pointed to the pitfalls of midwifery practice in hospital settings, but in two notable cases[98,99] nurse-midwifery activity has flourished since the publication of information about the problems of integrating midwives in those settings.[88,100] More recent reports about the use of nurse-midwives in teaching hospitals and managed-care set-

tings,[15,17,43,101,102] as well as in several rural health settings,[37,103] have broadened the information available about the potential impact of midwives in hospital practice and in medical education.

Two distinct nurse-midwifery models are used in the intrapartum setting: a comprehensive-care model and an episodic-care model.[17,40,91] The comprehensive-care model is used by midwives who have followed pregnant women prenatally and continue to manage their care during labor, birth, and the postpartum period. Using this model, the midwife often co-manages the woman's care in collaboration with physicians when complications arise. The episodic-care model is used by midwives who screen women in labor at the time of their admission and determine the appropriateness of nurse-midwifery management based on the assessment of their risk status. The comprehensive-care model is a model often used in settings that offer nurse-midwifery care as an alternative birth experience for women, whereas the episodic-care model has been used more often in high-volume clinical settings that serve underserved women of low-socioeconomic backgrounds, notably managed-care settings in which cost reduction is valued. In these settings the recipients of care are less likely to be presented with options about their intrapartum-care providers.

In a descriptive study of over 6,000 women, involving two nurse-midwifery caseloads in a tertiary setting with an overall cesarean birth rate of 17 percent, rates of cesarean delivery were found to be lower in the episodic-care group (1.3 percent) than in the comprehensive-care group (8.2 percent); the rate of outlet forceps use showed similar trends (1.8 percent and 3.8 percent, respectively). Similar results were found in another study of over 10,000 women in another inner-city hospital, in which the cesarean birth rate in episodic and comprehensive caseloads was 0.2 percent and 8.1 percent, respectively.[91] Both settings served predominantly low-income minority populations. These reports and others demonstrate that low operative intervention and complication rates are observed in episodic-care settings.[9,17]

When women are selectively screened at the time of their admission in labor, complications are evaluated and levels of care are determined accordingly. The levels of care are less clear-cut when the comprehensive-care model is used, especially for women who have specifically sought the care of a nurse-midwife. In the comprehensive-care setting the nurse-midwife remains with the woman through birth, despite problems that may have been identified or anticipated on admission. An increased level of co-management with physicians is practiced in the comprehensive-care model, and the outcomes tend to reflect the fact that more complex risk factors may be present for women in this model.

The foregoing are some of the many factors that make comparisons of intrapartum outcomes between physicians and nurse-midwives difficult to assess. However, two prospective studies comparing nurse-midwife and house-staff birth outcomes are notable in their attempts to control patient assignment. One study, reported nearly 20 years ago, demonstrated that low-risk women randomized to episodic house-staff care[9] had a threefold greater rate of low-forceps births than those randomized to epi-

sodic midwifery care; cesarean birth rates for the two groups were similar.

Another more recent study[102] randomized carefully selected women to either midwifery or house-staff care at the time of their admission in labor. There was no significant difference in cesarean birth rates between the two groups, but the house-staff group had significantly lower overall operative birth rates, attributed to more frequent use of forceps and vacuum extractions for births. In addition, there were significantly more episiotomies, third- and fourth-degree lacerations, and use of analgesics and oxytocic agents in the house-staff group. Both studies verified that intervention rates are higher among resident-physician-managed than in nurse-midwife-managed settings, even when population characteristics and cesarean birth rates are the same.

Out-of-Hospital Birth Models

Even though most births attended by CNMs occur in hospitals, nurse-midwives make a sizable contribution in the out-of-hospital birth setting. The characteristics of the populations served and some important geographic factors differ in the data for out-of-hospital births by CNMs. The highest percentage of CNM activity in free-standing birth centers takes place in the Southwest and the lowest percentage in the Central region of the United States. Most home-birth practices are located in the Northeast and Southwest, with such practices less common in the Southeast.[5]

Home birth has been attended by midwives throughout this century, but the numbers of CNM-attended home births have decreased over the past several years.[62] The primary reason for this decline is the decreasing availability of malpractice insurance for home-birth practitioners. By contrast, births in free-standing birth centers have risen steadily in the past several years. Since its inception at the Maternity Center Association in New York City in 1975, the free-standing birth center has gained popularity as an out-of-hospital birth setting.[27,28,38]

Broader interest in the free-standing birth center was bolstered by a 1989 *New England Journal of Medicine* report about 11,814 women admitted for labor and delivery in 84 free-standing birth centers in the United States.[41] Results indicated a below-average risk of a poor outcome in pregnancy among women giving birth at birth centers. Low rates of complications were reported, including a 2 percent emergency transfer rate in an overall transfer rate of 15.8 percent, a 4.4 percent cesarean birth rate, and no maternal deaths.[41,42] A number of other free-standing birth-center models are emerging throughout the country, providing a unique opportunity for nurse-midwives, physicians, nurses, and other midwives to provide innovative comprehensive care for women of all socioeconomic backgrounds.[104,105]

THE IN-HOSPITAL BIRTH CENTER

Providing what some call "the best of both worlds," the in-hospital birth center is gaining popularity among contemporary intrapartum practice settings.[106–109] A recent report from the Los Angeles County, University of California Women's Hospital Normal Birth Center—a nurse-midwife-managed birth unit serving predominantly low-income Hispanic women—represents the largest longitudinal

experience reported to date of nurse-midwifery collaborative practice[17] in a hospital-based birth center.

Adherence to the philosophy of midwifery care led to women at the Normal Birth Center having the support person(s) of their choice throughout labor and delivery; encouragement of ambulation; intermittent electronic fetal heart-rate monitoring; encouragement of oral fluids throughout labor; food being permitted in many circumstances; the use of primary pain-relief strategies such as showering, ambulation, position changes, and emotional support; labor-stimulation techniques such as ambulation, position changes and breast stimulation with the electric pump; hospital discharge occurring within 12 to 24 hours after delivery; and reminder phone calls. Newborns returned within 2 to 3 days after birth for a routine examination in the Normal Birth Center by pediatric nurse-practitioners. Consultation with a neonatologist or referral to a pediatric specialty clinic was available if needed. The clinical criteria used in 1992 for admission to the birth center, in-

---

Admission, Intra- and Postpartum Transfer, and Exclusion Criteria at the Normal Birth Center, 1992

Admission Criteria

Gestational age >36 to <42 completed weeks

Gestational age ≥43 weeks with reactive non-stress test and amniotic fluid index ≥10 cm

Estimated fetal weight 2,500 to 4,000 g

Low-risk class A1 diabetes
  1. Regular attendance at clinic with normal fasting blood sugar (FBS <105) documented in prenatal records within last month
  2. Without history of overt diabetes, antepartum stillbirth, or traumatic delivery due to macrosomia

One prior cesarean section with
  1. Documented low transverse uterine scar and patient desire for trial of labor at the Normal Birth Center

  2. Undocumented uterine scar with history of uncomplicated vaginal birth after cesarean

Exclusion Criteria for Admission

Anemia (hematocrit <28 percent)

Parity >8

Previous cesarean section with the following
  1. Undocumented uterine scar, no prior vaginal birth after cesarean
  2. Low vertical or classic uterine scar
  3. More than one cesarean section

Previous difficult delivery

Weight >225 lb

Hypertension 140/90 mm Hg

Proteinuria >2+

Positive syphilis serology, untreated

(Continues)

Client in custody

Spontaneous rupture of membranes
1. Not in labor
2. Signs or symptoms of amnionitis

At-risk class A1 diabetic patients, including history of
1. Previous overt diabetes
2. Prior antepartum stillbirth
3. Traumatic delivery due to macrosomia

Abnormal vaginal bleeding

Multiple gestation

Temperature >99.6°F

Unidentifiable presenting part

Station >-3 for multiparas; >-2 for primiparas

Thick meconium

Acute or chronic medical condition

Nonvertex presentation

Intrapartum and Postpartum Transfer Criteria

Fetal

Abnormal fetal heart rate pattern indicative of fetal distress that is unresponsive to alleviating interventions

Maternal:

Evidence of amnionitis
Development of pregnancy-induced hypertension/pre-eclampsia
Request or need for regional anesthesia
Hematocrit <28 percent on admission
Hemorrhage prior to delivery
Excessive blood loss at delivery or fourth stage—and symptomatic
Prolonged second stage (2 or 3 hours)
Failure to progress during active labor
Clients who, after evaluation, do not comply with admission criteria
Client request for medical management

Exclusion Criteria for 12-Hour Discharge

Abnormal physical examination

Medical, surgical, or psychiatric problem

Estimated blood loss >750 mL

Hematocrit <30 percent

Marked episiotomy discomfort; severe bruising or edema

Temperature >100.4°F during hospitalization or >99.4°F at 12 hours

Unable to ambulate easily and/or care for self and infant

Third- or fourth-degree laceration

(From Greulich et al,[17] with permission.)

trapartum and postpartum transfer, and exclusion for 12-hour discharge are provided in the boxed list.

Study results demonstrated the very impressive outcomes achieved during 36,410 birth center admissions and 30,311 nurse-midwife attended births at the Normal Birth Center from 1981 to 1992. No intrapartum maternal or fetal deaths occurred. The intrapartum transfer rate averaged 17 percent with a steady decline from 28 percent in 1982 to 7 percent in 1990, when changes occurred in the criteria for transfer. Resident-team care or transfer to the traditional high-risk labor and delivery ward was pro-

vided if labor complications occurred. Obstetric and pediatric residents responded within 3 to 5 minutes for emergencies. Among a subset of 25,890 admissions and 22,490 births, the overall primary cesarean birth rate was 1.8 percent and the operative birth rate was 4 percent; the overall hospital birth rate was 10 percent. Figure 5-6 shows how decreases in intrapartum transfers were associated with small but steady decreases in the rates of operative intervention.

Tables 5-4 and 5-5 give detailed information about 6,109 women who gave birth at the Normal Birth

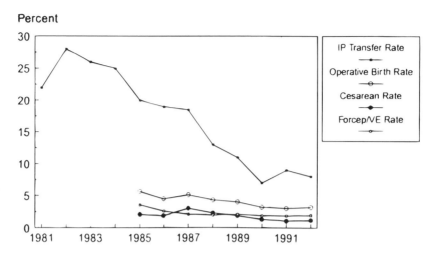

Fig. 5-6. Intrapartum transfer and operative birth rates among all Normal Birth Center admissions, 1981–1992. (From Greulich et al,[17] with permission.)

Table 5-4. Selected Demographic and Clinical Characteristics of Women Whose Births Occurred at the Normal Birth Center, 1990–1991[a]

Demographics	n	%
Age		
<18	409	6.7
18–34	5,329	87.2
≥35	371	6.1
Race		
Hispanic	5,771	95
Asian	85	1.0
Black	59	1.0
White	62	1.0
Unknown	132	2.0
Parity		
0	1,681	28
1	1,784	29
2–4	2,334	38
≥5	310	5
No prenatal care	579	9.5
Gestational age		
<38 wk	756	12.4
38–41 wk	5,021	82.2
≥42 wk	332	5.4

[a] n = 6,109.
(From Greulich et al,[17] with permission.)

Table 5-5. Selected Labor and Birth Outcomes at the Normal Birth Center, 1990–1991[a]

Labor and Birth Outcomes	n	%
Medications in labor		
None	5,683	93
Meperidine	259	4.3
Hydroxyzine	167	2.7
Perineum		
Intact	3,493	57.2
Episiotomy	311	5.1
1st- or 2nd-degree	2,128	34.8
laceration	109	1.8
3rd- or 4th-degree	68	1.1
laceration		
Unknown		
Meconium stained amniotic fluid		
None	4,684	77
Thin	870	14
Thick	514	8.3
Unknown	41	0.7
Apgar score		
<8 at 5 min	27	0.4
Birth weight		
<2,500 g	61	1
2,500–4,000 g	5,566	91
4,001–4,500 g	445	7.3
>4,500 g	37	0.7

[a] n = 6,109.
(From Greulich et al,[17] with permission.)

Center in 1991 and 1992. The nurse-midwifery practice in this setting allowed for the use of a wide variety of noninterventive methods, many of which are described earlier in this chapter as integral aspects of nurse-midwifery care. Outcomes reflected adherence to nurse-midwifery practice philosophies; for example, as seen in Table 5-4, over 90 percent of all labors were not medicated, and over half led to births without episiotomy or lacerations. Newborn outcomes were also very impressive. Data available from 1985 to 1992 reported a neonatal intensive care unit (NICU) admission rate of 1.5 percent and a 1-week newborn readmission rate of 1.3 percent among newborns discharged within 12 to 24 hours. Eighty-five percent of all newborns returned for follow-up care.

The Los Angeles County example confirms that excellent outcomes can be achieved when nurse-midwives, working collaboratively and cooperatively with obstetricians, neonatologists, resident physicians, pediatric nurse-practitioners, and nurses, provide episodic care in a hospital-based birth-center setting.[17] The report of the Normal Birth Center experience also offers important information about in-hospital birth center practices by nurse-midwives, and the importance of providing similar models for low-income populations as well as for childbearing families with the means for seeking childbirth alternatives.

REGULATORY OBSTACLES FACING NURSE-MIDWIVES

Despite the sizable body of literature in support of nurse-midwifery practice, barriers continue to exist for CNMs and those seeking to support them. While some improvements have been made, especially in the acceptance of nurse-midwifery by the medical community and heightened awareness of it by the general public, obstacles persist that preclude nurse-midwives from full-scope clinical practice and collaborative relationships with physicians.[110] Recent studies demonstrate that a higher number of CNMs are in practice in states in which the regulatory environment is supportive of nurse-midwives, and there is as much as a threefold increase in the proportion of births attended by CNMs.[7,50] Nurse-midwives and their colleagues will have to work together to achieve

regulatory environments that enhance practice opportunities for all members of the team while maximizing care opportunities for all child-bearing families.[7,50,56,59]

ROLE OF THE NURSE-MIDWIFE IN THE 21st CENTURY

Throughout this century, nurse-midwives have kept pace with the ever-changing health-care environment, and more recently have developed ways in which to integrate their practice into the broader health-care arena. As consumer demand for nurse-midwives increases, government officials have begun to emphasize the prospective roles of CNMs in health-reform plans and health-care work-force projections.[110]

Nurse-midwifery practice encompasses all aspects of care for pregnant women and newborns, as well as family planning and preventive gynecologic and primary care for women of all ages.[112,113] The CNM's range of practice settings and access to other health-care providers will be an important factor in determining the scope of the clinical services that CNMs provide and other roles they may assume in the future.[43] For example, in rural locations the CNM will provide a broader range of primary care and comprehensive health-care services than in the urban centers in which care is often provided by larger and sometimes more specialized teams. In all settings, CNMs will assume expanded roles in medical and obstetrics residency education, and the sites of medical education will shift from the hospital to the community settings in which nurse-midwives have played key roles in ambulatory service.

Advanced nurse-midwifery practice and expanded collaboration will flourish in the future as the national emphasis on partnership, team-building, and careful allocation of resources unfolds. Through a specific postgraduate process specified by the ACNM,[114,115] the CNM's role can be expanded to include advanced practice skills.[116] These include the skills of third-trimester ultrasonography,[117] advanced fetal assessment,[117,118] circumcision,[119] vacuum extraction,[120] home care for women at risk of preterm labor,[43] primary care of women (with special emphasis on at-risk populations such as women with human immunodeficiency virus infection and drug addiction),[120,121] and collaborative management of women with high-risk pregnancies.[43,94,95,122]

Perhaps the greatest opportunity for nurse-midwives lies in broadened leadership roles in administration, education, service, research, and advocacy.[43,124] These leadership roles would allow for the smooth integration of midwifery practice modalities into the health-care arena. Broader roles for nurse-midwives in intrapartum practice administration include the management of labor and delivery units in hospitals,[17,35] management of other in-hospital clinical services such as fetal assessment units,[117,118] and development and management of out-of-hospital birth centers in collaboration with hospitals and health centers.[40,105,106]

Broader roles for nurse-midwives in education include the coordination of continuing professional education activities[118]; coordination of intrapartum education for residents, medical students, midwives and nurses[43,100,125]; and training of community-health workers to improve community linkages, especially in communities with high infant mortality rates.[88] Broader intrapartum research roles for nurse-midwives include the design and implementation of research in technology assessment,[126] health-services research on access to care,[5–7,41] and a variety of collaborative clinical research projects.[127–130] Broader health-policy roles for nurse-midwives include the development of clinical-practice guidelines[131]; participation with policy-making agencies about care payment strategies and other issues related to childbirth[7,56,59]; and active participation in local, regional, or national organizations concerned with the quality of care for childbearing families in the United States[19,20,51,103,131,132] and around the world.[133]

Experts conferring about the role of the obstetrician/gynecologist in the 21st century concluded that a team approach [that includes nurse-midwives] is needed to meet the reproductive needs of all American women in a cost-effective manner.[23] As this century draws to a close, growing numbers of nurse-midwives, working in close collaboration with their colleagues in medicine and nursing, will provide balance to an intrapartum health-care team striving to meet the needs and desires of childbearing families in the United States today. Certified nurse-midwives

also have the capacity to extend care to underserved populations and provide both medical and preventive care to all women and infants.

REFERENCES

1. Summit II: Visionary Planning for Health Care of Women. American College of Nurse-Midwives, Washington, DC, 1993
2. Weidenbach E: Family-centered Maternity Nursing. GP Putnam's Sons, New York, 1958
3. Laird MD: Report of the Maternity Center Association Clinic, New York, 1931–1951. Am J Obstet Gynecol 60:178, 1955
4. Rooks J: American nurse-midwifery practice in 1976–1977: reflections of 50 years of growth and development. Am J Public Health 9:70, 1980
5. Scupholme A, DeJoseph J, Strobino DM, Paine LL: Nurse-midwifery care to vulnerable populations. Phase I. Demographic characteristics of the national CNM sample. J Nurse Midwifery 37:341, 1994
6. Scupholme A, Paine LL, Lang JL et al: Time associated with components of clinical services rendered by nurse-midwives: sample data from phase II of nurse-midwifery care to vulnerable populations in the United States. J Nurse Midwifery 39:5, 1994
7. Paine LL, DeJoseph JF, Strobino DM et al: Nurse-midwives: quality care for women and infants. American College of Nurse-Midwives, Washington, DC, 1994
8. Levy BS, Wilkinson PS, Marine WM: Reducing neonatal mortality rate with nurse-midwives. Am J Obstet Gynecol 109:51, 1971
9. Slome C, Wetherbee H, Daly M et al: Effectiveness of certified nurse-midwives: a prospective evaluation study. Am J Obstet Gynecol 124:177, 1976
10. Cherry J, Foster J: Comparison of hospital charges generated by certified nurse-midwives' and physicians' clients. J Nurse-Midwifery 27:7, 1982
11. Diers D, Burst H: Effectiveness of policy related research: nurse-midwifery as case study. J Nurs Scholarship 15:68, 1983
12. Leppert P, Namerow P: Costs averted by providing comprehensive prenatal care to teenagers. J Nurse Midwifery 30:285, 1985
13. Platt LD, Angelini DJ, Paul RH et al: Nurse-midwifery in a large teaching hospital. Obstet Gynecol 66:816, 1985
14. Thompson J: Nurse-midwifery care: 1925–1984. p. 153. In Wesley HH, Fitzpatrick JJ (eds): Annual Review of Nursing Research. Vol. 4. Springer, New York, 1984
15. Bell K, Mills J: Certified nurse-midwife effectiveness

in the health maintenance organization obstetric team. Obstet Gynecol 74:112, 1989

16. Minor AF: Research Bulletin: The Cost of Maternity Care and Childbirth in the United States, 1989. Health Insurance Association of America, Washington, DC, 1989

17. Greulich B, Paine LL, McLain C et al: Twelve years and over 30,000 nurse-midwife attended births: the LAC + USC Women's Hospital birth center experience. J Nurse Midwifery 39:185, 1994

18. Olivio LB, Freda MC, Piening S et al: Midwifery care: a descriptive study of patient satisfaction. J Women's Health 3:3, 1994

19. Committee to Study the Prevention of Low Birthweight: Preventing low birthweight. National Academy Press, Washington, DC, 1985

20. Committee to Study Outreach for Prenatal Care: Prenatal care. Reaching mothers, reaching infants. National Academy Press, Washington, DC, 1988

21. Office of Technology Assessment: Nurse-practitioners, physician assistants and certified nurse-midwives: a policy analysis (OTA, HCS [37]). United States Government Printing Office, Washington, DC, December, 1986

22. AGOG creates a Department of Collaborative Practice. ACOG Newsletter 37:10, 1993

23. The Obstetrician/Gynecologist in the Twenty-First Century—Meeting Society's Needs: Conference Summary. Josiah Macy Jr. Foundation, New York, 1993

24. Boschert S: California rides wave of the future: collaborative ob./nurse-midwife practices. Ob/Gyn News 29:18, 1994

25. Varney H: Nurse-Midwifery. 2nd Ed. Blackwell, Boston, 1987

26. Browne HE, Isaacs G: The Frontier Nursing Service: the primary care nurse in a community hospital. Am J Obstet Gynecol 124:14, 1976

27. Rooks J, Haas JE: Nurse-midwifery in America. A report of the ACNM Foundation Inc. American College of Nurse-Midwives, Washington, DC, 1986

28. Ulrich S: Revisiting an "old" solution to the high costs of maternity care. Med Interface October:106, 1994

29. Smith WE: Nurse-midwife Maude Callen eases the pain of birth, death, and life. Life Magazine December 3:134, 1951

30. Hogan A: A tribute to the pioneers. J Nurse Midwifery Summer 6, 1975

31. Mann R: San Francisco General Hospital nurse-midwifery practice: the first thousand births. Am J Obstet Gynecol 140:676, 1981

32. Baruffi G, Dellinger W, Strobino D et al: A study of

the pregnancy outcomes in a maternity hospital and a tertiary care hospital. Am J Public Health 74:9, 1984

33. Baruffi GS, Strobino DM, Paine LL: An investigation of institutional differences in primary cesarean rates. J Nurse Midwifery 35:274, 1990

34. Piechnik SL, Corbett MA: Reducing low birthweight among socioeconomically high-risk adolescent pregnancies: successful intervention with certified nurse-midwife-managed care. J Nurse Midwifery 30:88, 1985

35. Haire DB, Elsberry CC: Maternity care and outcomes in a high-risk service: the North Central Bronx Hospital experience. Birth 18:33, 1991

36. Murdaugh A: Experiences of a new migrant health clinic. Women Health 1:25, 1976

37. Bacchi D, Phillips D, Kessel W et al: Federal programs affecting rural perinatal health care. J Rural Health 5:413, 1989

38. Bennetts AB, Lubic RW: The free-standing birth center. Lancet 1:378, 1982

39. Laube DW. Experience with an alternative birth center in a university hospital. J Reprod Med 28:391, 1983

40. Scupholme A, McLeod AGW, Robertson EG: A birth center affiliated with the tertiary care center: comparison of outcomes. Obstet Gynecol 67:598, 1986

41. Rooks J, Weatherby N, Ernst E et al: Outcomes of care in birth centers. The national birth center study. N Engl J Med 321:1804, 1989

42. Rooks JP, Weatherby NL, Ernst EKM: The national birth center study. Part III. Intrapartum and immediate postpartum and neonatal complications and transfers, postpartum and neonatal care, outcomes, and client satisfaction. J Nurse Midwifery 37:361, 1992

43. Paine LL: Primary ob/gyn rounds at the Johns Hopkins Medical Institutions: the role of the nurse-midwife in primary ob/gyn. Fem Patient 17:129, 1992

44. Declercq ER: Where babies are born and who attends their births: findings from the revised 1989 United States Standard Certificate of Live Birth. Obstet Gynecol 81:997, 1993

45. Declercq E: The transformation of American midwifery: 1975 to 1988. Am J Public Health 82:680, 1992

46. Schappert SM: National ambulatory medical care survey: 1992 Summary. Advance Data-National Center for Health Statistics, Washington, DC, 253:1, 1993

47. McCormick B: Childbearing and nurse-midwives: A woman's right to choose. NYU Law Rev 58:661, 1983

48. Langton P, Kammerer D: Childbearing and women's

choice of nurse-midwives in Washington, DC hospitals. Women Health 15:49, 1989

49. Hoffman C: Medicaid payment for nonphysician practitioners: an access issue. Health Affairs 13:140, 1994

50. Sekscenski ES, Sansom S, Bazell C et al: State practice environments and the supply of physician assistants, nurse practitioners, and certified nurse-midwives. N Engl J Med 331:1266, 1994

51. National Commission on Nurse-Midwifery Education: Educating nurse-midwives: a strategy for achieving affordable, high-quality maternity care. Executive Summary. American College of Nurse-Midwives, Washington, DC, 1993

52. Roberts J: An overview of nurse-midwifery education and accreditation. J Nurse Midwifery 36:373, 1991

53. Whitfill KA, Burst HV: ACNM-accredited and pre-accredited nurse-midwifery education programs: program information. J Nurse Midwifery 39:221, 1994

54. Core competencies for basic nurse-midwifery practice. American College of Nurse-Midwives, Washington, DC, 1992

55. Rooks J, Carr K, Sandvold I: The importance of non-master's degree options in nurse-midwifery education. J Nurse Midwifery 36:124, 1991

56. Fennell K: Prescriptive authority for nurse-midwives, a historical review. Nurs Clin North Am 26:511, 1991

57. Bidgood-Wilson M, Barickman C, Ackley S: Nurse-midwifery today: a legislative update. Part I. J Nurse Midwifery 37:96, 1992

58. Pearson L: 1992–93 update: how each state stands on legislative issues affecting advanced nursing practice. Nurs Pract 18:23, 1993

59. Williams DR: Credentialing certified nurse-midwives. J Nurse Midwifery 39:4, 1994

60. Safriet BJ: Health care dollars and regulatory sense: the role of advanced practice nursing. Yale J Regul 2:9, 1992

61. Guidelines for obtaining hospital practice privileges including guidelines for medical staff bylaws. American College of Nurse-Midwives, Washington, DC, 1989

62. Centers for Disease Control and Prevention/National Center for Health Statistics: Advance report of final natality statistics, 1992. Monthly Vital Statistics Report, Suppl. 43, October 25, 1994

63. Philosophy of the American College of Nurse-Midwives. American College of Nurse-Midwives, Washington, DC, 1989

64. Eastman N: Briefs. The Johns Hopkins Hospital. Baltimore, 1953

65. Montgomery TA: A case for nurse-midwives. Am J Obstet Gynecol 105:309, 1969

66. Gatewood TS, Stewart RB: Obstetricians and nurse-midwives: the team approach in private practice. Am J Obstet Gynecol 1:35, 1975

67. Perry HB, Youngs DD, King TM: Patient acceptance of a nurse-midwife in a private group practice. J Reprod Med 16:1, 1976

68. Perry HB: Role of the nurse-midwife in contemporary maternity care. In Youngs DD, Ehrhardt AA (eds): Psychosomatic Obstetrics and Gynecology. Appleton-Century-Crofts, E. Norwalk, CT, 1980

69. Long WN, Sharp E: Relationships between professions: from the viewpoint of the physician and nurse-midwife in a tertiary center. Emory University School of Medicine-GYN/OB Dept Bull 3:184, 1991

70. Baruffi G, Dellinger W, Strobino D et al: Patterns of obstetric procedure use in maternity care. Obstet Gynecol 64:4, 1984

71. Strobino D, Baruffi G, Dellinger W et al: Variations in pregnancy outcomes and use of obstetrics procedures in two institutions with divergent philosophies of maternity care. Med Care 26 (4):333, 1988

72. Position statement on the use of technology in childbirth. American College of Nurse-Midwives, Washington, DC, 1992

73. Standards for the practice of nurse-midwifery. American College of Nurse-Midwives, Washington, DC, 1993

74. Continuing competency assessment. American College of Nurse-Midwives, Washington, DC, 1992

75. Peer review. American College of Nurse-Midwives, Washington, DC, 1992

76. Jenkins S: The myth of vicarious liability: impact on barriers to nurse-midwifery practice. J Nurse Midwifery 39:98, 1994

77. Marchese T, Coughlin J-H, Adams CJ: Childbirth. p. 115. In Adams C (ed): Nurse-Midwifery Health Care for Women and Newborns. Grune & Stratton, Orlando, FL, 1983

78. Thorp JM, Bowes WA: Episiotomy: can its routine use be defended? Am J Obstet Gynecol 160:1027, 1989

79. Banta HD, Thacker SB: The case for reassessment of health care technology: Once is not enough. JAMA 264:235, 1990

80. Chalmers I, Enkin M, Kierse MFNC (eds): Effective Care in Pregnancy and Childbirth. Vol. 1, 2. Oxford University Press, Oxford, 1989

81. Enkin M, Keirse NC, Chalmers I: A Guide to Effective Care in Pregnancy and Childbirth. Oxford University Press, New York, 1989

82. Hickson G, Clayton E, Githens P et al: Factors that prompted families to file medical malpractice claims following perinatal injuries. JAMA 267:1359, 1992
83. Lesser MS, Keane VR: Nurse-Patient Relationship in a Hospital Service. CV Mosby, St. Louis, 1956
84. American College of Nurse-Midwives, American College of Obstetricians and Gynecologists: Joint statement of practice relationships between obstetrician/gynecologists and certified nurse-midwives. American College of Nurse-Midwives, Washington, DC, 1982
85. Collaborative management in nurse-midwifery practice for medical, gynecological, and obstetrical conditions. American College of Nurse-Midwives, Washington, DC, 1992
86. Baldwin LM, Raine T, Jenkins L et al: Do providers adhere to ACOG standards? The case of prenatal care. Obstet Gynecol 84:4, 1994
87. Kong D, McNamara: Birth in the "death zones" (5-part series on infant mortality). Boston Globe, September 9–13, 1990
88. Maternal and Child Health Commission, 1991–1992 Annual Report. Boston Maternal and Child Health Commission, Boston, 1992
89. Rollins AJ, Kaplan JA, Ratkay ME et al: A homestyle delivery program in a university hospital. J Fam Pract 9:407, 1979
90. Scupholme A: Nurse-midwives and physicians: a team approach to obstetrical care in a perinatal center. J Nurse Midwifery 27:21, 1982
91. Sharp ES, Lewis LE: A decade of nurse-midwifery practice in a tertiary university-affiliated hospital. J Nurse Midwifery 29:353, 1984
92. Wingeier R, Bloch S, Kvale J: A description of a CNM-family physician joint practice in a rural setting. J Nurse Midwifery 33:86, 1988
93. DeVane DM, Richwald GA, Elftman S et al: Babies and mothers at risk: perinatal needs assessment for Los Angeles County. March of Dimes Birth Defects Foundation, Burbank, CA, October, 1990
94. Heins HC, Nance NW, McCarthy BJ et al: A randomized trial of nurse-midwifery prenatal care to reduce low birth weight. Obstet Gynecol 75:3, 1990
95. Butler J, Abrams B, Parker J et al: Supportive nurse-midwife care is associated with a reduced incidence of cesarean section. Am J Obstet Gynecol 168:1407, 1993
96. Capan P, Beard M, Mashburn M: Nurse-managed clinics provide access and improved health care. Nurse Pract 18:50, 1993
97. Davis L, Riedmann G, Sapiro M et al: Cesarean section rates in low-risk private patients managed by certified nurse-midwives and obstetricians. J Nurse Midwifery 39:91, 1994
98. Breece C, Israel E, Friedman L: Closing of the nurse-midwifery service at Boston City Hospital: what were the issues involved? J Nurse Midwifery 34:41, 1989
99. Graham SB: A structural analysis of physician-midwife interaction in an obstetrical training program. Soc Sci Med 32:931, 1991
100. Sedler KD, Lydon-Rochelle M, Castillo YM et al: Nurse-midwifery service model in an academic environment. J Nurse Midwifery 38:241, 1993
101. Barton JJ, Rovner S, Puls K et al: Alternative birthing center: experience in a teaching obstetric service. Am J Obstet Gynecol 137:377, 1980
102. Chambliss LR, Daly C, Medearis AL et al: The role of selection bias in comparing cesarean birth rates between physician and midwifery management. Obstet Gynecol 80:161, 1992
103. Rural Information Center Health Service: Nurse practitioners, physician assistants, and certified nurse-midwives: primary care providers in rural areas. Rural Health in Brief May 1, 1994
104. Wintemute K, Jackson DJ, Mateo M et al: A descriptive study of the co-management model at the BirthPlace, San Diego. OB/GYN Consultants, San Diego, CA, 1992
105. Dickinson CP, Jackson DJ, Swartz WH: Making the alternative the mainstream: maintaining a family-centered focus in a large free-standing birth center for low-income women. J Nurs Midwifery 39:197, 1994
106. Hewitt MA, Hangsleben KL: Nurse-midwives in a hospital birth center. J Nurse Midwifery 26:21, 1981
107. DeVries RG: Image and reality: an evaluation of hospital alternative birth centers. J Nurse Midwifery 28:3, 1983
108. Hoffman K, Lorkovic M, Rayburn W et al: Alternative birth centers: a four-year experience at the University of Nebraska Medical Center. Neb Med J 72(8):268, 1987
109. Survey of obstetric and newborn services—1989. p. 1. Hospital Data Center and the Section for Maternal and Child Health, American Hospital Association, Chicago, 1990
110. Office of the Inspector General: A survey of certified nurse-midwives. U.S. Department of Health and Human Services, Atlanta, GA, March 1992
111. Mullan F, Rivio ML, Politzer RM: Doctors, dollars, and determination: making physician work-force policy. Health Affairs 12:138, 1993
112. Definition of a certified nurse-midwife and nurse-

midwifery practice. American College of Nurse-Midwives, Washington, DC, 1992

113. Certified nurse-midwives as primary care providers. American College of Nurse-Midwives, Washington, DC, 1992

114. Expansion of nurse-midwifery practice beyond basic core competencies. American College of Nurse-Midwives, Washington, DC, 1992

115. Guidelines for the incorporation of new procedures in nurse-midwifery practice. American College of Nurse-Midwives, Washington, DC, 1992

116. Avery M, DelGiudice GT: High-tech skills in low-tech hands: issues of advanced practice and collaborative management. J Nurse Midwifery, suppl., 38:9s, 1993

117. Gegor CL: Third trimester ultrasound for nurse-midwives. J Nurse Midwifery, suppl., 38:49s, 1993

118. Gegor CL, Paine LL, Johnson TRB: Antepartum fetal assessment—a nurse-midwifery perspective. J Nurse Midwifery 36:153, 1993

119. Gelbaum I: Circumcision: refining a traditional surgical technique. J Nurse Midwifery, suppl., 38:18s, 1993

120. Johnson P, Pace S: Guide to the use of vacuum extraction. J Nurse Midwifery, suppl., 38:88s, 1993

121. DeFerrari E, Paine LL, Gegor CL et al: Midwifery care for women with HIV disease in pregnancy: a demonstration project at the Johns Hopkins Hospital. J Nurse Midwifery 38:97, 1993

122. DeFerrari E, Gegor CL, Summers L et al: Nurse-midwifery management of women with HIV disease. J Nurse Midwifery 38:86, 1993

123. Ellings JM, Newman RB, Hulsey TC: Reduction in very low birth weight deliveries and perinatal mortality in a specialized, multidisciplinary twin clinic. Obstet Gynecol 81:3, 1993

124. Paine LL: Midwifery education and research in the future. J Nurse Midwifery 36:199, 1991

125. Keleher K: Nurse-midwifery care in an academic health center. J Obstet Gynecol Neonatal Nurs 15:369, 1986

126. Paine LL, Benedict MI, Strobino DM et al: A comparison of the auscultated acceleration test and the nonstress test as predictors of perinatal outcome. Nurs Res 41:87, 1992

127. Paine LL, Greener DL, Strobino DM: Birth registration: nurse-midwifery roles and responsibilities. J Nurse Midwifery 33:107, 1988

128. Blakemore KJ, Qin N-G, Petrie RH et al: A prospective comparision of hourly and quarter-hourly oxytocin dose increase intervals for the induction of labor at term. Obstet Gynecol 75:757, 1990

129. Reddy U, Paine LL, Gegor C et al: Fetal movement in labor. Am J Obstet Gynecol 165:1073, 1991

130. Paine LL, Tinker DD: The effect of maternal bearing-down efforts on arterial umbilical cord pH and length of the second stage of labor. J Nurse Midwifery 37:61, 1992

131. Committee on Nutritional Status During Pregnancy and Lactation: Nutrition During Pregnancy and Lactation: An Implementation Guide. National Academy Press, Washington, DC, 1992

132. Merkatz IR, Thompson JE (eds): New perspectives on prenatal care. Elsevier, New York, 1990

133. Kwast B: Midwives role in safe motherhood. J Nurse Midwifery 36:366, 1991

Chapter 6

Normal Labor and Delivery

Thomas D. Shipp and John T. Repke

ANATOMY

The human female pelvis is not only indispensable in transmitting the weight of the upper body to the lower extremities, but also functions as the birth canal. Intimate knowledge of the structure and function of the pelvis is essential to the practice of obstetrics.

The bony pelvis is made up of two hip bones and the sacrum. Each hip bone, which usually completely ossifies by early adult life, is formed by the fusion of the ileum, ischium, and the pubic bones. The sacrum is formed as the fusion of the sacral vertebrae. The sacrum articulates superiorly with the fifth lumbar vertebra and inferiorly with the coccyx. Both hip bones articulate anteriorly at the pubic symphysis and posteriorly with the sacrum at the sacroiliac joints (Fig. 6-1).

The pelvic brim divides the pelvis into two portions. The pelvic brim is outlined by the sacral promontory, the anterior ala of the sacrum, the arcuate line of the ilium, the pectineal line of the pubic bone, the pubic crest, and the symphysis[1] (Fig. 6-1). The portion above the pelvic brim is termed the false, or greater pelvis, and the portion below the brim is termed the true, or lesser pelvis. This border is important in obstetrics because it is the most narrow portion of the pelvic inlet and leads into the true pelvis. The pelvic inlet is typically oval, which has significance for the fetus in that it allows easier en-trance of the fetal head at the narrow threshold of the birth canal.

OBSTETRIC PLANES AND DIAMETERS

Given the unique configuration of the human pelvis, a number of planes have obstetric significance. Obstetric planes have been characterized for the pelvic inlet, the midpelvis, and the pelvic outlet. The plane of the pelvic inlet makes an angle of about 60 degrees with the horizontal. The axis of the pelvis, which is approximated by the midpoints of the diameters of the pelvis from inlet to outlet, makes an unusually angled course as it descends through the pelvis[1] (Fig. 6-2).

The plane of the pelvic inlet accommodates two clinically useful diameters, the transverse and the anteroposterior. The transverse diameter is ordinarily the largest diameter of the pelvic inlet and is measured from the left to the right arcuate line (Fig. 6-3). A normal value for this diameter is greater than 12 cm. This diameter lies closer to the promontory of the sacrum than the pubic symphysis. The anteroposterior diameter cannot be directly measured clinically, but is closely estimated. The true conjugate is the distance from the promontory of the sacrum to the most superior portion of the pubic symphysis, yet this is not the limiting distance of the pelvic inlet. The obstetric conjugate, which represents the small-

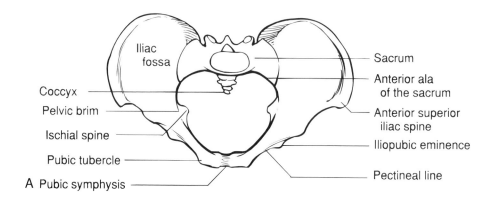

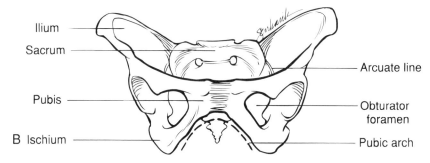

Fig. 6-1. **(A)** Superior view of the female pelvis. **(B)** Anterior view of the female pelvis.

est diameter through which the fetus must pass in the pelvic inlet, is the distance from the promontory of the sacrum to the nearest portion of the pubic symphysis. The lower limit of normal for the obstetric conjugate is 10 cm. We estimate the obstetric conjugate by measuring the diagonal conjugate from the sacral promontory to the most inferior portion of the pubic symphysis, and subtracting 1.5 to 2 cm (Fig. 6-4).

The midpelvis is distinguished as being the smallest plane in the pelvis, chiefly because of the transverse diameter, which lies between the ischial spines (Fig. 6-5). This diameter normally measures more than 10 cm. The anteroposterior diameter in this plane is not routinely measured.

The pelvic outlet is rarely of a profoundly contracted state without significant midpelvis or pelvic-inlet constriction. The two planes that describe the pelvic outlet are contiguous anterior and posterior

triangles that use the intertuberous diameter as their base. The apex of the anterior triangle is the pubic symphysis, and the apex of the posterior triangle is the coccyx. The anteroposterior diameter from the pubic symphysis to the coccyx typically measures approximately 13 cm.[1] The most important diameter of the pelvic outlet is the transverse diameter between the ischial tuberosities, which normally measures more than 8 cm[9] (Fig. 6-6).

Significant changes in the pelvis occur during pregnancy, and especially during labor. Simple widening of the symphysis pubis and sacroiliac joints is standard as the pelvis prepares for vaginal delivery. Rotation of the sacroiliac joints about a transverse axis, and sliding of the sacrum in its connection with the hip bones, also occur. An increase in the diameters of the pelvis, to a mean of 5 mm as documented radiologically, ensues during labor.[3] These changes lead to an increased capacity of the pelvis.

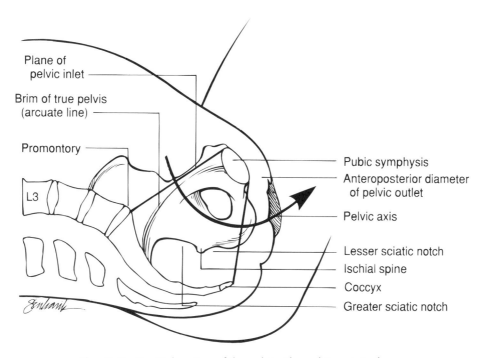

Fig. 6-2. Sagittal section of the pelvis. The pelvic axis is shown.

PELVIC SHAPES

The various types of pelves show considerable diversity. Over half a century ago, Caldwell and Moloy[4] categorized the female pelvis into four general classifications: gynecoid, android, anthropoid, and platypelloid (Fig. 6-7). The estimated frequency of these four types is gynecoid 50 percent, android 26 percent, anthropoid 18 percent, and platypelloid 5 percent.[2] It must be remembered that few women have pelves that fit exactly into each of the pelvic classes, instead being much more likely to have pelvic characteristics of two or more classes. Therefore, intimate knowledge about the possible variation in pelvic characteristics is requisite before reliable assessment is possible.

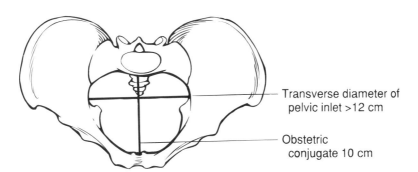

Fig. 6-3. Superior view of the pelvis demonstrating the anteroposterior and transverse diameters of the pelvic inlet.

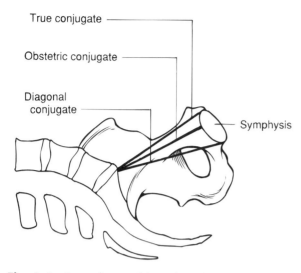

Fig. 6-4. Sagittal view of the pelvis. The three anteroposterior diameters of the pelvic inlet are demonstrated. The obstetric conjugate is estimated from clinical evaluation of the diagonal conjugate.

The gynecoid type is encountered most frequently and is the classic female type of pelvis. A more expansive anteroposterior diameter, coupled with the widest transverse diameter of the inlet being positioned more anterior to the sacral promontory than that noted in the male pelvis, results in the anterior and posterior portions of the pelvis occupying roughly the same commodious area. The walls originate from a circular rim and either run parallel to each other or diverge toward the roomy outlet. The sacrum is rounded and extends posteriorly. A wide, rounded sacrosciatic notch is present and gives an

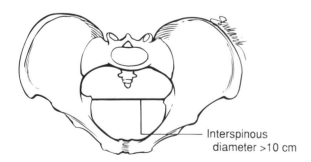

Fig. 6-5. Superior view of the pelvis demonstrating the transverse diameter of the midpelvis at the level of the ischial spines.

ample posterior pelvis, which is an identifying characteristic. There is also a long sacrospinous ligament and a wide subpubic angle[4,5] (Fig. 6-8).

The android type of pelvis has more male characteristics, especially at the posterior inlet, and is therefore often described as being heart shaped. There is an associated narrow forepelvis and a distinctively decreased capacity noted in the posterior portion of the pelvis despite the adequate anteroposterior diameter. The curves are more shallow and the stance more erect than with the more splayed and wide gynecoid pelvis. The walls commonly converge toward the outlet. The sacrum is usually wider and straighter than that seen in the gynecoid pelvis. There is a male-type sacrosciatic notch and an associated short sacrospinous ligament. The ischial spines are unusually palpable. A wide subpubic angle is commonly associated with a sufficient anterior inlet and may help compensate for the male-type posterior segment[4,5] (Fig. 6-9). The pure android pelvis is observed in as many as one-third of white women and in less than one-sixth of nonwhite women.[6] Difficulty can occur with engagement of the fetal head as a result of the limited pelvic capacity. Even if engagement occurs, there remains a risk of the arrest of labor, given the problematic midpelvis with prominent ischial spines and converging pelvic side-walls. Persistence of an occiput-posterior position can also result.[2]

Even with the extended anteroposterior diameter of the inlet, the anthropoid type pelvis can be unexpectedly limited. The transverse diameter of the inlet is relatively narrow, but the primary concern is the limited anterior capacity of the pelvis. If the subpubic angle is narrow, the anterior inlet is then triangular, and the anterior capacity of the pelvis is seriously limited. The side-walls of the pelvis are frequently convergent, and the ischial spines may be somewhat prominent. There is a wide, shallow sacrospinous notch with long sacrospinous ligaments. The sacrum is long and narrow and inclined posteriorly, but if it juts forward can hamper the pelvic outlet capacity[4,5] (Fig. 6-10). The anthropoid pelvis is the most common type of pelvis in nonwhite women, and constitutes roughly half of the pelves in this group.[6] Engagement generally does not present a problem with this pelvis type, nor is descent typically impeded. If the fetal head presents in the occiput-anterior position, labor commonly progresses

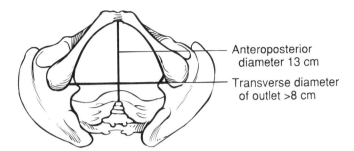

Fig. 6-6. Inferior view of the pelvis demonstrating the diameters of the pelvic outlet. The transverse diameter is assessed between the ischial tuberosities.

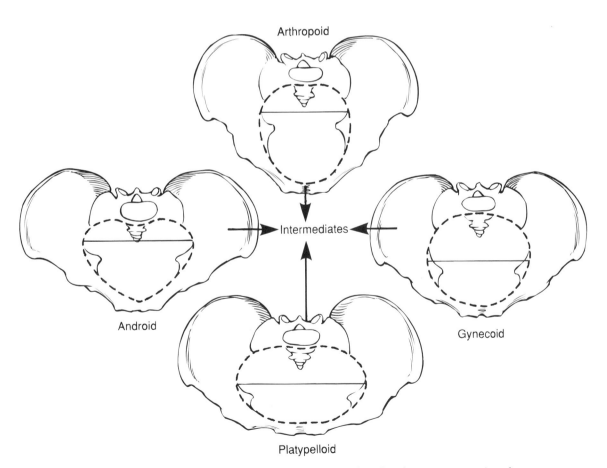

Fig. 6-7. The four true pelvic types according to the Caldwell-Moloy classification. Intermediate forms are more common than the four true types.

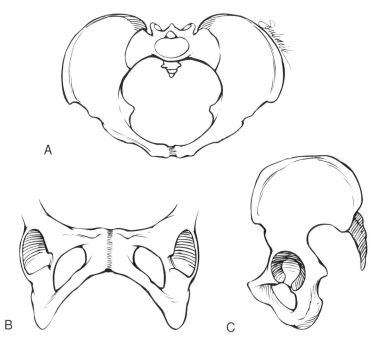

Fig. 6-8. Gynecoid pelvis. **(A)** Superior view demonstrating round inlet. **(B)** Frontal view demonstrating curved, open subpubic arch and outwardly flowing pelvic sidewalls. **(C)** Lateral view demonstrating spacious sacrosciatic notch. The sacrum has a gentle inward inclination. (Adapted from Steer,[5] with permission.)

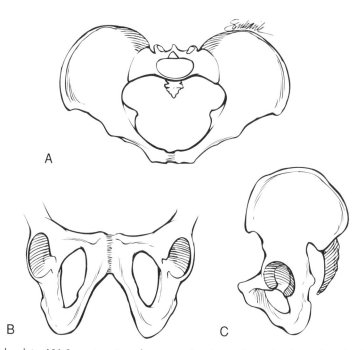

Fig. 6-9. Android pelvis. **(A)** Superior view demonstrating heart-shaped pelvic inlet. The forepelvis is narrow, but more prominent is the limited posterior pelvic capacity. **(B)** Frontal view demonstrating straight, narrow subpubic arch and convergent sidewalls. **(C)** Lateral view demonstrating narrow sacrosciatic notch and sharp inward inclination of the sacrum. (Adapted from Steer,[5] with permission.)

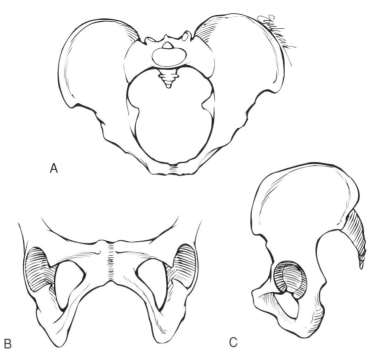

Fig. 6-10. Anthropoid pelvis. **(A)** Superior view demonstrating deep oval pelvic inlet with narrow, angled forepelvis. **(B)** Frontal view demonstrating an intermediate curvature of the subpubic arch and slight convergence of the pelvic sidewalls. **(C)** Lateral view demonstrating wide, shallow sacrosciatic notch and gentle inward inclination of the sacrum. (Adapted from Steer,[5] with permission.)

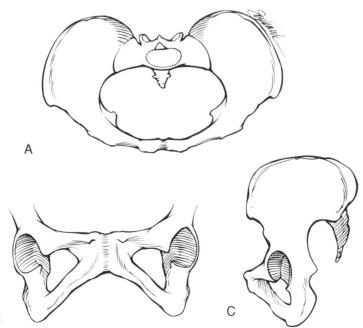

Fig. 6-11. Platypelloid pelvis. **(A)** Superior view demonstrating a wide, oval pelvic inlet. **(B)** Frontal view demonstrating a wide subpubic arch. **(C)** Lateral view demonstrating a narrow sacrosciatic notch and a flat sacrum. (Adapted from Steer,[5] with permission.)

without incident, whereas if it presents in the occiput-posterior position rotation is less likely to occur, and a persistent occiput-posterior position would likely follow.[2]

The rarest type of pelvis is the platypelloid, which is best described as being broad and flat. It is essentially the opposite of the anthropoid pelvis, with the elliptical shape of the pelvic inlet being located transversely. There is a short anteroposterior diameter of the inlet, with a more than ample transverse diameter. The sacrosciatic notch has a narrow aperture, and the sacrum is wide and flattened[4,5] (Fig. 6-11). Because the inlet is so irregularly shaped, engagement can present a significant obstacle to successful labor. Asynclitism often becomes necessary for labor to progress. Internal rotation can also occur later in labor secondary to the flat sacrum.[2]

CLINICAL PELVIMETRY

Clinical pelvimetry is today the most commonly used technique for assessment of the female pelvis. It should be performed during the initial prenatal visit and again when the patient presents in labor and delivery, since significant relaxation of the pelvic joints occurs during pregnancy through the effects of the hormone relaxin. Only through repeated critical assessments can clinical pelvimetry be sufficiently reliable to be valuable for patient management. Successful vaginal delivery can occur with all pelvic types but a greater rate of difficulties develop in labor with nongynecoid pelves. An important factor that must be considered when evaluating pelves is the size of the pelvis, since a small gynecoid pelvis can also present difficulties in labor.

One of the most important pelvic measurements is the obstetric conjugate of the inlet. As previously reported, this diameter cannot be directly assessed clinically; instead, it is necessary to quantify the length of the diagonal conjugate. To do this, the index and middle finger of the examination hand are inserted into the vagina and the sacral promontory is palpated. The distance between the sacral promontory and the lower edge of the pubic symphysis is the diagonal conjugate (Fig. 6-12A). Depending on the attitude of the pubic symphysis, from 1.5 to 2 cm is deducted from the diagonal conjugate to give the obstetric conjugate; an obstetric conjugate of 10 cm is generally considered adequate. The transverse diameter of the inlet is less commonly utilized, but can be estimated from palpation of the arcuate line of the ilium on the left and right, and is normally at least 12 cm. Assessment of the curve and prominence of the sacrum should not be omitted.

The midpelvis is best estimated by palpating the ischial spines and determining their prominence, and by estimating the distance between them (Fig. 12B), with the lower limit of normal being 10 cm. Although the true bi-ischial diameter can only be evaluated radiologically, critical assessment by an experienced examiner can give very useful clinical information about this diameter. Further assessment of the character of the sacrosciatic notch, the length of the sacrospinous ligament, the pelvic side-walls, and the lie of the sacrum are also meaningful in evaluation of the midpelvis.

Evaluation of the pelvic outlet cannot be overlooked. The subpubic arch is normally wide and is commonly predictive of the pelvic inlet. With nongynecoid pelves, the spaciousness of the outlet, and specifically the subpubic angle, can be pivotal in the capacity of the pelvis for the fetus. The intertuberous diameter can be assessed by placing the closed fist on the perineum and measuring the distance between the ischial tuberosities (Fig. 16-12C). A normal value is at least 8 cm.[2]

RADIOGRAPHIC PELVIMETRY

Over most of this century, radiographic pelvimetry has been used for further evaluating the maternal bony pelvis at or near the time of labor. Many different techniques have been devised as means for predicting cephalopelvic disproportion based on maternal pelvic diameters and, subsequently, fetal skull diameters.

Radiographic pelvimetry using anteroposterior and lateral roentgenograms was the first technique to be developed, and routinely provided measurements of the anteroposterior and transverse diameters of the pelvic inlet and measurement of the interspinous distance. Various correction factors were developed to account for the divergence caused by the distance between the film and the pelvis. Estimation of the fetal head volume was proposed as an

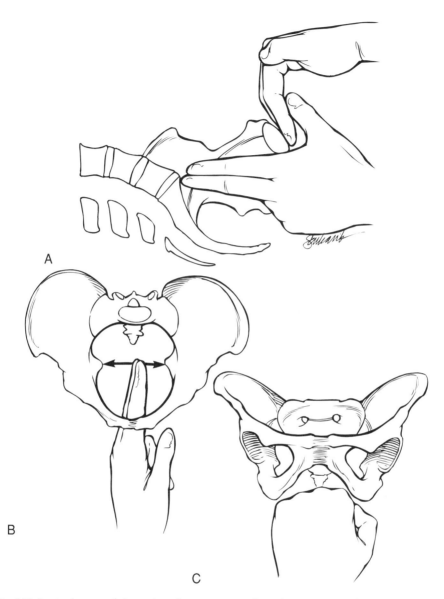

Fig. 6-12. **(A)** Sagittal view of the pelvis demonstrating clinical assessment of the diagonal conjugate. **(B)** Superior view of the pelvis demonstrating clinical assessment of the midpelvic interspinous diameter. **(C)** Frontal view of the pelvis demonstrating clinical assessment of the intertuberous diameter of the pelvic outlet.

adjunct in assessing the risk of cephalopelvic disproportion. Early studies of fetuses in the cephalic presentation documented higher rates of surgical deliveries in those cases judged to have a high risk of disproportion.[7] Measurements that have shown predictability of pelvic adequacy for breech-presenting labors are an anteroposterior diameter at the pelvic inlet of 11 cm, a transverse diameter of the pelvic inlet of 12 cm, and an interspinous diameter of 10 cm.[8–10]

The efficacy of radiographic pelvimetry in labors with fetuses presenting cephalically has been seriously questioned. The concerns about ionizing radiation and its modest fetal risk[11–13] were thought not to justify the insufficient information obtained from radiographic pelvimetry in the cephalically presenting fetus.[14-16] Because of its failure to provide information used to alter labor management, the use of radiographic pelvimetry in labor with a cephalic presentation has been all but abandoned. The inaccuracy of radiographic pelvimetry in predicting cephalopelvic disproportion (CPD) results from the myriad of factors that cannot be resolved by this technique and which are integral for achievement of a vaginal delivery. A partial list of such factors includes the uterine contraction force, pelvic soft tissues, ability of the fetal head to mold, and probably most importantly, the presentation, attitude, and position of the fetus.

Subsequent research has been primarily directed at decreasing fetal radiation exposure when radiographic pelvimetry has been used to evaluate the maternal pelvis for vaginal breech delivery. Computed tomographic (CT) pelvimetry has been shown to accomplish this by reducing the fetal dose of radiation to an estimated 2.3 mGy.[17] CT pelvimetry has also been shown to be an accurate method of assessing the maternal pelvis, and compares in this respect to conventional radiographic pelvimetry.[18,19] Magnetic resonance imaging (MRI) has also been shown to be as reliable as radiographic pelvimetry,[20] and has the added benefit of not using ionizing radiation. However, the use of these technologies for evaluation of the cephalically presenting fetus remains unclear. A recent study has documented fetal shoulder measurements with MRI that may help with the prediction of shoulder dystocia,[21] and another study has shown benefit from MRI in the management of an obese patient.[22] Much more work is required before the use of MRI with the cephalically presenting fetus is further defined.

LABOR AND DELIVERY

History

On initial evaluation in labor and delivery, as in all areas of medicine, assessment of the patient's chief presenting complaint will yield the most informative data, which will direct further interactions between the patient and her attendant. Because pregnancy can be a time of great emotional stress, and most patients will present in presumed labor or with some complication of pregnancy, a need for deep care and concern is paramount.

Routine assessment for the presence, strength, duration, and frequency of contractions from the patient's perspective will assist in discerning how labor is or is not progressing in a particular patient. The presence or absence of vaginal bleeding, and some quantitation if present, are vital prior to attempted physical examination, as is an appraisal of the status of the membranes. If the membranes are ruptured, the amount of fluid and the presence or absence of meconium should be investigated. Fetal activity during the pregnancy and any recent changes in such activity should be noted.

Any nonobstetric complaints or concerns demand evaluation. Women who are pregnant remain at risk of disorders of other body systems, and are at times at higher risk for such disorders. Therefore, a thorough medical and surgical history is essential. An assessment of the outcome of previous pregnancies and a gynecologic history can yield significant information that may affect care during the immediate pregnancy. Medicines taken, allergies, and any substance abuse should be queried. The presence of a fetus, although it should be noted and included in any risk assessment of evaluation and treatment, should not deter such evaluation and treatment if they are indicated.

The history should include obstetric factors such as dating criteria and the occurrence of, indications for, and results of any ultrasound examinations done prenatally. Complications during the pregnancy should be questioned and confirmed from patient-held obstetric care summaries, which should be updated at each visit or from the prenatal record (or both).

Physical Examination

A general physical examination and investigation of vital signs should be done on all women presenting in labor and delivery. Concentration on obstetric issues should predominate in those cases free of nonobstetric concerns. Assessment of fundal height and an estimated fetal weight are essential clinical data that must be carefully assessed in all parturients.

The presentation and position of the fetus can be clinically assessed through abdominal and vaginal examinations. Leopold and Sporlin in 1894 suggested four maneuvers useful during abdominal examination for appraisal of the fetal presentation and position. During these maneuvers the examiner is at the patient's side with the patient in the supine position. During the first three maneuvers the examiner faces the maternal upper body, while for the last maneuver the examiner faces the patient's lower body. The first maneuver entails palpation of the fundus of the uterus to determine which fetal pole is present at the fundus of the uterus. The fetal head feels hard and is round, whereas the breech feels more irregular and is less mobile. For the second maneuver, the examiner's hands are slid to the sides of the uterus, where deep pressure is used to palpate for the orientation of the fetus. The fetal back is hard, linear, and unyielding, whereas the extremities are irregular, with small parts frequently palpable. The third maneuver is performed with the thumb and fingers of the examiner's arm closest to the maternal abdomen. Just superior to the pubic symphysis, the presenting fetal part is palpated and the findings of the first maneuver are confirmed. Engagement of the presenting part is assessed. If the fetus is in a cephalic presentation, the attitude of the fetal head is judged by palpation of the cephalic prominence. If it is on the same side as the extremities, the head is considered to be flexed, whereas if it is on the same side as the back, the head is deemed to be extended. Useful information can be obtained with the fourth maneuver when the fetus is in a cephalic presentation. With the examiner facing the maternal feet, the fingers of both hands are used to palpate deeply in the direction of the pelvic axis. The ease of palpation of the cephalic prominence is used to assess descent of the fetal head into the pelvis[6] (Fig. 6-13).

Further information is obtainable in most cases from vaginal examination. If there are no contraindications to vaginal examination, such as known or suspected placenta previa with undiagnosed vaginal bleeding, the vaginal examination should be performed after amassing information from the history and the remainder of the physical examination, and sometimes from an ultrasound examination. In cases with suspected rupture of the membranes, a sterile speculum examination can be employed for further evaluation. Support for the diagnosis of ruptured membranes would be the presence of a pool of fluid in the vagina, a positive nitrazine test (the basic amniotic fluid will turn nitrazine paper blue), and the presence of ferning on a dried smear of fluid from the anterior fornix of the vagina (Fig. 6-14). An assessment of the cervix can be made visually, but is not comparable to the information that can be obtained by a digital examination.

A digital examination of the cervix can give extremely useful information in an evaluation of the parturient. It is sometimes withheld for women who are not "committed to delivery," such as those who are preterm with ruptured membranes but not in active labor. The dilatation, effacement, station, position, and consistency of the cervix are commonly assessed. The dilatation is estimated as anywhere from closed or fingertip dilated to 10 cm, which is by convention completely dilated. The effacement is usually rated from long to "paper thin" by the designation 0 percent to 100 percent effaced, respectively, and is subject to considerable observer bias. The station is rated using the ischial spines as landmarks. Zero station is the point at which the presenting part of the fetus is at the level of the ischial spines; a presenting part at or below this level is said to be engaged. When the presenting part is above the level of the ischial spines, the station is termed minus 1, minus 2, minus 3, or floating, depending on the distance of the part from the ischial spines, with floating being at the level of the inlet and the farthest position from the ischial spines. Divisions below the ischial spines are divided into centimeters (e.g., plus 1, plus 2, and so forth), with plus 5 designating that the fetal head is on the perineum, or "crowning" (Fig. 6-15). The position of the cervix is palpated, and usually indicated as posterior, midposition, or anterior. The consistency of the cervix, especially of the internal os, is judged and designated as firm, medium, or soft.

Evaluation of the position of the fetus is of utmost importance during the initial examination. The pelvic examination should be used as a confirmation of Leopold's maneuvers. Palpation for the sagittal suture should be performed first. A search for either the "diamond"-shaped anterior fontanelle or the triangular posterior fontanelle should follow (Fig. 6-16). The degree of flexion or extension should be

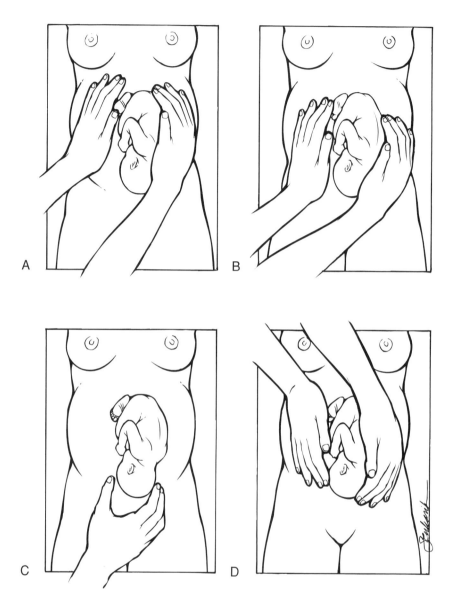

Fig. 6-13. (A–D) Leopold maneuvers with a longitudinal cephalic presentation. (Adapted from Cunningham et al,[6] with permission.)

noted, as well as the degree of asynclitism. It is important to assess the position of the fetus early in labor, since this can prove more difficult with descent of the fetal head. When the sagittal suture of the fetus lies midway between the pubic symphysis and the sacrum, the head is said to be synclitic. Normal labor is commonly associated with some degree of asynclitism, which is recognized when the sagittal suture lies anteriorly or is displaced posteriorly. Anterior asynclitism occurs when the sagittal suture is displaced posteriorly and the anterior parietal bone presents, whereas posterior asynclitism is noted when the sagittal suture is displaced anteriorly and the posterior parietal bone leads the presenting part (Fig. 6-17). The position of the fetus as well as the degree of asynclitism and flexion are important for

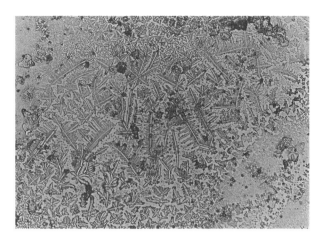

Fig. 6-14. Air-drying of amniotic fluid gives the characteristic ferning pattern.

evaluating the progress of labor, as is discussed below. During the pelvic examination, clinical pelvimetry should also be reassessed (see above).

Laboratory Studies

The laboratory tests obtained during the patient's prenatal course should be reviewed when the patient presents in labor and delivery. Standard prenatal tests include a blood-type and antibody screen, a serologic test for syphillis (rapid plasma reagin [RPR] or venereal disease research laboratory [VDRL], rubella titer, hepatitis B surface antigen (HbsAg), and complete blood count (CBC). In addition, many patients will have a Papanicolaou smear, glucose screen, or maternal serum α-fetoprotein (MSAFP) assay.

When a patient presents in labor and delivery, we routinely test the urine for protein and glucose and

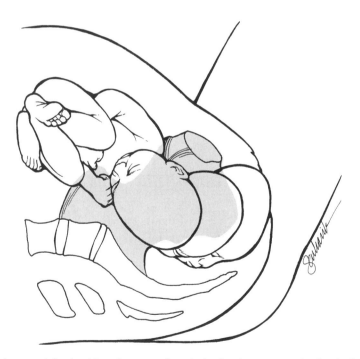

Fig. 6-15. Sagittal view of the fetal head engaged, with the leading part at the level of the ischial spines or 0 station. Further descent is estimated in centimeters until the head is crowning on the perineum, when it is at +5 station by convention.

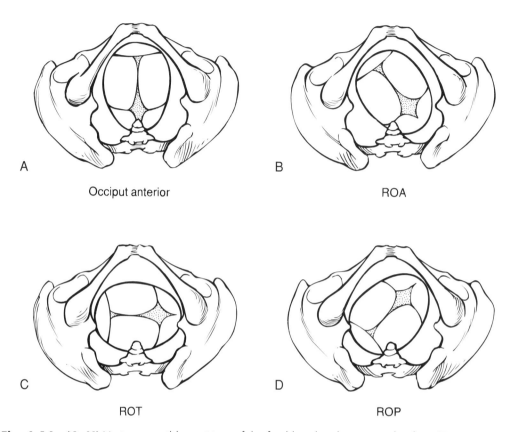

A Occiput anterior

B ROA

C ROT

D ROP

Fig. 6-16. (A–H) Various possible positions of the fetal head in the maternal pelvis. *(Figure continues.)*

recheck a CBC, blood type and antibody screen, and RPR. Other laboratory studies must be individualized to the parturient.

Monitoring and Evaluation

Some assessment of fetal well-being should be made on all patients who present after the time of fetal viability. This is most commonly done with external fetal monitoring. Evaluation for the presence of decelerations or an abnormal baseline heart rate may be all that are done on fetuses that are at an extremely early point in gestation. After 32 weeks of gestation, a reactive fetal heart-rate tracing would be reassuring, while its absence would demand further testing.

A primary reason for further monitoring of the patient presenting in seeming labor and delivery is to judge whether the patient is actually in labor. Re-

view of the external monitoring strip is only one part of this evaluation. A standard period of 1 to 2 hours is necessary in many cases to confidently reach a conclusion. Irregular, infrequent contractions; a stable, unfavorable cervical examination; and the absence of significant pain all point toward a diagnosis of "false labor," or may represent early latent-phase labor. Because of the difficulty that can arise with making this diagnosis, management options are discussed below.

Uterine Contraction Monitoring

Any endeavor into understanding labor should begin with an appreciation of the work of one of the most important factors in this cascade, the gravid uterus. Palpation has for many years been used for describing the strength, duration, and frequency of uterine contractions in the laboring patient. Al-

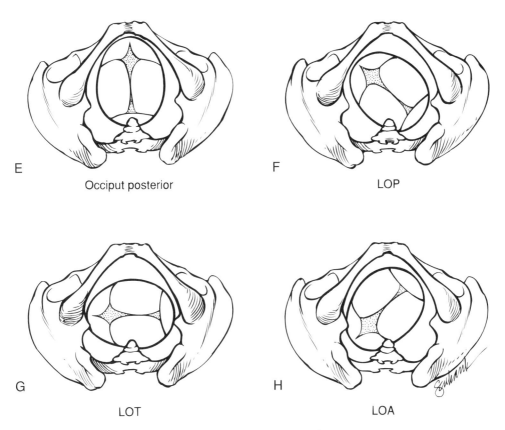

E Occiput posterior

F LOP

G LOT

H LOA

Fig. 6-16. *(Continued).*

though external monitoring of uterine contractions, as with palpation, can provide very useful information in the characterization of contractions, intrauterine monitoring is necessary for determining the strength of contractions. Schatz,[23] in 1872, is recognized as the first to have scientifically studied the pressure produced by the contracting, gravid human uterus. Since that time a number of investigators have advanced our knowledge in this area.

Early work by Caldeyro-Barcia et al[24] resulted in quantitation of the pressure produced during labor through use of the Montevideo unit, which is the mean pressure of uterine contractions above the baseline (in millimeters of mercury) multiplied by the number of contractions within 10 minutes. Notwithstanding that the Montevideo unit has weathered the test of time, a number of other measures of uterine activity have been proposed. The Alexandria

unit was suggested to account for the differential duration of contractions, and is calculated by multiplying the Montevideo unit by the mean duration of contractions (in minutes).[25] A number of other measures have also been proposed for more precise evaluation of uterine activity, and have been shown to correlate significantly.[26]

Contractions of the uterus during normal human pregnancy are anticipated findings. As illustrated in Figure 6-18), spontaneous uterine activity occurs from very early in gestation and is characterized by frequent, small, localized contractions intermingled with irregular, occasionally strong, Braxton–Hicks contractions.[27] Normal uterine activity at this time is less than 20 Montevideo units.[27] A recent study has confirmed the increase in uterine activity with increasing gestation, and has also shown an increase in uterine activity at night.[28] At roughly 30 weeks'

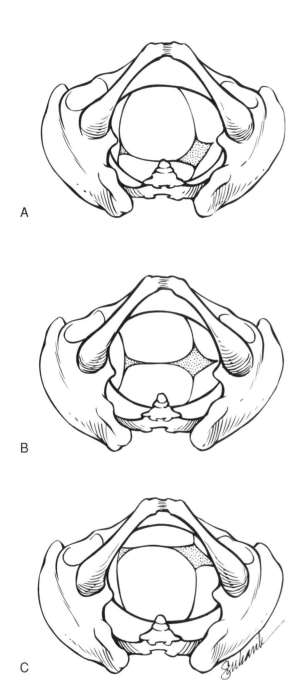

Fig. 6-17. The fetal head can occupy varied positions in the maternal pelvis. **(A)** Anterior asynclitism occurs when the anterior parietal bone is presenting. **(B)** Normal synclitism occurs when the sagittal suture lies midway between the pubic symphysis and sacrum. **(C)** Posterior asynclitism occurs with anterior displacement of the sagittal suture.

gestation, the frequency and strength of the Braxton–Hicks contractions increase in an almost logarithmic fashion until the beginning of labor, when a more coordinated and effective rhythm is observed. Although no absolute definition of labor with respect to uterine activity is possible, given the considerable variation, the onset of clinical labor is usually associated with an average of 80 to 120 Montevideo units.[27] Labor is characterized by a continued increase in uterine activity, which may reach levels of 250 Montevideo units. After delivery, uterine activity remains coordinated and exists at a level as high as or higher than at delivery before slowly abating with time.[27,29]

There is a progressive increase in uterine activity as labor progresses. Most of this occurs in the first stage, primarily in the active phase of labor, and has been estimated at 80 percent of the total uterine activity necessary to effect vaginal delivery after 3 cm dilatation.[30] A number of factors affect the amount of uterine activity required for labor to progress normally. A significantly greater uterine activity is necessary for nulliparous spontaneous labor to progress normally than is needed for multiparous spontaneous labor, especially before the latter part of the active phase of labor.[31] The position of the presenting fetal head is also important in the amount of uterine activity required for dilatation to progress, with fetuses in the occiput-anterior position requiring significantly less uterine activity than those in the occiput-transverse or -posterior positions.[32] Amniotomy can also lead to an increase in uterine activity as labor progresses.

Cervical Monitoring

Various methods of labor evaluation have been proposed since Schatz first scientifically studied the process of labor. Few have contributed as much as Friedman,[33] with his proposal of graphically following labor via cervical dilatation over time and his application of this information to individual patients so that abnormalities of labor could be further evaluated and treated. Friedman analyzed primigravidas at term and performed frequent evaluations of cervical dilatation, via rectal examination, during the peak of contractions. He plotted the change in cervical dilatation during labor versus time. The curves that he obtained had a sigmoid configuration; the

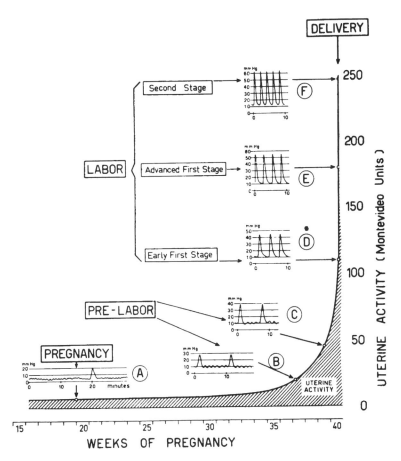

Fig. 6-18. Progression of uterine activity throughout pregnancy and the early puerperium. Selected points demonstrate uterine contractility at the corresponding selected times in pregnancy, labor, or soon after delivery. (From Caldeyro-Barcia and Poseiro,[27] with permission.)

most predictive portion of the curve was the area of maximal slope, which was inversely proportional to the total duration of the first stage of labor. Because of the correlation noted in this area of the curve, abnormalities of labor during the active phase can be easily determined, as discussed below. The sigmoid configuration of the "labor curve," and particularly the deceleration phase, has not subsequently been commonly encountered in normal labor.

Friedman[34] extensively scrutinized 500 labor curves derived from primigravida women. Applying the distinction that labor begins with regular uterine contractions, he found that the latent phase lasts a mean of 8.6 hours and a maximum of 20.6 hours (2 SD above the mean). The mean duration of the active phase was 4.9 hours and the statistical maximum was 11.7 hours. The maximum total duration of the first stage was 28.5 hours, and of the second stage 2.5 hours. When looking at the slope of the active phase, Friedman found that the 95th percentile lay at a minimum increment of 1.2 cm/hr, a figure that has been further verified. The average duration of labor as described above has been confirmed at the Chicago Lying-In Hospital.[35] Average cervical dilatation rates were tabulated for a cohort of 335 primigravida patients as related to fetal position, and are shown in Figure 6-19); the continued increase in rate with increasing dilatation and time is noteworthy.

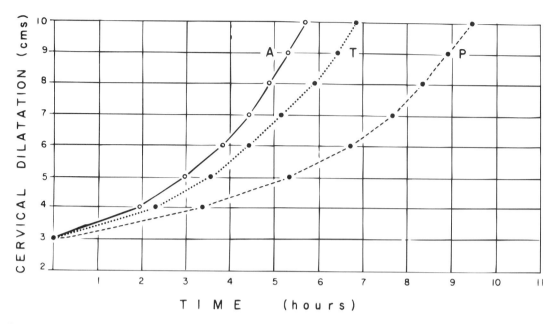

Fig. 6-19. Average cervical dilatation curves in the first stage of labor in primigravid women, arranged by position. Transverse and posterior positions were diagnosed at some point during the first stage, but may have converted to anterior positions after categorization. Anterior positions remained as such throughout labor. A, anterior; T, transverse; P, posterior. (From Cibils,[35] with permission.)

By contrast, and as expected, multiparas tend to have labors of shorter duration. Friedman also showed that the mean duration of multipara latent-phase labor is 5.3 hours, and maximally remains normal at 13.6 hours. The active phase has a mean duration of 2.2 hours and normally ends by 5.2 hours. The limit of normal for the phase of maximal dilatation is 1.5 cm/hr, although the mean is much higher, at 5.7 cm/hr.[36] Cibils,[35] who reviewed the labors of 550 multiparas, and reached results similar to those of Friedman, except for the absence of a deceleration phase in these normally progressing labors (Fig. 6-20); the differences as related to position are again noteworthy.

The mean cervical dilatation by deciles and quintiles, in multipara and nullipara women, respectively, is depicted graphically by Hendricks and associates[37] (Fig. 6-21). The absence of the sigmoid configuration in the labor curve is apparent in normally progressing labor, but it may be seen, as noted in Figure 6-21, in pregnancies with the slowest progression. Documentation of this finding has been limited

to few pregnancies with abnormal fetal head positions.[32] A number of authors have evaluated the labors of women who have reached the second stage, and have retrospectively measured the duration of the first stage of labor. Hendricks and associates[37] found no difference related to parity in duration of the active phase of labor (Fig. 6-22). Liu and Kerr-Wilson[38] found no difference in the duration of labor after 2 cm dilatation in nulliparous as opposed to parous women in whom labor was induced or spontaneous (Fig. 6-23). These findings are probably primarily related to the exclusion of abnormal labors; they also do not take into account the total duration of the latent phase, which is much longer than the active phase of labor, and thus contributes significantly to the duration of the first stage of labor. These studies do suggest a lack of any difference between nulliparous and parous women with normally progressing labors. The means and limits of normal for the various measures of labor are noted above.

Besides parity, there exists other easily obtainable

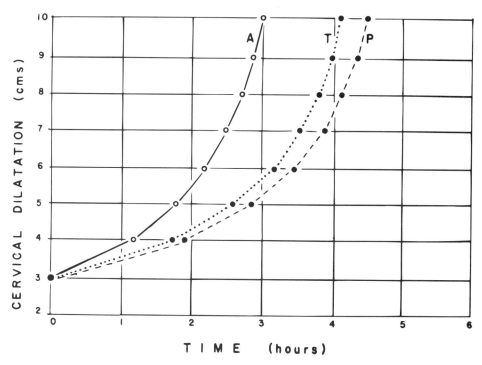

Fig. 6-20. Average cervical dilatation curves in the first stage of labor in multiparas, arranged by position as in Figure 6-19. A, anterior; T, transverse; P, posterior. (From Cibils,[35] with permission.)

information that permits the findings described above to be individualized to specific patients, of which three of the most important sources are the initial cervical examination, fetal head position, and state of the membranes. Uterine contractions, as shown, are present throughout pregnancy and assist in preparing the parturient for labor through ripening of the cervix. Prior to the onset of labor, the mean cervical dilatation has been shown to be 1.8 cm in nulliparas and 2.2 cm in multiparas.[37] Women who have riper cervices have shorter labors. A dramatic shortening of the latent phase is noted with increasing initial cervical dilatation, and a significant reduction in duration of the active phase has been well documented with increasing dilatation, especially in nulliparas. However, little change has been noted in duration of the second stage[39] (Table 6-1). Additionally, Cibils and Hendricks[32] have documented an increase in the uterine work needed to complete the first stage of labor in patients with unripe cervices. They also were able to demonstrate a significantly greater uterine-work requirement, pri-

marily through an increase in number of uterine contractions if the occiput was posterior or transverse rather than anterior; this prolonged the duration of the first stage. Therefore, the efficiency of labor was greater when the occiput was in an anterior position. Also noted has been a greater efficiency of uterine contractions when the membranes are ruptured.[32,40]

Position

From almost the beginning of time, women have undergone labor and delivery either in the standing or squatting position. Indeed, childbirth in by far the majority of non-European societies is accomplished in the upright position.[41] In the 17th century, Francois Mauriceau is generally credited with having been instrumental in converting the position of the laboring gravid woman to the supine position. The primary motivation for this appears to have been its benefit for the medical attendant, especially in the interest of forceps delivery. With time, this indoctrination became standard fare in the western

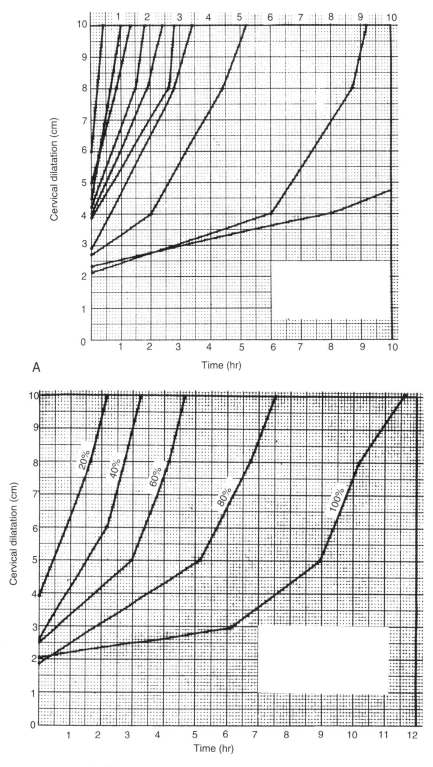

Fig. 6-21. (A) Mean cervical dilatation rates in multiparas initially in normal spontaneous labor, by deciles. Note the significant variation; the 10th percentile is incompletely shown due to space limitation. (From Hendricks et al,[37] with permission.) **(B)** Mean cervical dilatation rates in nulliparas initially in normal spontaneous labor, by quintiles. (From Hendricks et al,[37] with permission.)

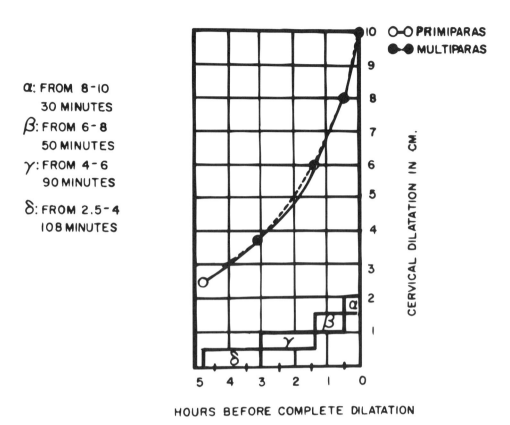

α: FROM 8-10
30 MINUTES
β: FROM 6-8
50 MINUTES
γ: FROM 4-6
90 MINUTES
δ: FROM 2.5-4
108 MINUTES

○-○ PRIMIPARAS
●-● MULTIPARAS

CERVICAL DILATATION IN CM.

HOURS BEFORE COMPLETE DILATATION

Fig. 6-22. Mean cervical dilatation rate in multiparous and primiparous women, graphed backward from 10 cm in women with normal labor (From Hendricks et al,[37] with permission.)

Table 6-1. Effect of Initial Cervical Dilatation on Duration of the Latent and Active phases of Labor in Nulliparas and Multiparas

Initial Cervical Dilatation (cm)	Nulliparas		Multiparas	
	Latent Phase (hr)	Active Phase (hr)	Latent Phase (hr)	Active Phase (hr)
0.0–0.5	11.6 ± 0.83 (19.2)[a]	6.4 ± 0.52 (11.4)	8.7 ± 1.30 (16.1)	2.4 ± 0.43 (5.0)
0.6–0.9	9.9 ± 0.91 (14.8)	6.0 ± 0.77 (10.7)	5.5 ± 0.90 (10.1)	2.3 ± 0.30 (3.9)
1.0–1.9	8.6 ± 0.29 (15.4)	4.9 ± 0.18 (8.8)	5.3 ± 0.20 (8.8)	2.2 ± 0.07 (3.3)
2.0–2.9	6.6 ± 0.64 (12.0)	4.1 ± 0.27 (6.0)	4.0 ± 0.42 (7.6)	1.9 ± 0.20 (3.5)
3.0–3.9	4.9 ± 0.60 (8.2)	3.6 ± 0.33 (5.2)	4.2 ± 0.28 (7.1)	1.9 ± 0.11 (2.9)
≥4.0	4.5 ± 0.91 (7.9)	3.1 ± 0.37 (4.1)	3.4 ± 0.39 (5.7)	1.5 ± 0.14 (2.3)

[a] Data in parentheses represent the upper 95 percent statistical limits. The numbers following ± are the standard error of the mean.
(From Friedman et al,[39] with permission.)

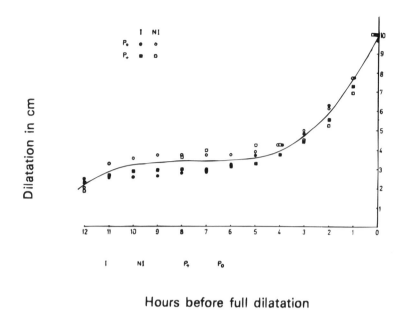

Hours before full dilatation

Fig. 6-23. Mean cervical dilatation rates in parturients having vaginal deliveries, graphed over time. Po, nulliparous; P+, parous; I, induced; NI, spontaneous labor. (From Liu et al,[38] with permission.)

world. However, significant questions have lately arisen about the benefits and utility of this obstetric dogma.

Caldeyro-Barcia and colleagues[42] have demonstrated a greater intensity and lesser frequency of contractions when the patient lies in a lateral recumbent than in a dorsal supine position, corresponding with the so-called law of position. These differences were greater in cases of spontaneously progressing labor than in those with oxytocin augmentation. The interpretation was that the stronger, more coordinated uterine contractions observed in the lateral recumbent position would be more efficient for labor to proceed.[42] Other investigators have also noted difference in uterine with different positions. A higher resting tone has been described in sitting gravid women, in association with a significantly shorter duration of the active phase of labor,[43] and stronger although not more frequent contractions have been noted in women in the standing as opposed to the supine position.[44] None of the available studies has shown a detrimental effect of the standing or sitting positions on uterine activity. Less clear is whether the sitting or standing position shortens the duration of labor. A number of studies have supported both sides of the issue,[45-48] but evidence that an upright position delays the duration of labor is lacking.

Apart from their effects on the progression of labor, various positions may have different fetal effects. The Poseiro effect, described in 1955 by that author, describes a decrease in femoral blood pressure with uterine contractions in laboring women in the supine position, which is thought to indicate hypoperfusion below the level of the gravid uterus.[49] Goodlin[49] was able to show an increased risk of this occurrence, to almost double its usual incidence, when conduction anesthesia was used, as opposed to complete elimination or a significant decrease in the Poseiro effect when the parturient was placed in the lateral or semilateral position. One-third of the fetuses of gravid women showing the Poseiro effect had abnormal heart rate tracings, which were found to resolve with lateral displacement. Aortocaval compression during uterine contraction was judged to be responsible for the hypoperfusion. Abitbol[50] made similar findings, including data to suggest that aortocaval compression contributes to one-fifth of cases of fetal distress, indicating a weighty role of maternal position in fetal well-being.

At delivery, position remains an important issue. Historically, women have been known to deliver from the squatting stance. It has been known for over a century that the capacity of the pregnant pelvis varies with position, and squatting has been shown to increase the capacity of the outlet.[51,52] Yet despite this the medical community has continued to overwhelmingly prefer the supine position for delivery, as previously stated, primarily to the advantage of the accoucheur. The conventional dorsal supine position has definite advantages for delivery, including the ease of instrumental vaginal delivery, improved ability to maintain a clean field, facility in examination, performance of episiotomy, and ease of delivery itself. However, a number of advantages have been ascribed to upright labor and delivery, including the advantage of gravity, less marked aortocaval compression, stronger contractions, and improved pelvic diameters, especially with squatting and kneeling.[53] Gravity may help appose the presenting part of the fetus to the posterior vaginal wall, stimulating Ferguson's reflex, causing the release of oxytocin and inciting the urge to push. In randomized studies with a birthing chair, acceptance of this technique seemed to be high, but neither mothers nor infants realized significant benefits from it, and the blood loss was greater in mothers who delivered in the chair.[54,55] Squatting has also been evaluated in the second stage of labor, but western women have shown difficulty in sustaining this seldom-assumed posture.[53] Assistance in maintaining this posture with the "birth cushion" has been well-accepted by parturients and has been shown to decrease the duration of the second stage of labor, as well as the incidence of forceps deliveries, and has not been associated with an increase in blood loss.[56]

Fetal effects are also influential in determining the delivery position. Humphrey and colleagues have shown that the left lateral tilt position would benefit some fetuses, as evidenced by Apgar score and umbilical artery blood gas valves.[57] More recently, further study has shown a lower umbilical artery pH for dorsally delivered gravid women than for those in the left lateral tilt position. When the second stage of labor lasted less than 15 minutes, the pH and base excess were similar for the two groups, but when the dorsally delivered women had a second stage lasting longer than 15 minutes, there was a progressive decline in pH and increase in base excess of the umbilical artery blood.[58] Neonatal outcome has been shown to be comparable with use of the obstetric chair,[55] birth cushion,[56] and delivery in the upright position,-whether-by kneeling, sitting, squatting, or standing,[53] all of which were better than delivery in the recumbent posture, as indicated by Apgar score or umbilical artery pH (or both).

Food and Fluid Management

American obstetricians currently express a general admonition against eating and drinking during labor, although this was not always so. DeLee, for most of the first half of the 20th century, encouraged food and drink during labor to guard against the faintness and weakness caused by starvation.[59] The past 50 years have witnessed the development of distinctly different ideas. Advances in anesthesia led to widespread use of general anesthesia for delivery, and the risk of Mendleson syndrome, or aspiration pneumonia, was described.[60] DeLee subsequently recommended the sparing use of nourishment and fluid during labor, except when labor was prolonged.[59] Subsequent educators have continued the teaching of prohibiting food during labor, and most have also refused the ingestion of fluid, fearful of the occurrence of Mendleson syndrome and its sequelae.

Concern has been generated primarily over the risk factors for development of Mendleson syndrome. Aspiration of particulate matter is much more serious than that of nonparticulate matter, and has led to the requirement by some clinicians that oral sustenance during labor be limited to clear liquids. A lower gastric pH has been associated with increased lung-tissue damage. Labor itself leads to delayed gastric emptying, as does narcotic analgesia, which also relaxes the lower esophageal sphincter, whereas epidural anesthesia is believed to have none of these effects.[61]

Intravenous fluid during labor can be associated with certain maloccurrences. Of note is that intravenous infusions are uncomfortable and limit mobility. Intravenous dextrose has been associated with neonatal hyperglycemia, hyponatremia associated with transient tachypnea, hyperinsulinemia, hypoglycemia, jaundice,[62] and metabolic acidosis[63]; accordingly, infusions of dextrose in doses of up to 6 g/hr have been advocated.[64] Because pregnancy is considered a starvation state, if enteral nutrition is denied, some parenteral nutrition is necessary to avert maternal starvation ketosis, which has been associated in animal models with a significant reduction in fetal arterial oxygen tension (PaO_2), and an increase in fetal lactate levels.[65]

We often find indications for intravenous lines during labor, such as for oxytocin stimulation, persistent maternal emesis and dehydration, and hydration prior to epidural anesthesia. When an indication such as these does not exist and immediate intravenous access is deemed necessary, a heparin lock can be easily placed prophylactically and can obviate many of the risks of intravenous fluid when the latter is not desired. With the well-documented risks associated with intravenous infusion, as well as the risks associated with ketonemia, increased use of regional anesthesia, development and use of new anesthetic techniques, and extensive use of antacids, the general prohibition of enteral nutrition in labor should be rethought, and consideration of its use should at least be individualized.

Amniotomy

Elective amniotomy has become a portentous weapon in the obstetric armamentarium. Its introduction early in this century was for the prevention of prolonged labor.[66] Sadly, little documentation of its benefit was offered until recently.[67–69] Common indications for amniotomy in labor are nonreassuring fetal testing, dystocia, an inadequate externally monitored fetal heart rate or poor findings on contraction monitoring, and when the second stage of labor is attained, to evaluate for the presence of meconium. The effect of amniotomy on the progress and outcome of labor has recently been evaluated.

A frequently cited concern with amniotomy and the progress of labor are the fetal effects resulting from it. Amniotomy decreases amniotic-fluid volume, which would be expected to increase the risk of cord compression. Transitory fetal heart rate abnormalities have been observed with amniotomy, the most common being a short-lived acceleration and less commonly a short-lived bradycardia, but no effect on fetal or neonatal well-being was recognized.[70] The well-recognized risk of umbilical cord prolapse with ruptured membranes should not be increased if amniotomy is judiciously performed. Maternal discomfort from the procedure has also been described, although lasting dissatisfaction was not noted.[71]

Recently, a few large, randomized trials have sought to evaluate the benefit of elective amniotomy. A Canadian trial using nulliparous women at term

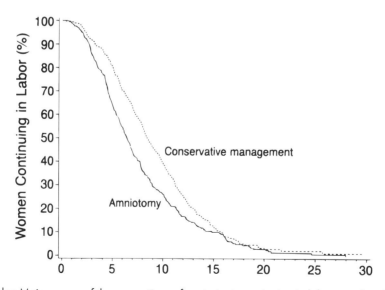

Fig. 6-24. Kaplan-Meier curves of the proportions of parturients continuing in labor as related to time (in hours) after randomization; $P < 0.001$ by the log-rank test for the comparison between the conservative management and amniotomy groups. (From Fraser et al,[72] with permission.)

Table 6-2. Mean Duration of Labor (in Minutes) in the Amniotomy and Intact Groups for Nulliparas and Multiparas

	Amniotomy Group (n = 235)	Intact Group (n = 224)	Significance
First stage			
All patients	276 ± 202	358 ± 236	$P < 0.05$
Nulliparous patients	347 ± 206	457 ± 233	$P < 0.05$
Multiparous patients	230 ± 186	284 ± 209	$P < 0.05$
Second stage			
All patients	47.6 ± 65	49.7 ± 61	NS
Nulliparous patients	83.6 ± 72	83.0 ± 58	NS
Multiparous patients	23.0 ± 45	26.2 ± 51	NS

(From Garite et al,[73] with permission.)

and in spontaneous labor evaluated the use of early elective amniotomy. Fifty-one percent of the conservatively managed control group required amniotomy in labor. Dystocia was diagnosed significantly less often in the amniotomy group, but the cesarean section rate was similar for the two groups. The duration of labor was significantly shorter in the amniotomy group (Fig. 6-24). Abnormal fetal heart rates or neonatal outcome were similar for the two groups.[72] A similar study involving multiparous in addition to nulliparous women had very comparable results. Again, no difference in the cesarean section rate or rate of operative vaginal delivery was seen, although the use of oxytocin was significantly more frequent in the intact group than in the amniotomy group. The duration of the second stage of labor was similar in both groups, but the duration of the first stage of labor was an average of 1 hour and 22 minutes longer in the intact group, and this significant difference between the two groups held up for multiparous as well as nulliparous women (Table 6-2). There was no difference in neonatal complications or outcome, notwithstanding a higher risk of mild to moderate variable decelerations in fetal heart rate of 66 percent versus 49 percent for the amniotomy and intact groups, respectively ($P = 0.0003$). No differences in severe variable decelerations, prolonged decelerations, or late decelerations in heart rate were observed in the two groups.[73] A large, multicenter English trial of spontaneous labor in nulliparous women at term found a median duration of labor of 8.4 hours in an early amniotomy group and 9.4 hours in a late rupture group ($P = 0.03$). No other statistically significant maternal or fetal effect was observed.[74]

Although we now have objective evidence of the benefit of early elective amniotomy, not all investigators are quick to espouse its routine use in spontaneous labor.[75] No significant adverse effect of this technique has been consistently demonstrated. The benefit of a shorter labor would probably be desired by most parturients, although as shown, no difference in outcome with elective amniotomy has been observed.

Social Support

Our need for social support is vital during the most stressful times of our lives, and labor is no exception. The labor and delivery experience should be one of joy. Emotional support has been shown to be beneficial for labor outcome as well as neonatal outcome.[76] The results of a recent study comparing the outcome of women provided with social support to those accompanied by a passive observer and those who received usual care are shown in (Table 6-3).[77] Remarkable benefits are realized solely with the provision of support during labor. These findings deserve further investigation, and may have implications for the way in which labor should be viewed and treated in the future.

DYSFUNCTIONAL LABOR
Prolonged Latent Phase

Dysfunctional labor in the latent phase of labor results in prolongation of this phase. As previously stated, the primigravid woman has a mean duration of the latent phase of 9 hours, and the multiparous woman a mean duration of 5 hours. The statistical maximum is 20 hours for the primigravid and 14 hours for the multiparous parturient.[78] Confirma-

Table 6-3. Effect of Emotional Support During Labor on Outcome

Outcome	Supported Group (n = 212)	Observed Group (n = 200)	Control Group (n = 204)
Duration of labor[a] (hr)	7.4	8.4	9.4
Cesarean section rate[b] (%)	8	13	18
Forceps rate[c] (%)	8.2	21.3	26.3
Oxytocin rate[d] (%)			
Total	17	23	43.6
SVD	14	13.1	37.4
Epidural rate[a] (%)			
SVD	7.8	22.6	55.3
Maternal fever[e] (%)	1.4	7.0	10.3
Abnormal neonatal course[f] (% hospitalized >48 hr for medical reasons)	10.4	17.0	24.0
Neonatal sepsis evaluations[g] (%)	4.2	9.5	14.7

SVD, spontaneous vaginal delivery.

[a] $P < 0.02$ for supported versus observed, supported versus control, and observed versus control.

[b] $P = 0.004$ for supported versus control.

[c] $P = 0.0006$ for supported versus observed and supported versus control.

[d] $P < 0.0001$ for supported versus control and observed versus control.

[e] $P = 0.009$ for supported versus observed, $P = 0.002$ for supported versus control.

[f] $P = 0.05$ for supported versus observed, $P = 0.001$ for supported versus control.

[g] $P = 0.05$ for supported versus observed, $P = 0.0005$ for supported versus control.

(Data from Kennell et al[77])

tion of the duration of the latent phase of labor was made over 20 years after Friedman's data set.[79] Notably, multivariate analysis and standard stepwise regression analysis showed that the most important variable affecting the duration of latent phase was cervical dilatation. Both parity and station had lesser effects on this duration,[79] findings best explained by the fact that multiparous women commonly begin labor and arrive at the hospital in a state of greater dilatation[37] than their primiparous counterparts.

Remaining in the latent phase for a prolonged period and having painful contractions from a dysfunctional labor can be frustrating and exhausting to the laboring woman. Despite the presumably similar etiologies for this disorder, a single mode of treatment is not recommended. Notwithstanding the statistical maxima for the duration of the latent phase, parturients clearly in dysfunctional labor will often require intervention, and awaiting the formal definition of a prolonged latent phase is neither in the best interest of the patient nor her attendant.

When the obstetrician faces a prolonged latent phase of labor, a search for possible etiologic factors is often successful. Excessive sedation and the use of latent-phase conduction anesthesia can account for almost half the cases seen.[80] Unripe cervices or dysfunctional contractions are also commonly encountered. False labor can also be responsible, but the diagnosis of this is difficult to make prospectively without an adequate period of observation. Because cervical dilatation is the most important factor in determining the duration of the latent phase, it should have a pivotal role in determining the optimal mode of therapy for the laboring woman. Treatment options are narcotically inducing resting, oxytocin with or without amniotomy, ambulation, or observation. The emotional state of the parturient is of utmost importance in the patient's tolerance of labor and her behavior during labor. Her wishes for therapy during such an exhausting time must be taken into account. The use of cesarean section should not be considered in this setting, and should be used only in the most extreme circumstances.

When, after a period of observation, it is clear that the patient has not entered the active phase of labor, administration of morphine (e.g., 15 mg subcutaneously) may be employed for induction of a narcotic rest. This will usually allow the parturient a chance to rest, although a repeat dose is sometimes necessary. Most of the patients medicated in this fashion will awaken having entered the active phase of labor. A small minority, approximately 5 percent, will awaken remaining in a dysfunctional pattern. An estimated 10 percent will be shown to have been in false labor, with the resolution of dysfunctional contractions.[81] A narcotically induced rest should be strongly considered, especially for patients with unfavorable cervices at the time a prolonged or dysfunctional latent phase is diagnosed. Most such patients will benefit from the rest afforded by the narcosis. Those with false labor will not be subjected to an oxytocin induction, and those with a persistent pattern of dysfunctional labor will probably be better able to tolerate their ensuing labor.

Oxytocin induction should be considered when the cervix is favorable or when postponement of delivery is not thought to be beneficial to the mother or fetus. Most women treated in this way will enter the active phase of labor in a timely fashion. Conversion to an effective labor contraction pattern can often be seen. Amniotomy can be helpful in cases in which the decision to effect delivery is made, although it cannot be recommended as a sole form of treatment. Ambulation can also be considered, but if no response is noted after a reasonable period, another form of therapy becomes necessary.

The fetal and neonatal effects of a prolonged latent phase are controversial. Most investigators do not believe that an isolated prolonged latent phase increases the risk of perinatal mortality.[80,81] Some have shown an increased risk of cesarean section and an increased risk of neonatal morbidity, although Chelmow and colleagues recently presented an unclear treatment regimen as a source of such morbidity.[82] In spite of this, a mechanism involving a longer latent phase and an unfavorable cervix with higher intrauterine pressures generated by oxytocin therapy has been offered to explain poorer neonatal outcome in this setting.[83]

Active Phase Disorders
Protracted Active Phase

The two active phase disorders of labor generally recognized are a protracted active phase and arrest of the active phase. Friedman initially described a

protracted active phase in the 1950s. This was also referred to as primary dysfunctional labor, and is characterized by less than the maximal rate of cervical dilatation of 1.2 cm/hr in nulliparous and 1.5 cm/hr in multiparous women after entry into the active phase of labor.[78] Most parturients will enter the active phase of labor by 4 cm of cervical dilatation, and roughly 90 percent by 5 cm dilatation. If the cervix is not progressing actively after this point, the labor is probably abnormal and a search for an etiology would be indicated.[84]

Protracted active-phase labor is a disorder defined by the graphicostatistical cervimetric method initially described by Friedman.[85] When it is encountered, a search for etiologic factors is necessary, since the risk of cesarean or midforceps delivery is greater in this condition, as is the perinatal mortality rate.[85] It is much more common for interacting multiple factors to create this abnormality of labor, and a thorough search for such factors is therefore indicted. Possible etiologic factors include malpresentation, especially breech presentation; malposition, especially an occiput-transverse or occiput-posterior position; cephalopelvic disproportion; early amniotomy; early heavy sedation, including conduction anesthesia; fatigue or exhaustion; and uterine hypotonia. Some of these factors are also etiologic in prolonged latent-phase labor, and it should therefore not be surprising that a significant proportion of patients experiencing a protracted active phase have come through a prolonged latent phase.[85]

After repeating a pelvic examination with clinical pelvimetry, Leopold's maneuvers, and/or ultrasonography, and an assessment of sedation and conduction anesthesia, a number of modes of therapy are possible for a protracted active phase of labor, although the most efficacious seems to be oxytocin stimulation. Observation and support are occasionally helpful to the parturient, but have not been shown to increase the rate of dilatation. Narcotic rest may also be helpful to the laboring patient at this point, but its use alone has not been shown to be effective for increasing the rate of cervical dilatation. When the decision to proceed with delivery is made, amniotomy should be performed if not already accomplished.[86] Assessment of the intensity of uterine contractions would be indicated, and treatment with oxytocin for hypotonic labor would then be recommended until at least 200 Montevideo units of uterine activity are attained. When the labor is no longer hypotonic, observation for secondary arrest, as discussed below, becomes imperative. Notably, one randomized study has shown that when the two procedures were used for a protracted active phase,[87] augmentation of labor with external tocography used to titrate the dosage of oxytocin was comparable to internal monitoring of uterine contractions in terms of the cesarean section rates, neonatal outcome, and incidence of hyperstimulation.

Friedman found little benefit of oxytocin stimulation to change a slow rate of dilatation.[85] In a recent randomized study in which it was compared to saline, oxytocin given empirically to women with a protracted active phase led significantly to a response defined as progressive cervical dilatation, and ultimately led to a significant reduction in cesarean section rate, although only 65 percent of nulliparous and 81 percent of multiparous women responded to the oxytocin infusion. There was no increase in the rate of cesarean section for fetal distress for women given oxytocin, although 13 percent of patients with a protracted active phase underwent a cesarean section for fetal distress. Neonatal outcome was similar for the two groups, but 15 percent of the infants required intubation.[88] Eight hours of oxytocin augmentation has been shown in another study to further increase the vaginal delivery rate to 80 percent for nulliparous and 90 percent for multiparous women. Adequate fetal heart rate monitoring led to a minimal risk of intrauterine asphyxia and a resultant good neonatal outcome, with only 2 of 319 neonates having a 5-minute Apgar score of 6 or less.[89]

Active Phase Arrest (Secondary Arrest of Labor)

When there is an arrest of dilatation during an otherwise normally progressing active phase of labor, a secondary arrest of dilatation is said to have occurred. The duration of arrest usually cited before assigning this diagnosis, as documented by serial vaginal examinations is at least 2 hours. The etiologies of this disorder are similar to those for a protracted active phase. Abnormal position, especially the occiput-transverse and occiput-posterior positions, is significantly more common in this disorder than in normally progressing parturients. An abnormal presentation, bony dystocia, and excessive seda-

tion, including conduction anesthesia, are all significantly associated with secondary arrest of labor, and the possible role of early amniotomy remains in question. As in the case of a protracted active phase, an interplay of etiologic factors is common and makes the evaluation of active phase arrest highly challenging, as its treatment can also be. There is an increased risk of cesarean and midforceps delivery. Overall, perinatal morbidity and mortality are not increased as they are in the related protracted active phase disorder,[90] except in those cases encompassing both disorders. Prolonged active phase disorders can adversely affect fetuses, who would exhibit abnormal fetal heart rate patterns,[91] and electronic fetal monitoring is therefore indicated in such cases. Treatment in these cases would be similar to that for active phase arrest, since the diagnosis of a combined disorder would not be possible until an arrest of progress is encountered.

When the diagnosis is made of no progress for two hours in the active phase, a search for etiologies becomes vital. Assessment of fetal presentation and position are important; clinical pelvimetry and a consideration of radiographic pelvimetry are in order; and an assessment should be made of the degree of sedation. Treatment options include rest, ambulation, sedation, or oxytocin stimulation.[90] In Friedman's series of nulliparous women, half of those who received no treatment subsequently delivered vaginally. Ambulation has been shown to be as effective as oxytocin for labor enhancement in cases of active phase arrest,[92] but deserves more study. Sedation was somewhat less effective, as was amniotomy (if not already performed), but should be considered in conjunction with oxytocin stimulation, which was the most effective maneuver for this situation.[90] Some obstetricians limit the use of oxytocin stimulation to patients with hypotonic labors,[93] although Friedman found that empirical use of oxytocin in this situation had an overall effectiveness of better than 85 percent, and produced an effect within 3 hours of the initiation of infusion.[90] When intrauterine contraction monitoring is being used, a goal of uterine contraction pressures of 200 Montevideo units should be reached. Neonatal outcome has been shown to be good after augmentation of labor at this level of uterine activity.[94] If there has been no response after 2 to 4 hours, and fetal testing is reassuring, delivery by cesarean section would be indicated.[93]

SECOND STAGE

Treatment of the second stage of labor has undergone a number of modifications over the past 2 centuries. In the early 1800s, Denman and others touted restricting the use of forceps until 6 hours of the second stage had elapsed and all other available means for effecting delivery were exhausted. This principle guided obstetrics for many years, until a few studies were published showing a decrease in maternal and neonatal mortality through the use of forceps to shorten the second stage of labor, which culminated in a paper by DeLee in 1920 on the "prophylactic" use of forceps.[95] Forceps deliveries were commonly performed to keep the duration of the second stage under 2 to 2.5 hours.[96]

Friedman showed that the mean duration of the second stage is 66 minutes and 23 minutes in nulliparous and multiparous women, respectively. The 95 percent limit of this stage was shown to be 2.9 hours and 1.1 hours for nulliparous and multiparous women, respectively.[78] Neonatal safety after a prolonged second stage, as evidenced by the lack of an increase in perinatal morbidity or mortality, has been shown.[97] Survival analysis has been used to evaluate the benefit of allowing the second stage of labor to proceed unimpeded after 3 hours in primigravida women. Of interest is the finding of a strong influence of birth weight and maternal age on the time required for spontaneous delivery, whereas maternal height, weight, or the need for augmentation in the first stage of labor had insignificant effects on

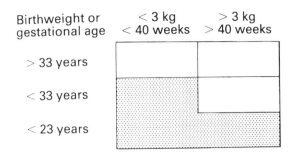

Fig. 6-25. Suggested criteria, as represented by the shaded area, for permitting the second stage of labor to proceed beyond 3 hours. (From Kadar et al,[98] with permission.)

this time. A high likelihood of spontaneous delivery following an allowed continuation of the second stage for 3 hours after an initial 3 hours had elapsed was found for women under 23 years of age and for those under 33 years of age with fetuses weighing less than 3 kg. All other parturients were unlikely to deliver spontaneously if allowed to labor beyond 3 hours after onset of the second stage[98] (Table 6-4 and Fig. 6-25). Epidural anesthesia prolongs the second stage of labor in nulliparous and multiparous women alike[99] (Fig. 6-26). There is limited convincing evidence that a prolonged duration of the second stage of labor significantly affects perinatal and long-term neonatal outcome,[99] with the caveat that adequate fetal monitoring is essential. Current recommendations of the American College of Obstetricians and Gynecologists (ACOG) for consideration of operative delivery in the absence of continuing progress analysis essential in all cases—are as shown (in Table 6-5).[100]

As can be seen from Table 6-4, primigravid women who are undelivered by 3 hours of the second stage will need varying ensuing periods to effect sponta-

Table 6-4. Additional Time (in Minutes) Necessary After 3 Hours in the Second Stage of Labor to Raise Cumulative Probability of Spontaneous Delivery From 40 to 60 Percent as Related to Maternal Age and Birth Weight

Maternal age (yr)	<3 kg	>3 kg
20	33	91
25	59	226
30	125	778
35	346	—

(From Kadar et al,[98] with permission.)

Table 6-5. ACOG-recommended Second Stage Limits for Consideration of Operative Delivery

	Nulliparous	Multiparous
Without regional anesthesia (hr)	2	1
With regional anesthesia (hr)	3	2

(Data from American College of Obstetricians and Gynecologists Technical Bulletin.[100])

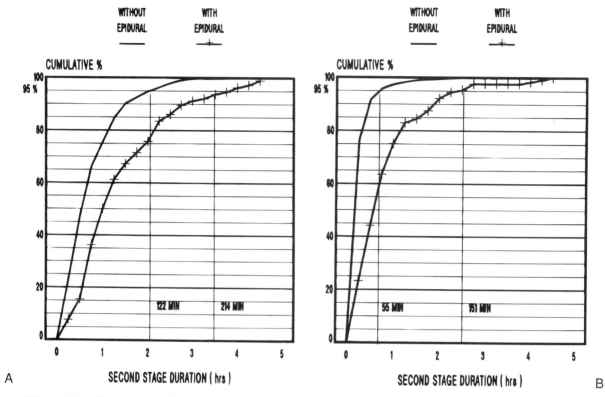

Fig. 6-26. **(A)** Cumulative delivery percentiles for spontaneously delivered infants after term spontaneous labor without augmentation, versus second-stage duration shown for primiparous women with and without epidurals. *(Figure continues).* **(B)** Cumulative delivery percentiles for spontaneously delivered infants after term spontaneous labor without augmentation, versus second-stage duration shown for multiparous women with and without epidurals. (From Derham et al,[99] with permission.)

neous vaginal delivery. The second stage of labor is at the very least a strain on both mother and fetus, and an indefinite open-ended approach to this stage cannot be recommended. Further study, using survival analysis and documenting the probabilities of delivery for various maternal and fetal risk factors (e.g., age and neonatal weight as above, fetal position, duration of pushing, station of the fetal head, and parity), would significantly benefit the approach to managing the second stage.

Disorders of the Second Stage

Protraction Disorders

An increase in the rate of active descent occurs during the active phase of labor with the maximum rate of dilatation. The cervix normally dilates rapidly until the standard 10-cm diameter is reached. The increased active descent continues until delivery. Protraction disorders are defined as a rate of dilatation of less than 1 cm/hr in nulliparas and less than 2 cm/hr in multiparas[101] (Table 6-6). As with the active phase of labor, uterine contractility plays a weighty role in successful termination of the second stage. When a protraction disorder is diagnosed, oxytocin would be recommended if contractions were not believed to be adequate. Continued adequate progress is the goal.[101] Maternal positioning may assist with the prevention or treatment of dystocia. Suggested alternative positions are (1) an upright posture, with a resultant reduction of lumbar lordosis and increase in the uterospinal drive angle, and production of stronger expulsive forces; (2) a sitting or squatting position to increase pelvic diameters; and (3) flexion

Table 6-6. ACOG-recommended Diagnostic Criteria and Treatment for Various Abnormal Labor Patterns

Labor Pattern	Nulligravida	Multipara	Treatment
Prolonged latent phase	>20/hr	>14 hr	Rest or oxytocin
Protraction disorders			
Dilatation	<1.2 cm/hr	<1.5 cm/hr	Oxytocin, if contractions are inadequate
Descent	<1.0 cm/hr	<2.0 cm/hr	
Arrest disorders			
Dilatation	>2 hr	>2 hr	Oxytocin, if contractions are inadequate
Descent	>1 hr	>1 hr	Forceps, vacuum, or cesarean delivery

(Data from American College of Obstetricians and Gynecologists Technical Bulletin.[101])

of the maternal spine to assist in rotating a fetus in the occiput-posterior position.[102] At times, oxytocin, support, alternate positioning, clear instruction in pushing techniques, or assistance with an operative vaginal delivery become necessary to overcome a protraction of active labor.

Arrest of Descent

As noted in Table 6-6, an arrest of descent is recognized when more than 1 hour passes with no further descent of the presenting part of the fetus. This can be seen with poor uterine contractility, excessive sedation, excessively dense conduction anesthesia, maternal exhaustion, and malposition (especially for the occiput-posterior position), and can be associated with a co-existing first stage labor disorder, (e.g., prolonged latent phase, protracted active phase, or arrest of dilatation).[103] Again, if contractions are thought to be insufficient, oxytocin is recommended. Time may be necessary if excessive sedation or a dense epidural anesthesia is deemed responsible for the second stage arrest. Malpositions can, not infrequently, be rectified with manual rotations. Maternal positioning may also assist with alleviating dystocia, as noted above.[102] Depending on the fetal position, degree of asynclitism, and station, an operative vaginal delivery may best serve both the mother and fetus. Cesarean section would be indicated if operative vaginal delivery is judged overly hazardous.

DELIVERY: CARDINAL MOVEMENTS OF LABOR

Successful progress during the first and second stages of labor sequentially effects specific motions of the fetus that lead to its delivery. These actions are termed the cardinal movements of labor. Although they are not discrete, distinct stages, their general pattern is noted in normally progressing labor. The cardinal movements are engagement, flexion, descent, internal rotation, extension, and external rotation (Fig. 6-27).

Engagement is the first cardinal movement to occur. It is said to occur when the widest diameter of the fetal head passes the pelvic inlet. The widest diameter is the biparietal diameter, which averages 9.5 to 10 cm at term.[104] Engagement of the fetal head gives assurance that the pelvic inlet is adequate. It is customary for nulliparous women to begin labor with an engaged fetal head, and less common for multiparous women, as they normally experience descent of the head somewhat later in labor. The fetal head commonly engages in the transverse position, given the longer transverse diameter as compared to the anteroposterior obstetric conjugate. Although abdominal examination was previously primarily used to detect the station of the head, the latter is now primarily determined with a pelvic examination. The distance from the ischial spines to the pelvic inlet is approximately 5 cm. If the station of the presenting part is at the level of the ischial spines, or zero station, the head is said to be engaged.

The uterine contractions force the fetus through the birth canal. This force, and the resistance it encounters from the maternal pelvic tissues, causes the fetus to present the smallest diameters possible for this passage. Flexion of the fetal head aids in offering these diameters to assist in projecting the fetus through the pelvis. The suboccipitobregmatic diameter, which is presented when the fetal head is flexed, is substantially smaller than the occipitofrontal diameter, which is presented when the fetal head is in the military position (Fig. 6-28).

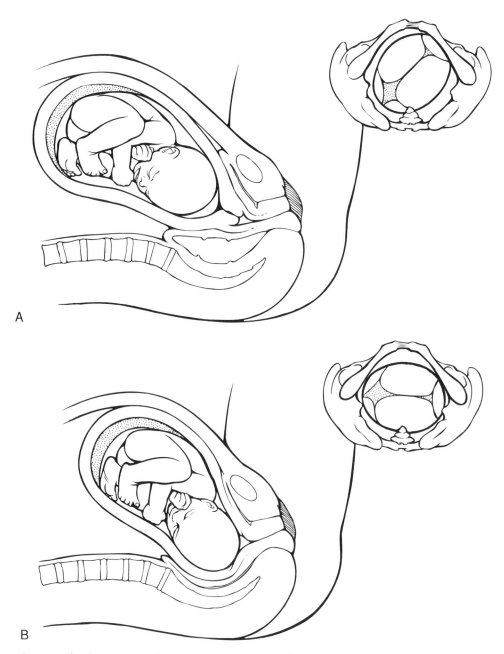

A

B

Fig. 6-27. Cardinal movements of labor. **(A)** Head floating, before engagement; **(B)** engagement with descent and flexion. *(Figure continues.)*

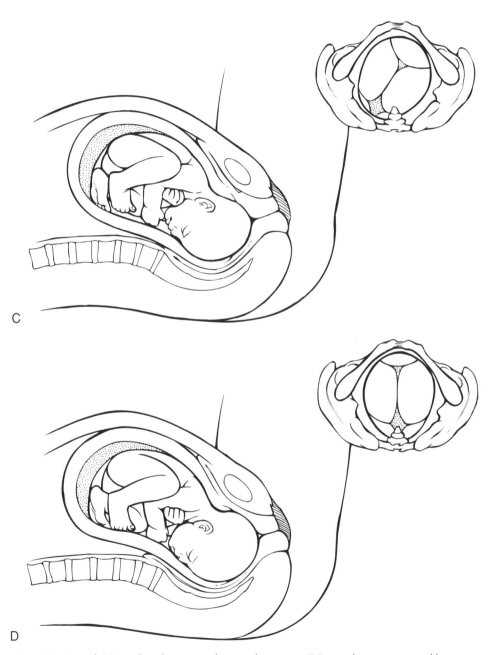

C

D

Fig. 6-27. *(Continued)* **(C)** Further descent and internal rotation; **(D)** complete rotation and beginning of extension. *(Figure continues.)*

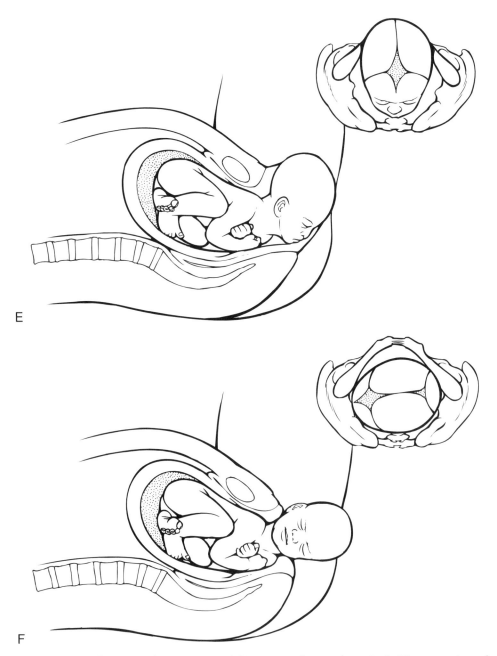

E

F

Fig. 6-27. *(Continued)* **(E)** Complete extension; **(F)** Restitution (external rotation). *(Figure continues.)*

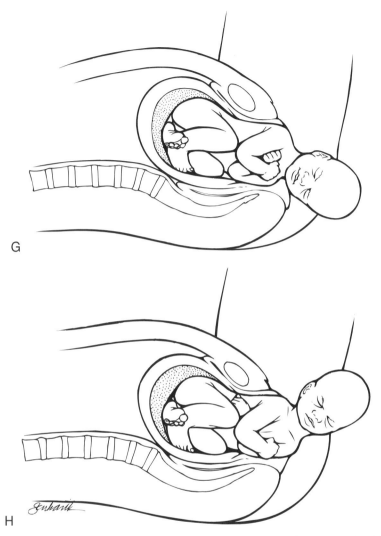

G

H

Fig. 6-27. *(Continued)* **(G)** Delivery of anterior shoulder; **(H)** delivery of posterior shoulder. (Adapted from Cunningham et al,[6] with permission.)

Descent occurs throughout labor and delivery. As previously noted, the rate of descent increases substantially in the late active phase and throughout the second stage. When the presenting fetal head diameters are the smallest that they are going to be, descent occurs much more efficiently. Assisting with the descent of the fetus are the uterine contractions and the maternal expulsion efforts through pushing.

The next cardinal movement is internal rotation.

As the fetus is driven through the pelvis, the pelvic floor muscles are instrumental in guiding this journey. Internal rotation occurs when the occiput, most commonly, is directed toward the pubic symphysis, primarily as the result of resistance generated by the pelvic floor muscles. Rotation is usually complete by the time the head reaches the pelvic floor,[105] but may occur slightly earlier in multiparous women.

When the fetus reaches the pelvic floor, and is visi-

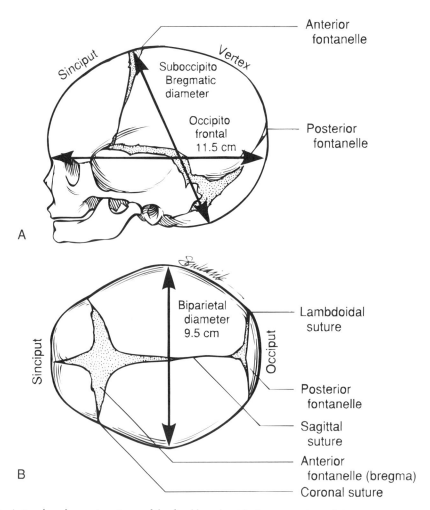

Fig. 6-28. Lateral and superior views of the fetal head, with demonstration of the various areas and diameters.

ble at the introitus, it is said to be crowning. As further force is used to expel the fetus, the head initially undergoes extension as it is delivered over the perineum. The fetal head uses the pubic symphysis as a fulcrum around which extension occurs. The motivation needed for this is the same as that which leads to flexion of the fetal head earlier in the labor process, but in extension, the axis of the pelvis changes and the pelvic outlet is directed upward and outward. The smallest part of the fetal head, at the suboccipitobregmatic diameter, can only be delivered by extension around the pubic symphysis.

After delivery of the fetal head, there is restitution of the former position held by fetus, which is usually in a transverse plane. Because the fetus is no longer constrained by the maternal pelvic floor musculature and bony pelvis, the fetal lie is more aligned than previously noted throughout the labor process.

ASSISTED VAGINAL DELIVERY

As the fetus is undergoing extension of the head, the accoucheur is in a position to assist with the delivery of the fetus, if the latter is a spontaneous delivery. The modified Ritgen maneuver can assist with introducing the smallest fetal head diameter through the introitus. With the protection of a sterile towel, the fetal chin is palpated through the perineum or rectum. Upward pressure on the fetal chin is used to effect further, continued extension of the fetal head about the pubic symphysis. After the fetal head is delivered over the perineum, a moment of respite is in order for the parturient in most circumstances. If there is concern about fetal shoulder dystocia, prompt attention to delivery of the anterior shoulder should be the first priority. Otherwise, allowing external rotation until the head is in a transverse position permits easy bulb suctioning of the fetal mouth and nares. In the setting of meconium, DeLee suctioning of the fetal mouth, oropharynx, and nasopharynx is strongly recommended. Palpation for a nuchal cord is usually mandated at this point. If encountered, a nuchal cord is customarily reduced if loose; if tight, the cord is doubly clamped and cut, although delivery "through" the loop of cord is also an option, and occasionally occurs with parturients who are unable to temporarily withhold their expulsive efforts.

When delivery of the remainder of the fetus is desired, the attendant gently places hands over both sides of the fetal head, overlying the parietal bones, taking care to avoid pressure over soft tissues of the neck. Gentle downward traction is used in conjunction with maternal pushing efforts to effect delivery of the anterior shoulder. (If there was a concern for shoulder dystocia, it is at this point that bulb suctioning and palpation for a nuchal cord can be done.) Upward traction is used for delivery of the posterior shoulder. Because the largest fetal diameters have at this point been delivered, no maternal assistance is subsequently needed normally. Gentle traction is all that is necessary for delivery of the remainder of the fetus. Supporting the occiput with one hand and placing additional gentle traction in the fetal axilla allows delivery to be completed with an easy transition of the baby to rest on the forearm of the occiput-supporting hand. Unless there is a dramatic need for transfer of the baby to an awaiting pediatrician, initial resuscitative efforts are the responsibility of the birth attendant. The infant's face should be dried, the baby kept warm, and the mouth and nares further suctioned. Further stimulation of the baby sometimes proves necessary. These efforts should occur prior to straightaway clamping of the umbilical cord.

CORD CLAMPING

Despite a multitude of opinions, there exists no precise knowledge about when the umbilical cord should be ligated after delivery. Although a number of postulated benefits of delayed clamping of the umbilical cord have been put forth for preterm neonates, its advantages are less clear for the normal term neonate.

With vaginally delivered term neonates, an average of 13 ml/kg of placental transfusion was observed when the umbilical cord was clamped after 30 seconds and the neonate held 10 to 20 cm below the level of the maternal introitus.[106] With infants delivered by cesarean section, the maximum placental transfusion occurred during the first 40 seconds of life, whereas a reversal of flow presumably occurred after that time. Vaginally delivered neonates had significantly higher transfusion rates when the umbilical cord was clamped at from 20 to 40 seconds of life than when it was clamped at less than 20 seconds of life (Fig. 6-29). Maternal blood pressure also had a significant positive influence on placenta-to-neonate

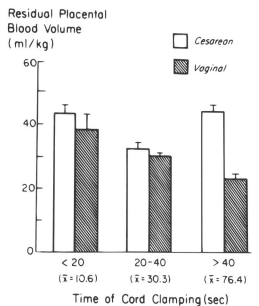

Fig. 6-29. Average residual blood volume, comparing elective cesarean section and vaginal delivery at various cord-clamping times. The average times shown are for the cesarean-delivered cases; the times for the vaginally delivered cases were not significantly different. For cesarean-delivered cases, comparing 20 to 40 seconds to both less than 20 and more than 40 seconds, $p < 0.01$. For vaginally delivered cases, comparing 20 to 40 seconds to less than 20 seconds, $p < 0.05$. (From Ogata et al,[107] with permission.)

transfusion.[107] An appealing postulate suggests that if the umbilical cord is clamped prior to expansion of the pulmonary circulation, the blood required for this circuit must come from systemic reserves rather than from the placental circulation.[108,109] The fact remains that for vigorous term neonates, the proper timing of umbilical-cord ligation remains obscure given the exceptional adaptability of a healthy individual.

THIRD STAGE

The third stage of labor begins with delivery of the neonate and ends with delivery of the placenta. Separation of the placenta is signaled when (1) the uterus becomes globular and more firm (this is usually the first sign to occur); (2) there is an abrupt gush of blood; (3) the uterus rises in the abdomen as the placenta descends into the lower uterine segment and vagina; and (4) there is lengthening of the umbilical cord as the separated placenta descends. These signs usually begin within 5 minutes after delivery of the infant.[6]

As recently as 50 years ago, maternal hemorrhage was a leading cause of maternal mortality in the United States. The introduction of oxytocic drugs for the treatment of postpartum hemorrhage has greatly reduced this risk.[110] A meta-analysis of available trials of the routine use of oxytocic drugs for the prevention of postpartum hemorrhage revealed that it reduced the risk of postpartum hemorrhage (defined as blood loss >500 ml) by about 40 percent, implying that for every 22 parturients given an oxytocic drug, one postpartum hemorrhage could be prevented.[111]

In addition to oxytocic agents, other factors may help to further reduce the risk of postpartum hemorrhage. In one randomized trial of active management of the third stage of labor, the use of an oxytocic agent after delivery of the anterior shoulder, attempted clamping of the umbilical cord by 30 seconds after delivery, and attempted delivery of the placenta by controlled cord traction with a hand on the abdomen to aid in shearing off the placenta and preventing uterine inversion was compared with physiologic management. In the latter protocol, no oxytocic agent was routinely given, no cord traction was attempted, and the cord was left attached to the neonate until delivery of the placenta. The incidence of postpartum hemorrhage, defined as an estimated blood loss of 500 ml or more, was 5.9 percent in the active management group and 17.9 percent in the physiologic group (odds ratio 3.13; 95 percent confidence interval, 2.3 to 4.2). A significant shortening of the third stage of labor was also seen, with a median of 15 minutes versus 5 minutes for the physiologic versus the active management group, respectively. There was no difference in need for manual removal of the placenta or evacuation for retained products of conception. A reduction in neonatal packed cell volume was also encountered in the active management group as compared with the physiologic management group.[112]

Routine use of oxytocin (10 IU IM) as the oxytocic as part of an active management regimen for the third stage of labor has been shown to be well tolerated and to compare favorably with other oxytocic regimens when used prophylactically.[113] Our standard regimen after delivery of the placenta is 20 IU of oxytocin (Pitocin) per liter of crystalloid, given intravenously at 100 to 150 ml/hr for as long as the patient remains in labor and delivery, or 10 IU oxytocin given intramuscularly to patients without intravenous access. Additional doses of oxytocics are sometimes necessary for the treatment of postpartum hemorrhage.

CONCLUSION

A thorough understanding of the normal labor and delivery process is essential for proper patient management. Such an understanding does our patients and the specialty of obstetrics a great service, and may lead to a better understanding of all labor, physiologic and pathologic, term and preterm.

REFERENCES

1. Langman J, Woerdeman MW: Atlas of Medical Anatomy. 1st Ed. WB Saunders, Philadelphia, 1978
2. Compton AA: Soft tissue and pelvic dystocia. Clin Obstet Gynecol 30:69, 1987
3. Ohlsen H: Moulding of the pelvis during labour. Acta Radiol Diagn 14:417, 1973
4. Caldwell WE, Moloy HC: Anatomical variations in the female pelvis and their effect in labor with a sug-

gested classification. Am J Obstet Gynecol 26:479, 1933

5. Steer CM: Moloy's Evaluation of the Pelvis in Obstetrics. 3rd Ed. Plenum, New York, 1975

6. Cunningham FG, MacDonald PC, Gant NF et al: William's Obstetrics. 19th Ed. Appleton & Lange, E. Norwalk, CT, 1993

7. Schwarz GS, Kirkpatrick RH, Tovell HMM: Correlation of cephalopelvimetry to obstetrical outcome with special reference to radiologic disproportion. Radiology 67:854, 1956

8. Todd WD, Steer CM: Term breech: Review of 1006 term breech deliveries. Obstet Gynecol 22:583, 1963

9. Gimovsky ML, Petrie RH, Todd WD: Neonatal performance of the selected term vaginal breech delivery. Obstet Gynecol 56:687, 1980

10. Gimovsky ML, Wallace RL, Schifrin BS, Paul RH: Randomized management of the nonfrank breech presentation at term: a preliminary report. Am J Obstet Gynecol 146:34, 1983

11. Stewart A, Webb J, Giles D, Hewitt D: Malignant disease in childhood and diagnostic irradiation in utero. Lancet 2:447, 1956

12. Stewart A, Kneale GW: Radiation dose effects in relation to obstetric x-rays and childhood cancers. Lancet 1:1185, 1970

13. Granroth G: Defects of the central nervous system in Finland, IV. Associations with diagnostic x-ray examinations. Am J Obstet Gynecol 133:191, 1979

14. Varner MW, Cruikshank DP, Laube DW: X-ray pelvimetry in clinical obstetrics. Obstet Gynecol 56:296, 1980

15. Barton JJ, Garbaciak JA Jr, Ryan GM Jr: The efficacy of x-ray pelvimetry. Am J Obstet Gynecol 143:304, 1982

16. Parsons MT, Spellacy WN: Prospective randomized study of x-ray pelvimetry in the primigravida. Obstet Gynecol 66:76, 1985

17. Moore MM, Shearer DR: Fetal dose estimates for CT pelvimetry. Radiology 171:265, 1989

18. Gimovsky ML, Willard K, Neglio M et al: X-ray pelvimetry in a breech protocol: A comparison of digital radiography and conventional methods. Am J Obstet Gynecol 153:887, 1985

19. Kopelman JN, Duff P, Karl RT et al: Computed tomographic pelvimetry in the evaluation of breech presentation. Obstet Gynecol 68:455, 1986

20. van Loon AJ, Mantingh A, Thijn CJP, Mooyaart EL: Pelvimetry by magnetic resonance imaging in breech presentation. Am J Obstet Gynecol 163:1256, 1990

21. Kastler B, Gangi A, Mathelin C et al: Fetal shoulder measurements with MRI. J Comput Assist Tomogr 17:777, 1993

22. Wright AR, Cameron HM, Lind T: Magnetic resonance imaging pelvimetry: A useful adjunct in the management of the obese patient. Br J Obstet Gynecol 99:852, 1992

23. Schatz F: Beitrage zur physiologischen Geburtskunde. Archiv Gynaekol 3:58, 1872

24. Caldeyro-Barcia R, Sica-Blanco Y, Poseiro JJ et al: A quantitative study of the action of synthetic oxytocin on the pregnant human uterus. J Pharmacol Exp Ther 121:18, 1957

25. El-Sahwi S, Gaafar AA, Toppozada HK: A new unit for evaluation of uterine activity. Am J Obstet Gynecol 98:900, 1967

26. Harbert GM, Jr: Assessment of uterine contractility and activity. Clin Obstet Gynecol 35:546, 1992

27. Caldeyro-Barcia R, Poseiro JJ: Oxytocin and contractility of the pregnant human uterus. Ann NY Acad Sci 75:813, 1959

28. Moore TR, Iams JD, Creasy RK et al: Diurnal and gestational patterns of uterine activity in normal human pregnancy. Obstet Gynecol 83:517, 1994

29. Hendricks CH, Eskes TKAB, Saameli K: Uterine contractility at delivery and in the puerperium. Am J Obstet Gynecol 83:890, 1962

30. Miller FC, Yeh S-Y, Schifrin BS et al: Quantitation of uterine activity in 100 primiparous patients. Am J Obstet Gynecol 124:398, 1976

31. Arulkumaran S, Gibb DMF, Lun KC et al: The effect of parity on uterine activity in labour. Br J Obstet Gynecol 91:843, 1984

32. Cibils LA, Hendricks CH: Normal labor in vertex presentation. Am J Obstet Gynecol 91:385, 1965

33. Friedman EA: The graphic analysis of labor. Am J Obstet Gynecol 68:1568, 1954

34. Friedman EA: Primigravid labor: a graphicostatistical analysis. Obstet Gynecol 6:567, 1955

35. Cibils LA: Electronic Fetal-Maternal Monitoring Antepartum/Intrapartum. 1st Ed. John Wright, PSG Inc., Boston, 1981

36. Friedman EA: Labor in multiparas: a graphicostatistical analysis. Obstet Gynecol 8:691, 1956

37. Hendricks CH, Brenner WE, Kraus G: Normal cervical dilatation pattern in late pregnancy and labor. Am J Obstet Gynecol 106:1065, 1970

38. Liu TY, Kerr-Wilson R: Cervical dilatation in spontaneous and induced labours. Br J Clin Pract 31:177, 1977

39. Friedman EA, Sachtleben MR: Determinant role of initial cervical dilatation on the course of labor. Am J Obstet Gynecol 84:930, 1962

40. Ledger WJ, Witting WC: The use of a cervical dilatation graph in the management of primigravidae in labour. J Obstet Gynaecol Br Commonw 79:710, 1972

41. Naroll F, Naroll R, Howard FH: Position of women in childbirth. Am J Obstet Gynecol 82:943, 1961

42. Caldeyro-Barcia R, Noriega-Guerra L, Cibils LA et al: Effect of position changes on the intensity and frequency of uterine contractions during labor. Am J Obstet Gynecol 80:284, 1960

43. Mitre IN: The influence of maternal position on duration of the active phase of labor. Int J Gynaecol Obstet 12:181, 1974

44. Mendez-Bauer C, Arroyo J, Garcia Ramos C et al: Effects of standing position on spontaneous uterine contractility and other aspects of labor. J Perinat Med 3:89, 1975

45. McManus TJ, Calder AA: Upright posture and the efficiency of labour. Lancet 1:72, 1978

46. Stewart P, Calder AA: Posture in labour: Patients' choice and its effect on performance. Br J Obstet Gynaecol 91:1091, 1984

47. Lupe PJ, Gross TL: Maternal upright posture and mobility in labor—a review. Obstet Gynecol 67:727, 1986

48. Johnson N, Johnson VA, Gupta JK: Maternal positions during labor. Obstet Gynecol Surv 46:428, 1991

49. Goodlin RC: Importance of the lateral position during labor. Obstet Gynecol 37:698, 1971

50. Abitbol MM: Supine position in labor and associated fetal heart rate changes. Obstet Gynecol 65:481, 1985

51. Russell JGB: Moulding of the pelvic outlet. J Obstet Gynaecol Br Commonw 76:817, 1969

52. Russell JGB: The rationale of primitive delivery positions. Br J Obstet Gynaecol 89:712, 1982

53. Gardosi J, Sylvester S, B-Lynch C: Alternative positions in the second stage of labour: A randomized controlled trial. Br J Obstet Gynaecol 96:1290, 1989

54. Stewart P, Hillan E, Calder AA: A randomised trial to evaluate the use of a birth chair for delivery. Lancet 1:1296, 1983

55. Stewart P, Spiby H: A randomized study of the sitting position for delivery using a newly designed obstetric chair. Br J Obstet Gynaecol 96:327, 1989

56. Gardosi J, Hutson N, B-Lynch C: Randomised, controlled trial of squatting in the second stage of labour. Lancet 2:74, 1989

57. Humphrey M, Hounslow D, Morgan S: The influence of maternal posture at birth on the fetus. J Obstet Gynaecol Br Commonw 80:1075, 1973

58. Johnstone FD, Aboelmagd MS, Harouny AK: Maternal posture in second stage and fetal acid base status. Br J Obstet Gynaecol 94:753, 1987

59. Broach J, Newton N: Food and beverages in labor. Part I. Cross-cultural and historical practices. Birth 15:81, 1988

60. Mendelson CL: The aspiration of stomach contents into the lungs during obstetric anesthesia. Am J Obstet Gynecol 52:191, 1946

61. McKay S, Mahan C: Modifying the stomach contents of laboring women: Why and how; success and risks. Birth 15:213, 1988

62. Keppler AB: The use of intravenous fluids during labor. Birth 15:75, 1988

63. Philipson EH, Kalhan SC, Riha MM, Pimentel R: Effects of maternal glucose infusion on fetal acid-base status in human pregnancy. Am J Obstet Gynecol 157:866, 1987

64. Kenepp NB, Shelley WC, Gabbe SG et al: Fetal and neonatal hazards of maternal hydration with 5% dextrose before caesarean section. Lancet 1:1150, 1982

65. Wasserstrum N: Issues in fluid management during labor: general considerations. Clin Obstet Gynecol 35:505, 1992

66. Kreis J: L'accouchement medical. Rev Fr Gynecol Obstet 24:604, 1929

67. Wetrich DW: Effect of amniotomy upon labor: a controlled study. Obstet Gynecol 35:800, 1970

68. Laros RK, Work BA, Witting WC: Amniotomy during the active phase of labor. Obstet Gynecol 39:702, 1972

69. Stewart P, Kennedy JH, Calder AA: Spontaneous labour: when should the membranes be ruptured? Br J Obstet Gynaecol 89:39, 1982

70. Smis B, Thiery M: Fetal heart rate pattern before, during and after amniotomy. Eur J Obstet Gynecol Reprod Biol 11:163, 1980

71. Fraser WD, Sokol R: Amniotomy and maternal position in labor. Clin Obstet Gynecol 35:535, 1992

72. Fraser WD, Marcoux S, Moutquin J-M et al: Effect of early amniotomy on the risk of dystocia in nulliparous women. N Engl J Med 328:1145, 1993

73. Garite TJ, Porto M, Carlson NJ et al: The influence of elective amniotomy on fetal heart rate patterns and the course of labor in term patients: a randomized study. Am J Obstet Gynecol 168:1827, 1993

74. The UK Amniotomy Group: A multicentre randomised trial of amniotomy in spontaneous first labour at term. Br J Obstet Gynaecol 101:307, 1994

75. Friedman EA, Sachtleben MR: Amniotomy and the course of labor. Obstet Gynecol 22:755, 1963

76. Kruse J: The physiology of labor and management of prolonged labor. Primary Care 20:685, 1993

77. Kennell J, Klaus M, McGrath S et al: Continuous emotional support during labor in a US hospital. JAMA 265:2197, 1991

78. Friedman EA: Labor: Clinical Evaluation and Management. 2nd Ed. Appleton-Century-Crofts, E. Norwalk, CT, 1978

79. Peisner DB, Rosen MG: Latent phase of labor in normal patients: a reassessment. Obstet Gynecol 66:644, 1985

80. Friedman EA, Sachtleben MR: Dysfunctional labor I. Prolonged latent phase in the nullipara. Obstet Gynecol 17:135, 1961

81. Koontz WL, Bishop EH: Management of the latent phase of labor. Clin Obstet Gynecol 25:111, 1982

82. Chelmow D, Kilpatrick SJ, Laros RK: Maternal and neonatal outcomes after prolonged latent phase. Obstet Gynecol 81:486, 1993

83. Olah KS, Gee H, Brown JS: Cervical contractions: the response of the cervix to oxytocic stimulation in the latent phase of labour. Br J Obstet Gynaecol 100:635, 1993

84. Peisner DB, Rosen MG: Transition from latent to active labor. Obstet Gynecol 68:448, 1986

85. Friedman EA, Sachtleben MR: Dysfunctional labor. II. Protracted active-phase dilatation in the nullipara. Obstet Gynecol 17:566, 1961

86. Seitchik J, Holden AEC, Castillo M: Amniotomy and oxytocin treatment of functional dystocia and route of delivery. Am J Obstet Gynecol 155:585, 1986

87. Chua S, Kurup A, Arulkumaran S, Ratnam SS: Augmentation of labor: does internal tocography result in better obstetric outcome than external tocography? Obstet Gynecol 76:164, 1990

88. Cardozo L, Pearce JM: Oxytocin in active-phase abnormalities of labor: a randomized study. Obstet Gynecol 75:152, 1990

89. Arulkumaran S, Koh CH, Ingemarsson I, Ratnam SS: Augmentation of labour—mode of delivery related to cervimetric progress. Aust NZ J Obstet Gynaecol 27:304, 1987

90. Friedman EA, Sachtleben MR: Dysfunctional labor III. Secondary arrest of dilatation in the nullipara. Obstet Gynecol 19:576, 1962

91. Ott WJ: Relationship of normal and abnormal late labor patterns to perinatal mortality. Clin Obstet Gynecol 25:105, 1982

92. Read JA, Miller FC, Paul RH: Randomized trial of ambulation versus oxytocin for labor enhancement: a preliminary report. Am J Obstet Gynecol 139:669, 1981

93. O'Brien WF, Cefalo RC: Abnormalities of the active phase: recognition and treatment. Clin Obstet Gynecol 25:115, 1982

94. Hauth JC, Hankins GDV, Gilstrap LC III: Uterine contraction pressures achieved in parturients with active phase arrest. Obstet Gynecol 78:344, 1991

95. DeLee JB: The prophylactic forceps operation. Am J Obstet Gynecol 1:34, 1920

96. Hellman LM, Prystowsky H: The duration of the second stage of labor. Am J Obstet Gynecol 63:1223, 1952

97. Cohen WR: Influence of the duration of second stage labor on perinatal outcome and puerperal morbidity. Obstet Gynecol 49:266, 1977

98. Kadar N, Cruddas M, Campbell S: Estimating the probability of spontaneous delivery conditional on time spent in the second stage. Br J Obstet Gynaecol 93:568, 1986

99. Derham RJ, Crowhurst J, Crowther C: The second stage of labour: durational dilemmas. Aust NZ J Obstet Gynaecol 31:31, 1991

100. American College of Obstetricians and Gynecologists Technical Bulletin: Operative Vaginal Delivery. No. 152. American College of Obstetricians and Gynecologists, Washington, DC, February, 1991

101. American College of Obstetricians and Gynecologists Technical Bulletin: Dystocia. No. 137. American College of Obstetricians and Gynecologists, Washington, DC, December, 1989

102. Fenwick L, Simkin P: Maternal positioning to prevent or alleviate dystocia in labor. Clin Obstet Gynecol 30:83, 1987

103. Friedman EA, Sachtleben MR: Station of the fetal presenting part VI. Arrest of descent in nulliparas. Obstet Gynecol 47:129, 1976

104. Callen PW: Ultrasonography in Obstetrics and Gynecology. 3rd Ed. WB Saunders Philadelphia, 1994

105. Calkins LA: Occiput posterior: incidence, significance, and management. Am J Obstet Gynecol 38:993, 1939

106. Kleinberg F, Dong L, Phibbs RH: Cesarean section prevents placenta-to-infant transfusion despite delayed cord clamping. Am J Obstet Gynecol 121:66, 1975

107. Ogata ES, Kitterman JA, Kleinberg F et al: The effect of time of cord clamping and maternal blood pressure on placental transfusion with cesarean section. Am J Obstet Gynecol 128:197, 1977

108. Redmond A, Isana S, Ingall D: Relation of onset of respiration to placental transfusion. Lancet 1:283, 1965

109. Moss AJ, Monset-Couchard M: Placental transfusion:

early versus late clamping of the umbilical cord. Pediatrics 40:109, 1967

110. Moir JC: The obstetrician bids, and the uterus contracts. Br Med J 2:1025, 1964

111. Prendiville W, Elbourne D, Chalmers I: The effects of routine oxytocic administration in the management of the third stage of labour: an overview of the evidence from controlled trials. Br J Obstet Gynaecol 95:3, 1988

112. Prendiville WJ, Harding JE, Elbourne DR, Stirrat GM: The Bristol third stage trial: active versus physiological management of third stage of labour. B M J 297:1295, 1988

113. McDonald SJ, Prendiville WJ, Blair E: Randomised controlled trial of oxytocin alone versus oxytocin and ergometrine in active management of third stage of labour. B M J 307:1167, 1993

Chapter 7

Induction of Labor: Indications and Techniques*

William F. Rayburn

Induction of labor is one of the most important and irrevocable interventions in obstetric practice. Induction implies stimulation of uterine contractions before the spontaneous onset of labor, with or without ruptured fetal membranes, for the purpose of accomplishing delivery. The most important decision to be made in relation to induction of labor does not concern the ease of the methods used to induce labor, but the justification for pre-empting the spontaneous onset of labor. Pelvic adequacy and underlying maternal and fetal conditions should be thoroughly evaluated beforehand.

Among other factors, induction of labor involves a complex interaction between oxytocin and prostaglandins. Safe and effective cervical ripening and induction of labor, although increasingly based on a firm scientific foundation, continue to require fine clinical judgment. This "art" of scientific obstetric management can only be gained through experience and careful attention to detail. A delicate balance between uterine activity, cervical dilatation rate, and response of the fetus should be sought to achieve this goal.

This chapter summarizes current practice in the stimulation of uterine contractions for labor induction. Indications and techniques for cervical ripening and induction of labor are described. The purpose is not to endorse a particular approach, but rather to describe a range of reported, acceptable methods for the management of labor.

INDICATIONS AND CONTRAINDICATIONS

Labor should be induced only after a thorough examination of both the mother and fetus. Indications for and methods of induction should be documented and understood by the patient. Contraindications to and precautions in the induction of labor should be sought in the case of each patient. A physician or qualified nurse should perform a cervical examination immediately before cervical ripening or oxytocin infusion. Personnel familiar with the effects of uterine-stimulating agents on both the mother and fetus should be in attendance.

Induction is warranted when the benefits to either the mother or fetus outweigh those of continuing the pregnancy. Indications may include, but not be limited to, the maternal or fetal conditions listed in Table 7-1 and approved by the American College of Obstetricians and Gynecologists (ACOG).[1] Postdates and hypertension are the most common indications.

A risk-benefit analysis is necessary before any induction of labor. There are few absolute contraindications to labor (Table 7-1) because there may be certain clinical situations in which an induction is appropriate (e.g., a prolapsed umbilical cord in the

* Adapted from Rayburn,[1] with permission.

Table 7-1. Conditions in Which Labor Induction is Indicated, Contraindicated, or Should Proceed With Caution

Indications	Contraindications	Proceed With Caution
Postdate pregnancy	Induction solely for convenience (elective)	Nonreassuring fetal status (not requiring emergent delivery)
Pregnancy-induced hypertension	Emergencies that require surgical intervention	Previous cesarean section or uterine surgery
Suspected fetal injury (e.g., several fetal growth retardation, abnormal heart rate pattern, isoimmunization)	Absolute cephalopelvic disproportion	Presenting part above the pelvic inlet
Maternal medical problems (e.g., diabetes mellitus, renal disease, chronic pulmonary disease)	Transverse fetal lie or compound presentation	Breech presentation Oligohydramnios
Premature rupture of membranes	Prolapsed umbilical cord	Severe hypertension
Chorioamnionitis	Placenta or vasa previa	Multifetal gestation
Fetal demise	Prior classical uterine incision	Polyhydramnios
Logistics factors (e.g., risk of rapid labor, distance from hospital, psychosocial indications)	Active genital herpes infection Pelvic structural deformities Invasive cervical carcinoma	Maternal cardiac disease (fixed cardiac output) Grand multiparity

(From Rayburn,[1] with permission.)

presence of fetal demise). By contrast, there are many situations in which induction of labor may proceed with caution.

A trial of labor is permitted in most women who have previously had a low transverse cesarean section (see Ch. 13). Risks of instrumental vaginal delivery, uterine-scar dehiscence, transfusion, birth trauma, or poor neonatal outcome are no greater with induced than with spontaneous labor as long as uterine activity is monitored closely.[1] Those women who have not previously delivered vaginally or who did not dilate to 4 cm in any prior pregnancy are less likely to deliver vaginally.[2] Chances for a vaginal delivery are improved by waiting for a more favorable cervix or spontaneous labor.

Premature rupture of the membranes without spontaneous uterine contractions occurs in 6 to 10 percent of term pregnancies.[3] Management of such cases generally includes stimulation of contractions when labor does not commence after 6 to 12 hours of observation. Physicians electing to observe beyond 12 hours must be careful that (1) no other obstetric or medical complication exists, (2) the patient is hospitalized until delivery, (3) there is frequent surveillance of the fetal heart rate, and (4) a careful search is made for infection. Observation is generally limited to women who are multiparous with unfavorable cervices.

CERVICAL RIPENING

The duration of labor induction is affected by parity and cervical status, and is predicted to only a minor degree by baseline contractions and uterine sensitivity to oxytocin. The state of the cervix is clearly related to the success of induction. In 1964, Bishop[4] designed a scoring system for elective induction (Table 7-2) and determined that when the cervical score exceeded 8, the incidence of vaginal delivery subsequent to labor induction was not significantly lower than that observed after spontaneous labor. ACOG later determined that a cervical score of at least 6 is considered favorable and likely to result in successful induction.[1] Induction with a poor cervical score has been associated with failure to induce labor, prolonged labor, and a high cesarean birth rate.[5]

Ripening is a complex process that culminates in the physical softening and distensibility of the cervix. In most pregnancies, some degree of cervical ripening is evidenced near term, and proceeds to spontaneous labor. However, in a significant proportion of

Table 7-2. Bishop Scoring System

Score	Dilation (cm)	Effacement (%)	Station	Consistency	Position of Cervix
0	Closed	0–30	−3	Firm	Posterior
1	1–2	40–50	−2	Medium	Midposition
2	3–4	60–70	−1,0	Soft	Anterior
3	≥5	≥80	+1,+2		

(From Bishop,[4] with permission.)

postdate pregnancies, the condition of the cervix is unfavorable. While the process of natural cervical ripening is associated with successful labor induction, effects of iatrogenic ripening are less well defined. It would appear reasonable that medically enhanced cervical ripening precedes contractions during an induction of labor, since it usually does in spontaneous labor.

The ideal cervical ripening agent should be simple, noninvasive, effective within 24 hours, not compromise the mother or fetus, and not stimulate labor excessively. Methods of ripening the cervix include osmotic dilators, extraovular catheters, and systemically or locally applied hormones such as prostaglandins (E_1, E_2, $F_{2\alpha}$), relaxin, RU486, and estrogens. While various hormones have been implicated, prostaglandins appear to play the most prominent role.

Prostaglandin E_2

Prostaglandin E_2 (PGE_2) gel applied locally is the most successful and widely used agent for cervical ripening. Histologic changes in the cervix after a low-dose application include a dissolution of collagen bundles and an increase in submucosal edema.[6] These changes in cervical connective tissue in the term pregnancy are similar to those observed in early labor.

The U.S. Food and Drug Administration (FDA) approved in December 1992 a PGE_2 gel for cervical ripening in pregnant women at or near term who have a medical or obstetric indication for induction of labor. The product contains 0.5 mg of dinoprostone (a form of PGE_2) per 3 g of triacetin gel; it is available in a syringe containing 2.5 ml of gel. This dose is the most commonly reported, and the intracervical route offers advantages over the larger intravaginal dose by prompting little uterine activity and greater efficacy in the very unripe cervix.

The greatest reported experience has been with delivering PGE_2 intravaginally in a higher-dose (2 to 5 mg) intravaginal gel. In the United States, an intravaginal gel prepared in hospital pharmacies by blending methylcellulose with 20 mg of PGE_2 has had widespread use. Its value in the face of a commercially available product can be debated, and it is often undesired by pharmacists.

A vaginal pessary providing sustained-release of PGE_2 was approved by the FDA in March 1995. Its advantage is its ease of removal with an attached net after uterine hyperstimulation or significant cervical change.[7] More widespread clinical experience is pending. Another product, prostaglandin E_1 (PGE_1), delivered as a gel or tablet, offers similar results at less cost.[8]

Clinical Effectiveness

The cumulative experience of more than 5,000 pregnancies in more than 70 prospective clinical trials in which an intracervical or intravaginal PGE_2 preparation has been used supports the belief that PGE_2 is superior to placebo or no therapy in enhancing cervical effacement and dilatation.[9] Part of the cervical-ripening process with this agent is initiation of labor.

Induction by PGE_2 gel mimics spontaneous labor. Although uterine-stimulating effects may not be clinically apparent, PGE_2 may enhance the myometrial sensitivity to oxytocin.[10] In general, use of a low-dose PGE_2 preparation has been reported to increase the chance of successful initial induction, decrease the incidence of prolonged labor, and reduce total and maximal doses of oxytocin.[5,9] Approximately one-half of treated patients are expected to enter labor, and one-half of nulliparous and more multiparous patients would be expected to deliver within 24 hours.

An important therapeutic end point is the rate of cesarean section. This parameter depends heavily on physician bias. A reduction in the rate of cesarean section is difficult to show without large patient enrollments. The rates of cesarean section resulting either from failed induction or fetal distress would be expected to be lower than or the same as for untreated control patients.[5,9,10]

Postdate gestation is the most common indication for cervical ripening, although significant perinatal morbidity or mortality in this group is too low to demonstrate any benefit of routinely ripening the cervix.[11] Cervical ripening with PGE$_2$ can be accomplished safely in pre-eclamptic women with an unfavorable cervical state.[12] Although not approved for this indication, intravaginal PGE$_2$ in a patient with prematurely ruptured membranes may be safe and beneficial.[13] Despite reports of its successful use, the safety of PGE$_2$ gel in patients with grand multiparity, history of cesarean delivery, or major uterine surgery has not been clearly determined.

An increase in the dose of PGE$_2$ gel does not increase the possibility of vaginal delivery but does reduce the requirement for oxytocin while minimally increasing the chance of uterine hyperstimulation. The higher dose of the intravaginal preparations is also easier to administer and often triggers early labor.[14]

Monitoring Protocol

Patients treated with PGE$_2$ should not be febrile, bleeding intravaginally, or allergic to prostaglandins. A Bishop score of 4 or less is considered to indicate an unfavorable cervix. Other prerequisites to PGE$_2$ therapy include a reassuring fetal heart rate tracing (preferably a reactive nonstress test), no regular uterine contractions (every 5 minutes or less), and a complete explanation to the patient of the reasons for and nature of the therapy. A nonreassuring fetal status does not contraindicate the use of cervical ripening, especially when realizing that the eventual need for oxytocin may be reduced.

The PGE$_2$ preparation is inserted either in or near the labor and delivery suite, where continuous uterine activity and fetal heart rate monitoring can be performed. Outpatient dosing offers more convenience and lower cost, but further study about its

safety is necessary. Intracervical application of PGE$_2$ gel is done through a specially designed catheter with a shield to avoid extra-amniotic infusion. The technique requires direct inspection with a speculum during insertion. The patient is expected to remain recumbent for 60 minutes, and may then be transferred elsewhere in the absence of uterine activity.

The onset of contractions, which are usually irregular and infrequent, is similar to that seen in spontaneous labor. The wide variation in contractions may be explained by differences in individual responsiveness, parity, PGE$_2$ dosage and absorption, initial Bishop score, and state of the membranes. Contractions usually become apparent within the first hour, show peak activity within the first 4 hours, and initiate labor in approximately one-half (25 to 76 percent) of all cases.[10,15] If any regular uterine contractions persist, electronic monitoring should be continued and maternal vital signs recorded at least hourly for the first 4 hours.

A minimum interval between dosing with PGE$_2$ and beginning the administration of oxytocin has not been established. Because effects of PGE$_2$ may be exaggerated by oxytocin, a postdosing observation period should be at least 4 to 6 hours.[5,15] The principal metabolite of PGE$_2$ is cleared from the blood within 6 hours, whereas drug-induced contractions subside within 4 hours if not sustained. Oxytocin should be used with caution and in low doses if the patient continues to have uterine activity from the PGE$_2$ gel.

In the presence of insufficient cervical change (Bishop score change ≤ 3) or inadequate uterine activity with PGE$_2$ therapy, an option may be a second dose of PGE$_2$. Less is known about the value of sequential PGE$_2$ dosing than about a single application followed by an equal period of observation. In the case of preterm cervix, at least two doses are needed before microscopic changes can be anticipated.[16] Prerequisites for the first dosing also apply for sequential dosing.

Side Effects

Uterine hyperstimulation is defined as contractions lasting 2 minutes or more (hypertonicity), or more than five contractions within 10 minutes (tachysystole).[1] The reported rates of uterine hyperstimulation are 1 percent with intracervical PGE_2 gel (0.5 mg) and 2 to 5 percent with the intravaginal gel (2 to 5 mg), and up to 15 percent with the sustained-release vaginal pessary (10 mg).[5,7,9,16] Hyperstimulation occurs more often in the presence of a predosing Bishop score of more than 4 or pre-existing labor, and often begins within the first hour after the gel is applied. Reversal of hyperstimulation by irrigation of the cervix and vagina is not helpful. A β-adrenergic-agonist (e.g., terbutaline 250 μg IV or SC) may be given without adverse effects, and rapid resolution of hyperstimulation can be expected in 98 percent cases without apparent untoward intrapartum effects.[17]

Maternal systemic effects (fever, vomiting, diarrhea) of PGE_2 gel are negligible. The manufacturers of the FDA-approved drug have advised caution in the use of any PGE_2 product in patients with glaucoma, severe hepatic dysfunction, renal impairment, or asthma. Bronchoconstriction or significant changes in blood pressure have not been reported after low doses of PGE_2. Physician discretion and individuality of patient care seem reasonable when using a low-dose PGE_2 preparation applied topically.

Neonatal outcomes among patients undergoing cervical ripening with PGE_2 compare favorably with those patients having induction with oxytocin alone. Infant follow-up to 5 years of age has shown no unusual sequelae from the use of the PGE_2 gel.[5]

Nonpharmacologic Methods

Stripping of Membranes

Induction of labor by stripping the amniotic membranes is a relatively common practice, although there are few reports documenting its efficacy. The technique carries the potential of infection, bleeding from an undiagnosed placenta previa or low-lying placenta, and accidental rupture of the membranes. Membrane stripping may be associated with a decreased incidence of postdate gestation, but this result has not been confirmed.[18] In most cases, the cervix is favorable and does not require another ripening agent.

Cervical Dilators

Cervical dilators may be effective for preinduction cervical ripening late in pregnancy, although much less has been reported about the use of these agents than PGE_2. Examples of dilators include Foley catheters, *Laminaria japonicum*, Dilapan, and Lamicel. As many of these dilators as possible (usually from 1 to 10) are placed in the endocervix without rupturing the membranes[19] (Fig. 7-1). Either the Dilapan or the Lamicel devices are removed the next morning.

Few randomized comparative studies of cervical dilators have been reported.[20,21] However, dilators are thought to significantly dilate the cervix, and may play a role in cervical ripening after a trial of PGE_2. Dilators have the disadvantage of requiring a speculum examination and the potentially uncomfortable requirement for ring forceps or a tenaculum placed on the anterior cervix for traction during their insertion. Their advantages include a reduced cost and convenience because of less need for subsequent monitoring of the uterus and fetus.

Amniotomy

Artificial rupture of the membranes is another nonpharmacologic method of inducing labor, when the cervix is favorable. Labor usually commences within 12 hours after membrane rupture. No randomized, controlled comparative studies of amniotomy versus oxytocin in totally unselected populations are available.[22]

Evidence indicates that amniotomy alone is often inadequate to induce effective contractions. Most studies of amniotomy involve patients in early labor after a spontaneous beginning of labor. However, the weight of evidence indicates that oxytocin infusion is more likely to be effective in achieving delivery within a reasonable time if it is combined with amniotomy then when it is used alone.

The timing of amniotomy during induction of labor is controversial. It seems reasonable for an amniotomy to be performed once the cervix is 3 cm dilated and the presenting fetal part is applied against the cervix. This permits a search for meconium and placement of an intrauterine pressure catheter and fetal scalp electrode.

Several precautions should be observed in the use of amniotomy. Care should be taken during the procedure to palpate for an umbilical cord and to avoid dislodging the fetal head. Rupturing the membranes with an assistant applying gentle fundal pressure toward the pelvis should reduce the risk of cord prolapse[19] (Fig. 7-2). The fetal heart rate should be

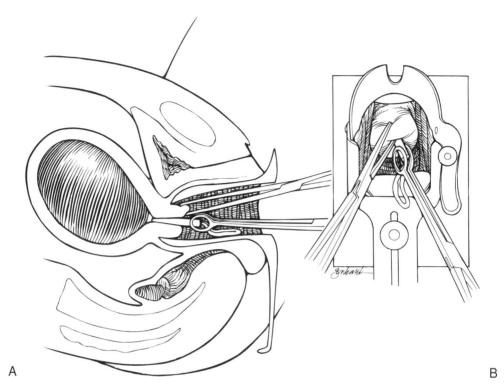

A

B

Fig. 7-1. Intracervical insertion of osmotic dilator. (From Rayburn,[19] with permission.)

recorded before and immediately after the procedure. Following amniotomy, it may be necessary to decrease the rate of any oxytocin infusion.

INDUCTION TECHNIQUES

Although it has not been consistently demonstrated that continuous electronic monitoring of uterine activity and the fetal heart rate with intermittent visits from professional personnel is better than palpation and auscultation performed by an educated attendant who is continuously present, the former practice is more common in the United States than the latter. Fetal and uterine monitoring similar to that recommended for high-risk patients in active labor should be employed when labor is induced.[23] A physician who has privileges to perform cesarean deliveries should be readily available.

Oxytocin

Oxytocin is an octapeptide first synthesized in 1953 by DuVigneaud.[24] The goal of its administration is to effect uterine activity sufficient to produce cervical

change and fetal descent while avoiding uterine hyperstimulation and a nonreassuring fetal heart rate pattern. A response to oxytocin, however, depends on pre-existing uterine activity and sensitivity, and on the cervical status, which are related to individual biologic differences and the duration of pregnancy. The increase in decidual oxytocin receptors appears to explain the increased sensitivity to oxytocin with advancing gestational age. The uterine response to oxytocin increases slowly from 20 to 30 weeks of gestation and is unchanged from 35 weeks until term, at which time sensitivity increases rapidly.[25]

Dosing

Oxytocin is usually diluted (10 U [USP]/ml) in 1,000 ml (10 mU/ml) of a balanced electrolyte solution (lactated Ringer's solution). To avoid bolus dosing, the infusion should be administered with a controlled infusion device and piggybacked through the main intravenous line, close to the venouspuncture site.

In the United States the prevailing obstetric practice is to use low-dosage oxytocin regimens, which

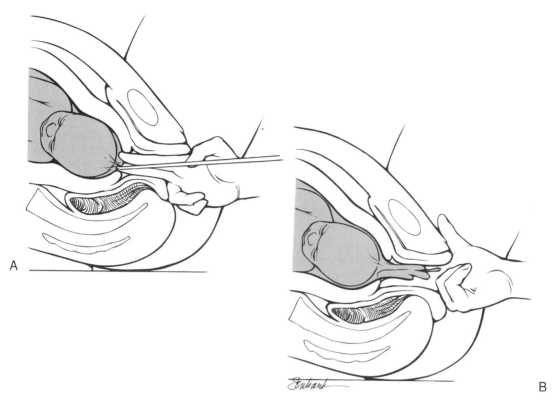

Fig. 7-2. Amniotomy. (From Rayburn,[19] with permission.)

are associated with fewer hazards. The infusion rates and dosages of oxytocin required for induction of labor are often significantly greater than those required for its augmentation. This is most likely because of the need for greater uterine forces to achieve delivery.

Examples of low-dose protocols for oxytocin administration are shown in Table 7-3. These protocols were considered to be better than another dosing regimen with which they were compared in a randomized, prospective manner. The method selected will depend on the individual physician's preference and experience, and may vary according to the patient's parity.

Based on a review of the literature and practical clinical experience, oxytocin should be started at a

Table 7-3.   Protocols of Oxytocin Infusion for Labor Induction

Reference	Initial Dose (mU/min)	Incremental Dose (mU/min)	Incremented Time Interval (min)
Blakemore et al[34] (1990)	0.5	2	60
Mercer et al[35] (1991)	0.5	Doubled	60
Chau et al[36] (1991)	2.5	2.5	30
Satin et al[37] (1992)	2	2	15
Muller[38] (1992)	1–2	1–2	30
Orhue[26] (1993)	2	2	45

low dose (0.5 to 2 mU/min). The initial dose should be no more than 2 mU/min until the contraction pattern is similar to that in normal labor. A slow arithmetic increase in dosage, in 1- to 2-mU/min dose increments every 30 to 60 minutes, is a rational choice. The slow increase is especially important for gravid multiparous patients.[26] Oxytocin infusion at 1 to 3 mU/min yields plasma levels similar to baseline values, whereas infusion at 4 to 6 mU/min gives levels similar to those in spontaneous labor.[27]

Another method of delivering oxytocin is by pulsatile infusion, which more closely simulates spontaneous labor. By giving oxytocin in 10-minute spurts under computer control, rather than continuously, the total amount of drug and duration of labor are slightly decreased.[28,29] This greater efficiency may be explained by an increase in transient oxytocin receptor saturation. Further study in humans is necessary to determine whether induction is more successful with this technique.

Uterine response

There is a physiologic difference between oxytocin-stimulated labor and natural labor. Following parenteral administration of oxytocin, a uterine response occurs within 3 to 5 minutes.[30] Continuous intravenous infusion shows first-order saturation kinetics, with a progressive, linear stepwise increase with each increase in the infusion rate. Drug concentrations at steady-state and at maximal end-organ response are directly proportional to the infusion rate and inversely proportional to systemic clearance. The time required to reach a steady-state concentration of oxytocin in plasma is 40 to 60 minutes after initiating or altering the infusion rate.[31] Increasing the rate of infusion at less than 30 minute intervals, increases the frequency of discontinuing or decreasing the oxytocin infusion by twofold because of hyperstimulation or a worrisome fetal heart-rate pattern.[32]

Minimal effective uterine activity has been characterized by three contractions with an average pressure exceeding 25 mm Hg, with intervals of less than 4 minutes between contractions. However, "adequate labor" describes a wide range of uterine activity. The pressure amplitude of each contraction may vary from 25 to 75 mm Hg, and combined durations of contractions occur over 2 to 4.5 minutes in every 10-minute window, achieving from 95 to 395 Montevideo units.[25]

Prediction of a given pregnancy's oxytocin requirement is difficult. The oxytocin levels required to produce effective contractions vary widely among individuals, most likely reflecting unpredictable individual uterine sensitivities and variabilities in oxytocin clearance rates. Predictors of the need for exogenous oxytocin also include cervical dilatation, parity, gestational age, and maternal body-surface area. The dosage is titrated against uterine contractions 1- to 2-mU/min increments every 30 to 60 minutes. There is no maximum rate of oxytocin infusion. However, a dose of more than 20 mU/min is usually unnecessary, and the uterine response generally will not improve if 30 mU/min or more is administered.[33]

A cervical dilatation rate of 1 cm/hr is another guide to the adequacy of oxytocin administration.[22] However, care must be taken not to resort to a cesarean section too quickly in disorders marked by a protracted latent phase of labor, since an unripe cervix may require additional contractions before dilatation. An increase in the dose of oxytocin after achieving a cervical dilatation of at least 1 cm/hr or maximal uterine activity may represent impatience. Instead, consideration should be given to reducing the dose with advanced cervical dilatation. Regardless of parity, an arrest of labor will be evident if there is either no cervical dilatation over a period of 2 hours (first stage) or a lack of descent over a period of 1 hour (second stage) despite adequate uterine contractions.[23]

Side Effects

Adverse effects of oxytocin are primarily dose-related, and may include uterine hyperstimulation or rupture. Decreasing the oxytocin dose may correct an abnormal pattern of contractions and prevent an unwarranted delay in delivery, although in the light of an unfavorable legal environment it may be prudent to stop the infusion. The half-life of oxytocin is approximately 10 to 15 minutes, and the duration of action is usually 20 minutes.[30,31] Additional measures for correcting unwanted effects of oxytocin include changing the patient's position, administering oxygen and more intravenous fluid, and injecting a β-adrenergic agonist, as described above. The oxytocin infusion may be restarted after re-evaluation. When restarting the oxytocin, it is recommended that it be infused at no more than one-half the previous rate, and that the interval at which the rate of infusion had been increased be lengthened.

Because oxytocin does not cross the placenta, no direct effects on the fetus have been observed. Uterine hyperstimulation or a resting tone above 20 mm Hg between contractions can lead to uteroplacental hypoperfusion and fetal distress from hypoxia. Cardiovascular problems in the mother are rare, since oxytocin is not given as a rapid intravenous injection. Rare electrocardiographic (ECG) changes include premature ventricular contractions, ST–T-wave changes, flattening of T waves, and prolongation of the QT interval. Hypotension from direct peripheral vasodilation may also occur when oxytocin is given rapidly in a concentrated solution in combination with a general anesthetic such as cyclopropane.

Both natural and synthetic oxytocin are structurally similar to antidiuretic hormone (ADH). To avoid delirium from water intoxication, large quantities of intravenous solutions should not be infused with high concentrations of oxytocin. The antidiuretic effect may be observed after a prolonged induction with the use of 40 U of oxytocin.[34]

Serial Inductions

Little is known about the value of repeated or serial inductions as opposed to committing the pregnancy to delivery within 48 hours. Although the practice of serial inductions is controversial, it appears to be widespread. Many patients do not have pressing indications for induction of labor, as evidenced by the high numbers of women who remain undelivered at 24 and 48 hours after the beginning of induction. Pregnancies must be re-evaluated for cephalopelvic disproportion, any worsening of the underlying complication, and infection, to ensure that further delay is safe for the mother and fetus. In doing so, the need for cesarean delivery with its accompanying surgical risks may be reduced. For example, serial inductions in cases of postdate pregnancy are advocated in the absence of other maternal or fetal mandates for imminent delivery. Most women undergoing induction of labor are exhausted, and it seems reasonable to allow them to rest overnight if they and the fetus are in stable condition. The oxytocin should be discontinued and the uterine activity monitoring continued until contractions subside.

Failure of a committed attempt at induction is especially common in preterm deliveries. In general, the preterm uterus is less sensitive to oxytocin than the full-term uterus, and may require larger doses or serial inductions. The response to uterine stimulants seems to increase slowly during pregnancy until becoming relatively stable after 33 weeks' gestation. Studies of oxytocin requirements in this situation are few and difficult to interpret, since the reason for induction may involve several variables, each of which alone can alter uterine sensitivity.

REFERENCES

1. Rayburn WF: Induction of labor. ACOG Technical Bulletin, American College of Obstetricians and Gynecologists, Washington DC (in press)
2. Molloy BG, Sheil O, Duignan NM: Delivery after cesarean section: review of 2,176 consecutive cases. BMJ 27:1645, 1987
3. Duff P, Huff R, Gibbs R: Management of premature rupture of membranes and unfavorable cervix in term pregnancy. Obstet Gynecol 63:697, 1984
4. Bishop EH: Pelvic scoring for elective induction. Obstet Gynecol 24:266, 1964
5. Brindley BA, Sokol RJ: Induction and augmentation of labor: basis and methods for current practice. Obstet Gynecol Surv 43:730, 1988
6. Rayburn W, Newland J, Lightfoot S et al: A model for investigating mircoscopic changes induced by prostaglandin E_2 in the term cervix. J Maternal Fetal Invest 4:137, 1994
7. Rayburn WF, Wapner RJ, Barss VA et al: An intravaginal controlled-release prostaglandin E_2 pessary for cervical ripening and initiation of labor at term. Obstet Gynecol 79:374, 1992
8. Fletcher H, Mitchell S, Frederick J et al: Intravaginal misoprostol versus dinoprostore as cervical ripening and labor-inducing agents. Obstet Gynecol 83:244, 1994
9. Rayburn WF: Prostaglandin E_2 gel for cervical ripening and induction of labor: critical analysis. Am J Obstet Gynecol 160:529, 1989
10. Bernstein P: Prostaglandin E_2 gel for cervical ripening and labour induction: a multicentre placebo-controlled trial. Can Med Assoc J 145:1249, 1991
11. The National Institute of Child Health and Human Development Network of Maternal-Fetal Medicine Units: A clinical trial of induction of labor versus expectant management in postterm pregnancy. Am J Obstet Gynecol 170:716, 1994
12. Rayburn W, Woods R, Ramadei C: Intravaginal prosta-

glandin E_2 gel and cardiovascular changes in hypertensive pregnancies. Am J Perinatol 8:233, 1991

13. Ray D, Garite T: Prostaglandin E_2 for induction of labor in patients with premature rupture of membranes at term. Am J Obstet Gynecol 166:836, 1992

14. Hales K, Rayburn W, Turnbull GL: Double-blind comparison of prostaglandin E_2 as a 0.5 mg intracervical gel or 2.5 mg intravaginal gel for cervical ripening and induction of labor. Am J Obstet Gynecol 171:1087, 1994

15. Miller AM, Rayburn WF, Smith CV: Patterns of uterine activity after intravaginal prostaglandin E_2 during pre-induction cervical ripening. Am J Obstet Gynecol 165:1006, 1991

16. Atkinson BD, Hales K, Lightfoot SA et al: Microscopic effects of sequential dosing of prostaglandin E_2 on the preterm and term rabbit cervix. J Soc Gynecol Invest (in press)

17. Egarter CH, Husslein PW, Rayburn WF: Uterine hyperstimulation after low-dose prostaglandin E_2 therapy: tocolytic treatment in 181 cases. Am J Obstet Gynecol 163:794, 1991

18. McColgin SW, Hampton HL, McCaul JF et al: Stripping membranes at term: can it safely reduce the incidence of post-term pregnancies? Obstet Gynecol 76:678, 1990

19. Rayburn WF: Cervical ripening. In Hankins GD, Clark SL, Lunninghan FG, Gilstrap L (eds): Operative Obstetrics. Appleton and Lange, E. Norwalk, CT, (in press)

20. Blumenthal PD, Ramanauskas R: Randomized trial of Dilapan and Laminaria as cervical ripening agents before induct of labor. Obstet Gynecol 75:365, 1991

21. Sanchez-Ramos L, Kaunitz AM, Connor PM: Hygroscopic cervical dilators and prostaglandin E_2 gel for preinduction cervical ripening. A randomized, prospective comparison. J Reprod Med 37:355, 1992

22. Bakos O, Backstrom T: Induction of labor: a prospective, randomized study into amniotomy and oxytocin as induction methods in a total unselected population. Acta Obstet Gynecol Scand 66:537, 1987

23. American College of Obstetricians and Gynecologists: Dystocia. ACOG Technical Bulletin 137, American College of Obstetricians and Gynecologists, Washington, DC, 1989

24. DuVigneaud V, Ressler C, Trippett S: The sequence of amino acids in oxytocin with a proposal for the structure of oxytocin. J Biol Chem 205:949, 1953

25. Calderyo-Barcia R, Poseiro JJ: Physiology of the uterine contraction. Clin Obstet Gynecol 3:386, 1960

26. Orhue AA: A randomized trial of 45 minutes and 15 minutes incremented oxytocin infusion regimens for the induction of labour in women of high parity. Br J Obstet Gynecol 10:126, 1993

27. Fuchs A, Goeschen K, Husslein P et al: Oxytocin and the initiation of human parturition. III. Plasma concentrations of oxytocin and 13, 14-dehydro-15-keto-prostaglandin F_2-alpha in spontaneous and oxytocin-induced labor at term. Am J Obstet Gynecol 141:694, 1981

28. Cummiskey KC, Dawood MY: Induction of labor with pulsatile oxytocin. Am J Obstet Gynecol 163:1868, 1990

29. Willcourt R, Payer D, Wendel J, Hale R: Induction of labor with pulsatile oxytocin by a computer-controlled pump. Am J Obstet Gynecol 170:603, 1994

30. Seitchik J, Castillo M: Oxytocin augmentation of dysfunctional labor. I. Clinical data. Am J Obstet Gynecol 144:899, 1982

31. Seitchik J, Amico J, Robinson AG, Castillo M: Oxytocin augmentation of dysfunctional labor. IV. Oxytocin pharmacokinetics. Am J Obstet Gynecol 150:225, 1984

32. Kruse J: Oxytocin: pharmacology and clinical application. J Fam Pract 23:473, 1986

33. Whalley PJ, Pritchard JA: Oxytocin and water intoxication. JAMA 186:601, 1963

34. Blakemore KJ, Qin NG, Petrie RH, Paine LL: A prospective comparison of hourly and quarter-hourly oxytocin dose increase intervals for the induction of labor at term. Obstet Gynecol 75:757, 1990

35. Mercer B, Pilgram P, Sibai B: Labor induction with continuous low-dose oxytocin infusion: a randomized trial. Obstet Gynecol 77:659, 1991

36. Chua S, Arulkumaran S, Kurup A et al: Oxytocin titration for induction of labour: a prospective randomized study of 15 versus 30 minute dose increment schedules. Aust NZ J Obstet Gynaecol 2:134, 1991

37. Satin AJ, Hankins GD, Yeomans ER: A prospective study of two dosing regimens of oxytocin for the induction of labor in patients with unfavorable cervices. Am J Obstet Gynecol 165:980, 1991

38. Muller PR, Stubbs TM, Laurent LS: A prospective randomized clinical trial comparing two oxytocin induction protocols. Am J Obstet Gynecol 167:373, 1992

Multiple Gestations

Lynn L. Simpson and Mary E. D'Alton

Despite the many advances in perinatal medicine, multiple gestations continue to pose a significant challenge to the practicing obstetrician. Because of the potential for serious maternal and perinatal complications, careful planning is required for the management of these high-risk pregnancies. Early diagnosis, optimization of the intrauterine environment, prevention of preterm delivery, close fetal surveillance, atraumatic labor and delivery, and provision of prompt neonatal care will lead to an improved perinatal outcome in multiple pregnancies.

INCIDENCE

Multiple gestation occurs in approximately 1 percent of pregnancies.[1] Most of these are twins, with triplets and higher-order pregnancies occurring much less frequently. It has been found that two-thirds of twins are dizygotic and one-third are monozygotic.[2] The dizygotic-twin rate varies widely, between 4 and 50 per 1,000 births.[3] Several factors are associated with an increased incidence of dizygotic twinning. A significant contribution to the increased incidence of dizygotic twins and higher-order gestations is the increased use of assisted-reproduction technology.[4] The incidence of multiple gestation ranges from 4 to 15 percent with induction of ovulation, and from 15 to 20 percent with in vitro fertiliza-

tion.[5] Between 1973 and 1990, when assisted reproduction was being used with increasing frequency, the number of twin births increased at twice the rate of singletons, and higher-order births increased at seven times the rate of singletons.[6] Unlike dizygotic twinning and higher-order gestations, the monozygotic twin rate of 3 to 5 per 1,000 births has been found to be relative constant.[3]

MATERNAL COMPLICATIONS

The maternal complications that occur in singleton pregnancies are observed more frequently in women with twins (Table 8-1). These include hyperemesis gravidarum, anemia, pyelonephritis, cholestasis, pre-eclampsia, antepartum hemorrhage, pre-term labor, premature rupture of membranes, operative delivery, and postpartum hemorrhage.[1] An operative delivery with its associated morbidity and mortality is one of the major risks to women with multiple pregnancies. Because the rate of cesarean-section for twins has increased significantly over the past 20 years, the complications of abdominal delivery continue to be a concern.

FETAL AND PERINATAL COMPLICATIONS

Prematurity poses a significant threat to the fetuses of multiple gestations. The perinatal mortality of twins is 5 to 10 times that of singletons.[2,7–9] The

---

Risk Factors for Dizygotic Twinning

Increased maternal age

Increased parity

Black race

Positive maternal family history

Ovulation induction

In vitro fertilization

---

increased incidence of perinatal morbidity and mortality in twin gestations is related primarily to prematurity and its complications. Between 40 and 50 percent of twin pregnancies will be less than 37 weeks at the time of delivery, compared with 8 to 10 percent of singleton pregnancies.[10–12] Although advances in neonatal care have improved the outlook for these premature infants, the overall incidence of preterm delivery for twins remains unchanged. Intrauterine fetal growth restriction, which occurs in up to one-quarter of twin pregnancies, also contributes to the poor perinatal outcome associated with multiple gestations.[10,13] Other fetal complications include congenital anomalies, polyhydramnios, twin-to-twin transfusion syndrome, intrauterine demise of one fetus, cord prolapse or entanglement, and malpresentation of one twin[1] (Table 8-2).

In the past, the mode of delivery was implicated as a major factor for increased perinatal morbidity and mortality in twin births. Although older obstetric literature has suggested that manipulative delivery is associated with a poor outcome, more recent reports challenge this concept.[14–16] The perinatal outcome in twin births may be most dependent on the degree of prematurity rather than on intrapartum events such as the route and mode of delivery. As a result, a major goal in the management of multiple pregnancies is to prevent preterm delivery.

ANTEPARTUM MANAGEMENT

Diagnosis

Before the use of ultrasonography, up to 50 percent of twin gestations were undiagnosed prior to labor and delivery.[7,17,18] In a large multicenter study, Berger and colleagues[19] found that poor perinatal outcomes were associated with late diagnosis of twin pregnancies. Unfortunately, the clinical detection of multiple gestation by symphysis fundal height, palpation, or detection of multiple fetal heart tones is unreliable. Despite the high index of suspicion associated with a positive maternal family history, ovulation induction, and increased maternal age and parity, multiple gestations have been underdiagnosed on historical and clinical grounds. However, with widespread use of triple screening in pregnancy, up to 57 percent of multiple gestations were identified during the evaluation of an elevated maternal serum α-fetoprotein concentration.[20] Since the early diag-

Table 8-1. Maternal Complications in Twin Gestations

Complication	Incidence (%)	References
Hyperemesis	10	Kauppila et al[124]
Anemia	11–24	Hall et al,[125] Jeffrey et al[126]
Pyelonephritis	18	Kauppila et al[124]
Cholestasis	4–10	Kauppila et al,[124] De Muylder et al[10]
Preeclampsia	18–20	Thompson et al,[77] De Muylder et al[10]
Antepartum hemorrhage	3–5	Jeffrey et al,[126] Farooqui et al[17]
Abruption	0.6–1.8	Kauppila et al,[124] Farooqui[17]
Previa	0.9–1.3	Kauppila et al,[124] De Muylder et al[10]
Preterm labor	50–70	Thompson et al,[77] Polin and Frangipane[55]
Premature rupture of membranes	5	De Muylder et al[10]
Operative delivery	50	Polin and Frangipane[55]
Postpartum hemorrhage	22	Farooqui et al[17]

Table 8-2. Fetal Complications in Twin Gestations

Complication	Incidence (%)	References
Prematurity	40–50	De Muylder et al,[10] Cetrulo[11]
Intrauterine growth retardation	16–26	De Muylder et al,[10] Chervenak et al[109]
Congenital anomalies	6	Polin and Frangipane[55]
Polyhydramnios	6–12	Farooqui et al,[17] Cetrulo et al[7]
Twin-to-twin transfusion	5–10	Burke[25]
Demise of one fetus	2–5	Fusi and Gordon,[67] Eglowstein and D'Alton[68]
Cord prolapse	4–6	Farooqui et al,[17] Hays and Smeltzer[1]
Malpresentation	55–60	Polin and Frangipane,[55] Adams and Chervenak[38]

nosis of multiple gestation has been shown to decrease perinatal morbidity and mortality, routine ultrasound examination to identify unsuspected multiple gestations also has its merits.[21]

Multiple gestation can be diagnosed early in the first trimester using ultrasound (Fig. 8-1). Interestingly, the incidence of twins in the first trimester is

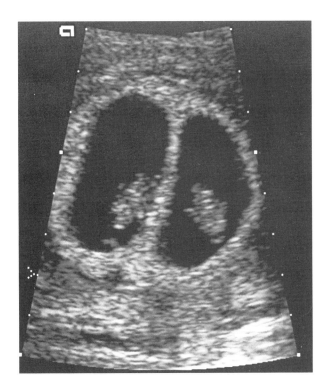

Fig. 8-1. Sonogram of a twin pregnancy in the first trimester. A thick separating membrane was observed between the two fetuses. This was a dichorionic diamniotic twin pregnancy conceived through in vitro fertilization.

about twice that at term.[22,23] The disappearance of one conceptus, termed the "vanishing twin," is often not recognized by the patient who goes on to have an uneventful pregnancy with delivery of a healthy singleton. With the routine use of ultrasound in midtrimester, over 95 percent of multiple pregnancies can be expected to be diagnosed.[24] The early detection of multiple gestation can lead to improved maternal and perinatal outcomes through proper management in the antepartum and intrapartum periods.

Chorionicity

The determination of chorionicity can be important in the management of twin pregnancies. Monochorionic twins are at greater risk than dichorionic twins, with a perinatal mortality of 26 percent compared to 9 percent.[25] It is estimated that 20 percent of twin pregnancies are monochorionic and 80 percent are dichorionic.[23] Chorionicity can usually be determined by a careful midtrimester ultrasound examination (Fig. 8-2). If two separate placentas are visualized or the fetuses are of opposite sex, the pregnancy is dichorionic (Fig. 8-3). If only one placenta can be identified and the fetuses are of the same sex, the separating membrane should be examined. If two layers are present, the placentation is monochorionic and diamniotic (Fig. 8-4A). If three or four layers are visualized, the placentation is dichorionic and diamniotic (Fig. 8-4B).

Although membrane thickness has been used to assess chorionicity, with thin membranes indicating monochorionicity and thick membranes indicating dichorionicity, there is some concern that a membrane may appear thin and thick at different times

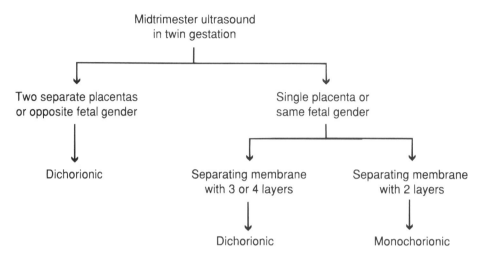

Fig. 8-2. Protocol to determine chorionicity of twin gestation by ultrasonography.

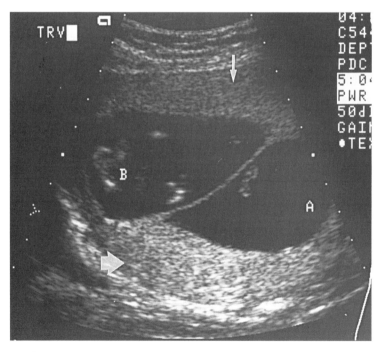

Fig. 8-3. Sonogram of a dichorionic gestation showing two separate placentas. Twin A had a posterior placenta (thick arrow) and twin B had an anterior placenta (thin arrow).

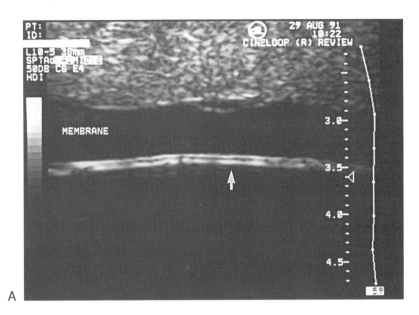

MEMBRANE

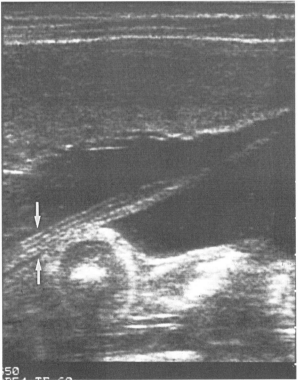

Fig. 8-4. (A) Sonogram of a monochorionic diamniotic gestation showing two layers within the dividing membrane (arrow). **(B)** Sonogram of a dichorionic diamniotic gestation showing four layers within the dividing membrane (arrows). (From D'Alton and Dudley,[28] with permission.)

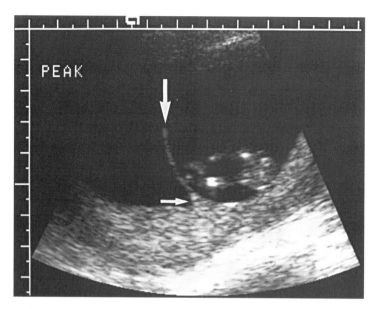

Fig. 8-5. Sonogram of the twin peak sign (small arrow). The triangular projection of placental tissue between the layers of the dividing membrane (large arrow) suggested a dichorionic gestation.

during the same ultrasound examination and at different gestational ages.[26–28] The "twin-peak" sign, identified on ultrasound examination by the presence of a triangular projection of placental tissue between the layers of the separating membrane, has been suggested as reliable evidence of dichorionic twinning with two fused placentas[29] (Fig. 8-5). However, the absence of the twin-peak sign does not help to determine chorionicity, which limits its usefulness as a clinical marker.[30]

The determination of chorionicity by ultrasonography is most easily accomplished late in the first trimester and early in the second trimester, and should be attempted in all multiple gestations. When ultrasound cannot establish chorionicity with certainty, amniocentesis for deoxyribonucleic acid (DNA) fingerprinting can be performed to accurately determine the zygosity.[31] This may be important in planning the management of twin pregnancies complicated by discordant growth, single intrauterine fetal demise, and discordant congenital anomalies.

Monoamniotic Twins

Monoamniotic twins occur in 1 percent of monozygotic gestations, and are associated with a 50 percent fetal mortality rate.[25,32,33] In a small series, Laros and Dattel[34] reported that 6 of 10 monoamniotic twins were stillborn or died in the neonatal period. Owing to the potential for a poor pregnancy outcome, early diagnosis with close fetal surveillance of monoamniotic twins is warranted.

A single amniotic sac is suspected when a separating membrane between twin fetuses cannot be visualized by ultrasound. The diagnosis is confirmed if entanglement of the two umbilical cords is identified by ultrasound examination.[35] This life-threatening complication develops in up to 70 percent of monoamniotic twins[36] (Fig. 8-6). Umbilical cord accidents appear to be the primary cause of fetal death in monoamniotic twins.[36] As a result, intensive antepartum fetal surveillance with nonstress testing and biophysical profiling is recommended.[36,37] The optimal frequency of fetal testing is unknown, but should be individualized according to gestational age, fetal growth, and previous test results. Because of the high incidence of fetal demise in monoamniotic twin pregnancies, serial amniocentesis for pulmonary maturity has been recommended at 32 to 36 weeks[1] gestation, with delivery when maturity is documented.[36,38] However, Carr and colleagues[39] in a review of 24 pairs of monoamniotic twins, and Tessen and Zlatnik[40] in a review of 20 monoamniotic

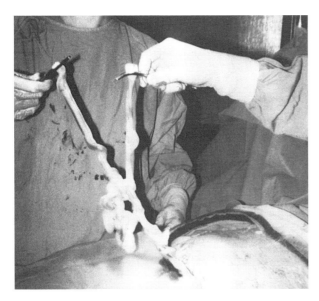

Fig. 8-6. Entangled umbilical cords found at cesarean section of monoamniotic twins. (Photograph provided by Dr. Gary Kaufman, New England Medical Center.)

pairs, found no intrauterine fetal deaths after 30 weeks and 32 weeks, respectively. Based on these retrospective observations, preterm delivery of monoamniotic twins may not be indicated in all cases.

Although monoamniotic twins have been born vaginally, cesarean section may be the safest route of delivery.[36,41,42] Inadvertent clamping of the second twin's umbilical cord with vaginal delivery of the first twin has been reported.[43] Rodis and colleagues[37] reported good outcomes in the cases of three consecutive monoamniotic twins delivered abdominally. By contrast, Tessen and Zlatnik[40] reported successful vaginal deliveries in 14 of 20 cases of monoamniotic twins, with only one emergent cesarean section being performed for fetal distress. The optimal route of delivery for monoamniotic twins remains uncertain, but labor with continuous fetal monitoring and vaginal delivery may be a reasonable option.

Conjoined Twins

Conjoined twins constitute a rare complication of monozygotic twinning, with an incidence of 1 in 50,000 births.[44] This complication should be suspected when the fetuses cannot be visualized separately on ultrasound examination. When the diagno-

sis is made early in pregnancy, termination by dilatation and evacuation or by induction of labor is possible and should be considered. Cesarean section has been recommended for the delivery of conjoined twins beyond 26 weeks' gestation.[1,9,42] Abdominal delivery may help to decrease fetal and maternal trauma caused by fetopelvic disproportion.[38]

Genetic Amniocentesis

Fetal karyotyping may be indicated for several reasons in a multiple gestation. The incidence of congenital anomalies is higher in dizygotic twins than in singletons.[23,45] Advanced maternal age, the most common indication for prenatal diagnosis, also increases the risk of dizygotic twinning. In addition, infertility and the use of assisted-reproduction technology are more common in women of advance maternal age. The risk of chromosomal abnormalities in a twin pregnancy is higher than that expected for a singleton. Rodis et al[46] calculated a mathematical risk of Down syndrome in one fetus of a 33-year-old woman with twins to be equivalent that for a singleton fetus of a 35-year-old woman. Unfortunately, triple screening is not helpful in providing a risk figure for chromosomal abnormalities in twin pregnancies. For these reasons, fetal karyotyping in women with twin gestations has been considered at a younger age than the traditional 35 years.

Amniocentesis of both gestational sacs in twin pregnancies is warranted and can be accomplished in more than 95 percent of cases.[47,48] Amniocentesis should be performed under continuous ultrasonographic guidance. On completion of the first aspiration, 1 to 2 ml of a 0.08 percent indigo carmine solution is injected into the first sac. This will help to confirm that amniotic fluid from the second sac is obtained during the subsequent aspiration, since this fluid should be clear.

The overall safety of genetic amniocentesis in twin gestations is uncertain. In a study of 339 cases of multiple gestation undergoing amniocentesis for prenatal diagnosis, there was a loss rate of 3.6 percent, compared with a 0.6 percent loss rate for singletons.[49] This increased risk may be partly explained by the higher spontaneous loss rate for twins. Coleman and co-workers[50] reported a rate of spontaneous loss of 5 percent in twins diagnosed after 20 weeks' gestation. With experience and only two needle insertions, it appears that genetic amniocentesis in twin gestations poses no greater risk than that for singleton pregnancies.[23,51]

Discordant Growth

A discordance of 15 to 25 percent, defined as the difference in birth weight expressed as a percentage of that of the larger twin, has been associated with increased perinatal mortality.[52] At present, there is no consensus about the definition of discordant growth.[53] However, a study by O'Brien et al[54] found that if the difference between the weights of the fetuses was less than 20 percent, intrauterine growth restriction was excluded more than 90 percent of the time. By contrast, when the discordance was greater than 20 percent, approximately 50 percent of the fetuses were growth-restricted.[54]

Discordant fetal growth may complicate 15 to 30 percent of twin pregnancies.[23] A difference in biparietal diameter of greater than 5 mm, a biparietal diameter of the smaller twin below 2 standard deviations (SD) of normal, or a head-circumference difference of greater than 5 percent have been found to be useful in the identification of discordant growth.[23] Uteroplacental insufficiency and twin-to-twin transfusion syndrome are the major etiologic factors in discordant fetal growth. Marginal and vela-

mentous insertion of the umbilical cord into the placenta, which have been associated with intrauterine growth restriction, are more frequent in twin gestations and may contribute to discordant fetal growth[55,56] (Fig. 8-7). Other causes of intrauterine growth restriction, including congenital anomalies, chromosomal abnormalities, and intrauterine infection, must also be considered.

In general, twin pregnancies complicated by discordant growth due to uteroplacental insufficiency are managed expectantly. Frequent antenatal assessments with serial nonstress testing, biophysical profiling, and Doppler velocimetry have been advocated on a daily to weekly basis depending on the individual case.[53] Ultrasonographic assessment of fetal biometry is recommended every 2 weeks to follow fetal growth. Delivery should be considered at term or with documented fetal lung maturity (Fig. 8-8). In a survey concerning the management of growth-discordant twins, Blickstein[53] reported that 87 percent of obstetricians did not consider discordancy to be an indication for cesarean section.

Twin-to-Twin Transfusion Syndrome

Despite vascular communications in virtually all monochorionic gestations, twin-to-twin transfusion syndrome is estimated to occur in only 5 to 10 percent

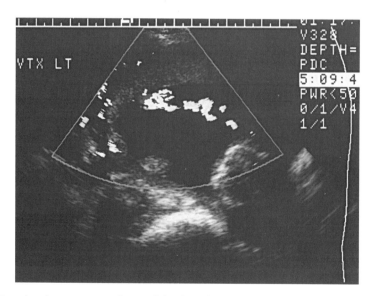

Fig. 8-7. Color Doppler ultrasonogram of an umbilical cord in a twin pregnancy, showing its marginal insertion into the placenta. (Color not shown.)

of twin pregnancies.[25] This may be an underestimation, owing to the wide spectrum of presentations observed with different degrees of clinical severity and at different gestational ages. Although the clinical manifestations of twin-to-twin transfusion syndrome are often not evident until 20 to 30 weeks[1] gestation, we have diagnosed a case of the condition as early as 17 weeks[57] (Fig. 8-9). The development of twin-to-twin transfusion syndrome is the result of a shared fetal circulation through arteriovenous communications within the placenta.[23,58] With the transfusion of blood through these channels, the donor twin becomes anemic and growth restricted and the recipient twin becomes polycythemic. Oligohydramnios tends to develop in the donor twin's sac and polyhydramnios in the recipient's sac. The oligohydramnios may become severe, with the effect that the fetus appears to be stuck in a fixed position between the dividing membrane and the adjacent uterine wall[59] (Fig. 8-9). In 10 to 25 percent of cases the recipient twin develops evidence of hydrops fetalis due to fluid overload and congestive heart failure.[59]

The prognosis in twin-to-twin transfusion syn-

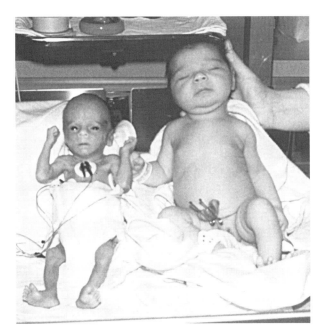

Fig. 8-8. Marked growth discordance in twin infants delivered at term.

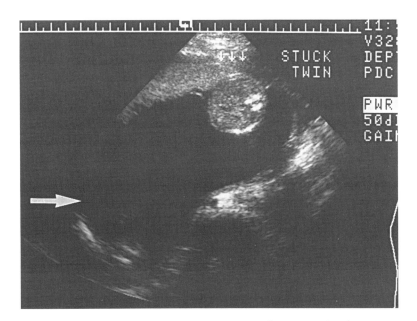

Fig. 8-9. Sonogram of a stuck twin at 17 weeks' gestation (small arrows). This fetus was in a fixed position between the separating membrane and the adjacent uterine wall. Severe oligohydramnios was present in the stuck twin's sac. Polyhydramnios was evident around the co-twin (large arrow).

drome is poor, with a mortality rate of 70 to 100 percent in untreated cases.[1,4] The decision to treat and the choice of treatment depend on the gestational age at the time of diagnosis, with the most aggressive interventions being reserved for cases of extreme prematurity. Serial amniocentesis to decompress the polyhydramnios has been shown to improve the prognosis.[60] Normalization of the amniotic-fluid volume in the sac containing the immobilized twin is observed following successful therapeutic amniocentesis. Reisner and associates[61] found a 54 percent reduction in perinatal mortality in 37 cases of "stuck-twin" syndrome managed with serial amniocentesis. From their data, serial amniocentesis in twin-to-twin transfusion syndrome was most beneficial in cases diagnosed at 20 to 30 weeks' gestation.[61] Although indomethacin has been used in the treatment of stuck-twin syndrome, it presents the potential for an adverse perinatal outcome. Jones et al.[62] reported two cases of severe twin-to-twin transfusion syndrome complicated by a single intrauterine fetal demise within 72 hours of starting indomethacin. Laser photocoagulation of the placental vessels has been utilized with some success in the management of twin-to-twin transfusion syndrome.[63] This approach has the disadvantage of requiring a laparotomy and insertion of a fetoscope into the uterus for visualization. Ligation of the umbilical cord and selective feticide have also been reported.[33,64] However, these procedures introduce the risk of neurologic injury and fetal death to the nonstuck twin, as in the case of the surviving twin of a monochorionic pregnancy complicated by single intrauterine demise.

Death of One Fetus

With the increasing use of ultrasound examination in early pregnancy, multiple gestations are being diagnosed earlier and more frequently. It is estimated that only 50 percent of twin pregnancies identified in the first trimester have successful deliveries of two live infants.[27,65] The intrauterine demise of one twin is most common during the first trimester. Although this may be associated with some vaginal spotting, the loss of one conceptus is often not clinically recognized. It appears that the prognosis for the surviving twin is excellent when the demise occurs early in pregnancy.[27,66]

Excluding early fetal loss, intrauterine demise of one fetus in twin gestations occurs in 2 to 5 percent of cases.[67,68] It is estimated that there is a threefold increase in intrauterine death with monochorionic twins as compared to dichorionic twins.[25] Demise of one fetus is also more common in triplet gestations, occurring in 14 to 17 percent of such cases.[69,70] Clinical management in this circumstance will depend on the gestational age, fetal lung maturity, and fetal or maternal complications. A major concern when fetal death occurs during the second half of twin pregnancies is the high incidence of morbidity and mortality in the surviving fetus. In a retrospective analysis of twin pregnancies complicated by the intrauterine death of one twin, Enbom[71] found that 46 percent of the surviving fetuses experienced major morbidity or mortality. Rydhstrom and Ingemarsson[72] reported a 27 percent perinatal mortality rate for the surviving twin after antenatal death of its co-twin. In this retrospective study, 4.6 percent of the surviving twins were handicapped by mental retardation or cerebral palsy at 8 or more years after birth.[72] In recent prospective studies, neurologic damage is reported in 5 to 19 percent of surviving twins.[67,68] The potential for injury appears to differ in monochorionic and dichorionic gestations. In monochorionic twin gestations, up to 20 percent of the surviving fetuses may experience neurologic injury.[73] Although the exact mechanism for the injury is uncertain, embolization of tissue thromboplastin through placental anastomoses to the surviving twin has been proposed.[25] Other possible mechanisms of neurologic injury include fetal hypotension with hypoxemia and fetal exsanguination. Unfortunately, immediate delivery has not prevented multicystic encephalomalacia in the surviving twin.[73] In dichorionic multiple gestations, the risk of major perinatal morbidity or mortality in the surviving twin appears to be negligible.[74] Fusi and Gordon,[67] in their review of eight dichorionic twins complicated by a single intrauterine death, found no neurologic defects in the survivors. The surviving twin may be protected from embolization by the rarity of vascular communications in dichorionic gestations. One of the greatest risks to the surviving co-twin is prematurity, with over 75 percent of cases delivering prior to term.[67,68]

In addition to possible harm to the surviving fetus, there is the potential for maternal consumptive coagulopathy in twin pregnancies complicated by a single intrauterine demise.[75] As in singleton pregnancies with retention of a dead fetus for 4 to 5 weeks, the incidence of maternal disseminated intravascular coagulation (DIC) is estimated at 25 percent when fetal demise occurs in multiple gestations.[76] However, only a few cases of maternal coagulopathy under these circumstances have been reported, and the 25 percent incidence figure may be an overestimation.[74,75] In a review of 16 pregnancies complicated by the intrauterine fetal death of one twin, Fusi and Gordon[67] found no cases of maternal DIC. Eglowstein and D'Alton[68] found transient fibrin split products and hypofibrinogenemia in 2 of 20 cases, neither of which required medical therapy. Because of the potential risk to the mother, serial coagulation profiles are recommended to detect the early development of this complication.

Although intensive antepartum assessment of multiple pregnancies complicated by the intrauterine demise of one fetus is required, fetal death should not be the sole indication for delivery.[70] It has been recommended that expectant management with close fetal and maternal surveillance be undertaken if prematurity is a concern.[74] In cases of documented fetal lung maturity or in pregnancies beyond 37 weeks' gestation, delivery should be considered.

Preterm Labor

Preterm labor poses the greatest threat to multiple pregnancies, complicating up to 70 percent of twin gestations.[77] Prematurity continues to be the primary cause of poor perinatal outcome in these cases. Only 50 percent of twin pregnancies reach 37 weeks' gestation and are delivered at term.[55] The exact etiology of preterm labor in multiple gestations is unknown. Both uterine distension and polyhydramnios are more common in twin pregnancies and have been implicated as possible underlying causes of preterm labor. Because of its frequent occurrence, patients with multiple gestations must be educated about the subtle signs and symptoms of preterm labor so that the diagnosis can be made early and the success rate of active intervention increased.

The management of preterm labor in multiple gestations is similar to that in singletons, with the use of steroids and short-term tocolysis to delay delivery for 24 to 48 hours if possible.[7,78] Despite pro-

phylactic measures, including bed rest, cervical cerclage, and tocolytic agents, the gestational age of twins at delivery remains relatively unchanged. The value of bed rest in the prevention of preterm labor in multiple gestations is controversial.[79] If bed rest is to be recommended to patients with multiple pregnancies, it should be instituted early in the pregnancy. Between 70 and 80 percent of perinatal deaths associated with twins occur before 30 weeks' gestation.[8,13] Therefore, bed rest may be most beneficial between 20 and 30 weeks' gestation. Although cervical cerclage has been tried in the past, multiple gestation is not an indication for cerclage, which has been shown to be ineffective in prolonging twin pregnancies.[80,81] Cervical cerclage in multiple gestation should be used only in patients with a history compatible with an incompetent cervix. While the therapeutic use of tocolysis for preterm labor is recommended, the prophylactic use of tocolytic agents in multiple pregnancy has not been shown to be effective.[7,82] The prevention of preterm delivery remains a major goal in the management of multiple gestations.

Antepartum Fetal Surveillance

Serial ultrasonographic assessments of fetal growth in multiple gestation are useful for the early diagnosis of intrauterine growth restriction and growth discordance between the fetuses. Monthly biometry is recommended, with more frequent assessments if poor fetal growth is detected. Routine nonstress testing of twins before birth has been suggested, beginning at 30 to 34 weeks' gestation.[55] Knuppel and colleagues[83] found that nonstress testing decreased the incidence of intrauterine fetal death in twins in the third trimester of pregnancy. However, in the absence of abnormal fetal growth, routine testing of twins may not be warranted.[84] Simultaneous monitoring of both fetuses is usually possible. Biophysical profile assessments can be used to determine fetal well-being when fetal heart rate tracings are inadequate or nonstress testing is nonreactive. In certain cases, such as twin-to-twin transfusion syndrome and discordant or abnormal fetal growth, Doppler flow-velocity studies of the umbilical artery can contribute to patient management. Although Doppler studies remain investigational, abnormal umbilical artery waveforms may be useful in determining the frequency of fetal testing and the need for hospital admission. Daily fetal assessment with nonstress tests and biophysical profiles is recommended in cases of absent or reversed end-diastolic flow in the umbilical artery.

Amniocentesis for Pulmonary Maturity

In selected multiple gestations, amniocentesis may be indicated for the determination of fetal lung maturity. It remains unclear whether obtaining fluid from both gestational sacs is required. If the fetuses are concordant in size, obtaining fluid from only one sac is probably adequate.[27,85] However, when the fetuses are of unequal size, both sacs should be sampled when possible. Although the smaller twin is expected to have accelerated lung maturity because of stress in utero, Leveno et al[86] found that in 9 of 15 discordant twin pairs, it was the larger twin that had the higher lecithin/sphingomyelin ratio. As a result of these findings, fetal pulmonary maturity studies should be performed on amniotic fluid from each sac whenever feasible.

INTRAPARTUM MANAGEMENT

There is considerable controversy about the optimal intrapartum management of multiple gestations. Unfortunately, large, well-designed prospective studies of the intrapartum management of twins have not been performed and may prove impractical. As a result, conflicting recommendations about the management of labor and delivery of twins are present in the literature.

In general, it is recommended that multiple gestations be delivered by 40 weeks.[84] Traditionally, the route of delivery has been determined by the presentation of the first twin. However, experience with vaginal twin delivery has become limited owing to changes in obstetric practice. Malpresentation of the second twin has become a common indication for operative delivery. This is in part due to decreased experience with vaginal breech delivery. In addition, second twins are known to have poorer outcomes than first twins. However, malpresentation of the second twin does not fully explain this difference, and delivery by cesarean section does not appear to significantly improve neonatal outcome.[87]

At present, one-half of all twin pregnancies are

delivered by cesarean section.[55] Although liberal use of cesarean section has been recommended, improved perinatal outcome has not been conclusively established and maternal morbidity may be substantial. Infectious morbidity is increased two- to fourfold and maternal mortality is increased four- to eightfold with cesarean section.[42] Because of the potential for maternal complications, and the observation that the route of delivery has little impact on perinatal outcome, a rational indication for abdominal delivery of twins should be identified. The major considerations affecting the mode of delivery in twin gestation include fetal presentation, relative size of the second twin to the first, and fetal well-being.[88]

General Preparations

When a woman with twins presents to the labor and delivery unit, a comprehensive assessment is required with preparation for possible delivery. This includes confirmation of fetal presentation, electronic monitoring of both fetuses, establishment of intravenous access with blood kept available, and notification of the neonatology and anesthesiology departments.

Regional anesthesia has significantly improved the intrapartum management of multiple gestations. Early continuous lumbar epidural anesthesia is recommended for labor and delivery of twin pregnancies.[89] The presence of an anesthesiologist in the delivery room should be requested when vaginal delivery of twins is anticipated. Despite careful

---

Requirements for Labor and Delivery in Twin Gestation

Determination of presentation and estimated fetal weights

Continuous electronic fetal monitoring of both twins

Intravenous access with blood available

Notification of anesthesiology and neonatology

Availability of intrapartum ultrasound

Obstetrician skilled in operative vaginal delivery

preparation, potential problems may arise during the course of delivery. General anesthesia for uterine relaxation may be required for delivery of the second twin. In one series, cesarean section was required for delivery of the second twin in 7.6 percent of cases.[89] Anesthesiology as well as neonatology personnel need to be available in the event of an emergency cesarean section. A neonatologist should also be present for vaginal births, since the second twin delivered vaginally frequently requires resuscitation.

Ultrasound equipment should be available in the delivery room for assessment of the second twin after the first is delivered. The presentation of the second twin may change in up to 20 percent of cases after delivery of the first twin.[42] The management of the second twin will depend on several factors, including the presentation, fetal heart rate tracing, and experience of the obstetrician.

Delivery Interval

With the advent of intrapartum fetal monitoring, the interval between the delivery of first and second twins has become less important than previously. In a review of 341 twin gestations, Thompson et al[77] found that the interval between the birth of the twins did not affect perinatal outcome. Chervenak and co-workers[21] reported that 5-minute Apgar scores did not correlate with the time interval between the delivery of the twins. Therefore, in the presence of a reassuring fetal heart rate tracing, there is no urgency to deliver the second twin. However, a sixfold increase in the cesarean section rate (from 3 to 18 percent) for delivery of the second twin has been observed when the delivery interval is greater than 15 minutes.[90] This observation supports active rather than expectant management for delivery of the second twin in the second stage of labor. This may include artificial rupture of the membranes, intravenous oxytocin, and total breech extraction in the case of a breech presentation or transverse lie of the second twin.

A failure of descent of the presenting part of the second twin has been associated with an increased risk of cesarean section.[42] Although the overall duration of labor is similar with twin and singleton pregnancies, dysfunctional labor is more common in multiple gestations.[91] Augmentation of labor with intravenous oxytocin is acceptable when uterine con-

Table 8-3. Intrapartum Fetal Presentation in Twin Gestations

Twin A	Twin B	Incidence %
Vertex	Vertex	40–45
Vertex	Nonvertex	35–40
Nonvertex	Vertex/nonvertex	20

(Data from Polin and Frangipane,[55] and Adams and Chervenak.[38])

traction are inadequate.[1,9] The use of oxytocin is often valuable during the second stage of labor to shorten the interval between delivery of twins.

Vertex-Vertex Presentation

The most common intrapartum presentation of twins is the vertex-vertex presentation, which occurs in 40 to 45 percent of cases[1,10] (Table 8-3). In an otherwise uncomplicated pregnancy, vaginal delivery should be anticipated with vertex-vertex presentation. In the past, it was recommended that cesarean section might be the optimal route of delivery for all twins weighing less than 1,500 to 2,000 g, irrespective of presentation.[14,92] However, more recent data support a trial of labor and vaginal delivery when both fetuses are in the vertex presentation regardless of gestational age.[21,93–96] Of 154 twin pregnancies with vertex-vertex presentations, Chervenak and associates[21] found that 81 percent had successful vaginal deliveries. Abdominal delivery of vertex-vertex twins should be reserved for standard obstetric indications such as failure to progress in labor or nonreassuring fetal testing remote from imminent vaginal delivery.

Vertex-Nonvertex Presentation

In 35 to 40 percent of twin gestations presenting in labor, the first twin will be in the vertex position and the second twin will be in the breech or transverse positions.[1,10] The appropriate route of delivery for vertex-nonvertex twins is one of the most controversial issues in the intrapartum management of multiple gestations (Fig. 8-10).

There have been three approaches to the delivery of twins when the second fetus is in a nonvertex position. Cesarean section can be done on the basis of malpresentation alone, the criteria for vaginal breech delivery of a singleton can be applied to the

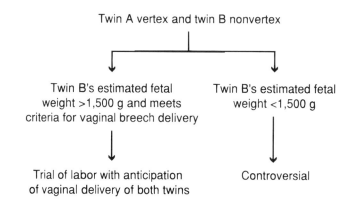

Fig. 8-10. Protocol for intrapartum management of vertex-nonvertex twins.

second twin and a trial of labor offered if the criteria are met, or a vaginal delivery can be planned based on vertex presentation of the first twin.

In the past, liberal use of cesarean section was advocated on the basis of reports of increased perinatal morbidity and mortality associated with breech delivery of the second twin and low-birth-weight singletons.[97,98] These studies have had a significant impact on the intrapartum management of twins, with an increased proportion of multiple pregnancies being delivered by cesarean section. However, a number of investigators have found that the high perinatal morbidity and mortality of both twins is related to prematurity and intrauterine growth restriction and not to the presentation of the second twin.[93–95,99] Increasing data suggest that routine cesarean section is not necessary when the second fetus is nonvertex. In fact, there are data suggesting that cesarean section does not improve the outcome of low-birth-weight singletons, including those in a breech presentation.[100,101]

Recent comparisons between vaginally delivered and cesarean-delivered nonvertex second twins have failed to show a significant difference in perinatal outcome (Table 8-4). Acker and colleagues[102] found no increase in low 5-minute Apgar scores or perinatal mortality when 76 second twins weighing 1,500 g or more were delivered vaginally in breech presentations. Comparing the mode of delivery on the outcome of 206 twin pregnancies, Laros and Dattel[34] found no significant difference in perinatal morbidity or mortality between twin pairs delivered vagi-

nally or abdominally. In a randomized study of 60 vertex-breech or vertex-transverse twin deliveries of 35 to 41 weeks' gestation, Rabinovici and associates[103] found that the route of delivery did not significantly affect neonatal outcome. By contrast, maternal febrile morbidity was significantly increased in the cesarean section group.[103]

Another approach when the presentation of the second twin is nonvertex is to determine whether this twin is a candidate for a vaginal breech delivery. Because of the potential for birth trauma and feto-pelvic disproportion, it has been recommended that infants who weigh less than 1,500 g or more than 3,500 g not be considered for vaginal breech delivery.[92,104] It is argued that there are insufficient data to recommend a specific mode of delivery for a second nonvertex twin with a birth weight of less than 1,500 g.[84] However, recent studies have failed to demonstrate that cesarean delivery improves perinatal outcome in twin pregnancies for fetuses in any weight group.[93–96,105] In a study of 416 sets of twins in four different weight categories (500 to 1,499, 1,500 to 1,999, 2,000 to 2,499, and 2,500 g or more) Greig et al[106] reported that the presentation and mode of delivery of the second twin were not associated with a significant difference in outcome except for lower 1-minute Apgar scores in nonvertex twins delivered vaginally.

A critical review of the available data suggests that vaginal delivery of the second twin is reasonable and appropriate in carefully selected cases. A trial of labor with anticipation of a vaginal delivery may be

Table 8-4. Route of Delivery of the Nonvertex Second Twin and Its Impact on Perinatal Outcome[a]

Authors	Year	Gestational Age (wk)	Weight (g)	Vaginal Breech Delivery	Cesarean Delivery	Perinatal Outcome
Davison et al[16]	1992		750–2,000	54	43	NS
Greig et al[106]	1992		500–1,499	9	44	NS
			1,500–1,999	12	24	NS
			2,000–2,499	21	31	NS
			>2,500	21	46	NS[b]
Adam et al[104]	1991		1,000–1,499	17	3	NS
			>1,500	99	32	NS
Rydhstrom[99]	1990		<1,500	154	73	NS
Gocke et al[15]	1989		>1,500	53	40	NS
Laros and Dattel[34]	1988	20–43	220–3,800	39	78	NS
Rabinovici et al[103]	1987	35–41	1,300–3,550	27	27	NS
Bell et al[93]	1986	>37		77	47	NS
		29–36		60	50	NS
Kelsick and Minkoff[127]	1982		>1,000	839	173	NS
Acker et al[102]	1982		>1,500	76	74	NS

[a] NS, not statistically significant. Includes studies that compared the perinatal outcome of nonvertex second twins delivered vaginally to nonvertex second twins delivered by cesarean section.

[b] Only statistically significant difference was a lower 1-minute Apgar score in nonvertex second twins delivered vaginally.

based on a vertex presentation of the first twin alone, provided that the second twin is of similar size. If the second, nonvertex twin is significantly larger than the first, cesarean section may be the most appropriate route of delivery.[55,105] However, intrapartum external version or assisted breech delivery, if the criteria for vaginal breech delivery are met, are reasonable alternatives. Of 139 twin pregnancies with vertex-nonvertex presentations, Chervenak and colleagues[21] found that 71 percent had successful vaginal deliveries. In this study there were 20 neonatal deaths among infants with birth weights between 500 and 1,000 g. All of these deaths, 12 involving the first twin and 8 the second twin, were due to complications of prematurity and not to the route of delivery.[21] At present, it is reasonable to offer a trial of labor in cases of vertex-nonvertex twins when the second twin has an estimated fetal weight above 1,500 g and is of similar size to the first twin. Recent literature suggests that this option may also prove appropriate for very low-birth-weight second twins in a nonvertex position. Because of the increased frequency of classic cesarean sections in preterm multiple gestations with malpresentation, vaginal delivery of vertex-nonvertex twins would de-

crease maternal morbidity associated with operative delivery and with repeat cesarean section in subsequent pregnancies.[107]

The approach to the vaginal delivery of the second twin after successful delivery of a first twin is also controversial. The options include external cephalic version and subsequent delivery as a vertex, assisted breech delivery, and total breech extraction. The management choice depends of the individual case and on the experience of the obstetrician. There exist instances of intrapartum complications such as cord prolapse, placental abruption, retraction of the cervix, and nonreassuring fetal testing in which vaginal delivery is not imminent and emergency abdominal delivery is the most appropriate management option. Cesarean section may also be the safest mode of delivery when the delivering obstetrician is not comfortable with external and internal version, breech extraction, and assisted breech delivery.

However, cesarean section does not eliminate possible birth trauma, and a less aggressive use of abdominal delivery of vertex-nonvertex twins may be justified. In a study of 136 pairs of vertex-nonvertex twins with birth weights above 1,500 g, there was no significant difference in perinatal morbidity or mortality with external version, breech extraction, or cesarean section.[15] Good perinatal outcomes have been reported with external cephalic version and vaginal breech delivery.[108–110] Chervenak et al[108] found that intrapartum external version was successful in over 70 percent of deliveries involving nonvertex second twins. However, in a review of 41 attempted external versions and 55 attempted breech extractions for the delivery of second twins, Gocke and associates[15] found a 46 percent rate of successful vaginal delivery in the external-version group as compared to a 96 percent rate of successful vaginal delivery in the breech-extraction group. Even with successful external version, cesarean section may be required for complications, including fetal decelerations or bradycardia, cord prolapse, failure to descend, or compound presentation.[15] Because it entails fewer complications and yields a greater number of successful vaginal deliveries, breech extraction may be preferred over external version for the delivery of second nonvertex twins.

The decision to use active intervention rather than expectant management for the delivery of a nonvertex second twin should be individualized. A fetus in frank or complete breech presentation with a reassuring heart rate tracing is a candidate for expectant management and an assisted vaginal delivery. In these cases, the membranes of the second sac should be left intact until the presenting part is in the pelvic inlet. Active intervention to facilitate vaginal delivery may be undertaken either electively or in situations in which immediate delivery is necessary and the vaginal route is considered the best option. When complete breech extraction is performed, both feet are identified and drawn into the pelvis. The membranes are then ruptured and the delivery completed. The potential advantages of intact membranes during a total breech extraction include increased mobility of the fetus and decreased risk of fetal injury.[88] Although infants delivered by breech extraction tend to be more depressed at delivery, most will respond to immediate resuscitative measures. The use of total breech extraction in low-birth-weight infants has been controversial. However, Davison and colleagues[16] reported no significant adverse outcome in 54 second twins delivered by breech extraction who weighed between 750 and 2,000 g. For a second twin in a transverse lie, internal

podalic version with intact membranes, followed by total breech extraction, is an appropriate approach for the experienced obstetrician.[111] Delaying rupture of the membranes until the feet are brought into the pelvis may increase the maneuverability of the fetus and success of the extraction.

It has been suggested that an emergency cesarean section for a second twin after vaginal delivery of the first twin should rarely, if ever, be done.[112] Before 1982, there were only nine cases of combined vaginal-abdominal delivery of twins reported in the literature.[113] At present, from 6 to 8 percent of second twins require cesarean section following vaginal delivery of a first twin.[89,114] Declining skill and experience of obstetricians with intrauterine manipulation have been implicated in the increased incidence of abdominal delivery for second twins.[115,116] With a trial of labor and vaginal delivery being recommended as the optimal method of management in carefully selected cases of vertex-nonvertex twins, it is important that obstetricians experienced with intrauterine maneuvers be involved in training future obstetricians who may require such skills to provide optimal care to pregnant women with twins.

Nonvertex First-Twin Presentation

Traditionally, cesarean section has been recommended when the first twin is in a nonvertex position, which occurs in 20 percent of cases.[1,10] This is based on the potential risk of interlocking twins.[21] It is estimated that interlocking twins occur in 1 of 1,000 twin gestations.[117] However, in a retrospective review of 34 vaginally delivered twin pregnancies in which the presenting twin was in the breech position, there were no cases of interlocking twins.[118] In fact, it has been suggested that if the presenting twin is in the breech position and is a candidate for vaginal birth by standard criteria, a trial of labor may be considered.[1] Using the same protocol for singletons in breech presentation, Blickstein et al[119] found no significant difference in perinatal outcome in 24 breech-vertex twins delivered vaginally compared with 35 breech-vertex twins delivered abdominally. Despite these observations, no prospective studies have been done to determine the optimal route of delivery when the first twin is in the breech position. As a result, it is generally agreed that cesarean section is indicated in cases in which the first twin is not in the vertex position.

Undiagnosed Twins

Despite the widespread use of ultrasound examination, a twin pregnancy may not be recognized until after the delivery of the first infant. It is estimated that 10 to 15 percent of all twin pregnancies will be unsuspected at the time of maternal presentation for labor and delivery, and that 5 to 10 percent will arrive in the delivery room before the diagnosis is made.[13,42] This is one of the most challenging situations faced by obstetricians. Without information about how the second fetus has tolerated labor, a prompt assessment of the fetus is necessary. The fetal heart rate and presentation must be determined immediately. Anesthesiology and neonatology personnel need to be notified and their presence requested in the delivery room. A logical approach to the delivery of the second twin must be formulated and executed in an efficient manner to make the best of a less-than-ideal situation.

Multifetal Gestations

The incidence of multifetal gestations has increased significantly with the widespread use of assisted-reproduction technology. As with twin gestation, prematurity is the most important determinant of perinatal morbidity and mortality in these high-risk pregnancies.[120] Approximately 75 percent of triplets are born before term, with an average gestational age of 33 to 35 weeks.[120]

The optimal route of delivery in multifetal pregnancies is uncertain. In a review of 16 triplet and higher-order deliveries, Thiery and colleagues[121] reported a vaginal delivery rate of 81 percent, and suggested that in selected cases, a trial of labor may be indicated. In a series of 35 multifetal pregnancies, Loucopoulos and Jewelewicz[122] found that the route of delivery did not affect the perinatal outcome. However, no large series exists to establish the safety of vaginal delivery. In addition, electronic monitoring of multiple fetuses during labor can be difficult. Therefore, although vaginal delivery of triplets and quadruplets has been reported, liberal use of cesarean section is recommended for a gestation of three or more fetuses.[123]

SUMMARY

Prematurity continues to be the primary cause of perinatal mortality in multiple gestations, irrespective of the route of delivery. As a result, early diagnosis and prevention of preterm labor are important objectives in the management of these high-risk pregnancies. Although obstetricians may have little impact on the factors that influence perinatal outcome, the provision of close fetal surveillance in the intrapartum period, with atraumatic labor and delivery, will give these infants the best possible start. The challenge of improving maternal and fetal outcomes in multiple pregnancies remains.

REFERENCES

1. Hays PM, Smeltzer JS: Multiple gestation. Clin Obstet Gynecol 29:264, 1986
2. Hollenbach KA, Hickok DE: Epidemiology and diagnosis of twin gestation. Clin Obstet Gynecol 33:3, 1990
3. MacGillivray I: Epidemiology of twin pregnancy. Semin Perinatol 10:4, 1986
4. Lantz ME, Johnson TRB: Multiple pregnancy. Curr Opin Obstet Gynecol 5:657, 1993
5. Ron-El R: Complications of ovulation induction. Baillieres Clin Obstet Gynecol 7:435, 1993
6. Luke B: The changing pattern of multiple births in the United States: maternal and infant characteristics, 1973 and 1990. Obstet Gynecol 84:101, 1994
7. Cetrulo CL, Ingardia CJ, Sbarra AJ: Management of multiple gestation. Clin Obstet Gynecol 23:533, 1980
8. Hawrylyshyn PA, Barkin M, Bernstein A, Papsin FR: Twin pregnancies—a continuing perinatal challenge. Obstet Gynecol 59:463, 1982
9. Zuidema L: The management of labor. Clin Perinatol 15:87, 1988
10. De Muylder X, Moutquin JM, Desgranges MF et al: Obstetrical profile of twin pregnancies: a retrospective review of 11 years (1969–1979) at Hospital Notre-Dame, Montreal, Canada. Acta Genet Med Gemellol 31:149, 1982
11. Cetrulo CL: The controversy of mode of delivery in twins: the intrapartum management of twin gestation. Part I. Semin Perinatol 10:39, 1986
12. American College of Obstetricians and Gynecologists: Preterm labor. (ACOG) Technical Bulletin No. 133. American College of Obstetricians and Gynecologists, Washington, DC, October 1989
13. Chervenak FA, Youcha S, Johnson RE et al: Twin

gestation. Antenatal diagnosis and perinatal outcome in 385 consecutive pregnancies. J Reprod Med 29:727, 1984

14. Gandhi J, Gugliucci CL: Intrapartum management of twin gestation: what is best for the second and the small? Bull NY Acad Med 59:358, 1983

15. Gocke SE, Nageotte MP, Garite T et al: Management of the nonvertex second twin: primary cesarean section, external version, or primary breech extraction. Am J Obstet Gynecol 161:111, 1989

16. Davison L, Easterling TR, Jackson JC, Benedetti TJ: Breech extraction of low birth weight second twins: can cesarean section be justified? Am J Obstet Gynecol 166:497, 1992

17. Farooqui MO, Grossman JH, Shannon RA: A review of twin pregnancy and perinatal mortality. Obstet Gynecol Surv 28:144, 1973

18. Keith L, Ellis R, Berger G, Depp R: The Northwestern University multihospital twin study: I. A description of 588 twin pregnancies and associated pregnancy loss, 1971–1975. Am J Obstet Gynecol 138:781, 1980

19. Berger GS, Keith LG, Ellis R, Depp R: The Northwestern University multihospital twin study: III. Obstetric characteristics and outcome. Prog Clin Biol Res 69A:207, 1981

20. Johnson JM, Harman CR, Evan JA et al: Maternal serum alpha-fetoprotein in twin pregnancy. Am J Obstet Gynecol 162:1020, 1990

21. Chervenak FA, Johnson RE, Youcha S et al: Intrapartum management of twin gestation. Obstet Gynecol 65:119, 1985

22. Socol ML, Tamura RK, Sabbagha RE: Multiple gestation. Clin Obstet Gynecol 27:352, 1984

23. D'Alton ME, Mercer BM: Antepartum management of twin gestation: ultrasound. Clin Obstet Gynecol 33:42, 1990

24. Grennert L, Persson PH, Gennser G: Benefits of ultrasonic screening of a pregnancy population. Acta Obstet Gynecol Scand 78:5, 1978

25. Burke MS: Single fetal demise in twin gestation. Clin Obstet Gynecol 33:69, 1990

26. Hertzberg BS, Kurtz AB, Choi HY et al: Significance of membrane thickness in the sonographic evaluation of twin gestations. AJR 148:151, 1987

27. Samuels P: Ultrasound in the management of the twin gestation. Clinc Obstet Gynecol 31:110, 1988

28. D'Alton ME, Dudley DK: The ultrasonographic prediction of chorionicity in twin gestation. Am J Obstet Gynecol 160:557, 1989

29. Finberg HJ: The "twin peak" sign: reliable evidence of dichorionic twinning. J Ultrasound Med 11:571, 1992

30. Kurtz AB, Wapner RJ, Mata J et al: Twin pregnancies: accuracy of first-trimester abdominal US in predicting chorionicity and amnionicity. Radiology 185:759, 1992

31. Machin GA: Definitive methods of zygosity determination in twins: relevance to problems in the biology of twinning. Acta Genet Med Gemellol 39:459, 1990

32. Mantoni M, Pedersen JF: Monoamniotic twins diagnosed by ultrasound in the first trimester. Acta Obstet Gynecol Scand 59:551, 1980

33. Benirschke K, Kim CK: Multiple pregnancy. Part I. N Engl J Med 288:1276, 1973

34. Laros RK, Dattel BJ: Management of twin pregnancy: the vaginal route is still safe. Am J Obstet Gynecol 158:1330, 1988

35. Nyberg DA, Filly RA, Golbus MS, Stephens JD: Entangled umbilical cords: a sign of monoamniotic twins. J Ultrasound Med 3:29, 1984

36. Lee CY: Management of monoamniotic twins diagnosed antenatally by ultrasound. Am J Gynecol Health 6:25, 1992

37. Rodis JF, Vintzileos AM, Campbell WA et al: Antenatal diagnosis and management of monoamniotic twins. Am J Obstet Gynecol 157:1255, 1987

38. Adams DM, Chervenak FA: Intrapartum management of twin gestation. Clin Obstet Gynecol 33:52, 1990

39. Carr SR, Aronson MP, Coustan DR: Survival rates of monoamniotic twins do not decrease after 30 weeks gestation. Am J Obstet Gynecol 163:719, 1990

40. Tessen JA, Zlatnik FJ: Monoamniotic twins: a retrospective controlled study. Obstet Gynecol 77:832, 1991

41. Colburn DW, Pasquale SA: Monoamniotic twin pregnancy. J Reprod Med 27:165, 1982

42. Trofatter KF: Management of delivery. Clin Perinatol 15:93, 1988

43. McLeod FN, McCoy DR: Monoamniotic twins with an unusual cord complication. Br J Obstet Gynecol 88:774, 1981

44. Hanson JW: Incidence of conjoined twinning. Lancet 2:1257, 1975

45. Schinzel A, Smith D, Miller J: Monozygotic twinning and structural defects. J Pediatr 95:921, 1979

46. Rodis JF, Egan JFX, Craffey A et al: Calculated risk of chromosomal abnormalities in twin gestations. Obstet Gynecol 76:1037, 1990

47. Elias S, Gerbie AB, Simpson JL et al: Genetic amniocentesis in twin gestations. Am J Obstet Gynecol 138:169, 1980

48. Tabsh KM, Crandall B, Lebherz TB, Howard J: Genetic amniocentesis in twin pregnancy. Obstet Gynecol 65:843, 1985

49. Anderson RL, Goldberg JD, Golbus MS: Prenatal diagnosis in multiple gestation: 20 years experience with amniocentesis. Prenat Diagn 11:263, 1991

50. Coleman BG, Grumbach K, Arger PH et al: Twin gestations: monitoring of complications and anomalies with US. Radiology 165:449, 1987

51. Lynch L: Twins in older women: amniocentesis detects Down syndrome. Contemp Obstet Gynecol 37:33, 1992

52. Blickstein I, Lancet M: The growth discordant twin. Obstet Gynecol Surv 443:509, 1988

53. Blickstein I: The definition, diagnosis, and management of growth-discordant twins: an international census survey. Acta Genet Med Gemellol 40:345, 1991

54. O'Brien WF, Knuppel RA, Scerbo JC, Rattan PK: Birth weight in twins: an analysis of discordancy and growth retardation. Obstet Gynecol 67:483, 1986

55. Polin JI, Frangipane WL: Current concepts in management of obstetric problems for pediatricians. II. Modern concepts in the management of multiple gestation. Pediat Clin North Am 33:649, 1986

56. Wenstrom KD, Gall SA: Incidence, morbidity and mortality, and diagnosis of twin gestations. Clin Perinatol 15:1, 1988

57. Benirschke K: The placenta in twin gestation. Clin Obstet Gynecol 33:18, 1990

58. Robertson EG, Neer KJ: Placental injection studies in twin gestations. Am J Obstet Gynecol 147:170, 1983

59. Patten RM, Mack LA, Harvey D et al: Disparity of amniotic fluid volume and fetal size: problem of the stuck twin—US studies. Radiology 172:153, 1989

60. Wax J, Callan N, Perlman E et al: The stuck twin phenomenon: experience with serial therapeutic amniocenteses. J Matern Fet Med 1:239, 1992

61. Reisner DP, Mahony BS, Petty CN et al: Stuck twin syndrome: outcome in thirty-seven consecutive cases. Am J Obstet Gynecol 169:991, 1993

62. Jones JM, Sbarra AJ, Dilillo L et al: Indomethacin in severe twin-to-twin transfusion syndrome. Am J Perinatol 10:24, 1993

63. DeLia JE, Rogers JG, Dixon JA: Treatment of placental vasculature with a neodymium-yttrium-aluminum-garnet laser via fetoscopy. Am J Obstet Gynecol 151:1126, 1985

64. Wittman BK, Farquharson DF, Thomas WDS et al: The role of feticide in the management of severe twin transfusion syndrome. Am J Obstet Gynecol 155:1023, 1986

65. Varma TR: Ultrasound evidence of early pregnancy failure in patients with multiple conceptions. Br J Obstet Gynecol 86:290, 1979

66. Landy HJ, Weiner S, Corson SL et al: The "vanishing twin": ultrasonographic assessment of fetal disappearance in the first trimester. Am J Obstet Gynecol 155:14, 1986

67. Fusi L, Gordon H: Twin pregnancy complicated by single intrauterine death. Problems and outcome with conservative management. Br J Obstet Gynecol 97:511, 1990

68. Eglowstein M, D'Alton ME: Intrauterine demise in multiple gestation: theory and management. J Matern Fet Med 2:272, 1993

69. Gonen R, Heyman E, Asztalos E, Milligan JE: The outcome of triplet gestations complicated by fetal death. Obstet Gynecol 75:175, 1990

70. Borlum KG: Third-trimester fetal death in triplet pregnancies. Obstet Gynecol 77:6, 1991

71. Enbom JA: Twin pregnancy with intrauterine death of one twin. Am J Obstet Gynecol 152:424, 1985

72. Rydhstrom H, Ingemarsson I: Prognosis and long-term follow-up of a twin after antenatal death of the co-twin. J Reprod Med 38:142, 1993

73. D'Alton ME, Newton ER, Cetrulo CL: Intrauterine fetal demise in multiple gestation. Acta Genet Med Gemellol 33:43, 1984

74. Carlson NJ, Towers CV: Multiple gestation complicated by the death of one fetus. Obstet Gynecol 73:685, 1989

75. Anderson RL, Golbus MS, Curry CJR et al: Central nervous system damage and other anomalies in surviving fetus following second trimester antenatal death of co-twin. Prenat Diagn 10:513, 1990

76. Landy HJ, Weingold AB: Management of a multiple gestation complicated by an antepartum fetal demise. Obstet Gynecol Surv 44:171, 1989

77. Thompson SA, Lyons TL, Makowski EL: Outcomes of twin gestations at the University of Colorado Health Sciences Center, 1973–1983. J Reprod Med 32:328, 1987

78. National Institutes of Health Consensus Conference: Effect of Corticosteroids for Fetal Maturation on Perinatal Outcomes, JAMA 273:413, 1995

79. Saunders MC, Dick JS, Brown IM et al: The effects of hospital admission for bed rest on the duration of twin pregnancy: a randomised trial. Lancet 2:793, 1985

80. Dor J, Shalev J, Mashiach S et al: Elective cervical suture of twin pregnancies diagnosed ultrasonically in the first trimester following induced ovulation. Gynecol Obstet Invest 13:55, 1982

81. Sinha DP, Nandakumar VC, Brough AK, Beebeejaun MS: Relative cervical incompetence in twin pregnancy. Assessment and efficacy of cervical suture. Acta Genet Med Gemellol 28:327, 1979

82. Marivate M, Norman RJ: Twins. Clin Obstet Gynecol 9:723, 1982

83. Knuppel RA, Rattan PK, Scerbo JC, O'Brien WF: Intrauterine fetal death in twins after 32 weeks of gestation. Obstet Gynecol 65:172, 1985

84. American College of Obstetricians and Gynecologists: Multiple gestation. American College of Obstetricians and Gynecologists, Washington, DC, ACOG Technical Bulletin No. 131. August 1989

85. Spellacy WN, Cruz AC, Buhi WC, Birk SA: Amniotic fluid L/S ratio in twin gestation. Obstet Gynecol 50:68, 1977

86. Leveno KJ, Quirk JG, Whalley PJ et al: Fetal lung maturation in twin gestation. Am J Obstet Gynecol 148:405, 1984

87. Sureau C, Leroy F: Multiple pregnancy: current obstetric and pediatric aspects. Eur J Obstet Gynec Reprod Biol 15:261, 1983

88. Depp R, Keith LG, Sciarra JJ: The Northwestern University twin study. VII. The mode of delivery in twin pregnancy, North American considerations. Acta Genet Med Gemellol 37:11, 1988

89. Redick LF: Anesthesia for twin delivery. Clin Perinatol 15:107, 1988

90. Rayburn W, Lavin J, Miodovnik M, Varner M: Multiple gestation: time interval between delivery of the first and second twins. Obstet Gynecol 63:502, 1984

91. Friedman EA, Sachtleben MR: The effect of uterine overdistention on labor. Obstet Gynecol 23:401, 1964

92. Barrett JM, Staggs SM, Van Hooydonk JE et al: The effect of type of delivery upon neonatal outcome in premature twins. Am J Obstet Gynecol 143:360, 1982

93. Bell D, Johansson D, McLean FH, Usher RH: Birth asphyxia, trauma, and mortality in twins: has cesarean improved outcome? Am J Obstet Gynecol 154:235, 1986

94. Rydhstrom H, Ingemarsson I, Ohrlander S: Lack of correlation between a high cesarean section rate and improved prognosis for low birth weight twins (<2500 g). Br J Obstet Gynecol 97:229, 1990

95. Rydhstrom H: Prognosis for twins with birth weight <1500 gm: the impact of cesarean section in relation to fetal presentation. Am J Obstet Gynecol 163:528, 1990

96. Rydhstrom H, Ingemarsson I: A case-control study of the effects of birth by cesarean section on intrapartum and neonatal mortality among twins weighing 1500–2499 g. Br J Obstet Gynecol 98:249, 1991

97. Taylor ES: Editorial. Obstet Gynecol Surv 31:535, 1976

98. Duenhoelter JH, Wells E, Reisch JS et al: A paired controlled study of vaginal and abdominal delivery of the low birth weight breech fetus. Obstet Gynecol 54:310, 1979

99. Mazor M, Leiberman JR, Dreval D et al: Management and outcome of vertex-breech and vertex-vertex presentation in twin gestation: a comparative study. Eur J Obstet Gynecol Reprod Biol 22:69, 1986

100. Worthington D, Davis LE, Grausz JP, Sobocinski K: Factors influencing survival and morbidity with very low birth weight delivery. Obstet Gynecol 62:550, 1983

101. Olshan AF, Shy KK, Luthy DA et al: Cesarean birth and neonatal morbidity in very low birth weight infants. Obstet Gynecol 64:267, 1984

102. Acker D, Lieberman M, Holbrook H et al: Delivery of the second twin. Obstet Gynecol 59:710, 1982

103. Rabinovici J, Barkai G, Reichman B et al: Randomized management of the second nonvertex twin: vaginal delivery or cesarean section? Am J Obstet Gynecol 156:52, 1987

104. Adam C, Allen AC, Basket TF: Twin delivery: influence of the presentation and method of delivery on the second twin. Am J Obstet Gynecol 165:23, 1991

105. Blickstein I, Schwartz-Shoham Z, Lancet M, Borenstein R: Vaginal delivery of the second twin in breech presentation. Obstet Gynecol 69:774, 1987

106. Greig PC, Veille JC, Morgan T, Henderson L: The effect of presentation and mode of delivery on neonatal outcome in the second twin. Am J Obstet Gynecol 167:901, 1992

107. McCarthy BJ, Sachs BP, Layde PM et al: The epidemiology of neonatal death in twins. Am J Obstet Gynecol 141:252, 1981

108. Chervenak FA, Johnson RE, Berkowitz RL, Hobbins JC: Intrapartum external version of the second twin. Obstet Gynecol 62:160, 1983

109. Chervenak FA, Johnson RE, Berkowitz RL et al: Is routine cesarean section necessary for vertex-breech and vertex-transverse gestations? Am J Obstet Gynecol 148:1, 1984

110. Tchabo JG, Tomai T: Selected intrapartum external cephalic version of the second twin. Obstet Gynecol 79:421, 1992

111. Rabinovici J, Barkai G, Mashiach S: Intrapartum management of second twin: internal podalic version

with unruptured membranes. Am J Obstet Gynecol 155:914, 1986

112. Taylor ES: Editorial. Obstet Gynecol Surv 42:565, 1987

113. Evrard JR, Gold EM: Cesarean section for delivery of the second twin. Obstet Gynecol 57:581, 1981

114. Rattan PK, Knuppel RA, O'Brien WF, Scerbo JC: Cesarean delivery of the second twin after vaginal delivery of the first twin. Am J Obstet Gynecol 154:936, 1986

115. Olofsson P, Rydhstrom H: Twin delivery: how should the second twin be delivered? Am J Obstet Gynecol 153:479, 1985

116. Blickstein I, Zalel Y, Weissman A: Cesarean delivery of the second twin after the vaginal birth of the first twin: misfortune or mismanagement? Acta Genet Med Gemellol 40:389, 1991

117. Cohen M, Konl SJ, Rosental AH: Fetal interlocking complicating twin gestation. Am J Obstet Gynecol 91:407, 1965

118. Oettinger M, Ophir E, Markovitz J et al: Is cesarean section necessary for delivery of a breech first twin? Gynecol Obstet Invest 35:38, 1993

119. Blickstein I, Weissman A, Ben-Hur H et al: Vaginal delivery of breech-vertex twins. J Reprod Med 38:879, 1993

120. Alvarez M, Berkowitz R: Multifetal gestation. Clin Obstet Gynecol 33:79, 1990

121. Thiery M, Kermans G, Derom R: Triplet and higher-order births: what is the optimal delivery route? Acta Genet Med Gemellol 37:89, 1988

122. Loucopoulos A, Jewelewicz R: Management of multifetal pregnancies: sixteen years' experience at the Sloane Hospital for Women. Am J Obstet Gynecol 143:902, 1982

123. Feingold M, Cetrulo C, Peters M et al: Mode of delivery in multiple birth of higher-order. Acta Genet Med Gemellol 37:105, 1988

124. Kauppila A, Jouppila P, Koivisto M et al: Twin pregnancy: a clinical study of 335 cases. Acta Obstet Gynecol Scand 44:5, 1975

125. Hall MH, Campbell DM, Davidson RJ: Anemia in twin pregnancy. Acta Genet Med Gemellol 28:279, 1979

126. Jeffrey RL, Bowes WA, DeLaney JJ: Role of bed rest in twin gestation. Obstet Gynecol 43:822, 1974

127. Kelsick F, Minkoff H: Management of the breech second twin. Am J Obstet Gynecol 144:783, 1982

Malpresentation*

Jerome N. Kopelman, Arthur S. Maslow, Glenn R. Markenson, and Katherine S. Foley

Malpresentation is a broad term used to describe all fetal presentations other than vertex. Included are both nonvertex cephalic (face, brow) and noncephalic (breech, transverse/oblique) lies.

The discovery of an abnormally presenting fetus is anxiety provoking, and the management of these cases remains highly controversial. It is our goal in this chapter to present the obstetric practitioner with an understanding of the incidence, diagnosis, etiology, mechanism of labor, and means of management in each type of malpresentation. This knowledge will allow the obstetrician to select the means of delivery most likely to result in optimal maternal and neonatal outcomes.

BREECH PRESENTATIONS

Incidence and Etiology

As gestational age increases, the incidence of breech presentation decreases. More than 25 percent of pregnancies of less than 28 weeks' duration involve fetuses in the breech position, declining to approximately 8 percent of pregnancies at 33 weeks and 3 to 4 percent of term labors.[1,2] Factors other than gestational age that may predispose to breech presentation include anything that distorts normal intrauterine contour (i.e., large myomas), multiple fe-

tuses, fetal malformations (both anatomic and genetic), fundal placentations, and abnormalities of amniotic fluid volume.[3,4] The fetus in the breech presentation occupies a more-or-less longitudinal axis, with the head in the uterine fundus. The three types of breech presentation are the frank, complete, and incomplete, representing 48 to 73 percent, 4.6 to 11.5 percent, and 12 to 38 percent of the overall proportion of breech presentations,[5,7] respectively. The fetus in the frank breech position is flexed at the hips and extended at both knees, while the fetus in the complete breech position is flexed at both the hips and knees, and that in the incomplete (footling) position has one or both hips extended (Fig. 9-1). The risk of cord prolapse increases dramatically for the respective presentations, being cited as 0.5 percent for the frank breech presentation and increasing to approximately 5 percent for the complete breech presentation and dramatically to 15 to 18 percent for the incomplete breech presentation.[8]

Thus, conditions related to gestational age, fetal and uterine muscular tonus, intrauterine configuration, and fetal mobility affect the frequency and perhaps the type of breech presentation. These same conditions, and other confounding variables such as practitioner bias, experience, and literature evaluation, may affect the mechanism of labor and management of the breech presentation. Diagnosis of the breech position can be established clinically by abdominal palpation, vaginal examination, and auscultation. Confirmation can be achieved using radiography or ultrasonography.

---

* The opinions expressed in this chapter are solely those of the authors and do not reflect those of the Department of the Army or the Department of Defense.

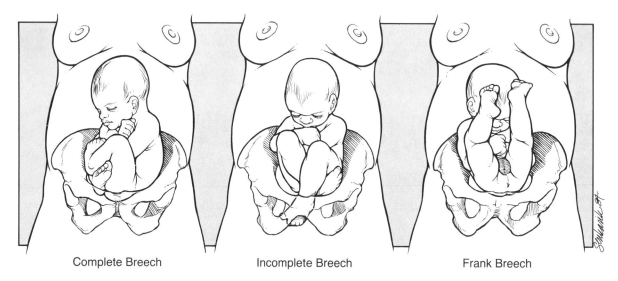

Complete Breech   Incomplete Breech   Frank Breech

Fig. 9-1. Three possible breech presentations. The complete breech demonstrates flexion of the hips and flexion of the knees. The incomplete breech demonstrates intermediate deflexion of one hip and knee. The frank breech shows flexion of the hips and extension of both knees. (From Seeds,[89] with permission.)

Mechanism of Labor

The fetus in the frank breech position typically enters the pelvis with the bitrochanteric diameter in one of the maternal pelvic diagonal diameters. Engagement, defined as passage of the fetal bitrochanteric diameter through the maternal pelvic inlet, can be appreciated clinically by palpation of the presenting part at the −1 or −2 station relative to the maternal ischial spines. With further descent, resistance of the pelvic floor is met and internal rotation of the bitrochanteric diameter to the anteroposterior (AP) axis of the maternal pelvis usually occurs. Continued descent results in bulging of the perineum, and crowning occurs when the bitrochanteric diameter passes under the pubic rami. As the breech emerges, external rotation begins, usually in a sacrum-anterior direction, drawing the shoulders into one of the diagonal diameters of the pelvis. Descent and internal rotation of the shoulders bring the bisacromial diameter of the infant into the AP axis. Further descent brings the flexed head quickly into one of the diagonal diameters of the maternal inlet, and subsequent internal rotation occurs in such as way as to bring the head into an occipito-anterior position.

Atypical labor mechanisms occur in which the breech may become engaged in the transverse as op-posed to a diagonal maternal pelvic diameter. Infrequently, external rotation of the bitrochanteric diameter proceeds toward the sacrum-posterior position and predisposes to extensions of the fetal head as it descends into the pelvis, particularly if excessive traction is applied.

Management

In 1959, Wright[9] proposed that all breech presentations be delivered by cesarean section. Indeed, this practice is so ubiquitous that the cesarean delivery rate in many hospitals is greater than 90 percent for breech presentations at all gestational ages, and virtually 100 percent for fetuses weighing less than 2,000 g.[10]

What confluence of circumstances occurred that encouraged the virtually complete adoption of cesarean delivery, which carries a 1:5000 maternal mortality rate[11] and a marked increase in maternal morbidity,[8,12] for breech presentations? The rationale for cesarean delivery is based on the higher corrected perinatal mortality rate, of 7 to 16 percent, for all breech presentations than for the vertex fetus.[13,14] By extension, it is argued that the mechanics of vaginal delivery are responsible for the disproportionately high perinatal mortality in cases of breech presentation. Is this assumption correct?

In general, the national and international literature divide vaginal delivery in breech presentations between issues related to the breech presentation of term fetuses 1,500 g or more and those of the low-birth-weight breech-presenting fetus (<1,500 g). A recent review of the English-language literature from 1966 to 1992 evaluated 82 articles about singleton breech presentation at term.[15] Thirty-nine studies that made comparisons between actual method of delivery without differentiating between elective cesarean sections and those performed for failed trial of labor were excluded. Likewise, six other reports were excluded for comparing two different protocols of management of labor and delivery rather than planned vaginal delivery versus elective cesarean section. An additional 13 reports were excluded for a variety of other reasons. Among the 24 remaining reports, only two randomized trials were found.[8,12] In the trial that included frank breech presentations only,[8] 93 patients were planned for cesarean section and 115 for vaginal delivery, casting doubt on the randomization process, which was not reported. Notwithstanding this potential deficiency, no difference was found between the vaginal and cesarean routes of delivery.

In the United States, the appropriateness of a procedure is defined by the caliber of the reported prospective randomized controlled studies to which it is subjected. For the term breech presentation, we are left with Gimovsky's prospective randomized trial,[12] which demonstrated no difference in neonatal mortality or morbidity in the vaginal versus cesarean group among nonfrank breech presentations. In evaluating the reports of nonrandomized studies, many others have confirmed the lack of a difference in perinatal mortality or morbidity for fetuses weighing more than 2,500 g delivered vaginally or by cesarean section.[8,16–22] If prospective randomized controlled studies of a particular procedure are not readily available, the next most reliable information can be derived from prospective observational studies. Brown's recent report is the most thorough analysis to date.[23] Seven hundred seventy-two singleton and 71 first-twin breech cases were collected prospectively and without exclusions. The data were corrected for stillborns, anomalies, gestational age, fetal weight, and, importantly, for cesarean section performed for fetal distress versus

planned cesarean delivery. Other than greater average weights among the infants in the cesarean group, no significant differences were observed in neonatal outcome. These results confirm the poor perinatal outcome for breech deliveries, but show that this is an association and not the cause-and-effect relationship implied in other reports.[24,25] This finding is in agreement with another observational study,[17] which included a 4-year follow-up of neonates and found no difference in the relative risk for long-term sequelae among those delivered vaginally or by cesarean section. Likewise, observational studies of neurologic development following different routes of delivery have also failed to find differences in outcome.[20,26]

Thus, with regard to the term breech delivery, there appears to be a contradiction between the results reported in most of the pertinent literature and the practice of most clinicians.

The literature and clinical conduct in managing the low-birth-weight (LBW) fetus (<1,500 g) presenting in the breech position is also curious. That delivery of such fetuses by cesarean section is entrenched in the United States[2] is clear. The classic teaching that breech presentation is dangerous for the fetus, and that the more preterm or smaller the fetus the worse the prognosis for vaginal delivery, appears to be unproved. No prospective randomized controlled trials of these issues are available for review, and the obstetric community is therefore forced to rely on nonexperimental data for decision analysis. In nonexperimental studies of therapeutic intervention, selection bias can be a major problem,[27] as are other confounding variables.

The literature attempting to account for a variety of confounding variables and which supports the classical teaching with regard to the breech-presenting LBW fetus essentially begins with a small comparative study by Tejani and colleagues.[28] This group evaluated the effect of vaginal delivery on the subsequent development (within 24 hours of birth) of periventricular/intraventricular hemorrhage (PV/IVH) in 92 consecutive cases of breech-presenting fetuses with birth weights of less than 2,000 g. Among those studied, 67 were delivered by cesarean section and 25 were delivered vaginally. Nine infants in each of the two groups experienced early PV/IVH. Because the groups with both types of hemorrhage were so small, the grading system for PV/IVH was not reported, and no analysis of cord-blood gases was done after delivery. Moreover, the cause of death among nonsurvivors was not provided. Therefore, it is difficult to determine whether the PV/IVH was in any way related to the mechanics of the breech delivery, and whether it truly resulted in long-term morbidity or mortality among the groups defined by mode of delivery. A much larger comparative multicenter study,[29] with appropriate and adequate corrections for maternal disease, gestational age, fetal distress, malpresentation, and grade of PV/IVH, concluded that cesarean delivery is not associated with a lower risk of either mortality or PV/IVH for the LBW breech-presenting infant. This was confirmed in a later study by Shaver and associates.[30] Contradicting results with regard to short- and long-term morbidity have been reported in the form of retrospective observational and population-based studies and those of small or large matched series.[25,31–33]

The largest and most recent prospective observational study by Cibil's group[34] confirms that it is not the mechanics of the vaginal breech delivery that are responsible for the poor perinatal outcomes of breech-presenting LBW infants. Rather, the poor outcomes are related to antenatal deaths, extreme LBW, congenital malformations, and prematurity. After appropriate adjustments, the odds of neonatal death or other poor-outcome measures for vaginal delivery compared with cesarean delivery were not significantly different. The study did, however, reveal that the subgroup of fetuses in the footling position had a higher neonatal mortality when delivered vaginally.

Our summary of the literature shows that the more recent and appropriately designed studies (short of prospective randomized controlled trials) confirm the exceedingly poor perinatal outcomes for breech-presenting LBW infants. It does not, however, support the notion that these poor outcomes are due to vaginal breech delivery. Indeed, it appears not to matter what route of delivery is chosen, with the single exception of the footling breech presentation. Why, then, are so many cesarean sections being performed for this group of patients?

Social Forces

As succinctly put by Paul,[35] the large number of cesarean sections in current practice is related partially to the unrealistic expectations ingrained in the public mind and reinforced constantly by the medicolegal climate that exists in the United States. Although most often unjustified, the continual threat of medicolegal action and the unjust assumption that compensation is due whenever an outcome is less than perfect provoke and catalyze the increased use of cesarean birth. Because the notion that breech vaginal delivery is more "dangerous" for the infant is now ingrained in the medical profession, there is at least one entire generation of obstetrician/gynecologists who are either uncomfortable or completely inexperienced in vaginal breech birth. Moreover, since the potential decrease in the percentage of cesarean sections that might be associated with vaginal delivery of breech-presenting fetuses is probably in the range of 1 to 2 percent, the professional societies have not strongly endorsed any significant attempt to rekindle this area of operative obstetrics. Equally devastating to the general acceptance of vaginal breech delivery may be the indirect incentives of cesarean section for both mothers and physicians. Not only does cesarean delivery take less time to accomplish, but its financial benefits to hospitals and professional personnel clearly reward this approach.

All these considerations have had an effect at the level of professional investigation of the subject. It would appear that prospective randomized studies of vaginal versus cesarean delivery are all but impossible to perform at this time. A prospective randomized controlled trial[36] was discontinued after 5 months when it was discovered that over 40 percent of eligible patients were withdrawn from the trial before randomization. After review, the conclusion was that a critical shift in obstetric practice toward cesarean delivery for LBW infants had already occurred, making it impossible to conduct a randomized trial. Interestingly, obtaining patient consent for participation in the trial, which had been the main predicted problem, was not difficult. In 1990,[37] as assessment was undertaken of the feasibility of performing a randomized control trial of vaginal versus cesarean delivery for preterm infants in England. In 25 of 36 hospitals there was universal support, whereas in the remaining 11, universal support was not obtained. Reasons given for nonparticipation included the time-consuming nature of the consent process, anxiety over requisite skill levels, medicolegal considerations, and disagreements about the desirability of the trial among consultant members. A second survey confirmed these findings.[38] Closer to home, Amon[39] reported on a questionnaire regarding management of the breech presentation that was answered by 405 maternal-fetal medicine subspecialists. Approximately 75 percent of the respondents allow a trial of labor in selected frank breech presentations at term. Moreover, 43 percent of this latter group, usually augment hypotonic contractions with pitocin. There was little agreement about management of the preterm breech-presenting fetus, but despite this lack of consensus, more than 90 percent of those responding answered that they perform cesarean sections in this clinical setting. Interestingly, only 14 percent of the respondents believed that there is adequate scientific documentation demonstrating a benefit to cesarean section for the term or near-term uncomplicated frank breech presentation in the face of spontaneous labor. More importantly, 63 percent of the respondents agreed that the medicolegal environment compelled them to perform cesarean sections for this group of patients.

Taking these observations together, we conclude that the best available literature demonstrates no benefit to cesarean delivery over vaginal birth for the selected breech-presenting fetus, regardless of gestational age. Social trends, however, have become more significant than the available scientific documentation. Finally, it appears to be the particular circumstances of each pregnancy yielding a breech presentation (anomalies, multiple fetuses, prematurity) that are responsible for the poor perinatal outcomes, and not the mechanics of how the infant is delivered.

External Cephalic Version

External cephalic version (ECV) refers to the conversion of a breech presentation to a cephalic presentation by manual manipulation through the maternal abdomen. This technique has long been used in an attempt to decrease both the perinatal morbidity and mortality associated with breech delivery, and more recently to decrease the maternal morbidity associated with cesarean birth.

In 1973, Ranney[40] described his own experience with 860 patients in whom weekly ECV attempts were performed from 23 weeks on. He reported a breech-presentation rate at term of 0.56 percent, with no increase in perinatal morbidity or mortality. However, this technique of early initiation of serial attempted ECV cannot be recommended. Several cross-sectional and longitudinal population studies[41-43] of ultrasonically determined fetal position show a 65 to 75 percent reduction in breech presentation between 32 and 37 to 40 weeks, as well as an overall 95 percent spontaneous cephalic version rate. Similarly, two randomized studies of serial version attempts beginning at 32 weeks demonstrated either a spontaneous version rate equal to the successful manual version rate, or no change in the incidence of breech presentation at term. Neither study identified a decrease in the rate of cesarean sections for breech deliveries, and one study demonstrated significant perinatal mortality as a result of preterm version attempts.[44,45]

In 1991, Van Dorsten[46] evaluated the combination of ultrasonography electronic fetal monitoring and β-mimetic tocolysis as adjuncts to the safety and efficacy of ECV.[46] This method rapidly set the standard for this technique in the United States, even though the benefit of tocolysis was not confirmed in a subsequent randomized controlled trial.[47]

Studies of ECV at term typically show a success rate of 50 to 75 percent. Various factors such as breech type, fetal-spine position, amniotic, fluid volume, parity, maternal obesity, and descent of the presenting part have all been shown to affect this rate,[48-50] as has the experience of the operator.[40] Spontaneous return to the breech position occurs in up to 3 to 5 percent of cases, and is often associated with uterine anomalies.[51]

Although generally shown to be safe, the technique of ECV is not without risk. Fetal bradycardia[52] rates of 11 percent, fetomaternal hemorrhage rates of 6 to 28 percent,[53,54] and isolated case reports of severe neurologic[55,56] injury have been reported.

Despite the popular and widespread use of ECV,[39] only five randomized controlled studies of the technique have been reported.[44-46,57,58] An earlier meta-analysis of four of these studies,[59] as well as our updated meta-analysis, show no significant decrease in the cesarean section rate when ECV is used in conjunction with selective vaginal breech delivery. This renders the claim that ECV can decrease maternal morbidity and mortality suspect (Table 9-1) One also

Table 9-1. Meta-Analysis of Randomized Controlled Trials of ECV[a]

	Method of Delivery		Total
	Vaginal	Cesarean	
ECV	359	75	434
Control	378	106	484
Total	737	181	918

ECV, external cephalic version.

[a] χ^2, 2.80; P, 0.094.

finds an excessive perinatal mortality of 6.2 per 1,000 associated with ECV, but only among those fetuses who verted before term.

Clearly, if a trial of vaginal delivery is not planned, ECV may be of benefit to the mother. There are no reports of improved neonatal or developmental outcome among infants successfully verted from the breech position. The well-known predisposition of the breech-presenting infant to increased morbidity and mortality, regardless of the method of delivery, is unlikely to be altered by version.

Technique

Prerequisites for ECV of the term breech fetus include an estimated gestational age of 37 weeks or more, ultrasonographic evaluation revealing a normal fetus and normal amniotic fluid volume, intact secundines, a reactive nonstress test (NST), a presenting part not yet descended into the pelvis, capability of immediate cesarean section, and informed consent.

The use of tocolytic agents as an adjunct to ECV is optional, but is recommended in cases with uterine activity or early labor. Ultrasonsongraphy and electronic fetal monitoring should be used throughout the procedure to monitor fetal position and heart rate. Decelerations and bradycardias are common and usually benign, but their occurrence may require abandonment of the procedure.[51,52]

The patient is positioned supine, with a left lateral tilt displacing the uterus, and is advised to avoid straining against a closed glottis during the procedure. A pillow beneath the knees and placement of the hands on the chest may decrease tension on the anterior abdominal wall. The fetal poles are identified and the breech is elevated out of the pelvis and

moved to the side of the maternal abdomen. At the same time the fetal head is directed toward the pelvis in either a forward or backward roll maneuver. ECV is a one-person procedure. If two operators are involved for training purposes, care must be taken not to exert excessive force, both to avoid injury and to avoid pinning the fetus against the maternal spine. The procedure must be abandoned if excess maternal discomfort is encountered. If the version is successful the fetal head is held over the inlet for a few minutes as the uterus reconforms. A postprocedure NST is required, and Rh-negative patients must be given Rh immunoglobulin. If tocolytic agents were not used initially, and attempted ECV is unsuccessful, they may be used subsequently with a 10 percent greater success rate.[47]

Successfully verted fetuses should receive weekly NSTs, and their mothers may be allowed to enter labor spontaneously or may be considered for induction. Unsuccessfully verted fetuses are likewise followed with NSTs and their mothers are instructed to report early in labor for evaluation for vaginal breech delivery.

Evaluation and Selection Criteria for Vaginal Breech Delivery

As discussed above, cesarean section offers no demonstrable benefit over vaginal delivery for selected breech presentations. Recent cesarean section rates of 80 to 90 percent for breech-positioned fetuses are unwarranted.[10,23]

Certain prerequisties, however, must be met before undertaking a vaginal breech delivery. Labor must be undergone in a hospital with capabilities for emergency cesarean section. Pediatric and anesthesia support must be readily available during labor and present at delivery. The capabilities for ultrasonography and electronic fetal monitoring are also essential. The most critical factor, however, is the presence of two obstetricians experienced in the evaluation and management of vaginal breech deliveries.

Selection Criteria

Initial evaluation of the breech-presenting fetus must include a thorough ultrasonographic evaluation to estimate fetal weight, rule out fetal anomalies, determine the type of breech position, and attempt to identify extension of the fetal head.

Fetal Weight

The risks attendant on the vaginal delivery of a macrosomic fetus have long been known,[13,61] and the excess morbidity and mortality in fetuses weighing more than 4,000 g make cesarean section imperative in such cases. The benefit of cesarean section for LBW fetuses, other than the those weighing less than 1,500 g and in the incomplete or footling breech position, has not been established.[29,34,62,63]

Fetal Anomalies

Ultrasound examination should allow identification of large anomalies that may obstruct or hinder labor (i.e., hydrocephaly, sacrococcygeal teratoma, or giant omphalocoele). Knowledge of lethal abnormalities, such as anencephaly, or known severe aneuploidy (trisomy 13 or 18) may prevent unwarranted cesarean delivery.

Type of Breech Position

Both frank and nonfrank breech presentations are appropriate for vaginal delivery. Prospective data from randomized studies indicate that the increased risk of cord prolapse in the case of fetuses weighing more than 2,000 g who are in the nonfrank breech position can be managed safely. Cord prolapse is managed by cesarean section in the first stage of labor. If the second stage of labor, which must be undergone in the delivery room with standby anesthesia and pediatric support, is complicated by cord prolapse, total breech extraction should be performed.[12] The recent review by Ciblis and associates[34] recommends a cesarean birth only for fetuses under 1,500 g and in the footling breech position. Should ultrasound examination not allow identification the type of breech presentation, low-dose computed tomographic (CT) imaging should be performed (Fig. 9-2).

Fetal Head Position

Extreme degrees of deflexion or hyperextension of the fetal head, the so-called stargazing fetus, have been associated with significant fetal trauma, including dislocation of cervical vertebrae and cord transection.[64,65] Mild degrees of deflexion, including the so-called neutral or military position, however, appear to be safe and appropriate for vaginal breech deliveries (Fig. 9-3).

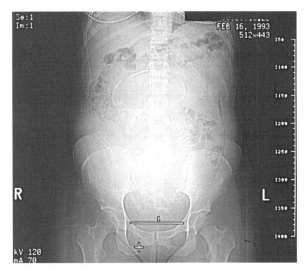

Fig. 9-2. Anteroposterior digital radiograph demonstrating a frank breech-presenting fetus with a well-flexed head. Line 1 measures the transverse (bispinous) diameter of the midpelvis, which along with the transverse diameter of the pelvic inlet, can be measured from this image.

Pelvimetry

Although never tested critically by means of a randomized trial, the use of roentgenologic pelvimetry is supported by two bodies of evidence. Todd and Steer's review[67] in 1963 of the breech experience at Columbia-Presbyterian Hospital identified pelvic-inlet diameters (AP ≥11.0 cm, transverse ≥12 cm) above which safe fetal progress in a normal, well-formed pelvis was likely. A bispinous diameter of 10 cm or more was included by Gimovsky and Petrie[68] in a 1980 retrospective study at the same institution, which demonstrated increased fetal morbidity for patients managed outside a strict pelvimetry-based protocol. These pelvimetry values were used subsequently in the only prospective randomized trial of breech-presentation management at term.[8,12,69,70]

A second set of pelvimetric criteria (AP inlet ≥10.0 cm, transverse inlet ≥11.5 cm, bispinous >9.5 cm, posterior sagittal ≥4.0 cm) was established in 1966 by Beischer.[71] Based on data from Melbourne, Australia, these values have subsequently been applied safely for over 20 years, first by Benson[72] at Tripler Army Medical Center in Honolulu, and later at Madigan Army Medical Center, retrospectively by

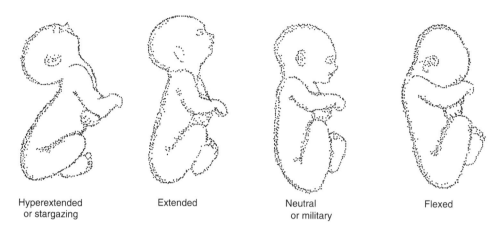

| Hyperextended or stargazing | Extended | Neutral or military | Flexed |

Fig. 9-3. Fetal head positions.

Watson[73] and prospectively by Kopelman[74] and Christian,[78] in over 380 patients with breech-presenting fetuses.

Over the past decade, classic radiographic pelvimetry has become a lost art and has been replaced by CT[74,75] (Figs. 9-2 and 9-4 to 9-6.) The latter technique is easier to perform, read, and interpret, subjects the fetus to far less radiation,[76] and appears to be more accurate and reproducible[77] than standard radiographic pelvimetry. CT pelvimetry has the unique ability of allowing direct axial measurement of the crucial midpelvic bispinous diameter by imaging through the level of the fovea capitalis (Fig. 9-6). Nevertheless, Aronson[78] recently reported that this technique may in fact overestimate the bispinous

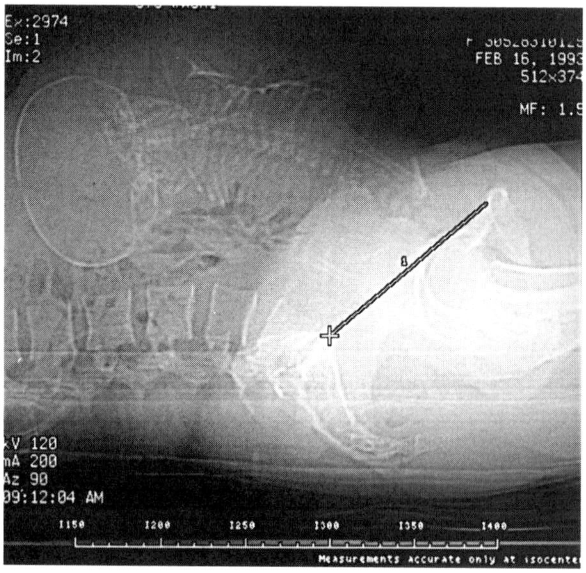

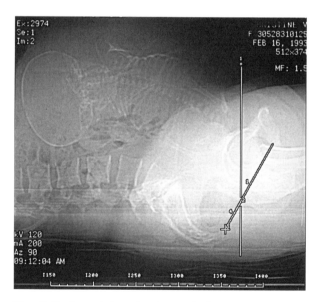

Fig. 9-5. Lateral digital radiograph demonstrating a perpendicular line projected through the level of the ischial spines. This line divides the anteroposterior diameter of the midpelvis into anterior sagittal and posterior sagittal segments, and was used to localize the axial slice shown in Fig. 9-6.

Fig. 9-4. Lateral digital radiograph demonstrating the AP diameter of the pelvic inlet.

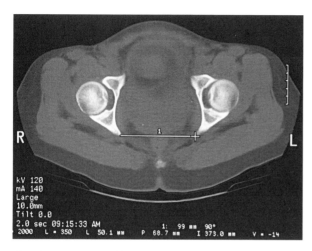

Fig. 9-6. Computed CT image at the level of the ischial spines and fovea capitalis, measuring the transverse (bispinous) diameter of the midpelvis.

diameter by 1.0 cm in 65 percent of cases, and advised identifying the spines directly on the scout films before selecting the level of the axial cut. Magnetic resonance imaging (MRI) has also been advocated as an accurate and radiation-free technique for pelvic mensuration.[79,80]

One must keep in mind that the goal of pelvimetry is not to guarantee a safe delivery, but rather to establish a cutoff below which vaginal delivery should not be attempted, and above which careful, prudent management of labor, in association with other strict selection criteria, appears to be a safe alternative to cesarean section.

One recent retrospective study in Australia compared results among three consultants who either always (n = 125), occasionally (n = 65), or never (n = 72) used radiographic pelvimetry.[81] The use of radiographic pelvimetry was associated with a greater initial cesarean section rate. Among candidates selected for a trial of labor, no difference in cesarean section rate or perinatal outcome was seen. Clearly, this is an area in which large-scale multicenter randomized trails are needed.

Conduct of Labor

Anesthesia

Anesthesia support should be available throughout the first stage of labor. We agree with the recommendation of Gimvosky and Petrie[82] and favor the use of epidural anesthesia, as it keeps the mother relaxed and may lessen maternal efforts at bearing down until such time as the cervix is fully dilated. This in turn may decrease the risk of cord or body prolapse.[82] The patient should be moved to the delivery room just before or at the onset of the second stage of labor, where anesthesia staff must continue to be present, since the need for rapid-sequence general endotracheal anesthesia (GETA) may arise. Uterine relaxation may be required to facilitate delivery. If the patient is under GETA, halothane may be used. In an awake patient with a functional epidural, a β-mimetic drug or nitroglycerine may be used.[83]

Induction and Augmentation

Candidates for induction of labor who present with fetuses in the breech position and otherwise meet selection criteria may be considered for a judicious trial of induction. Keeping in mind the tendency for the labor in the breech presentation to begin at a high station, as well as the increased risk of cord prolapse, amniotomy is best delayed until the presenting part is well seated.

Should labor be found to be desultory, cautious

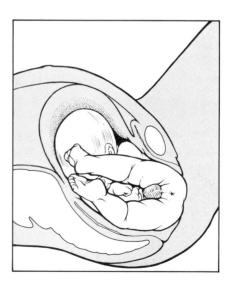

Fig. 9-7. Fetus emerging from the vaginal outlet spontaneously while the uterine contraction maintains flexion of the fetal head. (From Seeds,[89] with permission.)

oxytocin augmentation to optimize uterine activity is reasonable. However, if regular adequate contractions do not result in steady progress of at least 1 cm/hr in active-phase labor, oxytocin must not be used to correct arrest.[68,82]

Conduct of the Second Stage

As previously mentioned, the second stage of labor must be undergone in the delivery room with full anesthesia and pediatric and obstetric teams in place.

There are three general methods of vaginal breech delivery. The rarest, spontaneous breech delivery, refers to delivery of the fetus without any traction or manipulation other than supporting the fetus's body. At the other extreme, and rarely used other than at cesarean section, during cord prolapse in second-stage labor, or at delivery of a second twin, is the total breech extraction, in which the entire body of the fetus is extracted by the obstetrician. The most commonly used technique is the partial breech extraction, in which the fetus delivers spontaneously to the umbilicus, and the remainder of the body is then extracted.

Calm, patience, and gentle manipulation are essential for a successful vaginal breech delivery. The duration of the second stage in nulliparous breech labors is no different from that of nulliparous vertex presentations. In multiparous patients with breech-presenting fetuses the second stage is 50 percent longer than for vertex presentations, and a rapid second stage should therefore not be anticipated.[84]

Spontaneous delivery to the umbilicus assures that pressure from above maintains fetal head flexion and allows maximum sustained cervical dilatation, thereby decreasing the likelihood of entrapment of the aftercoming head. Premature traction may allow deflexion of the fetal head or predispose to nuchal arm entrapment.

As labor progresses, "crowning" occurs as the fetal bitrochanteric axis passes beneath the pubic symphysis (Fig. 9-7). A generous midline, mediolateral, or as recently described, modified median episiotomy[85] should be performed. Rotation to the sacrum-anterior position should occur spontaneously or with minimal assistance.

Once the umbilicus appears over the perineum, the operator may perform the Pinard maneuver, advancing two fingers along the fetal thigh to just behind the knee, and pushing laterally. This maneuver causes external rotation of the thigh, flexion of the knee, and delivery of the lower leg and foot.

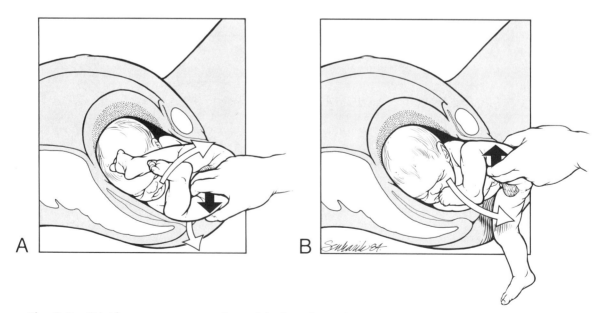

Fig. 9-8. **(A)** After spontaneous expulsion of the breech, **(B)** lateral rotation of the thighs on the hips should result in easy delivery of the legs. (From Seeds,[89] with permission.)

Once both legs are delivered, the body of the infant should be wrapped in a towel and supported with the help of the obstetric assistant (Fig. 9-8.)

Further progress of labor should occur only with maternal expulsive efforts. If traction is required it may be applied in a gentle downward direction. The thumbs of the operator must be placed over the infant's sacrum, and the hand in front of the hip. Care must be taken not to apply pressure above the pelvis, as the fetal kidneys and adrenal glands may be injured.

Once the lower halves of the scapulae pass through the introitus, the accoucheur should pass two fingers over the fetal shoulders to evaluate for nuchal arm entrapment. If none is found, the arms are delivered by following along the humerus and sweeping the arms laterally and across the fetus's chest, one after the other. If necessary the fetal trunk may be gently rotated clockwise for the left arm and counterclockwise for the right arm to aid in delivery of the arms (Figs. 9-9 and 9-10).

Should nuchal arm entrapment be encountered, the fetal trunk must be rotated so that friction from the birth canal will cause the entrapped elbow to move toward the front of the fetal neck and chest, from whence it may be delivered (i.e. clockwise for a nuchally entrapped left arm and counterclockwise for an entrapped right arm). Great care must be taken to splint the freed arm prior to delivery to decrease the risk of clavicular or humeral fractures. After both arms are safely delivered and wrapped in a towel, the fetus's chin and face should appear at the perineum. The assistant's abdominal hand must assure that head flexion is maintained at all times.

Spontaneous delivery of the head may occur, or the extraction may be completed with the Mariceau-Smellie-Veight (MSV) maneuver, or with Piper forceps applied to the aftercoming head. The MSV maneuver is performed by placing two fingers of one hand on the fetal maxillae (not the mandible) and flexing the fetal head while supporting the body of the fetus with the palm and wrist and allowing the infant's legs to straddle the forearm. The operator's other hand is placed along the neck at the infant's shoulders, and gentle downward traction and flexion are exerted in concert with maternal expulsive efforts and gentle suprapubic pressure from the assistant's abdominal hand (Fig. 9-11).

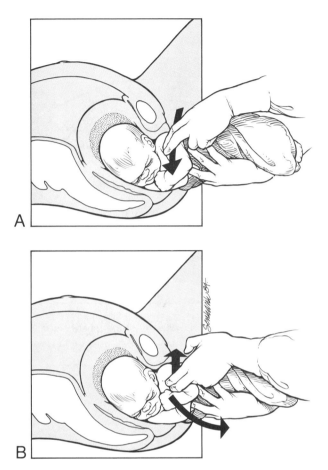

Fig. 9-9. After delivery of the legs, the operator **(A)** medially rotates the infant's left arm across the chest for **(B)** delivery of the left arm. (From Seeds,[89] with permission.)

Alternatively, and in the opinion of many, preferably, or if the MSV maneuver should fail, Piper forceps should be placed.[86] For this procedure the assistant supports and elevates the fetus to the horizontal position, taking care to avoid hyperextension of the fetal neck. Next, the operator, kneeling on one knee, applies the Piper forceps in a direct pelvic application from a 45-degree angle below the horizontal. The handle of the left blade of the forceps is held in the left hand while the right hand is introduced into the vagina beside the fetal head. The blade is then introduced diagonally upward and across the perineum, and is guided by the fingers of the right hand into the pelvis alongside the parietal bone. The right blade is then placed analogously, assuring that

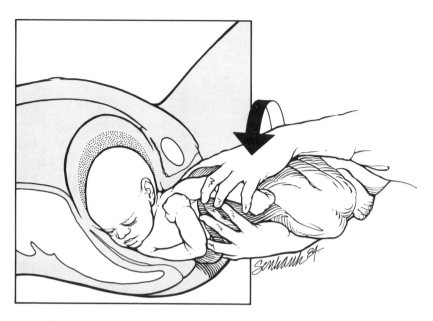

Fig. 9-10. After delivery of the anterior arm, the fetus may be rotated counterclockwise, facilitating delivery of the right arm. (From Seeds,[89] with permission.)

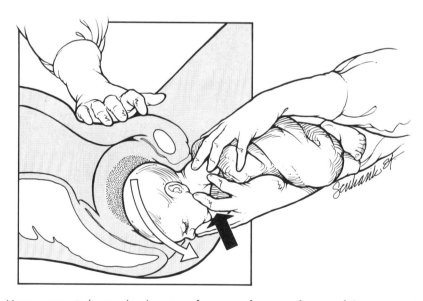

Fig. 9-11. Heavy arrow indicates the direction of pressure from two fingers of the operator's right hand on the fetal maxilla. This maneuver assists in maintaining appropriate flexion of the fetal vertex, as does moderate suprapubic pressure from an assistant, along with optimal maternal expulsive forces. (From Seeds,[89] with permission.)

the handles overlap so as to allow articulation. The operator's right hand is placed on the finger guards and handles, and secures the infant's legs. The operator's left hand is placed on the fetal neck and shoulders. Flexion and delivery are effected by a combination of gentle downward traction and elevation of the forceps handles toward, but never beyond, the horizontal. As the fetus's chin, mouth, and nose pass over the perineum, care must be taken to prevent the head from falling through the flexible blades[86] (Figs. 9-12 and 9-13).

Emergencies

Cord prolapse in the second stage of labor may be managed by cesarean section, or safely and more rapidly by total breech extraction.[12] Adequate anesthesia and uterine relaxation must be immediately available. The operator's hand is introduced into the vagina and both feet of the fetus, or one and then the other foot, are grasped and delivered to the introitus. If the hips are flexed, the breech may be decomposed by the Pinard maneuver, or gentle traction in the groin may be applied. Steady, gentle traction is employed until the fetus is delivered to the umbilicus, after which the delivery proceeds as for a partial breech extraction.

Entrapment of the aftercoming head is a rare[34] but truly terrifying complication. Gentle traction and the MSV maneuver may result in delivery, but abdominal rescue via the Zavanelli maneuver, augmented by the use of a vacuum extractor, may be

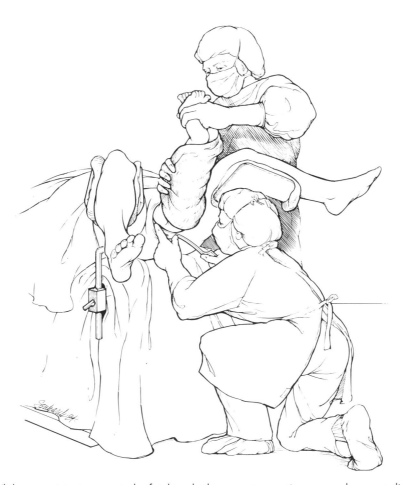

Fig. 9-12. While an assistant supports the fetal trunk, the operator, resting on one knee, applies Piper forceps to the fetal vertex directly. (From Seeds,[89] with permission.)

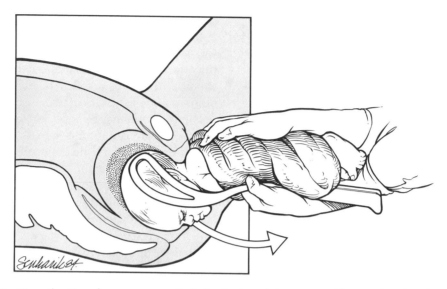

Fig. 9-13. Once the Piper forceps are applied, the fetal trunk is supported by one hand and gentle traction on the forceps, as illustrated by the arrow, in the direction of the pelvic axis results in a controlled delivery. (From Seeds,[89] with permission.)

required.[87,88] Older methods, such as Duhrssen's incision or symphysiotomy, may be considered as well.

Cesarean Section

Cesarean birth is not a guarantee of safe delivery for either mother or fetus. Great care must be paid to the type of incision chosen, and to gentle decomposition and extraction. The lower uterine segment is rarely well developed in the preterm breech-presenting fetus, and low vertical incisions are recommended to avoid head entrapment. The same maneuvers used to safely deliver the legs, arms, and head of the breech-presenting fetus delivered vaginally must also be used in cesarean delivery.

Recommendations

Given the lack of supporting data to the contrary, we would suggest that fetuses in all types of breech positions, save the footling breech position, be considered for vaginal delivery. The usual discriminators in our practice continue to be a fetal weight above 4,000 g; extension of the fetal head; and inadequate radiographic pelvimetric parameters. The physician's experience and comfort level must neces-

sarily remain part of the decision process. We believe it essential that a large-scale, nationwide, multicenter study be conducted. We anticipate that such a study will confirm our position and allow the reversal of the current trend toward cesarean delivery of breech presentations. The art of the vaginal breech delivery should not be lost.

TRANSVERSE AND OBLIQUE LIE

When the fetal long axis intersects the maternal spine at an angle of 90 degrees, the fetus is considered to be in a transverse lie. Any other intersection results in an oblique lie. In either case the fetal shoulder or arm will be presenting.[89] Because the complications in management of these nonlongitudinal lies are similar, they are discussed jointly (Fig. 9-14).

Incidence

The incidence of women presenting in labor in the United States with fetuses in a transverse or oblique lie is 0.4 percent.[90] Gestational age at the time of labor influences the occurrence of an abnormal axial lie. Prior to 30 weeks' gestation, as many as 15 per-

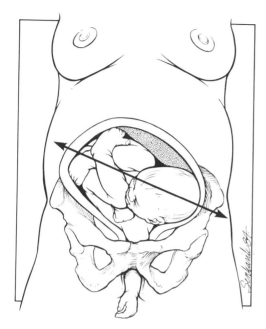

Fig. 9-14. Frontal view illustrating a fetus in an oblique lie with a shoulder or arm presenting. (From Seeds,[89] with permission.)

cent of fetuses are found in a transverse lie.[1] Populations containing a large proportion of multiparous women report an increased incidence (e.g., in Ireland the incidence has been reported to be 2.7 percent of all deliveries[91]).

Etiology

Numerous factors that distort the usual vertical polarity of the uterus have long been associated with the nonlongitudinal lie.[89] Women of high parity may develop a pronounced diastasis recti that allows the uterus to fall forward and become distorted. In one review, 87 percent of all patients with fetuses in a transverse lie were gravida 3 or greater, and 50 percent were grand multigravidas.[92] Other conditions involving an altered uterine topography can increase the risk of a transverse lie. These include a contracted pelvis, placenta previa, uterine anomalies, and uterine leiomyomata. Situations that increase the mobility of the fetus, such as polyhydramnios and prematurity, may also allow the fetus to assume a transverse lie, as may fetal anomalies that prevent engagement of the head.[91,92,95–97]

Diagnosis

On visual inspection, the maternal abdomen is elongated transversely instead of longitudinally. Palpation usually reveals the absence of the head or breech in the lower pole of the uterus. The abdomen, however, may be so tense secondary to the fetal position as to interfere with Leopold's maneuvers. Whenever the fundus is found near the umbilicus at term, and the fetal parts are difficult to palpate, a transverse lie should be suspected.[93]

On vaginal examination, the diagnosis of a transverse or oblique lie in labor should be suspected when an irregular presenting part is felt, or when the sutures of the vertex or the anal orifice of a breech presentation are not detected. Palpation of the gridiron or washboard texture of the fetal ribs is pathognomonic.[94] Ultrasound examination should be employed whenever there is a question about the identification of the presenting part.

Mechanism of Labor

There is no true mechanism of labor for a transverse lie. Typically, impaction of the shoulder occurs if these pregnancies are allowed to enter labor. Further labor results in elongation of the fetal neck, while the head and breech remain above the pelvic brim (Fig. 9-14). As labor continues, a contraction ring will develop and the lower uterine segment will become markedly dilated, possibly eventuating in uterine rupture.[98]

If spontaneous resolution to a longitudinal lie does not occur in labor, delivery is achieved either by spontaneous expulsion or spontaneous evolution. Spontaneous expulsion is successful only when a small, premature, or macerated fetus is present. The fetal back becomes bent on itself and is delivered, while the head is pressed into the abdomen. The remainder of the compressed and doubled up fetus (conduplicatio corpore) is then delivered.[93]

Spontaneous evolution rarely occurs. It has been described as "nature's last, least likely, and most dangerous effort." After impaction of the shoulder, the neck becomes extended enough to allow the shoulders to enter the vagina, followed by the arms. The fetus then rolls on itself, allowing the chest, body, breech, and finally the head to deliver. The extreme compression and stretching are usually incompatible with neonatal survival.[94]

Management

The diagnosis of transverse lie at term in a nonlaboring patient requires action. Although more than 80 percent of transverse-lying fetuses at 32 weeks will move to a longitudinal lie before labor, those who remain in the transverse lie are subject to significant excess morbidity and mortality from cord prolapse, traumatic delivery, or neglected labor. These patients are best managed by attempted ECV at 37 weeks, followed by cesarean section if ECV is unsuccessful.[99,100]

Before modern advances in obstetrics, internal podalic version was the method of choice for managing a transverse lie in labor. Owing to the high rate of maternal and infant morbidity and mortality, this technique has been abandoned.[91,92]

If a patient presents in labor with a suspected transverse lie, ultrasonography should be used to confirm the diagnosis. If confirmed, the location of the placenta should be determined and a careful anatomic survey of the fetus should be performed. A quantifiable assessment of the amniotic fluid is also required.

Once the transverse presentation is confirmed, placenta previa is excluded, and an adequate amount of fluid is ascertained to be present, external cephalic version should be considered. Continuous electronic heart rate monitoring should be employed. If there is no evidence of fetal compromise, tocolytic agents should be administered until uterine contractions have halted. Administration of epidural anesthesia at this time may be advantageous. If the version is successful, epidural anesthesia can be used for labor. If fetal distress results from the version, an immediate cesarean section can be performed without resorting to general anesthesia. No increase in complications has been noted when epidural anesthesia is in effect during versions. Also, there is evidence that epidural anesthesia may increase the success of ECV.[101] If the version is successful, the vertex should be held in the pelvis with suprapubic pressure to facilitate seating of the presenting part. Intrapartum ECV has been shown to be a safe and effective procedure, with a reported success rate of 83 percent in achieving a longitudinal lie.[90]

If a version is not successful or the patient is not a candidate for version, a cesarean section should be performed. The optimum choice of uterine incision is controversial. A low vertical incision has been recommended because of the high probability of having to vertically extend the low transverse incision in order to complete delivery.[89] In an attempt to avoid the complications of a vertical uterine incision, an "intra-abdominal version technique" has been proposed. In this procedure a cesarean section is begun in the usual manner. Before the uterus is entered, the operator grasps both poles of the fetus and then gently guides what will become the presenting part into the pelvis. Once the version is accomplished, the fetus is held in place and the cesarean section is completed. Either a cephalic or podalic version can be employed.[102]

If intra-abdominal version is unsuccessful, the choice of uterine incision should be individualized. If the fetus is in a back-down transverse lie, a classic incision may be necessary. When the shoulder is wedged into the pelvis or the lower uterine segment is not well developed, a vertical incision should be used. If, however, the lower uterine segment is well formed and the fetus is floating with its small parts accessible, a low transverse incision should be considered.[102,104] Even under these optimum conditions, difficulties can be encountered in extracting the fetus. Often, an intrauterine version is required,[103] and, as the uterus may contract tightly after the incision, intrauterine manipulation is often difficult. If problems are encountered, uterine relaxation can be achieved. Intravenous nitroglyerine is an attractive intraoperative agent because of its rapid onset and short duration of action.[105]

BROW PRESENTATION

A fetus is said to be presenting by the brow when it is in a longitudinal lie and the attitude of the head is midway between full flexion (vertex) and full extension (face). Since brow presentations occur infrequently, most series include cases identified before the advent of electronic fetal heart rate monitoring, relatively low-risk cesarean section, and antibiotics. Historical management included high- or midforceps delivery after forceps conversion to a face or vertex position, podalic version and extraction at term, and cranioclasty after intrapartum fetal death. Recommendations from studies that included these methods are difficult to apply to modern obstetric practice.

Incidence

The reported incidence of brow presentation has ranged from a high of 1 in 667 deliveries[106] to a low of 1 in 3,543.[107] In the sole study that reviewed cases after 1960, the incidence was 1 in 675.[108] The higher incidence found in several of the more recent studies may reflect the increased accuracy of vaginal over rectal examination.

Etiology

In 29 to 93 percent of cases, the cause of a brow presentation cannot be identified.[108,109] Of possible etiologies, cephalopelvic disproportion (i.e., factors that prevent or interfere with engagement) is most commonly cited. In Kovacs' review[109] of nine studies involving 291 brow presentations, 43 percent of parturients had relative or absolute cephalopelvic disproportion, 21 percent demonstrated a contracted pelvis, and 22 percent were delivered of an infant weighing in excess of 3,636 g. Four additional studies of 273 cases of brow presentation show a 15 percent incidence of contracted pelvis as well.[92,110–112] In three of these studies (n = 117), fetal weight exceeded 4,000 g 18 percent of the time.[92,110,111] Premature rupture of membranes also contributes to brow presentation by trapping the fetal head in an extended position. Overall, premature rupture of membranes precedes brow presentation in approximately 27 percent of cases.[109,111,113,114]

Diagnosis

The brow position is usually diagnosed during vaginal examination late in the first stage or during the second stage of labor. Often the cervix has failed to dilate or the fetal head has failed to engage or descend. On palpation, the area of the head between the supraorbital ridges and the anterior fontanelle is identified. Early diagnosis may be made by Leopold's maneuvers. The abdominal signs of a brow presentation include palpation of the cephalic prominence on the same side as the fetal back, a deep furrow at the fetal neck, an S-shaped curvature of the fetal back, and a high-riding occiput.[115]

Mechanism of Labor

Labor in the case of a brow-presenting fetus is referenced to the frontal bones, with the term *frontum* replacing *occiput* when describing fetal position. In the term fetus, the largest cephalic diameter, the occipitomental diameter (OMD), averages 13.5 cm. In the brow-presenting fetus, the OMD presents to and must negotiate through the pelvic inlet, midplane, and outlet diameters, which in the average pelvis are 2 to 3 cm smaller than the OMD. During labor, the average brow-presenting fetus can engage and descend only with significant molding. If the bony pelvis cannot accommodate the molded head, the head will remain unengaged or at a high station. Labor may be protracted, and arrest of dilatation or descent may occur.

With brow presentation, the fetal head, if it engages, often engages in the frontum-transverse position. Descent and internal rotation to the frontum-anterior position occur if the maternal pelvis is adequate and the face can fit behind or under the pubic arch. In most cases the brow position converts. Labor forces, if directed against the fetal occiput, flex the head and pivot the face under the pubic arch, converting the frontum-anterior to the occiput-posterior position (Fig. 9-15). Alternatively, if the occiput lies in the hollow of the sacrum, the forces of labor push against the fetal chin and face, causing the neck to

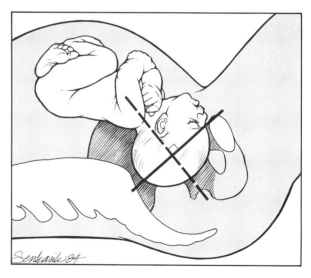

Fig. 9-15. This fetus demonstrates the intermediate deflexion attitude known as the brow presentation. The occipitofrontal plane of the fetal cranium describes a right angle with the axis of the cervical spine. This fetus is in a frontum-anterior position. (From Seeds,[89] with permission.)

further extend, and delivery occurs as a face presentation (see below) in the mentum-anterior position. Occasionally a fetus that is small relative to the maternal pelvis may deliver in the mentum-posterior position or in a persistent brow position.

Management

As noted above, unless the fetus is small or the maternal pelvis is large, a fetus that persists in the brow position will not deliver vaginally. Labor abnormalities are common in brow presentations, and are manifested primarily as prolongation of the decelerative and second stages of labor.[84] However, because a spontaneous conversion to a face or vertex presentation usually occurs, expectant management is acceptable if labor is progressing and fetal monitoring is normal. Historic techniques, such as manual or forceps conversion followed by forceps delivery, or internal podalic version and extraction, are no longer used because of the associated excessive perinatal mortality and maternal morbidity. If the pelvis is adequate, up to 90 percent of brow presentations will convert.[7] Overall 25.8 percent of 697 brow presentations were found to convert spontaneously and deliver vaginally.[92,108,109,111–113]

FACE PRESENTATION

Incidence

A fetus is said to be presenting by the face when it is in an attitude of full extension (i.e., with the fetal occiput lying in opposition to the fetal spine, the chin being the presenting part). Caveats noted in the discussion of brow presentations with respect to extrapolation of old data apply here as well. The incidence of face presentation in reported series ranges from 1 in 333[116] to 1 in 690.[117]

Etiology

As in the case of brow presentation, the factors most commonly associated with face presentation are prematurity,[116–123] fetal anomalies such as anencephaly,[107,116,117,119,121–126] and cephalopelvic disproportion from either a small pelvis or a large fetus.[116,117,119,122,124,126–129] Other, less commonly cited factors include premature rupture of membranes,[118,120,129] multiparity,[116,118,126,128,131] multiple gestation,[119,128] and a nuchal cord.[107,126]

Diagnosis

Although face presentation is rarely diagnosed by abdominal examination, several findings are suggestive of it. These findings include a high presenting part, cephalic prominence on the same side as the fetal back, a prominent groove between the fetal vertex and back, a concave fetal back, prominent small parts, loud fetal heart tones heard on the same side as fetal small parts, and a long, ovoid uterus.[107,116,124,125,131]

On vaginal examination, the fetal mouth, nasal bridge, and orbits are recognizable unless obscured by facial edema.[107] These irregular contours may be mistaken for a breech presentation.[117] However, the anus and ischial tuberosities lie in a straight line, while the mouth and malar eminences form a triangle.[132] The examiner may also be able to identify the soft tissues of the gums or sucking movements of the mouth.

Mechanism of Labor

The point of reference in a face presentation is the chin or mentum. The face is not truly engaged even when the presenting part is palpable at the ischial spines, as the distance from the biparietal diameter to the chin is greater than the distance to the occiput. The chin may present at the vulva without the trachelobregmatic and biparietal diameters having passed the pelvic inlet.[107] The findings of a hollow sacrum on vaginal examination, and an easily palpable fetal head suprapubically, suggest that engagement has yet to occur in the face presentation.[119]

Descent in labor occurs as the chin points toward one side, and the head, dolichocephalic through molding, enters the pelvic inlet. The chin will rotate anteriorly only after the elongated back of the head passes the sacral promontory,[125,131] and the chin descends low enough to meet soft tissue resistance sufficient to effect internal rotation.[107] Anteriorward internal rotation then brings the chin under the symphysis pubis, and the head delivers by flexion (Fig. 9-16).

Unless the fetus is very small, delivery from the mentum-posterior position will not occur. In a term infant in the mentum-posterior position, the fetal

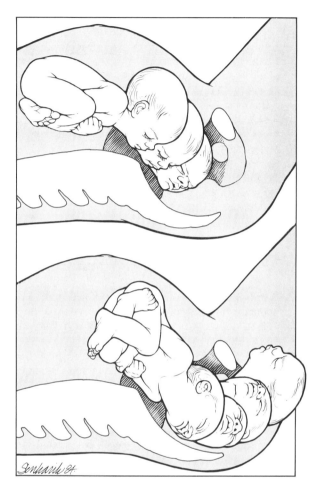

Fig. 9-16. Descent and delivery of a fetus in a face presentation. The fetus may engage and descend in a mentum-anterior position or engage in a mentum-posterior position as illustrated here, internally rotating for delivery from the mentum-anterior position. (From Seeds,[89] with permission.)

neck is shorter than the maternal sacrum and cannot stretch sufficiently to fill the hollow of the sacrum. Therefore, delivery of the mentum-posterior fetus by extension cannot take place.

Management

Most studies report that the duration of labor in the face presentation is generally the same as that in the vertex presentation.[117,118,122–124] Rare exceptions demonstrate prolongation of the first stage[107] and second stage,[1] as well as an overall shortening of

labor.[129] In approximately 50 percent of cases the diagnosis of face presentation is not made until the second stage of labor.[117,119]

As long as the progress of labor and the fetal heart rate tracing are normal, no specific intervention is required in the face presentation. Continuous fetal heart rate monitoring is, however, recommended, as these fetuses may be at increased risk of severe variable or late decelerations.[131–134] Most fetuses in the mentum-anterior position will have an uncomplicated spontaneous vaginal delivery. Rarely, low forceps, either of the Kjelland or a classic type, may be used.[86] A percentage of mentum-transverse or mentum-posterior presentations will rotate spontaneously, the anterior rotation tending to occur late in the second stage. Midforceps rotation, elevation, and conversion to an occiput position, and internal podalic version and breech extraction, are no longer practiced. Cesarean section is appropriate for standard obsteric indications such as suspected fetal distress, arrest of dilatation, or arrest of descent.

REFERENCES

1. Scheer K, Nubar J: Variation of fetal presentation with gestational age. Am J Obstet Gynecol 125:269, 1976
2. Cunningham FC, MacDonald PC, Gant NF et al: Williams' Obstetrics. 19th Ed. Appleton and Lange, E. Norwalk, CT, 1993
3. Braun FHT, Jones KL, Smith DW: Breech presentations as an indicator of fetal abnormality. J Pediatr 86:419, 1975
4. Fianu S, Vaclavinkova V: The site of placental attachment as a factor in the aetiology of breech presentation. Acta Obstet Gynecol Scand 57:371, 1978
5. Adams CM: Review of breech presentation. SD J Med 32:15, 1979
6. Collea JV: Current management of breech presentation. Clin Obstet Gynecol 23:525, 1980
7. Graves WK: Breech delivery in twenty years of practice. Am J Obstet Gynecol 137:229, 1980
8. Collea JV, Rabin SC, Weghorst GR, Quilligan EJ: The randomized management of term frank breech presentation-vaginal delivery versus cesarean section. Am J Obstet Gynecol 131:186, 1978
9. Wright RC: Reduction of perinatal mortality and morbidity in breech delivery through routine use of cesarean section. Obstet Gynecol 14:758, 1959
10. Green JE, McLean F, Smith LP, Usher R: Has an

increased cesarean section rate for term breech delivery reduced the incidence of birth asphyxia, trauma, and death? Am J Obstet Gynecol 142:643, 1982

11. Petitti DB: Maternal mortality and morbidity in cesarean section. Clin Obstet Gynecol 28:763, 1985

12. Gimovsky ML, Wallace RL, Schifrin BS, Paul RH: Randomized management of the non-frank breech presentation at term: a preliminary report. Am J Obstet Gynecol 146:34, 1983

13. Rovinsky J, Miller JA, Kaplan S: Management of breech presentation at term. Am J Obstet Gynecol 115:497, 1973

14. Fianu S: Fetal mortality and morbidity following breech delivery. Acta Obstet Gynaecol Scand, suppl. 56:1, 1976

15. Cheng M, Hannah M: Breech delivery at term: a critical review of the literature. Obstet Gynecol 82:605, 1993

16. Oian P, Skramm I, Hannisdal E, Bjoro K: Breech delivery. An obstetrical analysis. Acta Obstet Gynaecol Scand 67:75, 1988

17. Croughan-Minihane MS, Petitti DB, Gordis L, Golditch I: Morbidity among breech infants according to method of delivery. Obstet Gynecol 75:821, 1990

18. Christian SS, Brady K, Read JA, Kopelman JN: Vaginal breech delivery: a five-year prospective evaluation of a protocol using computer tomographic pelvimetry. Am J Obstet Gynecol 163:848, 1990

19. Wisestankora W, Herabutya Y, Prasertsawat P, Thanantaseth C: Fetal outcome in term frank breech primipara delivered vaginally and by elective cesarean section. J Med Assoc Thai, suppl. 73:47, 1990

20. Luterkort M, Polberger S, Persson PH, Bjerre I: Role of asphyxia and slow intrauterine growth in morbidity among breech delivered infants. Early Hum Dev 14:19, 1986

21. Flanagan TA, Mulchahey KM, Korenbrot CC et al: Management of term breech presentation. Am J Obstet Gynecol 156:1492, 1987

22. Barlow K, Larsson G: Results of a five-year prospective study using a fetopelvic scoring system for term singleton breech delivery after uncomplicated pregnancy. Acta Obstet Gynaecol Scand 65:315, 1986

23. Brown L, Karrison T, Cibils LA: Mode of delivery and perinatal results in breech presentation. Am J Obstet Gynecol 171:28, 1994

24. Cahill DJ, Turner MJ, Stronge JM: Breech presentation: is a reduction in traumatic intracranial hemorrhage feasible? J Obstet Gynaecol 11:417, 1991

25. Kiely JL: Mode of delivery and neonatal death in 17,587 infants presenting by the breech. Br J Obstet Gynaecol 98:898, 1991

26. Otamiri G, Berg G, Ledin T et al: Influence of elective cesarean section and breech delivery on neonatal neurological condition. Early Hum Dev 23:53, 1990

27. Chalmers I: Scientific inquiry and authoritarianism in perinatal care and education. Birth 10:151, 1983

28. Tejani N, Verma U, Shiffman R, Chayen B: Effect of route of delivery on periventricular/intraventricular hemorrhage in the low-birth-weight fetus with a breech presentation. J Reprod Med 32:911, 1987

29. Malloy MH, Onstad L, Wright E et al: The effect of cesarean delivery on birth outcome in very low birth weight infants. Obstet Gynecol 77:498, 1991

30. Shaver DC, Bada HS, Korones SB et al: Early and late intraventricular hemorrhage: the role of obstetric factors. Obstet Gynecol 80:831, 1992

31. Weissman A, Blazer S, Zimmer EZ et al: Low birth weight breech infant: short term and long term outcome by method of delivery. Am J Perinatol 5:289, 1988

32. Davidson S, Cohen WR: Influence of presentation on neonatal outcome of vaginally delivered low birth weight infants. A matched pair analysis. J Perinatol 10:38, 1990

33. Main DM, Main EK, Maurer MM: Cesarean section versus vaginal delivery for the breech fetus weighing less than 1500 grams. Am J Obstet Gynecol 146:580, 1983

34. Cibils LA, Karrison T, Brown L: Factors influencing neonatal outcomes in the very-low-birth-weight fetus (less than 1500 gms) with a breech presentation. Am J Obstet Gynecol 171:35, 1994

35. Phalen JP, Clark SL: Cesarean Delivery. Elsevier, New York, 1988

36. Lumley J, Lester A, Renon P, Wood C: A failed RCT to determine the best method of delivery for very low birth weight infants. Controlled Clin Trials 6:120, 1985

37. Penn ZJ, Steer PJ: Reasons for declining participation in a prospective randomized trial to determine the optimum mode of delivery of the preterm breech. Controlled Clin Trials 11:226, 1990

38. Penn ZJ, Steer PJ: How obstetricians manage the problem of preterm delivery with special reference to the preterm breech. Br J Obstet Gynaecol 98:531, 1991

39. Amon E, Sabai BM, Anderson GD: How perinatologists manage the problem of the presenting breech. Am J Perinatol 5:247, 1988

40. Ranney B: The gentle art of external cephalic version. Am J Obstet Gynecol 116:239, 1973

41. Hill LM: Prevalance of breech presentation by gestational age. Am J Perinatol 7:92, 1990

42. Hughey MJ: Fetal position during labor. Am J Obstet Gynecol 153:885, 1985

43. Westgreen M, Edvall H, Norstrom L et al: Spontaneous C.V. of breech presentation at term. Br J Obstet Gynaecol 92:19, 1985

44. Kasule J, Chimbira THK, McL. Brown I: Controlled trial of external cephalic version. Br J Obstet Gynaecol 92:14, 1985

45. Van Veelen AS, Cappellen AW, Flu PK et al: Effect of external cephalic version in late pregnancy on presentation of delivery: a randomized controlled trial. Br J Obstet Gynaecol 96:916, 1989

46. Van Dorsten JP, Schifrin BS, Wallace RL: Randomized control [*sic*] trial of external cephalic version with tocolysis in late pregnancy. Am J Obstet Gynecol 141:417, 1981

47. Robertson AW, Kopelman JN, Read JA et al: External cephalic version at term: is a tocolytic necessary? Obstet Gynecol 70:896, 1987

48. Donald WL, Barton JJ: Ultrasongraphy and external cephalic version at term. Am J Obstet Gynecol 162:1542, 1990

49. Hellstrom AC, Nilsson B, Stance L, Nylund L: When does external cephalic version succeed? Acta Obstet Gynaecol Scand 69:281, 1990

50. Fortunato SJ, Mercer LS, Guzick DS: External cephalic version with tocolysis: factors associated with success. Obstet Gynaecol 72:59, 1988

51. Stine ES, Phelan JP, Wallace R et al: Update on external cephalic version performed at term. Obstet Gynecol 65:642, 1985

52. Phelan JP, Stine LE, Mueller E: Observations of fetal heart characteristics related to external cephalic version and tocolysis. Am J Obstet Gynecol 149:658, 1984

53. Marcus RG, Crewe-brown H, Krawitz S, Katz J: Fetomaternal haemorrhage following successful and unsuccessful attempts at external cephalic version. Br J Obstet Gynaecol 82:578, 1975

54. Gjode P, Bremholm Rasmussen TN, Jorgensen J: Fetal maternal bleeding during attempts at external version. Br J Obstet Gynaecol 87:571, 1980

55. Petrikovsy BM, DeSilva HN, Fumia ED: Erb's palsy and fetal bruising after external cephalic version: case report. Am J Obstet Gynecol 157:258, 1987

56. Chapman GP, Weller RO, Normand KS, Gibbins D: Spinal cord transection in utero. BMJ 2:398, 1978

57. Brock V, Philipssen T, Secher NJ: A randomized trial of external cephalic version with tocolysis in late pregnancy. Br J Obstet Gynaecol 91:653, 1984

58. Hofmyer GJ: Effect of external cephalic version in late pregnancy on breech presentation and cesarean section rate: a controlled study. Br J Obstet Gynaecol 90:392, 1983

59. Weiner CP: Vaginal breech delivery in the 1990's. Clin Obstet Gynecol 35:559, 1992

60. Placek PL, Taffel SM, Moien M: 1986 C-section rise: VBACS inch upward. Am J Public Health 78:562, 1988

61. Neilson DR: Management of the large breech infant. Am J Obstet Gynecol 107:345, 1970

62. Myer SA, Gleicher N: Breech delivery: why the dilemma? Am J Obstet Gynecol 155:6, 1986

63. Karp LE, Doney JR, McCarthy T et al: The *premature breech*: trial of labor or cesarean section. Obstet Gynecol 53:88, 1979

64. Behrman SJ: Fetal cervical hyperextension. Clin Obstet Gynecol 5:1018, 1962

65. Abroms IF, Bressnan MJ, Zuckerman JE et al: Cervical cord injuries secondary to hyperextension of the head in breech presentations. Obstet Gynecol 41:369, 1973

66. Westgren M, Grundsell H, Ingemarson I et al: Hyperextension of the fetal head in breech presentation. A study with long term follow-up. Br J Obstet Gynaecol 88:101, 1981

67. Todd WD, Steer CM: Term breech: review of 1006 term breech deliveries. Obstet Gynecol 22:583, 1963

68. Gimovsky ML, Petrie RH, Todd WD: Neonatal performance of the selected term breech. Obstet Gynecol 56:687, 1980

69. Collea JV, Quilligan EJ: The management of the breech position. J Reprod Med 23:258, 1979

70. Collea JV, Chein C, Quilligan ET: The randomized management of term frank breech presentation: a study of 208 cases. Am J Obstet Gynecol 137:235, 1980

71. Beischer NA: Pelvic contraction in breech presentation. J Obstet Gynaecol Br Commonwealth 73:421, 1966

72. Benson WL, Boyce DC, Vaughn DL: Breech delivery in the primigravida. Obstet Gynecol 40:417, 1972

73. Watson WS, Benson WL: Vaginal delivery for the selected frank breech infant at term. Obstet Gynecol 64:638, 1984

74. Kopelman JN, Duff P, Karl RT et al: Computed tomographic pelvimetry in the evaluation of breech presentation. Obstet Gynecol 68:455, 1986

75. Federle MP, Cohen HA, Rosenwein MD et al: Pelvimetry by digital radiography: a low dose examination. Radiology 143:733, 1981

76. Kitzmiller JL, Mall JC, Gin GD et al: Measurement of fetal shoulder width with computed tomography in diabetic women. Obstet Gynecol 70:941, 1987

77. Gimovsky ML, Willard K, Neglio M et al: X-ray pelvimetry in a breech protocol: a comparison of digital radiography and conventional methods. Obstet Gynecol 153:887, 1985

78. Aronson D, Kier R: CT pelvimetry: the foveae are not an accurate landmark for the level of the ischial spines. AJR 156:527, 1991

79. Van loon AJ, Mantingh A, Cornelis JP et al: Pelvimetry by magnetic resonance imaging in breech presentation. Am J Obstet Gynecol 163:1256, 1990

80. Stark DS, McCarthy SM, Filly RA et al: Pelvimetry by magnetic resonance imaging. AJR 144:947, 1985

81. Biswas A, Johnstone MJ: Term breech delivery: does x-ray pelvimetry help? Aust NZ J Obstet Gynecol 33:150, 1993

82. Gimovsky ML, Petrie RJ: The intrapartum management of the breech presentation. Clin Perinatol 16:975, 1989

83. Douglas JM, Ward EM: Current pharmacology and the obstetric anesthesiologist. Int Anesthesiol Clin 32:1, 1994

84. Friedman EA: Labor: Clinical Evaluation and Management. Appleton Century-Crofts, E. Norwalk, CT, 1978

85. May JL: Modified median episiotomy minimizes the risk of third degree tears. Obstet Gynecol 83:156, 1994

86. O'Grady JP: Modern Instrumental Delivery. Williams & Wilkins, Baltimore, 1988

87. Sandberg EC: The Zavanelli maneuver extended: progression of a revolutinary concept. Am J Obstet Gynecol 158:1347, 1988

88. Landy HJ, Zarate L, O'Sullivan MJ: Abdominal rescue using the vacuum extractor after entrapment of the aftercoming head. Obstet Gynecol 84:644, 1994

89. Seeds J: Malpresentations. p. 539. In Gabbe SG, Niebyl JR, Simpson JL (eds): Obstetrics: Normal and Problem Pregnancies. 2nd Ed. Churchill Livingstone, New York, 1991

90. Phelan JP, Stine LE, Edwards MD et al: The role of external version in the intrapartum management of transverse lie presentation. Am J Obstet Gynecol 151:724, 1984

91. Hourihane MJ: Etiology and management of oblique lie. Obstet Gynecol 37:512, 1968

92. Cruikshank DP, White CA: Obstetric malpresentations: twenty years' experience. Am J Obstet Gynecol 116:1097, 1973

93. Beck AC: Obstetrical Practice. 3rd Ed. Williams & Wilkins, Baltimore, 1942

94. McCormick C: A Textbook on Pathology of Labor, the Puerperium and the Newborn. 2nd Ed. CV Mosby, St. Louis, 1947

95. Holmes R, Evans BS: Breech, transverse and compound presentations, multiple pregnancy, prolapse of cord, fetal anomalies. In Davis CH (ed): Gynecology and Obstetrics. 1st Ed. WF Hager, Hagerstown, MD, 1936

96. Gemor O, Segal S: Incidence and contribution of predisposing factors to transverse lie presentation. Int J Gynaecol Obstet 44:219, 1994

97. Kawathekar P, Kasturilal M, Spinivas P: Etiology and trends in the management of transverse lie. Am J Obstet Gynecol 117:39, 1973

98. Piper EB: Anomalies of the passenger. p. 83. In Curtis AH (ed): Obstetrics and Gynecology. WB Saunders, Philadelphia, 1933

99. Phelan JP, Mueller E, McCart D et al: The non-laboring transverse lie: a management dilemma. J Reprod Med 31:184, 1986

100. Hankins GDV, Hammond TL, Snyder RR, Gilstrap LC: Transverse lie. Am J Perinatol 7:66, 1990

101. Carlan S, Dent M, Huckaby T et al: The effect of epidural anesthesia on safety and success of external cephalic version at term. Anesth Analg 79:525, 1994

102. Pelosi MA, Apuzzio J, Friccione D, Gowda VV: The "intra-abdominal version technique" for delivery of transverse lie by low-segment cesarean section. Am J Obstet Gynecol 135:1009, 1979

103. Yasin SY, Walton DL, O'Sullivan MJ: Problems encountered during cesarean delivery. In Plauche WC, Morrison JC, O'Sullivan MJ (eds): Surgical Obstetrics. WB Saunders, Philadelphia, 1992

104. Zuspan FP, Quilligan EJ: Douglas-Stromme Operative Obstetrics. 5th Ed. Appleton Lange, E. Norwalk, CT, 1988

105. Abouleish A, Corn S: Intravenous nitroglycerin for intrapartum external version of the second twin. Anesth Analg 78:808, 1994

106. Moore ED, Dermen EH: Management of persistent brow presentation. Obstet Gynecol 6:186, 1955

107. Posner AC, Buch IM: Face and persistent brow presentations. Surg Gynecol Obstet 77:618, 1943

108. Abell DA: Brow presentation. S Afr Med J 47:1315, 1973

109. Kovacs SG: Brow presentation, Royal Hospital for Women, Paddington, 1950–1965, and review of literature. Med J Aust 2:820, 1970

110. Jennings PN: Brow presentation with vaginal delivery. Aust NZ J Obstet Gynaecol 8:219, 1968

111. Mostar S, Akaltin E, Babuna C: Deflexion attitudes. Obstet Gynecol 28:49, 1966

112. Meltzer RM, Sachtleben MR, Friedman EA: Brow presentation. Am J Obstet Gynecol 100:255, 1968

113. Ingolfsson A: Brow presentations. Acta Obstet Gynecol Scand 48:486, 1969

114. Skalley TW, Kramer TF: Brow presentation. Obstet Gynecol 15:616, 1960

115. Bednoff SL, Thomas EB: Brow presentation. NYS J Med 67:803, 1967

116. Chen HY, Wei PY: Facial presentation and pelvic type. J Int Coll Surg 34:756, 1960

117. Cucco UP: Face presentation. Am J Obstet Gynecol 94:1085, 1966

118. Magid B, Gillespie CF: Face and brow presentations. Obstet Gynecol 9:450, 1957

119. Posner AC, Friedman S, Posner LB: Modern trends in the management of face and brow presentations. Surg Gynecol Obstet 104:485, 1957

120. Salzmann B, Soled M, Gilmour T: Face presentation. Obstet Gynecol 16:106, 1960

121. Tancer ML, Rosanalli P: Face and persistent brow presentations. Obstet Gynecol 10:632, 1957

122. Dede JA, Friedman EA: Face presentation. Am J Obstet Gynecol 87:515, 1963

123. Jacobson LJ, Johnson CE: Brow and face presentations. Am J Obstet Gynecol 84:1881, 1962

124. Reinke T: Face presentation. Am J Obstet Gynecol 66:1185, 1958

125. Gomez HE, Denner EH: Face presentation. Obstet Gynecol 8:103, 1956

126. Hillman LM, Epperson JWW, Connally F: Face and brow presentation. Am J Obstet Gynecol 59:831, 1950

127. Posner CA, Cohn S: Analysis of 45 face presentations. Am J Obstet Gynecol 62:592, 1951

128. Posner LB, Rubin EJ, Posner AC: Face and brow presentations. Obstet Gynecol 21:745, 1963

129. Rudolph SJ: Face presentation. Am J Obstet Gynecol 54:987, 1947

130. Prevedourakis CN: Face presentation. Am J Obstet Gynecol 94:1092, 1966

131. Reddock JW: Face presentation. Am J Obstet Gynecol 56:86, 1948

132. Duff P: Diagnosis and management of face presentation. Obstet Gynecol 57:105, 1981

133. Benedetti TJ, Towersohn RI, Truscott AM: Face presentation at term. Obstet Gynecol 55:199, 1980

134. Watson WJ, Read JA: Electronic fetal monitoring in face presentation at term. Mil Med 152:324, 1987

Chapter 10

Forceps and Vacuum-Assisted Delivery

Ronald T. Burkman

Operative vaginal delivery is in a process of evolution relative to the modern practice of obstetrics. Like a pendulum, opinion over the past 25 years has swung from a highly favorable viewpoint, with rather widespread use of both forceps and vacuum extraction, to a cautious, even restrictive approach, with a more recent return toward greater openmindedness about both modalities. Unfortunately, many of our opinions are based on anecdotal evidence or case series, as the result of a paucity of well-controlled data about the efficacy and safety of operative vaginal delivery. Additionally, concern about medicolegal ramifications of unsuccessful or difficult vaginal deliveries and the presence of relatives at the delivery has significantly influenced practice. Finally, with lower numbers of operative deliveries available for house officers in training, there is a lower level of overall skill with vacuum extraction and particularly with the use of forceps than was formerly the case,[1] at a time when the usefulness of these approaches is regaining acceptance among obstetricians.

HISTORY

Obstetric Forceps

The history of the development of obstetric forceps is interesting because it encompasses both intrigue as well as the application of firm principles related to the introduction of new medical technology.

Readers interested in this subject should read Das' recently reprinted book or Laufe's textbook on forceps techniques.[2,3] The earliest versions of the obstetric forceps date back to antiquity. Based on Hindu, Greek, and Arabian writing, it appears that the early instruments were used to perform destructive operations in cases of fetal demise. The invention of conservative obstetric forceps designed to preserve fetal viability has been traced to a remarkable family of physicians, the Chamberlens, who practiced obstetrics in England between 1600 and 1728. Their forceps were probably the first to include separable blades. Each blade was about a foot long, with a cephalic curve and a fenestration. After insertion, the blades crossed, somewhat like a scissors, and were held together either by a rivet or some type of tie. The actual instruments and the techniques for their application were passed down a line of family members. Almost as remarkable as their invention was that this family was able to conceal the design for many decades, since nondisclosure of "trade secrets" was a practice quite common in that era. In the 1700s a number of physicians made modifications to obstetric forceps that were being independently developed at that time. The most important advance during this era was the development, nearly simultaneously, of instruments with pelvic curves by Pugh, Levret, and Smellie. Until the mid 1800s, little substantive design change occured despite the introduction of many different models. However, several authors of that era did point out that injudicious use of these instruments was to be condemned.

During the latter half of the 19th century, Tarnier, Simpson, and Elliott introduced modifications of obstetric forceps based on a better understanding of the function for which they were designed. Tarnier, a French physician, developed a forceps that may be the best overall prototype of traction instruments. His instrument was designed to allow easy traction through the maternal pelvis along the axis of the pelvic planes, while minimizing rotation of the fetal head. Simpson of Edinburgh, who was also famous for the introduction of chloroform anesthesia, designed an instrument with long, tapered blades to provide better application to a molded head, along with parallel shanks and a simple lock. Around 1858, Elliott of New York introduced a forceps with shorter blades, an increased cephalic curve, and overlapping shanks. In addition, there was an adjustable pin in the handle that was used to vary the pressure on the fetal head. Subsequently, the obstetric forceps of Simpson and Elliott have become the prototypes from which most low or outlet forceps have been developed. Also, in the late 19th century, McLane and other obstetricians introduced the first solid blades; however, it was not until 1937 that Luikart introduced the pseudofenestrated blade design. Other innovators of the early 20th century included Kielland's forceps, used today for midpelvic rotations; the unusually shaped forceps of Lyman Barton of Plattsburg, New York, which were designed to manage transverse arrest; and the elongated forceps of Piper, with a pronounced perineal curve designed to manage the aftercoming head at a breech delivery. Others, such as Bill and Dewey, designed instruments for the application of axis traction. Although there were some modifications in forceps after the 1930s, most of the changes were modest variations of existing instrumentation.

In the 1960s, although a number of obstetricians contributed to knowledge of obstetric forceps, two individuals, Leonard Laufe of Pittsburgh and Edward Dennen of New York, stand out. Laufe introduced a divergent forceps consisting of Luikart-type blades with a pivot lock at the very end of the handles or shanks for use in outlet deliveries, and a shortened version of the Piper forceps for application to

an aftercoming head during a breech delivery. In addition, he wrote extensively about the advantages and disadvantages of various forceps models and the types of forces generated by their use. In 1931, Dennen, working with Hawks, also designed a traction forceps (Hawks–Dennen forceps) that allowed fixed-axis traction by incorporating a backward bend of the proximal shanks and handles. Dennen is best remembered, however, for his classic textbook on forceps techniques, which has been used by several generations of house officers.[4] The 1970s, saw the beginning of a steady decline in the use of vaginal operative deliveries, particularly with obstetric forceps. Major factors in this decline included reports of adverse infant outcomes with the use of midforceps, concern about potential litigation, increased utilization of cesarean section to solve obstetric problems, and a significant reduction in the overall experience in forceps delivery by most young obstetricians.[1] For example, data from the United States National Hospital Discharge Survey on trends in the use of obstetric forceps, vacuum extraction, and cesarean section between 1980 and 1987 demonstrated that while the rate of forceps procedures declined by 43 percent, the rate of cesarean section increased by 48 percent in the same period.[5]

Vacuum Extraction

Although a number of authors from the 1600s onward discussed the use of some type of vacuum device to treat depressed skull fractures or to affect vaginal delivery, it was James Simpson in 1848 who described an instrument for this purpose consisting of a cup directly attached to a piston-like pump.[6] While Simpson made some modifications in this device and discussed its use in his writings, within a period of a year or two he apparently devoted most of his energies to forceps development. Witkowski in 1887 and McCahey in 1890 designed devices that separated the cup from the pump device. In 1912, Vakuumhelm was the first to incorporate a pressure gauge into such a device. During the ensuing 40 years, although a number of obstetricians developed various types of instruments, it was not until the introduction of the vacuum extractor designed by Tage Malmstrom of Gothenburg, Sweden, in 1953 that the use of this device in obstetrics began to gain any widespread acceptance.

The important elements of the Malmstrom design included various-sized metal cups with incurved margins to produce an artificial caput succedaneum or chignon, a chain attached to the cup through the vacuum hose to allow traction, a vacuum bottle interspersed between the vacuum hose and the pump, and a separate pump with a pressure guage.[6,7] In many institutions, particularly in Europe, this device largely displaced forceps. In some less developed countries, even midwives were trained in its use. The major reasons for the widespread acceptance of the Malmstrom extractor by some institutions was the relative ease in learning its use as compared with learning the wide variety of forceps operations used at that time, and the decrease in frequency of maternal morbidity with the device as compared with forceps delivery. However, these advantages were somewhat counterbalanced by the need for several minutes to safely achieve adequate vacuum pressure, a feature that was a disadvantage when rapid delivery was indicated. Further, some infants occasionally suffered either scalp trauma or even cranial injury with the Malmstrom device. In 1973, Kobayashi introduced a silicone rubber cup that by its design did not produce an unsightly chignon and appeared to be associated with less scalp trauma.[8] In the 1980s, a number of disposable soft-cup silicone vacuum extractors were introduced.[9,10] The major advantages of these instruments included reduced scalp trauma as a result of the cup design, and the ability to rapidly and safely achieve a negative pressure through the use of either hand or electronic pumps. These newer designs of extractors, like the Malmstrom device before them, have also significantly displaced the use of obstetric forceps in many institutions around the world. Thus, for example, although the previously noted National Hospital Discharge Survey described a 43 percent decline in forceps deliveries in the United States between 1980 and 1987, the use of vacuum extraction experienced more than a fivefold increase during that same period.[5] However, by 1987, vacuum extraction was still performed in only 3.3 percent of all deliveries.

CLASSIFICATION OF FORCEPS OPERATIONS

The classification of forceps operations is based on the station of the fetal head in the bony pelvis, and on the position of the head. Until recently, the use of forceps to perform any rotation was automatically classified as a midforceps procedure. Moreover, a station ranging from engagement to location of the fetal vertex just superior to the perineum was also classified as a midforceps procedure. In older nomenclature, high forceps procedures were operations performed when the fetal head was unengaged. Any procedures not fulfilling the definition of high or midforceps were classified as low forceps; no distinction was made between low and outlet forceps procedures. In 1988, obstetric forceps operations were reclassified by the American College of Obstetricians and Gynecologists (ACOG)[7] (Table 10-1). In the new classification, the station is defined as the distance of the leading bony part of the fetal skull

Table 10-1. American College of Obstetricians and Gynecologist Classification of Forceps Operations

Type of Procedure	Classification
Outlet forceps	Scalp is visible at the introitus without separating the labia Fetal skull has reached the pelvic floor Sagittal suture is in anteroposterior diameter or right or left occiput-anterior or -posterior position Fetal head is at or on the perineum Rotation does not exceed 45 degrees

Low forceps	Leading point of the fetal skull is at station of $\geq +2$ cm and not on the pelvic floor
	    Rotation ≤ 45 degrees (left or right occiput-anterior to occiput-anterior, or left or right
	        occiput-posterior to occiput-posterior)
	    Rotation >45 degrees

Midforceps	Station $> +2$ cm but head engaged
High	Not included in classification

(From American College of Obstetricians and Gynecologists,[7] with permission.)

from the maternal ischial spines in centimeters, from 0 to +5, as opposed to the former method of 0 to +3 to divide the lower pelvis into thirds. Although this new approach may appear more precise, one needs to always recognize that there is considerable inter- and intraoperator variation when following a patient with pelvic examinations. The major substantive change in the classification was the allowance of some degree of rotation even for operations classified as low or outlet, the inclusion of outlet operations in the classification, and the elimination of high forceps from the classification. Certainly this last decision is warranted, since attempting a forceps or vacuum-assisted delivery in the presence of an unengaged head is associated with a considerably increased risk of maternal and fetal morbidity.

INDICATIONS AND CONTRAINDICATIONS FOR OPERATIVE VAGINAL DELIVERY

Operative vaginal delivery with either forceps or vacuum extraction is indicated for almost any condition that might adversely affect the mother or fetus. However, this rather broad indication is in order only if the procedure can be accomplished with minimal risk to the mother or infant. Because of the potential for increased trauma, as well as the paucity of experienced operators, the use of midforceps is probably not indicated unless there are exceptional circumstances. Standard maternal indications for operative delivery include cardiopulmonary conditions such as congenital heart disease or cystic fibrosis, intrapartum infection such as chorioamnionitis, exhaustion of the mother, or a prolonged second stage of labor.

Fetal indications for operative vaginal delivery include terminal placental abruption or an abnormal fetal heart rate pattern. In addition, there has been some debate about the use of "prophylactic forceps" to accomplish preterm vaginal delivery. For example, data from the Collaborative Perinatal Projects in 1965 indicated a better mental and motor performance after 1 year among low-birth-weight infants delivered by forceps than in those delivered vaginally.[11] However, studies by Haesslein and Goodlin[12] and by O'Driscoll and colleagues[13] suggested that such infants suffered greater risk of intracranial hemorrhage when delivered by forceps than spontaneously. Other studies, by Fairweather[14] and

Schwartz and colleagues[15] demonstrated no significant differences in outcome for low-birth-weight infants delivered spontaneously or by forceps. However, since intracranial hemorrhage occurs more often in preterm infants, including those who deliver spontaneously, one should minimize potential trauma to the head through well-controlled deliveries (with or without forceps) and with the use of generous episiotomies if needed. Although one can safely use vacuum extraction with some preterm deliveries, particularly with the new soft-cup devices, the technique is contraindicated for use with infants of extremely low birth weight.

A final issue of some controversy involves the elective use of either forceps or vacuum extraction. This practice is often used in situations in which epidural anesthesia appears to be prolonging the second stage of labor. However, one needs to keep in mind that the current ACOG definition of a prolonged second stage of labor for nulliparous and multiparous patients not given regional anesthesia is a second stage that exceeds 2 hours and 1 hour, respectively; for nulliparas and multiparas receiving regional anesthesia, the second stage must exceed 3 hours and 2 hours, respectively, to be defined as prolonged.[7] However, these definitions should not be interpreted rigidly. For example, if a patient appears to have no evidence of cephalopelvic disproportion and the fetus is not exhibiting a worrisome fetal heart rate pattern, one can quite safely allow a labor to progress. The performance of a difficult low forceps or even a midforceps procedure without evidence of a maternal or fetal problem cannot be justified. Furthermore, there continues to be debate about whether operative vaginal delivery, even as an elective outlet procedure, increases the risk of maternal or fetal trauma. However, some data do suggest that the use of the soft-cup vacuum extractor may be associated with less maternal and perhaps less fetal trauma than obstetric forceps in this situation.[9,10]

The contraindications to operative vaginal delivery are failure to meet the prerequisites described subsequently. Other contraindications to vacuum-extraction procedures are abnormal presentations (face, breech, brow), extreme prematurity, previous scalp sampling, known fetal coagulopathies or thrombocytopenia, and macrosomia.

OBSTETRIC FORCEPS AND VACUUM EXTRACTORS TYPES

Obstetric Forceps

Obstetric forceps are essentially levers. Those in current use have two branches or vecti that either cross like an X or diverge at the end of the handle or shank like a V. The basic parts of obstetric forceps are detailed in Figures 10-1, and 10-2. Figure 10-2 also demonstrates the major differences between the two traction-forceps prototypes, the Elliott and Simpson instruments. The Elliott forceps have overlapping shanks and blades, with less tapered cephalic curves than the Simpson variety. By contrast, the Simpson forceps have parallel shanks and long, tapered blades, a design that makes them particularly suited for use with molded heads. The two parts (branches or vectors) of obstetric forceps are referred to as left or right, according to their orientation to the maternal pelvis after application.

The forceps locks in current use are the English lock, a modified sliding lock with notches on each shank that keep the instrument articulated; the sliding lock, used primarily in instruments designed for rotation, which has a clamp on one of the blades to maintain articulation; and the pivot lock, which allows the divergent forceps to vary the distance of apposition of the blades on the fetal head. Figure 10-3 demonstrates these three lock designs.

The blades of obstetric forceps can be fenestrated or open, as with the classic versions of the Elliott or Simpson instruments; nonfenestrated, as with the Tucker–McLane forceps; or pseudofenestrated, having a depression on the cephalic side that is known as the Luikart modification. Figure 10-4 demonstrates the Tucker–McLane instrument and the Laufe divergent forceps (which has a Luikart modifi-

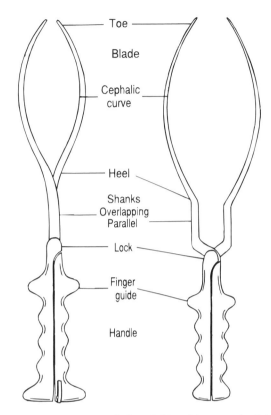

Fig. 10-2. Anatomy of Elliott (left) and Simpson (right) obstetric forceps (superior view). (From Laufe,[3] with permission.)

cation to its blades) along with several other versions of obstetric forceps instrumentation. The shanks of the various forceps can vary in length from as short as 4 cm with the short versions of the Elliott instruments to as long as 15 cm with the Piper forceps.

There are also a number of special instruments designed to accomplish rotation, for use with an af-

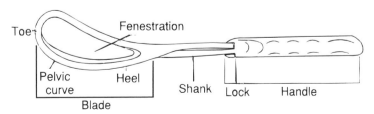

Fig. 10-1. Anatomy of obstetric forceps (lateral view). (From Laufe,[3] with permission.)

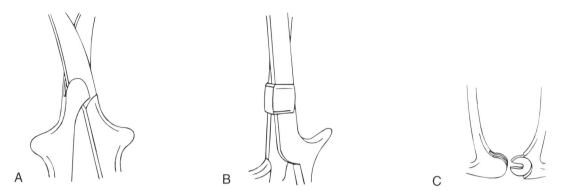

Fig. 10-3. Locking mechanisms for obstetric forceps. **(A)** English lock. **(B)** Sliding lock. **(C)** Pivot lock. (From Laufe,[3] with permission.)

tercoming head with a breech delivery, and for managing a deep transverse arrest. The classic Kielland forceps or the Luikart adaptation of the Kielland forceps have a slight or even backward pelvic curve, a sliding lock that allows them to correct asynclytism, and buttons on the handles for orientation during application. The Luikart version replaces the fenestrated blade with one that is pseudofenestrated and has a handle designed to fill the gap between the handles that exists in the Kielland instrument. The primary function of this instrument is for rotation. Figure 10-4 demonstrates the Luikart version of the Kielland forceps and its minimal pelvic curve as compared to an Elliott model. The Piper forceps, also shown in Figure 10-4, consists of tapered, fenestrated blades and parallel shanks with a marked perineal curve. These instruments are specifically designed for application on the aftercoming head during a breech delivery. One of the more unusual instruments is the Barton forceps, designed specifically for managing a transverse arrest. As shown in Figure 10-4, it consists of a hinged anterior blade and a rigid posterior blade with a marked cephalic curve. Although of historic interest, the Barton forceps is an instrument that is probably infrequently used in today's obstetrics, owing to concern about the safety of midforceps operations as well as most operators' lack of experience with this instrument. The last part of instrumentation in obstetric forceps deliveries is the axis-traction handle. The Bill handle shown in Figure 10-4 can be attached to almost any instrument and allows the operator to more readily maintain traction in the appropriate direction, rather than relying on less precise maneuvers.

Vacuum Extractors

In its basic design, an obstetric vacuum extractor consists of a cup that is attached to the fetal head through suction, connecting tubing, a handle to accomplish traction, and a pump to achieve the vacuum or suction within the cup. As noted earlier, the first modern vacuum extractor was designed by Malmstrom in the 1950s.[6] Its metal cups come in four sizes with internal diameters of 30, 40, 50, and 60 mm. A perforated plate and chain connect the cup to the traction handle. Using either a hand pump or an electronic pump, the operator reaches a negative pressure of 0.6 to 0.8 kg/cm^2, which is equivalent to 18 to 24 cm Hg. However, to achieve a satisfactory artificial caput succedaneum or "chignon" and keep the instrument attached to the infant without increased risk of trauma, one needs to reduce pressure gradually over about 5 or 6 minutes. This need for a slow achievement of a negative pressure in nonemergent situations is one of the distinguishing features of the Malmstrom instrument as compared with newer versions of the vacuum extractor.

More recent has been the introduction of vacuum extractors that use flexible silastic or plastic cups varying from 60 to 65 mm in diameter. As shown in Figure 10-5, these instruments, although somewhat similar in design to the Malmstrom device, disengage at lower pressure, a feature thought to reduce fetal morbidity.[16] Many of the newer instruments are

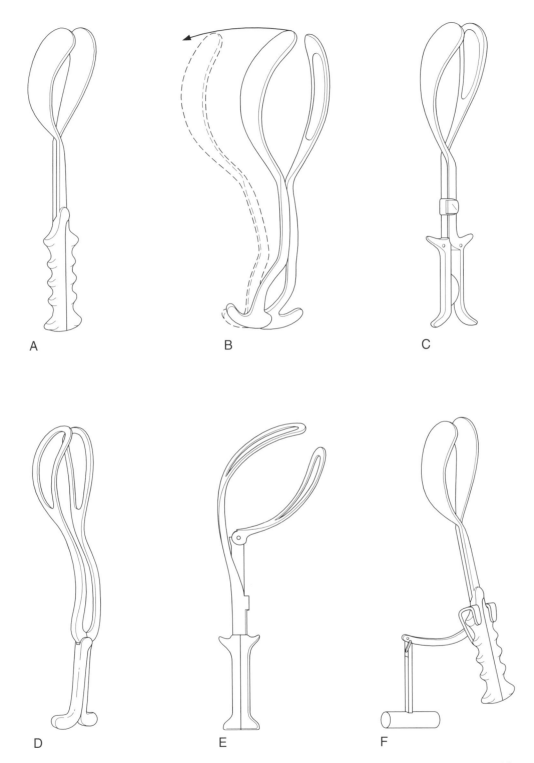

Fig. 10-4. **(A)** Tucker-McLean forceps, **(B)** Laufe divergent forceps, **(C)** Kielland forceps (Luikart modification), **(D)** Piper forceps, **(E)** Barton forceps, and **(F)** Bill traction handle. (Courtesy of Sklar Instruments, West Chester, PA.)

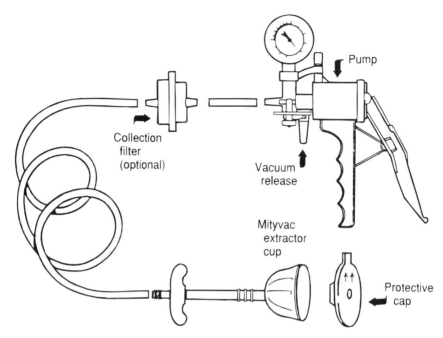

Fig. 10-5. Mityvac vacuum extractor. (Courtesy of Neward Enterprises Inc., Cucamonga, CA.)

lightweight and disposable except for their pump devices.

TECHNIQUES OF FORCEPS OPERATIONS

Prerequisites

A number of prerequisites must be met before initiating a forceps operation. From a fetal standpoint, the presentation must be vertex, the position known, and engagement must exist. With regard to the latter point, one must carefully evaluate each patient to determine the fetal station, since severe molding, asynclitism, and posterior positions may suggest more descent than is actually present. From a maternal standpoint, the cervix must be fully dilated and the membranes ruptured. In addition, a clinical assessment of the pelvis must have been undertaken at some point before forceps application to exclude cephalopelvic disproportion. Additional prerequisites include adequate anesthesia, suitable operator experience, and the ability to proceed immediately to cesarean section should the forceps operation fail. Failure to meet all these prerequisites substantially

increases the risk to both mother and infant. Finally, the operator must understand the anatomy of the pelvis and the cardinal movements of delivery. In spontaneous delivery, uterine contractions and the mother's pushing efforts guide the fetus through the planes of the pelvis. With operative delivery, the ability of the operator to mimic these movements will

---

Essential Prerequisites for Forceps Delivery

Fetal requirements
  Vertex presentation
  Position known
  Engagement present and station known

Maternal requirements
  Full cervical dilation with membranes ruptured
  No indication of cephalopelvic disproportion

Other requirements
  Adequate anesthesia
  Operator experience
  Ability to proceed to cesarean section

substantially determine whether the delivery will proceed smoothly and without problems, or whether it will be difficult, with increased morbidity.

Outlet and Low-Forceps Operations

Occiput-Anterior Fetuses

Once the decision to undertake a forceps operation has been made, the next step is selection of the appropriate instrument. In the case of molded heads, as are usually seen in the fetuses of primipara patients, the Simpson-type forceps offers a long, tapered cephalic curve that better fits the fetal head. With less-molded heads, Elliot-type forceps, such as the Tucker–McLane forceps with or without the Luikart modification, are often selected, since the cephalic curve is less tapered and the overlapping shanks cause less distension of the perineum. However, it should be noted that many skilled operators will use only one type of forceps for most operations throughout their career, with results equivalent to those who tend to routinely vary their instrumentation. The major reasons for success in both circumstances are adherence to the prerequisites listed above, gentle and appropriate application of the forceps to the fetal vertex, and traction that follows the actual vectors through the planes of the maternal pelvis.

After selecting an appropriate forceps, one should ensure emptying of the patient's bladder if it is full, ensure that there is adequate anesthesia, and lubricate the forceps blades. Holding the forceps articulated in the position they will assume in front of the perineum before beginning the operation will serve as a quick reminder of the proper application. In general, one inserts the blade of the left branch first to facilitate articulation. If the right blade is inserted initially, one must manipulate and uncross the shanks to achieve articulation. There are two methods of insertion of the forcep blades: (1) a "direct" insertion along the side of the fetal skull, in front of the ear and over the maternal ischial spines, and (2) an "indirect" insertion into the hollow of the sacrum, followed by "wandering" or moving the blade to its proper position.

With the "direct" approach, the shank of the left branch is held nearly vertical by the operator's left hand, with the handle inclined somewhat toward the

right maternal groin. One places the index and middle finger of the right hand between the fetal head and vaginal wall to guide the insertion of the forceps blade, create a space between the fetal head and vagina, and reduce the chance of soft-tissue trauma to either mother or infant. The blade is then cradled between the fingers and the thumb. As the handle is dropped and the shank slides over the operator's thumb, the blade usually slides almost effortlessly between the fetal head and vaginal wall to achieve a bimalar-biparietal cephalic forceps application. If needed, the thumb of the vaginal hand is used to exert pressure toward the fetal head to guide the insertion. One should not exert pressure through manipulation of the forceps handle. Figure 10-6 demonstrates the initial insertion of the left branch. Figure 10-7 shows an appropriate application.

Occasionally, prominent ischial spines may make the direct approach technically difficult, prompting the decision to proceed with the indirect insertion method. In this procedure, the shank of the left for-

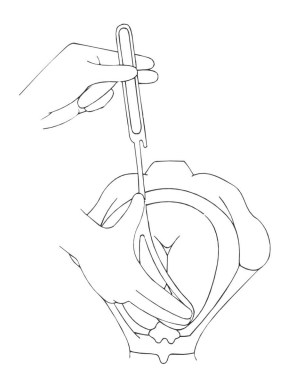

Fig. 10-6. Occiput-anterior position, insertion of the left forceps branch. (From Laufe,[3] with permission.)

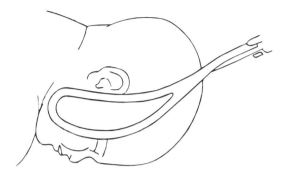

Fig. 10-7. Cephalic (bimalar-biparietal) forceps application. (From Laufe,[3] with permission.)

ceps blade is also held nearly vertical, but in this case, to facilitate insertion into the hollow of the sacrum, the handle is inclined toward the left maternal groin. As the shank is depressed during insertion, one also circumscribes the handle in a wide counterclockwise arc to "wander" or position the blade appropriately on the fetal skull. In this approach it is necessary for the handles to describe a wide arc in order to avoid trauma. If one remembers that for-

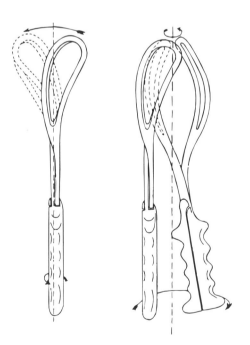

Fig. 10-8. Rotation of forceps. (From Laufe,[3] with permission.)

ceps are essentially levers, minimizing trauma calls for the toe of the blades to be the point of rotation or fulcrum, rather than the distal shanks, as shown in Figure 10-8. Alternatively, after insertion of the left forceps blade into the sacral hollow, one can use the fingers of the right hand to gently push the blade into proper position.

After initial application, one can adjust the blade by depressing the handle further and using the fingers of the right hand to exert most of the force needed to properly position it along the fetal skull. The right blade is then inserted in a similar manner, but with reversal of the hands and positions described above. If necessary, the left branch can be held in place by an assistant while the right branch is inserted. At this point the branches are articulated or locked. If the blades are properly applied, this is a simple maneuver. When difficulty is encountered, it is usually necessary to adjust the application of one or the other branches; the locking of the branches should not be used as the means of adjustment.

Once the forceps branches are locked, one must assure that proper application has been achieved before proceeding further. The three cardinal points that indicate proper application are (1) the sagittal suture is equidistant between the branches; (2) with fenestrated blades, a finger can be inserted between the fetal head and the heel of the blade, while with

---

Cardinal Points in Appropriate Application of Outlet or Low Forceps to the Fetal Head

1. The sagittal suture is equidistant between the branches of the forceps.
2. With fenestrated blades, a finger can be inserted between the heel and fetal head; with solid blades, the space between the heel and head is equivalent on both sides.
3. The posterior fontanelle is one finger's width above the plane of the shanks.

Points 1 and 2 ensure that the forceps application is symetric, while point 3 provides assurance that the forceps blades are in a proper position in relation to the fetal head.

solid blades the space between the fetal head and heels should be equivalent on each side; and (3) the posterior fontanelle is about one finger's width above the plane of the shanks.

Traction on the forceps is the next step in the operation. Depressing the shanks below the horizontal initially helps correct deflexion of the fetal head and often improves the ease of delivery. The operator should be seated, with the forearms flexed, so that the instrument can be grasped from beneath. Traction must be applied in such a way as to follow the curve of the pelvis or, more accurately, the vectors through the planes of the pelvis. The use of the Saxtorph-Pajot maneuver, as shown in Figure 10-9, allows one to achieve the appropriate angle of traction. Alternatively, one can utilize an axis-traction handle. Traction should essentially mimic the forces generated by labor, and should be applied with steady, continuous efforts rather than jerking motions. Side-to-side motions or "wiggling" should be avoided, since such movement serves only to increase the risk of vaginal laceration. Between traction efforts, the forceps should be unlocked to reduce skull compression. In most cases the initial traction effort is in a downward direction at an angle of 45 degrees or greater below the horizontal, in order to bring the fetal occiput under the maternal symphysis pubis. During this step, one must closely observe the descent or check the descent using the fingers of one hand (or both). Once the occiput is below the symphysis, one proceeds to traction that will assist the extension of the head. To accomplish this, the operator maintains outward traction while slowly elevating the forceps handles as further descent occurs, with the symphysis acting as the fulcrum of the movement. At the end of this step, as the fetal occiput presents through the vulvar ring, the forceps handles will be above the symphysis, pointing toward the maternal abdomen. If needed, an episeotomy can be done before application of the forceps, immediately after application, or near the end of the traction effort. Once the fetal head presents at the vulvar ring, the forceps can be removed in a reverse manner to that of their application; as the branches are removed, the shanks should be vertical with the handles inclined to their position at initial application. One should never force the removal of the forceps branches; if necessary, the fetal head can be delivered with the forceps still applied. While the forceps are removed, the head can be held in place with the Ritgen maneuver, which can then be used to finish the delivery.

Rotation Operations of 45 Degrees or Less

Fetal rotations of 45 degrees or less can be done with instruments primarily designed for traction; special instrumentation, such as the Kielland forceps, is not usually needed. The basic steps of application are followed as described above, with some modifications. When inserting the forceps, one should insert the posterior branch first to prevent the fetal head from rotating to a transverse or even posterior position during the forceps application. With a left occiput-anterior position, one inserts the left branch initially; with a right occiput-anterior position one inserts the right branch first. With oblique positions,

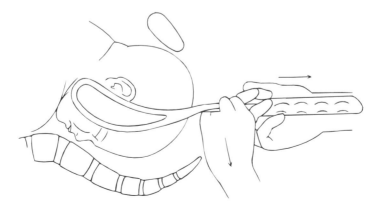

Fig. 10-9. Saxtorph–Pajot maneuver. (From Laufe,[3] with permission.)

the handle will be almost opposite the maternal groin when positioned just prior to insertion. One still utilizes the fingers of the opposite hand to guide the blade to a position in front of the fetal ear while the shank and handle descend. The anterior branch is then inserted into the hollow of the sacrum as described previously, and the blade is wandered over the fetal brow and into position. After articulating the branches together, one should check the cardinal points. To accomplish the rotation, the handles are swung through a moderate arc toward the midline and elevated. This approach minimizes the movement of the blades as the toes of the blades become the fulcrum for the rotation, as illustrated in Figure 10-8. After ascertaining that the rotation has been successful, traction is exerted in the previously described manner.

Occiput-Posterior Fetuses

Delivery of a fetus in the occiput-posterior position without rotation requires some modification of the technique described for the occiput-anterior presentation. The basic insertion technique is the same. However, when the forceps are applied, the toes of the blades curve toward the fetal mouth. Therefore, use of the Simpson-type instruments with their more tapered blades ensures a better fit and reduces the chance of fetal trauma. The cardinal points of proper application are the same, except that the posterior fontanelle should be one finger's width below the plane of the shanks. Traction is applied so as to follow the curve of the pelvis. However, during delivery, the fetal head undergoes flexion rather than extension. Therefore, the initial traction vector is usually only slightly below the horizontal until the brow has been pulled under the symphysis pubis. After this point has been reached, one flexes the fetal head to achieve delivery. However, since a larger diameter of the head passes through the perineum than with an occiput-anterior delivery, one should utilize a liberal episiotomy to avoid undesired perineal lacerations.

Midforceps Operations

Rotation Operations of Greater Than 45 Degrees

Rotations of greater than 45 degrees require that the operator be experienced in forceps operations. Although traction instruments can be used to accom-plish such rotations, many operators elect to use instruments more specifically designed for rotation. Before initiating rotation operations of this degree, however, one must be assured the prerequisites have been met. In particular, the fetal position must be known, and cephalopelvic disproportion should be ruled out as a likely reason for the fetal cephalic position. In a 1983 review of midforceps operations by Richardson and colleagues,[17] the authors suggested that the comparative standard is cesarean section, and that midforceps procedures must be examined from the standpoint of improvement or lack of an increase in either maternal or fetal morbidity. Because this review was published before the 1988 reclassification of forceps operations, these "standards" should be considered before proceeding with a low or midforceps procedure (under the current classification), such as is described in this section. Additionally, a recent survey indicates that many teaching institutions have essentially abandoned midforceps or extensive rotation procedures.[1] Therefore, the overall frequency of these procedures is likely to diminish markedly over the next decade.

For more extensive rotation operations, the Luikart modification of the Kielland forceps is ideal because of its minimal pelvic curve, sliding lock, and applicability for traction following the rotation. However, since rotation is from a transverse or near transverse position to an anterior position, use of the Luikart-modified Kielland forceps when the pelvic type is android or platypelloid is ill advised, since the rotation results in a fetal position that is unlikely to result in a successful, nontraumatic vaginal delivery.

When beginning the operation, aligning the Kielland forceps' branches outside the perineum in the position of final application will avoid confusion and errors during insertion. The buttons on the handles should be pointing toward the fetal occiput. The branch that will become anterior is inserted first. In the case of a left occiput-transverse position, for example, it is the right branch that is inserted first; with a right occiput-transverse position, the left branch is inserted first. Although various methods have been described for inserting and positioning the anterior branch, the safest approach is to insert the blade laterally over the fetal brow or face, then wander it into position around the face anteriorly, using the fingers of the vaginal hand. During this maneuver, the handle is aligned to the opposite maternal buttock to minimize movement of the blade's toe. Alternatively, the branch can be held upside down (the guide buttons pointing toward the floor), inserted to the side of the pelvis containing the occiput, and then wandered over the occiput into proper position. When considering these two approaches to wandering the anterior blade into position, one can clearly appreciate the utility of positioning the articulated forceps before insertion, and the usefulness of the directional buttons. The posterior branch is then inserted into the sacral hollow. To avoid uncrossing, it should be introduced in front of the anterior blade. The vaginal hand should guide the blade along the fetal head and inside the cervix. Occasionally, gentle up-and-down motions, while keeping the blade closely applied to the side of the fetal head with the vaginal hand, will assist in insertion.

Because of the sliding lock of the Luikart-modified Kielland forceps, the shanks can usually be readily articulated. However, asynclitism may cause the handles to not be aligned. After checking to be sure the posterior fontanelle is posterior to the plane of the shanks, one can pull on the trigger-like projection of the handle closest to the perineum while pushing on the opposite trigger to correct the asynclitism. Moving the handles horizontally toward the fetal face will correct any deflexion. The rotation is then accomplished by essentially pronating one's hand while grasping the forceps handles. Because of the minimal pelvic curve of the instrument, the handles do not have to circumscribe a wide arc. Occasionally, slight upward pressure on the shanks will facilitate the rotation. Traction can be exerted after the rotation has been done. However, the shanks must be lowered well below the horizontal plane to compensate for the forceps's limited pelvic curve. The direction of traction follows the vectors of the pelvic planes, as described previously. For descriptions of other types of forceps rotations or midforceps applications, interested readers should consult the specialized textbooks by Laufe or Dennen.[3,4]

Use of Piper Forceps to Deliver an Aftercoming Head With a Breech Presentation

The use of Piper forceps to deliver an aftercoming head may be the only legitimate pelvic application of forceps in modern obstetrics. With an assistant holding the fetus in a horizontal plane, one usually introduces the left branch first to avoid uncrossing the branches during articulation. The handle of the left branch is positioned opposite the maternal right groin, while the shank is held below the horizontal. With the right hand guiding the blade into the vagina, the operator circumscribes a wide arc while raising the handle upward and toward the midline. The opposite branch is applied similarly, although the hands and positions are obviously reversed. The assistant can usually facilitate application of the branches by swinging the fetus's body away from the side of application. Once the branches are articulated, traction is essentially exerted in a horizontal to slightly downward direction while elevating the handles to encourage flexion of the fetal head. Since delivery is usually accomplished with the forceps applied, the operator must be prepared to support the head after delivery through the perineum.

Vacuum-Extraction Operations

The definitions, indications, and prerequisites for the use of vacuum extraction to effect a vaginal delivery are the same as for forceps operations. Although some authors have reported use of this type of procedure in a fairly high proportion of deliveries classified as midforceps operations, it should be stressed that apart from exceptional circumstances, it should not be used with high fetal stations, owing to the potential risks involved.

In performing a vaginal delivery by vacuum extraction, one should check the system carefully before using it, to ensure that all parts are present and that the delivery team knows how to assemble them, and to be certain that suitable vacuum pressure can be obtained once the instrument is applied. Regardless of the type of cup to be used, the operator must ensure that the cervical lip or vaginal tissue is not entrapped within the cup after application. One should wipe the fetal scalp clean prior to application of the cup to ensure that a proper seal will be obtained. If using metal cups, one should use the largest cup possible. When applying any type of cup, it should be positioned as far posterior as possible, ideally over the posterior fontanelle. Insertion is done in a manner quite similar to that for inserting a contraceptive diaphragm. Plastic cups have the advantage of enabling the operator to flex their edges to ease insertion beyond the vaginal introitus. Once the cup is brought into position on the fetal head, the operator should sweep a finger around the circumference of the cup to be sure that vaginal or cervical tissue has not become trapped. After checking the application of the cup, one can produce a vacuum of about 4 in Hg to initiate adherence of the cup.

Vacuum extractors are designed only for traction; they cannot be utilized for active rotation. However, with these devices, the fetal head is free to rotate to the position that has the least resistance, which will usually enhance delivery. Positioning the cup posteriorly corrects deflexion and allows descent and "natural" rotation. Traction should be perpendicular to the cup and in the axis of the pelvis, as with forceps deliveries. Traction should be exerted during contractions; maternal pushing efforts should be encouraged. The operator should use one hand to perform traction while the other hand is used to check the fetal station and progress of the traction efforts. Before initiating traction, one must achieve an adequate vacuum. A pressure of 15 to 24 in Hg provides adequate adherence of the cup while reducing the risk of fetal trauma. Unlike the newer soft-cup instruments, the Malmstrom device requires 5 or 6 minutes to achieve vacuum. Between contractions, one can reduce the vacuum with the newer systems to about 4 in Hg. In general, one should not allow the system to remain at maximum allowable pressures for more than 10 accrued minutes while attempting delivery. The pulling off of the cups with loss of suction, which occurs at forces of less than 22 kg with the newer devices, should be considered a safety feature.[16] When the cup pulls off repeatedly, the operator should consider the possibility of relative cephalopelvic disproportion or a more serious condition, which may make vaginal delivery infeasible or unsafe. Once the vertex presents at the introitus, one exerts traction upward so as to complete extension of the fetal head. The vacuum can then be released, the cup removed, and delivery completed in the usual manner.

Trial Forceps and Failed Forceps Delivery

The terms *trial forceps delivery* and *failed forceps delivery* have been somewhat controversial, since they imply that operators who have attempted such deliveries

on a trial basis, which failed, have not met the basic prerequisites for attempting operative vaginal delivery. However, it must be accepted that the determination of both fetal size and pelvic dimensions is at best subjective. Therefore, it is appropriate to attempt operative delivery provided that one can proceed expeditiously to cesarean section if the attempt is unsuccessful. Several authors have documented the lack of an increased risk of neonatal morbidity if either forceps or vacuum extraction is attempted in this manner.[18–20]

MORBIDITY WITH OPERATIVE VAGINAL DELIVERY

With the increased use of cesarean section to manage many of the obstetric problems listed as indications for forceps deliveries, the comparative standards of today are whether operative vaginal delivery can be accomplished with less risk to the mother, and whether fetal outcome can either be improved or not be worsened with vaginal delivery as compared to cesarean section. In addition, a corollary to any morbidity analysis is whether forceps procedures have a greater risk than vacuum extraction.

Maternal Morbidity

There is little question that cesarean section is associated with greater maternal morbidity than forceps operations. As shown in Table 10-2, a study compar-

Table 10-2. Frequency of Maternal Events, Midforceps versus Cesarean Section, UCLA Medical Center, 1981–1988[a]

	Midforceps (n = 358)	Cesarean Section (n = 486)
Mean length of stay (days)	2.5	5.0
Lacerations		
Cervicovaginal	64 (18%)	15 (3%)
Third-degree	52 (14.5%)	0
Fourth-degree	43 (12%)	0
Uterine extension	0	102 (21%)
Bladder	0	3 (0.6%)
Febrile morbidity	14 (4%)	122 (25%)
Transfusion	7 (2%)	29 (6%)
Thromboembolism	0	7 (1.4%)

[a] Old midforceps definition.
(Adapted from Bashore et al,[21] with permission.)

ing all non-repeat cesarean section deliveries and all midforceps deliveries (old definition) between 1981 and 1988 at the University of California, Los Angeles Medical Center found that midforceps deliveries were generally associated with less significant maternal morbidity.[21] One can reasonably assume that outlet and low-forceps deliveries are also associated with no greater or, more likely, with less morbidity than seen with midforceps deliveries.

When one compares forceps deliveries with vacuum extraction, the literature generally suggests that vacuum extraction is associated with less trauma. Table 10-3 presents the results of four randomized clinical trials examining the differences between forceps and vacuum extraction.[9,10,22,23] The British study by Vacca and colleagues evaluated the use of a modification of the Malmstrom instrument versus forceps operations.[22] Operators with varied experience participated in the trial; the study did not provide a classification of the type of operative delivery (e.g., outlet, low, or midforceps). Another British study, by Johanson and co-workers, compared a silicone-cup vacuum extractor with forceps.[23] As with the Vacca study, there was no classification of the operative deliveries in the report of the study. The American study by Williams and co-workers compared the CMI Soft Touch vacuum extractor with forceps applications.[10] In this study the vast majority of applications in both groups were either classified as low forceps or outlet forceps. Furthermore, by contrast with what was done in prior studies, women whose deliveries were completed on a basis other than initial randomization were evaluated separately. However, Table 10-3 includes only those women who completed delivery by the initial method in this study. In the study by Dell and associ-

Table 10-3. Randomized Clinical Trials Comparing Vacuum Extraction to Forceps Deliveries: Maternal Mortality[a]

Study	Vacuum Extraction		Forceps
Vacca et al[22] (1983)			
(152 Bird cup, 152 forceps)			
Lacerations			
Third- and fourth-degree	9 (5.9%)		26 (17.1%)
Vaginal	5[a] (3.3%)		10 (13.2%)
Cervical	1 (0.7)		0
Hematoma	0		2 (1.3%)
Uterine rupture	0		1 (0.7%)
Johanson et al[23] (1989)			
(132 Silicone cup, 132 forceps)			
Lacerations			
Third- and fourth-degree	6 (4.5)		16 (12.1%)
Vaginal	8 (6.0%)		24 (18.2%)
Williams et al[10] (1991)			
(41 CMI Soft Touch cup, 40 forceps)			
Lacerations			
Third- and fourth-degree	12 (29.3%)		12 (30%)
Vaginal	6 (14.6%)		7 (17.5)
Postpartum hemorrhage	3 (7.3%)		5 (12.5%)
Endometritis	3 (7.3%)		6 (15%)
Dell et al[9] (1985)	Silastic	Mityvac	
(36 Silastic cup, 37 Mityvac cup, 45 forceps)			
Lacerations			
Third- and fourth-degree	12 (33.3%)	6 (16.2%)	10 (22.2%)
Vaginal	2 (5.6%)	3 (8.1%)	17 (37.8%)
Cervical	5 (13.9%)	3 (8.1%)	7 (15.6%)
Hematoma	0	0	1 (2.2%)

[a] All crossed over to another method to effect delivery.

ates in New Orleans, the investigators compared a silastic and Mityvac vacuum extractor to forceps.[9] All deliveries were completed by second-year house officers, and all deliveries were low-forceps procedures according to the old classification. Although Table 10-3 suggests that vacuum extraction may be associated with less morbidity than forceps operations, the two American studies of these procedures also indicate that with low- or outlet-forceps classifications, the difference in morbidity with the two approaches may not be as great as some authors suggest. Thus, proper timing of a forceps operation, coupled with adequate knowledge of the technique of application should result in little difference in morbidity when using forceps or vacuum extraction to accomplish a simple low or outlet procedure.

Additionally, operators should be aware of several recent studies that document the association of midline episiotomy with an increased risk of third- and fourth-degree perineal laceration, and which show that the use of forceps independently increases the risk of such lacerations over that in spontaneous vaginal deliveries.[24–31] For example, Shiono and coworkers, in examining the Collaborative Perinatal Project data, showed that mediolateral episiotomy reduced the frequency of such lacerations by about 2.5-fold in nulliparous women; midline episiotomy was associated with a 4.2-fold increase in the same group of women.[31] In addition, forceps deliveries increased the risk of third- and fourth-degree perineal lacerations by about eightfold over that with spontaneous delivery. Data from Crawford and colleagues[24] and Helwig and associates[25] also suggest that forceps carry a somewhat greater risk of causing laceration than does vacuum extraction. In addition to the immediate discomfort associated with such laceration and the need for a meticulous repair, Crawford and colleagues' study documented that 17 percent of women experiencing a third- or fourth-degree laceration complained of incontinence of flatus at 6 to 9 months after delivery.[24] Several European studies have also documented that such tears may ultimately be associated with pelvic-floor dysfunction, including fecal incontinence.[27–30] Such literature indicates that operators may wish to utilize mediolateral episiotomies when extensions seem likely on beginning an operative delivery (e.g., in cases of macrosomia or a short perineum). Further,

such data would also argue against the routine use of operative delivery procedures, particularly in nulliparous women.

Perinatal Morbidity

A critical analysis of perinatal morbidity associated with operative vaginal delivery is complicated by multiple confounders, including varying indications for delivery, changing definitions for operative delivery, operator experience, type of anesthesia, parity, duration of follow-up, differences in either assessment or treatment of infants during the long periods encompassed by many of these studies, frequent use of retrospective case reviews as opposed to prospective observational or randomized study designs, and lack of appropriate control groups. Therefore, most of the conclusions reached in studies of operative vaginal delivery require some subjective interpretation to put the various findings into a clinically useful perspective.

When one examines the information available about midforceps deliveries with either the older or newer definitions, it is clear that such operations, if done at a relatively high station, may carry significant neonatal risk.[17] For example, Hughey and coworkers,[32] using a perinatal morbidity index, demonstrated an unfavorable immediate fetal outcome in 30 percent of midforceps deliveries, as compared with no morbidity in a small cesarean section comparison group.[32] A study by Bowes and Bowes[33] in 1980 also suggested that midforceps deliveries caused more neonatal morbidity. However, their comparison group was normal spontaneous deliveries, a comparator that is not the most appropriate for this type of analysis. Chiswick and James[34] also compared infants delivered by midforceps with those undergoing vaginal delivery. Evidence of birth trauma was noted in 15 percent of the forceps group, including three neonatal deaths from tentorial tears. In addition, 17.4 percent of the infants delivered by forceps had delayed respiration and 23.4 percent had abnormal neurologic behavior. Gilstrap and associates' study found no significant differences in neonatal morbidity when midforceps deliveries were compared to both spontaneous delivery and cesarean section after adjusting for indication.[35] It should be noted that in this study, the station at the time of forceps application was probably lower than reported in earlier studies. More recently, when stratifying immediate neonatal morbidity according to either the new or old classification of forceps deliveries, Hagadorn-Freathy and co-workers[36] demonstrated that deliveries with higher stations were associated with increased morbidity. Two recent studies have also indicated that forceps deliveries may be associated with increased risk of either transient[21] or permanent seventh-nerve palsy.[37] In summary, review of the available literature suggests that the performance of difficult midforceps deliveries increases the risk of significant neonatal morbidity. Therefore, such operations are to be avoided. Although there are fewer data on low- or outlet-forceps deliveries, the study by Hagadorn-Freathy et al[36] did suggest that neonatal trauma was less frequent with such deliveries than with midforceps deliveries. As previously discussed in the section on indications for forceps delivery, data on the use of this technique with premature infants are conflicting.

The four randomized clinical trials comparing vacuum extraction to forceps delivery showed little difference in immediate neonatal morbidity with the two approaches.[9,10,22,23] The studies by Dell et al[9] and Williams et al[10] reported a greater number of superficial skin changes with forceps than with vacuum extraction, Johanson and co-workers[23] suggested that vacuum extraction produced more changes of this type, and Vacca et al[22] reported no differences. The study by Dell et al[9] also suggested that cephalhematoma might be more common with vacuum extraction, although the other three studies did not have such findings. Major morbidity did not appear to be a significant occurrence in any of these trials; however, the small sample sizes do not permit a satisfactory analysis of this question. Furthermore, prolonged follow-up was not included in these studies. Despite these shortcomings, the data suggest that with low-station deliveries, as reported primarily in the American studies, there appears to be little significant difference in the occurrence of immediate fetal trauma with forceps or vacuum-extraction procedures, and that the frequency of major trauma with the two procedures appears to be low.

Relative to long-term morbidity, many of the studies are conflicting. Several earlier studies suggested an increased risk of cerebral palsy with midforceps deliveries[38–40]; other studies did not demonstrate such an association.[41,42] Recent reviews of cerebral palsy suggest that it is a complex process, with most cases probably resulting from events preceding the intrapartum period.[43] Therefore, given the multiplicity of potential risk factors, it is difficult to assign any significant risk to forceps operations in most cases of this disorder. Similarly, data from examinations of intellectual development are also conflicting. For example, as discussed in a review by Richardson et al[17] of midforceps deliveries, two studies comparing such deliveries to spontaneous deliveries, using data from the Collaborative Perinatal Project, showed no differences in mental development or intelligence quotient (IQ) score,[11,44] while a third study showed lower IQ scores among infants delivered by midforceps.[45] All three studies had methodologic flaws with the potential for bias. Furthermore, a subsequent reanalysis of much of the same data also showed lower IQ scores following midforceps deliveries but no significant impact on IQ scores with low-forceps procedures (old definition).[46] A more recent study of Israeli draftees provides little evidence of substantive differences in IQ scores according to method of delivery.[47]

In summary, operative vaginal delivery is associated with neonatal risks. However, it appears that avoidance of difficult operative deliveries and or deliveries with high stations reduces such morbidity to an acceptable level.

CONCLUSION

Although the use of operative vaginal delivery remains controversial, it is an important part of the armentarium of modern obstetricians. As with most technical skills, attention to detail, coupled with practice, will result in better outcomes. With today's concerns about the appropriateness of many cesarean sections, operative techniques for vaginal delivery offer an opportunity to facilitate such delivery without resorting to major surgery. However, ultimate success requires both the application of technical skills and the use of sound judgment.

REFERENCES

1. Ramin SM, Little BB, Gilstrap LC: Survey of forceps delivery in North America in 1990. Obstet Gynecol 81: 307, 1993

2. Das K: Obstetric Forceps—Its History and Evolution. Medical Museum Publishing, Leeds, 1929

3. Laufe LE: Obstetric Forceps. Hoeber Medical Division, Harper & Row, New York, 1968

4. Dennen PC: Dennen's Forceps Deliveries. 3rd Ed. FA Davis, Philadelphia, 1989

5. Zahniser SC, Kendrick JS, Franks AL et al: Trends in obstetric operative procedures, 1980–1987. Am J Public Health 82:1340, 1992

6. Chalmers JA: The Ventouse—The Obstetric Vacuum Extractor. Year Book Medical Publishers, Chicago, 1971

7. American College of Obstetricians and Gynecologists: Operative vaginal delivery. ACOG Technical Bulletin No. 152, Washington, DC, February, 1991

8. Maryniak GM, Frank JB: Clinical assessment of the Kobayashi vacuum extractor. Obstet Gynecol 64:431, 1984

9. Dell DL, Sightler SE, Plauche WC: Soft cup vacuum extraction: a comparison of outlet delivery. Obstet Gynecol 66:624, 1985

10. Williams MC, Knuppel RA, O'Brien WF, et al: A randomized comparison of assisted vaginal delivery by obstetric forceps and polyethylene vacuum cup. Obstet Gynecol 78:789, 1991

11. Bishop EH, Israel SL, Briscoe CL: Obstetrical influences on the premature infant's first year of development—a report from the Collaborative Study of Cerebral Palsy. Obstet Gynecol 23:549, 1980

12. Haesslin H, Goodlin R: Survey of the tiny newborn. Am J Obstet Gynecol 134:192, 1979

13. O'Driscoll K, Meagher D, MacDonald D et al: Traumatic intracranial haemorrhage in firstborn infants and delivery with obstetric forceps. Br J Obstet Gynaecol 88:577, 1981

14. Fairweather D: Obstetric management and follow-up of the very low-birth weight infant. J Reprod Med 26:387, 1981

15. Schwartz DB, Miodovnik M, Lavin JP: Neonatal outcome among low birth weight infants delivered spontaneously or by low forceps. Obstet Gynecol 62:283, 1983

16. Duchon MA, DeMund MA, Brown RH: Laboratory comparison of modern vacuum extractors. Obstet Gynecol 71:155, 1988

17. Richardson DA, Evans MI, Cibils LA: Midforceps delivery: a critical review. Am J Obstet Gynecol 145: 621, 1983

18. Boyd ME, Usher RH, McLean FH et al: Failed forceps. Obstet Gynecol 68:779, 1986

19. Lowe B: Fear of failure: a place for the trial of instrumental delivery. Br J Obstet Gynaecol 94:60, 1987

20. Berkus MD, Ramamurthy RS, O'Connor PS et al: Cohort study of silastic obstetric vacuum cup deliveries. II. Unsuccessful vacuum extraction. Obstet Gynecol 68:662, 1986

21. Bashore RA, Phillips WH, Brinkman CR: A comparison of the morbidity of midforceps and cesarean delivery. Am J Obstet Gynecol 162:1428, 1990

22. Vacca A, Grant A, Wyatt G et al: Portsmouth operative delivery trial: a comparison vacuum extraction and forceps delivery. Br J Obstet Gynaecol 90:1107, 1983

23. Johanson R, Pusey J, Livera N et al: North Staffordshire/Wignan assisted delivery trial. Br J Obstet Gynaecol 96:537, 1989

24. Crawford LA, Quint EH, Pearl ML et al: Incontinence following rupture of the anal sphincter during delivery. Obstet Gynecol 82:527, 1993

25. Helwig JT, Thorp JM, Bowes WA: Does midline episiotomy increase the risk of third- and fourth-degree lacerations in operative vaginal deliveries? Obstet Gynecol 82:276, 1994

26. Walker MPR, Farine D, Rolbin SH et al: Epidural anesthesia, episiotomy, and obstetric laceration. Obstet Gynecol 77:668, 1991

27. Snooks SJ, Henry MM, Swash M: Faecal incontinence due to external anal sphincter division in childbirth is associated with damage to the innervation of the pelvic musculature; a double pathology. Br J Obstet Gynaecol 92:824, 1985

28. Sorensen SM, Bondesen H, Istre O et al: Perineal rupture following vaginal delivery-long-term consequences. Acta Obstet Gynecol Scand 67:315, 1988

29. Haadem K, Dahlstrom JA, Lingman G: Anal sphincter function after delivery: a prospective study in women with sphincter rupture and controls. Eur J Obstet Gynecol Reprod Biol 35:7, 1990

30. Haadem K, Ohrlander S, Lingman G: Long-term ailments due to anal sphincter rupture caused by delivery—a hidden problem. Eur J Obstet Gynecol Reprod Biol 27:27, 1988

31. Shiono P, Klebanoff MA, Carey JC: Midline episiotomies: more harm than good? Obstet Gynecol 75:765, 1990

32. Hughey MJ, McElin JW, Lussky R: Forceps operations in perspective: I. Midforceps rotations operations. J Reprod Med 20:253, 1978

33. Bowes WA, Bowes C: Current role of the midforceps operation. Clin Obstet Gynecol 23:549, 1980

34. Chiswick ML, James DK: Kielland forceps: association with neonatal morbidity and mortality. BMJ 1:7, 1979

35. Gilstrap LC, Hauth JC, Schiano S et al: Neonatal acidosis and method of delivery. Obstet Gynecol 63:681, 1984

36. Hagadorn-Freathy AS, Yeomans ER, Hankins GDV: Validation of the 1988 ACOG forceps classification system. Obstet Gynecol 77:356, 1991
37. Falco NA, Eriksson E: Facial nerve palsy in the newborn: incidence and outcome. Plast Reconstr Surg 85:1, 1990
38. Chefetz MD: Etiology of cerebral palsy: role of reproductive insufficiency and the multiplicity of factors. Obstet Gynecol 25:635, 1965
39. Eastman NJ, Kohl SG, Maisel JE et al: The obstetrical background of 753 cases of cerebral palsy. Obstet Gynecol Surv 17:459, 1962
40. Fuldner RV: Labor complications and cerebral palsy. Am J Obstet Gynecol 74:159, 1957
41. Amiel-Tison C: Cerebral damage in full-term newborns, tiological factors, neonatal status and long-term follow-up. Biol Neonat 14:234, 1969
42. Steer CM, Boney W: Obstetric factors in cerebral palsy. Am J Obstet Gynecol 83:526, 1962
43. Kuban KCK, Leviton A: Cerebral palsy. N Engl J Med 330:187, 1994
44. Broman SH, Nichols PL, Kennedy WA: Preschool IQ: Prenatal and Early Development Correlates. Lawrence Erlbaum Associates, Hillsdale, NJ, 1975
45. Friedman EA, Sachtleben MP, Bresky PA: Dysfunctional labor. XII. Long-term effects on infant. Am J Obstet Gynecol 127:779, 1977
46. Friedman EA, Sachtleben-Murray MR, Dahrouge D et al: Long-term effects of labor and delivery on offspring: a matched-pair analysis. Am J Obstet Gynecol 150:941, 1984
47. Seidman DS, Laor A, Gale R et al: Long-term effects of vacuum and forceps deliveries. Lancet 337:1583, 1991

Shoulder Dystocia

Peter E. Nielsen and Bernard Gonik

Shoulder dystocia is an infrequent, unexpected, and potentially catastrophic obstetric emergency that occurs at a time when expert consultation may be unavailable and which may result in serious complications for both mother and fetus. Therefore, all clinicians engaged in the practice of obstetrics should understand the need to have a clinical management plan that may be instituted in the delivery room to decrease maternal and fetal morbidity.

EPIDEMIOLOGY

The overall incidence of shoulder dystocia is reported to be 0.15 to 0.63 percent, or about 1 in 300 vaginal deliveries.[1] However, the incidence of this complication varies greatly and depends upon a variety of clinical factors, including clinician awareness. Langer and colleagues[2] retrospectively reviewed 75,979 women who delivered vaginally, and determined the incidence of shoulder dystocia according to the presence or absence of maternal diabetes and fetal birth weight. The incidence of dystocia in fetuses of diabetic gravid women was found to be significantly increased when the birth weight exceeded 4,250 g (when stratified in 250-g categories from 2,500 to more than 5,000 g). In this study the incidence of shoulder dystocia in infants weighing more than 4,000 g in the presence of maternal diabetes was 15 percent, and in the absence of maternal dia-

betes was only 5 percent. In addition, the incidence of dystocia in those fetuses that weighed more than 4,500 g at birth, and whose mothers had diabetes, was 42 percent, while in the absence of maternal diabetes it was 10 percent. Eighty percent of shoulder dystocias occurred in the maternally diabetic group when the fetal birth weight was more than 4,250 g. By contrast, only one-third of the shoulder dystocias in the maternally nondiabetic group occurred when the fetal birth weight was more than 4,250 g, and only 2.5% occurred when birth weight exceeded 5,000 g. Langer and colleagues included both pregestational and gestational diabetic women in their diabetic group. Figure 11-1 displays combined data from this and the only other retrospective study that stratified the incidence of shoulder dystocia by infant birth weight and the presence or absence of maternal diabetes.[2,3] This figure shows that most shoulder dystocias in fetuses of nondiabetic patients occur at nonmacrosomic birth weights. By contrast, in the presence of maternal diabetes, most shoulder dystocias occur in macrosomic infants. Data from the study by Langer and colleagues is displayed in Figure 11-2 and clearly indicates that the increase in the incidence of shoulder dystocia as birth weight increases occurs disproportionally more often in the presence of maternal diabetes than in nondiabetic parturients at fetal birth weights beyond 4,250 g.[2]

Keller and colleagues noted that in gestational dia-

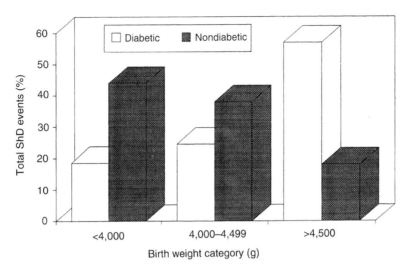

Fig. 11-1. Fraction of total shoulder dystocia (ShD) events related to birth weight category in diabetic and nondiabetic patients. (Data from Langer et al[2] and Acker.[3])

betic patients (class A1 and A2), the incidence of shoulder dystocia was 17 percent among infants with a birth weight of more than 4,000 g.[4] These data are quite similar to those in the previous study[2] that combined pregestational and gestational diabetic patients (incidence of 15 percent). However, fetuses of patients with one abnormal glucose tolerance test value had no significant difference in the incidence of shoulder dystocia compared with patients with a normal test.[5] Interestingly, the prophylactic use of insulin in class A1 diabetic patients (typically not treated with insulin) has been suggested in one report to be a method of decreasing the incidence of birth trauma, including the incidence of shoulder dystocia.[6]

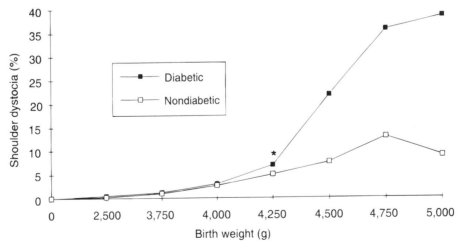

Fig. 11-2. Shoulder dystocia related to birth weight in diabetic and nondiabetic gravid women. *$P < 0.05$. (From Langer et al,[2] with permission.)

MATERNAL AND FETAL MORBIDITY

Delivery complicated by shoulder dystocia may result in a variety of maternal complications. These complications have anecdotally included fourth-degree perineal lacerations, cervical and vaginal lacer-ations, bladder injury and dysfunction, post-partum hemorrhage, and endometritis. In one report, 68 percent of parturients with fetuses having shoulder dystocia had an estimated blood loss in excess of 1,000 ml at delivery. Thirty-seven percent of these patients also had a vaginal laceration requiring repair.[7] In addition, when significant perineal lacer-ations occur in conjunction with shoulder dystocia, they are frequently associated with increased delayed morbidity, such as dehiscence, infection, and fistula formation.[8]

Fetal morbidity associated with shoulder dystocia is often more severe than maternal morbidity. Neonatal injury has certainly been associated with uncomplicated labor courses; however, some intrapartum events are more strongly associated with certain types of neonatal injury. Levine et al,[9] in a retrospective study of 13,870 full-term, consecutive live births, investigated the frequencies of brachial plexus injury, clavicular fracture, and facial nerve injury in newborns. Brachial plexus injury occurred in 2.6 per 1,000 newborns; clavicular fracture in 2.0 per 1,000; and facial nerve injury in 7.5 per 1,000. A variety of factors were found to be associated with an increased risk of fetal injury, including mid- and low-forceps delivery, shoulder dystocia, birth weight greater than 3,500 g, and a second stage of labor exceeding 60 minutes. The authors developed a risk-assessment profile that was applied retrospectively to patients (based on antepartum and delivery data) to assist in the prediction of each of these neonatal injuries. However, using this profile, the authors were only able to correctly predict slightly over 50 percent of the neonatal injuries.[9] These data suggest that, although neonatal injuries are associated with certain intrapartum events such as shoulder dystocia, they may be unpredictable (and therefore unavoidable) in many cases.

The possibility of permanent injury to the infant following shoulder dystocia is the obstetrician's greatest concern when considering neonatal morbidity. The degree of injury is related empirically to both the severity of the shoulder dystocia and the procedure or procedures necessary to resolve it. For example, fundal pressure, when used as the sole method of treating shoulder dystocia, resulted in a 75 percent complication rate, and was strongly associated with orthopedic and neurologic damage when evaluated in one study, although the duration of injury was not reported.[10]

Brachial plexus injuries, among the most common neonatal injuries resulting from shoulder dystocia, are categorized according to the cervical nerve roots affected. Upper brachial plexus injuries involve the C5-C6 nerve roots and are known as Erb's palsies. Lower brachial plexus injuries, known as Klumpke's palsies, involve the C7-C8 nerve roots and are significantly less common than Erb's palsies.

Because acute brachial plexus injury usually resolves within the early neonatal period, the rate of persistent injury has been investigated in several studies, all noting approximately a 5 percent persistence rate.[11,12] For example, an incidence of brachial plexus injury of 1 in 526 births, as reported by the 7-year prospective Collaborative Perinatal Project,[11] with a 5 percent persistence rate, results in one permanent injury in 10,520 births. If this rate is extrapolated to other studies not reporting persistence, the incidence of persistent injury ranges from 1 in 7,500 to 1 in 40,000 births. Interestingly, several studies have suggested that intrauterine maladaptation may play a role in brachial plexus injury as well as in clavicular fracture, and that these injuries may occur before the onset of labor in some patients and spontaneously during the course of labor in others.[13,14] In a study of 57 infants with clavicular fracture, only 3 cases (5 percent) of ipsilateral Erb's palsy were identified, all of which recovered by 3 months of age without neurologic sequelae.[15]

Maternal diabetes also has a special relationship with neonatal injury following shoulder dystocia. Acker and associates[16] found a significantly increased risk of fetal injury associated with delivery involving a diabetic gravid woman. In their review of 32,468 patients, the incidence of Erb's palsy among infants delivered from nondiabetic gravid women was 0.56 per 1,000, while among diabetic gravid women it was 10.5 per 1,000. This significant difference emphasizes the importance of screening for diabetes in pregnancy, since in this study, one in six infants of diabetic gravid women whose deliveries were complicated by fetal shoulder dystocia experienced Erb's palsy.

Central nervous system (CNS) injury may also be a consequence of shoulder dystocia. However, studies that conclude an association with neonatal asphyxia are confounded by a variety of factors, including vaginal delivery methods, fetal heart rate and labor abnormalities, the presence of meconium, and differences in fetal birth weight. Among 245 macrosomic neonates delivered vaginally and reported in three retrospective studies 20 (8.2 percent) manifested evidence of what the authors termed neonatal CNS compromise.[3,17,18] This CNS injury was variably defined as "severe perinatal asphyxia" (although no Apgar scores or cord gas evaluations were provided), uncontrollable seizures, abnormal CNS signs, or 5-minute Apgar scores of less than 7. No long-term follow-up was available for any of these infants; therefore, conclusions regarding the association between neonatal CNS injury and shoulder dystocia cannot be made with certainty.

Finally, fetal death resulting from shoulder dystocia has been reported, and appears to be related to the interval from the diagnosis of dystocia to delivery, as well as to the difficulty involved in reducing the dystocia.[19] However, diagnosis-to-delivery intervals of up to 70 minutes, as well as "difficult" deliveries, have been reported to result in good neonatal outcome.[19,20]

RISK FACTORS

Obstetricians have anecdotally identified many historical, antepartum, and intrapartum risk factors in an effort to predict and prevent shoulder dystocia. Some risk factors historically associated with shoulder dystocia include maternal birth weight, prior shoulder dystocia, prior macrosomia, diabetes, maternal obesity, multiparity, and advanced maternal age. Antepartum risk factors include maternal diabetes, excessive maternal weight gain, fetal macrosomia, short maternal stature, and post-term gestation. Suggested intrapartum risk factors include protraction disorders of the first and second stages of labor, arrest disorders of the second stage, precipitous second-stage labors, fetal molding, midpelvic

delivery (forceps or vacuum extractor), and oxytocin induction and augmentation of labor.

Because few of these purported risk factors have been rigorously evaluated to validate their relationship to the shoulder dystocia event, a recent review of 14,297 parturients with 12,532 vaginal deliveries was undertaken to assess some of these factors.[14] A total of 204 maternal and infant charts related to shoulder dystocia or neonatal injury were evaluated. The incidence of shoulder dystocia in this study was 1.4 percent of all vaginal deliveries, a figure higher than many studies report. Evaluation of the data revealed two subgroups. Charts coded specifically for shoulder dystocia were compared with those without specific coding but with evidence of neonatal injury at birth. When compared with the group coded for shoulder dystocia, the noncoded group had injuries of a significantly different nature; a higher proportion of neonates in the noncoded group had evidence of clavicular fracture at delivery. In addition, this group had a lower mean birth weight (3,528 g) compared with the shoulder dystocia group, whose mean birth weight was 4,112 g ($P<0.01$). Underreporting of shoulder dystocia may have explained some of the difference in injuries between these groups. However, the authors suggested that underreporting did not explain all the injuries, and that clavicular or brachial plexus injury may have occurred spontaneously, and may not have been directly precipitated by shoulder dystocia. Similar findings were reported by Gonik and associates,[21] who speculated that the failure to recognize shoulder dystocia may have contributed to a higher neonatal injury rate through failure to use appropriate corrective maneuvers.

The most important independent risk factors associated with a risk of shoulder dystocia determined by Nocon et al[14] were fetal macrosomia and a maternal history of bearing a previous large infant. Conditions such as diabetes and midforceps delivery after a prolonged second stage of labor became significant risk factors only in the presence of a large fetus. This study concluded that most of the traditional risk factors for shoulder dystocia have no predictive value, since shoulder dystocia in itself is an unpredictable event. Unrelated antepartum or intrapartum risk factors reported by Nocon and co-workers[14] include maternal obesity, multiparity, post-term gestation, oxytocin use, low forceps, episiotomy, and type of anesthesia utilized. Furthermore, it was virtually impossible to predict which infants were at risk of permanent injury, as evidenced by the case of the one nonmacrosomic infant who subsequently had a permanent brachial plexus injury.

Acker and associates[22] evaluated risk factors for shoulder dystocia in nondiabetic mothers with nonmacrosomic fetuses. In their study, infants with birth weights of 3,000 to 3,499 g whose mothers had disorders involving an arrest of labor experienced a significantly greater incidence frequency of shoulder dystocia. In cases in which fetal birth weight ranged from 3,500 to 3,999 g, however, disorders involving both protraction and arrest of labor were associated with a significant increase in the incidence of shoulder dystocia. The use of forceps in the latter group augmented this incidence. Arrest disorders were defined as cessation of dilatation for at least 2 hours in the active phase of labor, a prolongation of the deceleration phase to more than 3 hours in nulliparous women and 1 hour in multiparous women, or cessation of fetal descent for at least 1 hour in the second stage of labor. A protraction disorder was characterized by an active phase rate of dilatation of less than 1.2 cm/hr in the nulliparous and 1.5 cm/hr in the multiparous woman, or a second stage maximum slope of descent of less than 1.0 cm/hr in the nulliparous and 2.0 cm/hr in the multiparous woman.

Precipitous descent of the fetus during the second stage of labor is probably not a significant risk factor for shoulder dystocia, but may be a risk factor for the development of Erb's palsy, especially in the fetuses of diabetic patients. Acker et al reviewed 32,088 deliveries and found that only 6.7 percent of all fetuses with shoulder dystocia had mothers who had a precipitous second stage. However, 32 percent of all infants who sustained a shoulder dystocia and who developed Erb's palsy had been born to mothers who had a precipitous second stage.[16] In addition, all the infants of diabetic gravid women who developed an Erb's palsy had been born to women with a precipitous second stage. Interestingly, all but one of the reported palsies in this study were associated with spontaneous vaginal birth, illustrating the observation that spontaneous delivery is not fully protective against brachial plexus injury.

PREDICTION AND PREVENTION

It is apparent that fetuses at risk of shoulder dystocia cannot be reliably predicted by most maternal history or most antepartum or intrapartum events. Maternal diabetes and fetal macrosomia, however, are two of the best markers for risk. Therefore, the antenatal diagnosis of maternal diabetes and fetal macrosomia is an important goal of prenatal care. The antenatal diagnosis of maternal diabetes is usually straightforward and reliable. However, the prediction of infant birth weights above 4,000 g (macrosomia) is difficult, because most investigators have shown a poor correlation between ultrasonographically estimated fetal weight and actual birth weight in macrosomic infants.[23]

When clinical, sonographic, and parous patient estimates of fetal birth weight were evaluated prospectively, the maternal estimate had the lowest mean error and highest percentage of accuracy to within 10 percent of the actual birth weight (70 percent).[24] The small numbers in this study precluded statistically significant differences between the groups. However, based on these data, maternal estimation of infant birth weight is at least as accurate as clinical and sonographic methods.

In one study that included both diabetic and nondiabetic patients, antepartum ultrasonographic evaluation of estimated fetal weight had a sensitivity of 61 percent, specificity of 70 percent, positive predictive value of 65 percent, and negative predictive value of 67 percent for infants of birth weights over 4,000 g.[25] Therefore, 40 percent of macrosomic infants were missed by ultrasonography, and the latter technique was accurate in detecting macrosomia in just over one-half of these infants.

Because of the modest ability of ultrasound examination to detect macrosomia, a variety of techniques have been promoted to improve the ability to predict a macrosomic infant. Landon and associates[26] evaluated the rate of fetal abdominal growth as a predictor of macrosomic infants in patients with diabetes. A growth rate in abdominal circumference of more than 1.2 cm/wk between 32 and 39 weeks had a sensitivity of 84 percent and specificity of 85 percent for predicting infants with a birth weight exceeding 4,000 g.[26] For improved prediction of fetal macrosomia at term, Landon and colleagues recommended serial ultrasonography during the third trimester in patients with diabetes. Elliott et al used a macrosomia index, derived by subtracting the biparietal diameter from the chest diameter, to predict macrosomia in fetuses of diabetic patients. Using this measurement, 87 percent of macrosomic infants will have a macrosomia index of 1.4 cm or greater.[27] In addition, a prospective study by Modanlou et al[17] evaluating anthropometric measurements in the macrosomic neonate revealed that neonates experiencing shoulder dystocia had a significantly greater shoulder-to-head and chest-to-head disproportion than did either macrosomic neonates delivered by cesarean section because of arrest disorders or macrosomic neonates delivered without shoulder dystocia. This study also noted an increased incidence of shoulder dystocia in neonates whose mean macrosomia index was 1.6 cm. This value dramatically contrasts with that of infants who had no evidence of shoulder dystocia, whose mean macrosomia index was 0.2 cm.[17]

Another method for predicting the birth of macrosomic infants to diabetic mothers is the use of computed tomography (CT) to measure the width of the fetal shoulders. In a study by Kitzmiller and co-workers[28] all infants with an intrapartum fetal shoulder width of 14 cm as measured by CT had birth weights exceeding 4,200 g. Taking 14 cm as a positive test value, and a birth weight of 4,200 g as an abnormal result, the positive predictive value of the CT technique was determined to be 78 percent and the negative predictive value was 100 percent.[28] As expected, the value of this approach in the clinical setting is limited.

Maternal characteristics that may be predictive of fetal macrosomia include multiparity, advanced maternal age, a prepregnancy weight of more than 70 kg, a ponderal index (weight/height^3) above the 90th percentile, a weight gain in pregnancy of more than 20 kg, 41 or more weeks' gestation, and the presence of maternal diabetes.[18]

The liberal use of labor induction and cesarean section for suspected macrosomic fetuses has been advocated for the prevention of shoulder dystocia. However, no prospective, randomized, controlled trials of induction or cesarean section versus expectant management have been performed to validate this practice. A recent retrospective study by Combs and associates[25] found that patients with sonographic evidence of fetal macrosomia who were managed expectantly had a lower risk of cesarean delivery. No difference in the incidence of shoulder dystocia was found when compared with the induction group. However, patients were not stratified into diabetic and nondiabetic groups, and macrosomia was defined as a sonographic estimated fetal weight at or above the 90th percentile for gestational age (in contrast to a weight exceeding 4,000 g). In addition, the mean infant birth weight in the spontaneous labor (expectant management) group was 3,887 g, as compared with 4,162 g in the elective induction group ($P<0.01$).[25] Does elective induction of labor for a fetus with an estimated birth weight of more than 4,000 g decrease the rate of maternal and fetal morbidity and cesarean section? Currently available data cannot answer this question because of the lack of randomized trials and the many confounding variables present in other studies. Further studies are necessary to answer this very clinically relevant question.

A recent randomized trial of active induction of labor versus expectant management of insulin-dependent diabetic patients with nonmacrosomic fetuses found that in uncomplicated class A2 or B diabetic gravid women, expectant management did not decrease the cesarean section rate but was associated with an increased incidence of shoulder dystocia. This study randomized patients to either induction of labor or expectant management beginning at 38 weeks of gestation.[29]

Several thresholds of estimated fetal weight have been used to recommend primary or repeat cesarean section for both diabetic and nondiabetic patients bearing fetuses with suspected macrosomia. However, no absolute recommendations are widely accepted. Langer and associates[2] noted that primary cesarean section for delivery of a fetus whose birth weight was 4,250 g or more in the presence of maternal diabetes would have reduced the incidence of shoulder dystocia by 75 percent and increased the cesarean section rate by less than 1 percent in their study population. For the nondiabetic patient, Langer and colleagues[2] advocate a trial of vaginal delivery for fetuses with a birth weight of more than 4,000 g. A trial of labor may even be considered for nondiabetic gravid women with fetuses having birth weights up to 5,000 g, provided the clinician and patient accept the approximate 10 percent risk of shoulder dystocia that occurs in these vaginal deliveries. Elective cesarean section in nondiabetic gravid women at these upper limits of infant birth weight would reduce the incidence of shoulder dystocia by only 2.5 percent.[2] These recommendations should be interpreted with caution, since they are based on data evaluated retrospectively, using actual infant birth weights. Definitive data that prospectively apply many different clinical parameters to the problem of shoulder dystocia are still needed.

In the extremely large infant (birth weight 5,700 to 6,900 g), a poor outcome may be anticipated with vaginal delivery. A review of over 1-million deliveries between 1973 and 1984 identified 110 infants with birth weights above 5,700 g. Eight fetal deaths were reported (perinatal mortality rate 73 per 1,000), one-half of which were related to shoulder dystocia. Shoulder dystocia occurred in 40 percent of all infants in this birth weight range who were delivered vaginally, and brachial plexus injury occurred in 10 percent of these infants. In this report, over 70 percent of these patients underwent vaginal delivery because of the inability to identify the extremely large fetus during antepartum evaluation. No reliable or accurate combination of variables was identified to assist in the prediction of these extraordinary birth weights.[30]

Finally, even though infant birth weight is an important independent risk factor for shoulder dystocia, many studies report that from 30 percent to more than 50 percent of all shoulder dystocia events occur in infants with birth weights of less than 4,000 g.[2,31,32] Therefore, an overemphasis on infant birth weight estimation as the most critical factor in predicting the risk of shoulder dystocia should be tempered by the entire clinical picture. As always, patients should be allowed to make informed management decisions with their obstetricians on the basis of available data.

MECHANISM OF THE SECOND STAGE

The ability to identify and treat shoulder dystocia is based on a complete understanding of the normal as well as the abnormal mechanism of labor in the occiput-anterior presentation. The cardinal movements of labor occur as a coordinated combination of movements in the following sequence: extension, external rotation, and expulsion.

The course of the fetal shoulders during these movements is an important aspect in understanding the mechanism of shoulder dystocia. During engagement, descent, and flexion, as the fetal biparietal diameter (BPD) enters the pelvis in the anterior-posterior plane, the bisacromial diameter is also maintained in the anterior-posterior plane. On completion of internal rotation, the BPD is in the transverse position with the bisacromial diameter at an oblique angle (Fig. 11-3). Further descent of the fetal vertex, with extension and restitution, results in the occiput returning to its original position prior to descent (Fig. 11-4). The anterior shoulder is then delivered under the apex of the pubic arch in an oblique position. The pubic arch acts as a pivot for delivery of the posterior shoulder, and the remainder of the trunk follows.[33]

The persistent anterior-posterior rather than oblique location of the shoulders at the pelvic brim does not allow the anterior shoulder to enter the pelvis with the correct orientation. This abnormal orientation of the shoulders at the pelvic brim may be attributable to several factors that interfere with the easy rotation of the trunk at a time when fetuses in occiput-lateral or occiput-posterior positions undergo long rotations. Failure of trunk rotation with descent of the head into the pelvis may therefore contribute in large part to a shoulder dystocia event. Failure of trunk rotation may be caused by an increase in resistance between the fetal skin and the vaginal wall (i.e., maternal obesity), a large fetal chest (relative to fetal BPD), or a precipitous course of labor that allows no time for trunk rotation. In addition, arrests with the fetus in the deep transverse position or the fetal vertex in impacted posterior positions when manually rotated may produce no rotation of the fetal trunk, and therefore no rotation of the bisacromial diameter from an anterior-posterior to an oblique position. The anterior-posterior position of the bisacromial diameter results in an impaction of the anterior shoulder with the pubic symphysis, and is clinically represented by the well-known "turtle sign." The inward retraction of the fetal head toward the perineal body (i.e., turtle sign)

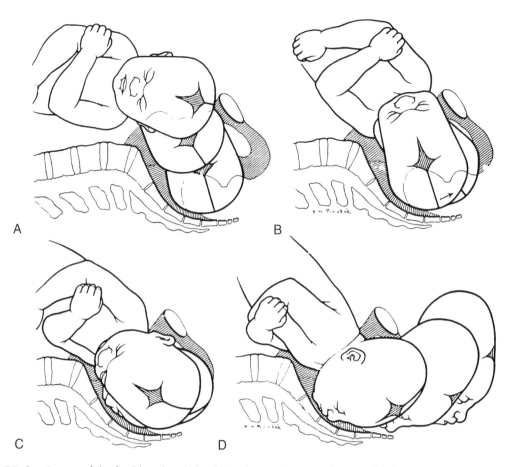

Fig. 11-3. Course of the fetal head and shoulders during the second stage of labor. **(A & B)** The shoulders enter the pelvis in the anterior-posterior plane. **(C & D)** On completion of internal rotation, the shoulders are oblique. (From Steele and Javert,[54] with permission.)

may be the first sign to the delivering obstetrician that a shoulder dystocia has occurred.

The previously described mechanisms for the second stage of labor make it clear why both macrosomic and nonmacrosomic fetuses are capable of experiencing shoulder dystocia. In the first case, the excessive amount of fetal tissue fills all available space within the pelvis, obstructing normal rotational movements. In the second case a relative disproportion between the bisacromial diameter and maternal pelvis occurs as a result of abnormal positioning of the fetal shoulder. Understanding these normal and abnormal mechanisms of labor should also help the clinician in understanding and implementing logical interventions.

CLINICAL MANAGEMENT/MANEUVERS

As previously stated, a well-rehearsed clinical management plan must be immediately instituted following recognition of shoulder dystocia. Assistance should be immediately requested; however, initial steps can be instituted even in the absence of consultation. One report has suggested the severity of the shoulder dystocia, as a means for determining the maneuver used for its reduction.[34] The grades of severity of dystocia included mild, moderate, severe, and undeliverable. However, since the degree of severity of shoulder dystocia may not be initially apparent, a routine set and order of procedures should be immediately instituted when the diagnosis of shoulder dystocia has been made. Since the fetal pH de-

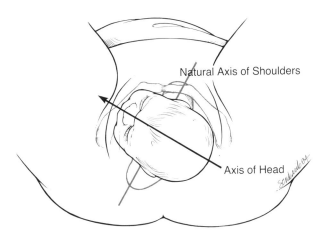

Fig. 11-4. Normal position of the fetal head and shoulders after restitution and before delivery of the shoulders. (From Seeds,[55] with permission.)

clines at a rate of 0.04 U/min between the delivery of the fetal head and that of the trunk, there is adequate time to proceed in a well-organized manner.[35]

Following recognition and request for assistance, a generous episiotomy is strongly recommended to allow for posterior descent of the fetal shoulders. At this time, initial maneuvers to be considered include suprapubic pressure applied by an assistant, as steady downward traction is applied to the fetal head, as advocated by Resnik[1] (Fig. 11-5). In addition, the McRoberts maneuver, initially described by Gonik and associates,[36] should be considered next, owing to its relative ease of performance. The procedure is performed by sharp flexion of the mother's thighs against her abdomen as mild traction is applied to the fetal head to free the impacted shoulder (Fig. 11-6). The McRoberts maneuver in conjunction with suprapubic pressure may be applied immediately and with the use of only one additional assistant. In most cases these maneuvers may be expected to result in disimpaction of the fetal shoulder,[37] and produce a lower incidence of fetal injury than other maneuvers.[14]

The use of the McRoberts maneuver alone, when compared with the lithotomy position, has been associated with a decrease in the force needed for delivery of the fetal shoulders, as well as a decrease in the force applied to the brachial plexus, especially for fetuses with moderately large bisacromial diameters (11 to 12 cm).[38] In addition, the rate at which this force is applied to the fetus is probably an impor-

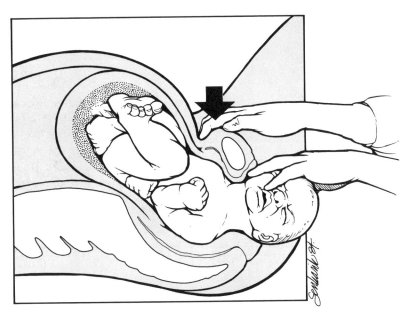

Fig. 11-5. Suprapubic pressure used initially can be expected to result in a majority of disimpactions of the fetal shoulder. (From Seeds,[55] with permission.)

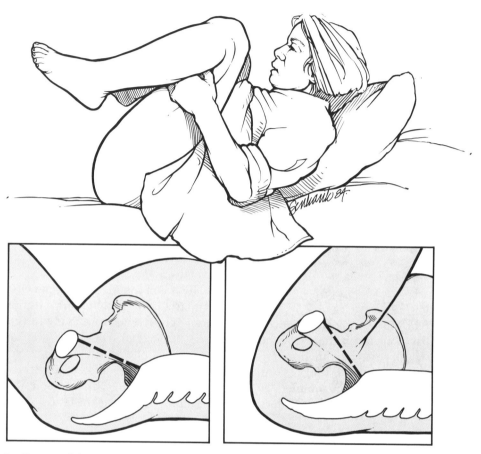

Fig. 11-6. Flexion of the maternal thighs (McRoberts maneuver) produces a more favorable position of the pelvic inlet and outlet, facilitating delivery of the fetal shoulders. (From Seeds,[55] with permission.)

tant consideration during a difficult delivery, since it is directly associated with the vulnerability of the fetus to injury. Because typical clinician-applied peak forces for a delivery involving shoulder dystocia are twice those applied during a routine delivery, jerking motions should be avoided, owing to the additional increase in peak forces applied in the region of the fetal brachial plexus.[39]

Despite the association of the McRoberts maneuver with a decrease in the clinically applied peak forces during a shoulder dystocia delivery, less than 50 percent of residency programs surveyed in the United States instructed house staff members in this maneuver, and less than one-third advocated it as a first-line approach.[37] Increasing house staff exposure to this maneuver should be considered, since it

involves only maternal manipulation and the potential for decreased fetal morbidity.

Should the procedures mentioned above be unsuccessful in resolving the dystocia, the choice of the next set of maneuvers should be based on clinician experience. The Woods corkscrew maneuver was originally described as a downward thrust made with the left hand on the buttocks of the baby (*without maternal expulsive forces*).[40] At the same time, two fingers of the right hand are placed on the anterior aspect of the posterior shoulder, producing a gentle clockwise motion upward around the circumference of the pubic arch and past the twelve o'clock position. This rotation delivers the posterior shoulder and places the anterior shoulder in precisely the same position as previously occupied by the posterior shoulder. Next, two fingers are inserted between the baby's head and shoulders on the anterior aspect of the remaining shoulder, and again with pressure applied downward from above with the left hand, the two fingers of the right hand are used to produce a counterclockwise motion upward to the twelve o'clock position, delivering the remaining shoulder. The Woods maneuver empirically results in abduction of both the posterior and anterior shoulders. Consequently, this maneuver may create a larger shoulder circumference and transverse diameter.[41]

As an alternative to the Woods maneuver, Rubin[41] recommended adduction of the most accessible shoulder by placement of two fingers on the posterior aspect of the shoulder with subsequent rotation. This "reverse Woods corkscrew maneuver" tends to reduce the circumference and transverse diameter of the shoulders during the delivery[41] (Fig. 11-7). In addition, Rubin advocated an alternative maneuver to disimpact the anterior shoulder by rocking it from side to side, first pushing off from one side of the mother's abdomen and then the other. This procedure attempts to move the shoulders into an oblique position rather than the impacted anterior-posterior position.[41]

Delivery of the posterior fetal arm is an additional procedure to consider when alternate methods have been unsuccessful. The maneuver requires the delivering obstetrician's hand to be passed posteriorly, within the vagina, identifying the fetal arm.[42] The fetal elbow is then flexed and the hand swept across the chest. With the posterior shoulder delivered, the anterior shoulder should be dislodged from beneath the pubic symphysis (Fig. 11-8A–D). If the dystocia persists, rotation of the fetus in a manner similar to the method of Rubin will resolve the dystocia and permit completion of the vaginal delivery (Fig. 11-8E & F). The delivery of the posterior arm has been associated with a higher incidence of neonatal injury, but is the maneuver that most often permits resolution of the dystocia when others have failed.[14]

Finally, the failure to resolve a severe shoulder dystocia using any of the aforementioned maneuvers requires the clinician to consider a more invasive maneuver to save the fetus. To resolve this severe degree of dystocia, a relatively new maneuver has been advocated. This procedure, known as the Zavanelli maneuver, was first described by Sandberg[43] in

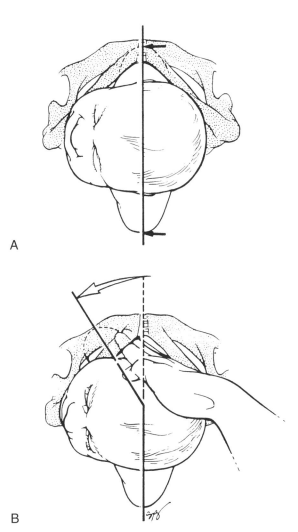

Fig. 11-7. Rubin maneuver. **(A)** Bisacromial diameter is shown as the distance between the arrows. **(B)** Adduction of the most accesible shoulder, with rotation, tends to reduce the bisacromial diameter and facilitates delivery. (From Cunningham et al,[56] with permission.)

1985. The Zavanelli maneuver requires a reversal of the cardinal movements of labor, with complete cephalic replacement and subsequent abdominal delivery.

In 1988, a registry for reporting the use of this procedure was initiated to evaluate both neonatal and maternal complications.[19] Fifty-nine patients were evaluated. Maternal complications associated with shoulder dystocia requiring resolution with the

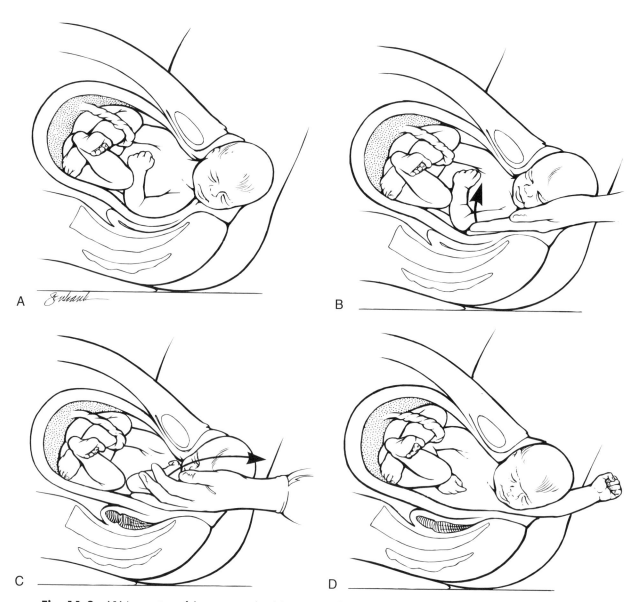

Fig. 11-8. **(A)** Impaction of the anterior shoulder against the symphysis pubis. **(B)** Flexion of the fetal forearm brings the wrist within reach. **(C)** The fetal forearm is swept across the chest and delivered. **(D)** The posterior arm has been delivered and delivery of the trunk usually follows easily. *(Figure continues.)*

Zavanelli maneuver included two (3.4 percent) cases of ruptured uterus. Both were secondary to a Bandl ring and required hysterectomy as definitive therapy. Three (5.1 percent) patients sustained a lacerated lower uterine segment. Six patients (10 percent) required transfusion, and eight patients (13.5 percent) had postoperative morbidity. Neonatal compli-

cations reported in this study included two deaths (both of macrosomic fetuses), one of which was secondary to a gastric hemorrhage and the second of which was due to hypoxic ischemic encephalopathy. Of the 59 patients evaluated, 12 (20 percent) sustained an Erb's palsy; however, in 5 (42 percent) of these cases the palsy was persistent. One stillbirth

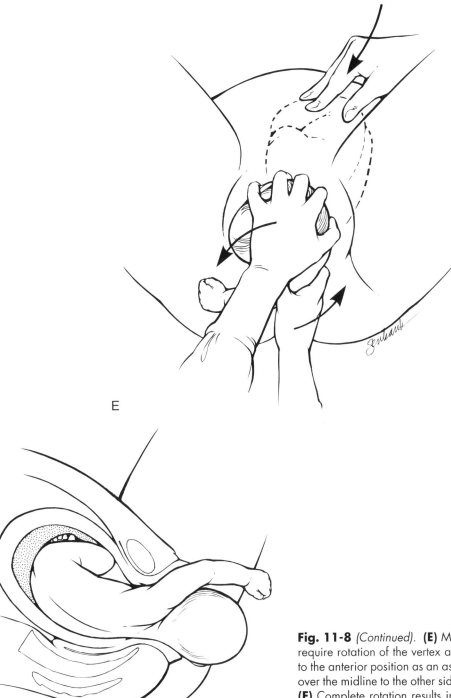

E

F

Fig. 11-8 *(Continued).* **(E)** More difficult impactions may require rotation of the vertex and of the posterior shoulder to the anterior position as an assistant pushes the fetal back over the midline to the other side of the maternal abdomen. **(F)** Complete rotation results in disimpaction and delivery of the trunk. (From Barnum,[42] with permission.)

was reported, secondary to an occult cord prolapse after a second cephalic replacement was required, and 4 of 59 (6.8 percent) neonates sustained seizure activity during the early neonatal period, with 2 infants developing cerebral palsy. It should be recognized that some of these complications may have preceded the attempt at cephalic replacement. Therefore, the observations described above need to be viewed within the clinical course of the events involved in resolving the dystocia.

The six failed cephalic replacements noted by O'Leary,[19] as well as case reports describing the difficulty involved in attempting the Zavanelli maneuver, show that this procedure is not as easily performed as one might assume from the original description. Difficulties with the Zavanelli maneuver have included the inability to completely reverse the cardinal movements of labor without administration of either a tocolytic agent or a general anesthetic agent to achieve uterine relaxation.[44] In addition, one case report describes a failed Zavanelli maneuver followed by the use of a low transverse hysterotomy to perform a manual rotation of the anterior shoulder

to the oblique position, producing further descent of the posterior shoulder and delivery of the posterior arm and fetus vaginally.[20]

Several procedures for the management of shoulder dystocia remain of historical but not clinical interest because of the potentially severe maternal and fetal injury they may produce. One of these procedures is the Hibbard maneuver, first described in 1969.[45] This maneuver involves the application of pressure against the infant's jaw and upper neck, carrying the head and neck posteriorly and upward to facilitate the release of the anterior shoulder. As this pressure is being applied on the fetus, an assistant applies strong fundal pressure to allow descent of the shoulder below the pubic symphysis. As previously mentioned, fundal pressure has been associated with significant fetal neurologic injury.[10] Therefore, the Hibbard maneuver cannot be recommended.

An obstetric instrument developed and reported in 1979 by Chavis,[46] was described as a shoulder horn, and consisted of a long-handled concave blade that was placed between the impacted anterior

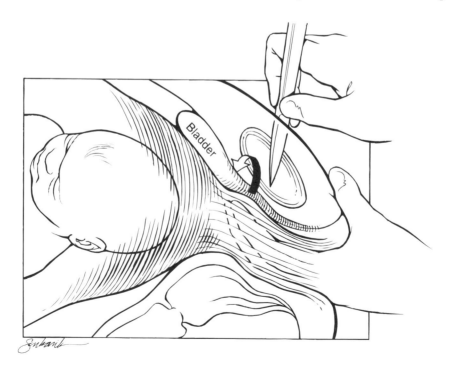

Fig. 11-9. The index and middle fingers displace the urethra and bladder neck laterally during symphysiotomy. (From Crichton and Seedat,[57] with permission.)

shoulder and the pubic symphysis. The blade was then used to posteriorly displace the anterior shoulder to allow its delivery. A pair of forceps described by Shute,[47] applied to the ventral and dorsal surface of the fetus, were used for rotation of the shoulder without the application of fundal, suprapubic, or maternal expulsive forces. Once rotation occurred, the forceps were removed and the delivery completed with gentle traction.[47] The use of these instruments is not currently recommended because of the potential for maternal and fetal injuries.

Deliberate fracture of the clavicle, either by pressing the anterior clavicle against the pubic ramus or cutting the clavicle with scissors (cleidotomy), has been described as a means of resolving severe episodes of shoulder dystocia.[48] Symphysiotomy has also been used to complete vaginal delivery complicated by shoulder dystocia, often after many other maneuvers have been attempted.[19]

In addition, the use of subcutaneous symphysiotomy[49] (Fig. 11-9) in some African countries has been shown to be associated with a lower rate of maternal morbidity and mortality than cesarean section in cases of cephalopelvic disproportion.[50] Although symphysiotomy is unlikely to be used in developed countries where cesarean section carries a low risk of maternal morbidity, this procedure may be a consideration elsewhere. These data show the need for appropriately utilizing symphysiotomy in managing labor complicated by cephalopelvic disproportion and shoulder dystocia in certain clinical situations.

MEDICOLEGAL CONSIDERATIONS

Negligence involves conduct that falls below the standard of care established by law for the protection of others against unreasonable risk of harm. To establish that a physician is negligent, the plaintiff's attorney must prove by a preponderance of the evidence the four elements of negligence. These elements include duty, breach, causation, and injury.[51]

The physician's duty, or obligation to the patient, may be demonstrated in a variety of ways, including (1) obtaining an appropriate degree of training (i.e., board certification); (2) using an appropriate standard of care; (3) using diligence and the physician's best judgment; and (4) through the foreseeability of harm. Foreseeability of harm indicates the ability to

predict, within reason, the risks or consequences a physician of ordinary prudence would expect from a particular action.[51] Because few risk factors are useful in accurately predicting adverse outcome in the case of shoulder dystocia, accountability for foreseeability of harm may be limited to identifying those risk factors that may increase the risk of a shoulder dystocia event. These risk factors include identification of parturients with diabetes (gestational or pregestational), a history of a macrosomic infant, abnormalities of active-phase or second-stage labor (especially with concomitant use of midpelvic delivery), and infant birth weights above 4,000 g. The difficulty with this final risk factor, as previously mentioned, is the inability to accurately predict infant birth weight. However, should macrosomia be suspected, appropriate clinical evaluation and patient counseling are essential.

Despite these risk factors, the obstetric literature clearly shows that more than one-half of all cases of shoulder dystocia occur in nonmacrosomic infants, and that these cases remain completely unpredictable in this group. The remainder of cases (in macrosomic infants), as well as subsequent neonatal injuries, are not predictable with any significant degree of accuracy using maternal history or antepartum or intrapartum risk factor evaluation.[9,14,52] Therefore, the failure to predict shoulder dystocia or prevent any resulting neonatal injury should not be construed as medical malpractice. Indeed, one cannot be held accountable for failing to predict the unpredictable.

Assuming, however, that a permanent injury results from a shoulder dystocia event, negligence may be proven if there is little or no effort to identify the risk factors mentioned previously, or if an inappropriate procedure is chosen in an attempt to resolve the event (i.e., fundal pressure, persistent traction on the fetal head, or failure to perform an episiotomy).[51] Adverse outcomes may also be interpreted as negligence if the physician fails to involve the patient in the decision-making process by requesting informed consent. Therefore, recognition of risk factors, informed consent, and timely and appropriate use of corrective measures to resolve shoulder dystocia are keys to improving maternal and neonatal outcome and the patient–physician relationship, as well as to decreasing the opportunity for litigation.

Shoulder Dystocia Intervention Form

The shoulder dystocia intervention form recommended by Acker[53] contains the following important data:

1. Anesthesia utilized
2. Episiotomy
3. Application of forceps or vacuum extractor; type of forceps operation (with indications)
4. Delivery times of head and complete infant
5. Degree of initial traction utilized
6. Maneuvers (in the order performed and duration of each)
7. Force required to effect delivery
8. Estimated fetal weight and actual birth weight
9. Personnel assisting with the delivery

Conversely, the presence of neonatal injury does not always indicate negligence. In fact, if basic standards of practice are followed, negligence may be a difficult argument for the plaintiff to win.

However, because litigation may result from an adverse neonatal outcome following delivery, all clinically significant details of complicated deliveries should be well documented in the patient's record. These records should be legible and should accurately reflect times and dates of events. Dictated notes may be preferable to hand-written documents.

Acker has recommended the use of a shoulder dystocia intervention form that arranges pertinent data in a logical format following a delivery complicated by shoulder dystocia.[53]

Other important data that should be included are umbilical cord blood gas (arterial and venous) values, Apgar scores, and the condition of the neonate in the delivery room. The importance of documentation cannot be overemphasized because, as the saying has it, "if you did not document it, you did not do it."

SUMMARY

Shoulder dystocia is an infrequent and unpredictable obstetric emergency that may result in serious injury to both the mother and infant. Independent risk factors for shoulder dystocia include maternal diabetes, fetal macrosomia (infant birth weight >4,000 g) and a maternal history of bearing a previous large infant. Other risk factors include arrest and protraction disorders of labor, especially in large fetuses undergoing forceps deliveries. However, because shoulder dystocia events are impossible to predict (mainly because of the inability to reliably predict macrosomic infant birth weights), infants at risk of permanent neonatal injury from such events are also unpredictable.

Early recognition and immediate institution of corrective maneuvers will help to decrease the maternal and neonatal morbidity and mortality associated with fetal shoulder dystocia. In addition, the liberal use of cesarean section in diabetic patients with fetuses having expected birth weights of more than 4,250 g should substantially reduce the risk of shoulder dystocia in this subgroup of patients, and cause only a small increase in the overall cesarean section rate. A trial of labor for nondiabetic parturients with suspected macrosomic fetuses is still recommended because predicting actual birth weights in this group of patients is difficult, and because a large number of cesarean sections would be required to affect the small number of dystocic events.

REFERENCES

1. Resnik R: Management of shoulder girdle dystocia. Clin Obstet Gynecol 23:559, 1980
2. Langer O, Berkus MD, Huff RW, Samueloff A: Shoulder dystocia: should the fetus weighing ≥4000 grams be delivered by cesarean section? Am J Obstet Gynecol 165:831, 1991
3. Acker DB, Sachs BP, Friedman EA: Risk factors for shoulder dystocia. Obstet Gynecol 66:762, 1985
4. Keller JD, Lopez-Zeno JA, Dooley SL, Socol ML: Shoulder dystocia and birth trauma in gestational diabetes: a five-year experience. Am J Obstet Gynecol 165:928, 1991
5. Lindsay MK, Graves W, Klein L: The relationship of one abnormal glucose tolerance test value and pregnancy complications. Obstet Gynecol 73:103, 1989
6. Coustan DR, Imarah J: Prophylactic insulin treatment of gestational diabetes reduces the incidence of macrosomia, operative delivery, and birth trauma. Am J Obstet Gynecol 150:836, 1984
7. Benedetti TJ, Gabbe SG: Shoulder dystocia: a compli-

cation of fetal macrosomia and prolonged second stage of labor with midpelvic delivery. Obstet Gynecol 52:526, 1978

8. Goldaber KG, Wendel PJ, McIntire DD, Wendel GD: Postpartum perineal morbidity after fourth-degree perineal repair. Am J Obstet Gynecol 168:489, 1993

9. Levine MG, Holroyde J, Woods JR et al: Birth trauma: incidence and predisposing factors. Obstet Gynecol 63:792, 1984

10. Gross SJ, Shime J, Farine D: Shoulder dystocia: predictors and outcome. A five-year review. Am J Obstet Gynecol 156:334, 1987

11. Gordon M, Rich H, Deutschberger J, Green M: The immediate and long-term outcome of obstetric birth trauma. Am J Obstet Gynecol 117:51, 1973

12. Sandmire HF, Halloin T: Shoulder dystocia: it's incidence and associated risk factors. Int J Gynaecol Obstet 26:65, 1988

13. Jennett RJ, Tarby TJ, Kreinick CJ: Brachial plexus palsy: an old problem revisited. Am J Obstet Gynecol 166:1673, 1992

14. Nocon JJ, McKenzie DK, Thomas LJ, Hansell RS: Shoulder dystocia: an analysis of risks and obstetric maneuvers. Am J Obstet Gynecol 168:1732, 1993

15. Oppenheim WL, Davis A, Growdon WA et al: Clavicle fractures in the newborn. Clin Orthopaed Rel Res 250:176, 1990

16. Acker DB, Gregory KD, Sachs BP, Friedman EA: Risk factors for Erb-Duchenne palsy. Obstet Gynecol 71:389, 1988

17. Mondanlou HD, Komatsu G, Dorchester W et al: Large-for-gestational-age neonates: anthropometric reasons for shoulder dystocia. Obstet Gynecol 60:417, 1982

18. Boyd ME, Usher RH, McLean FH: Fetal macrosomia: prediction, risks, proposed management. Obstet Gynecol 61:715, 1983

19. O'Leary JA: Cephalic replacement for shoulder dystocia: present status and future role of the Zavanelli maneuver. Obstet Gynecol 82:847, 1993

20. O'Leary JA, Cuva A: Abdominal rescue after failed cephalic replacement. Obstet Gynecol 80:514, 1992

21. Gonik B, Hollyer VL, Allen R: Shoulder dystocia recognition: differences in neonatal risks for injury. Am J Perinatol 8:31, 1991

22. Acker DB, Sachs BP, Friedman EA: Risk factors for shoulder dystocia in the average-weight infant. Obstet Gynecol 67:614, 1986

23. Sandmire HF: Whither ultrasonic prediction of fetal macrosomia? Obstet Gynecol 82:860, 1993

24. Chauhan SP, Lutton PM, Bailey KJ et al: Intrapartum clinical, sonographic, and parous patient's estimates of newborn birth weight. Obstet Gynecol 79:956, 1992

25. Combs CA, Singh NB, Khoury JC: Elective induction versus spontaneous labor after sonographic diagnosis of fetal macrosomia. Obstet Gynecol 81:492, 1993

26. Landon MB, Mintz MC, Gabbe SG: Sonographic evaluation of fetal abdominal growth: predictor of the large-for-gestational-age infant in pregnancies complicated by diabetes mellitus. Am J Obstet Gynecol 160:115, 1989

27. Elliott JP, Garite TJ, Freeman RK et al: Ultrasonic prediction of fetal macrosomia in diabetic patients. Obstet Gynecol 60:159, 1982

28. Kitzmiller JL, Mall JC, Gin GD et al: Measurement of fetal shoulder width with computed tomography in diabetic women. Obstet Gynecol 70:941, 1987

29. Kjos SL, Henry OA, Montoro M et al: Insulin-requiring diabetes in pregnancy: a randomized trial of active induction of labor and expectant management. Am J Obstet Gynecol 169:611, 1993

30. Rydhstrom H, Ingemarsson I: The extremely large fetus: antenatal identification, risks, and proposed management. Acta Obstet Gynecol Scand 68:59, 1989

31. Morrison JC, Sanders JR, Magann EF, Wiser WL: The diagnosis and management of dystocia of the shoulder. Surg Gynecol Obstet 175:515, 1992

32. Al-Najashi S, Al-Suleiman SA, El-Yahia A et al: Shoulder dystocia: a clinical study of 56 cases. Aust NZ J Obstet Gynaecol 29:129, 1989

33. Morris W: Report of societies: Newcastle-Upon-Tyne Obstetrical and Gynecological Society address on shoulder dystocia. J Obstet Gynaecol Br Commonw 62:302, 1955

34. O'Leary JA, Leonetti HB: Shoulder dystocia: prevention and treatment. Am J Obstet Gynecol 162:5, 1990

35. Wood C, Ng KH, Hounslow D, Benning H: Time: an important variable in normal delivery. J Obstet Gynaecol Br Commonw 80:295, 1973

36. Gonik B, Stringer CA, Held B: An alternate maneuver for management of shoulder dystocia. Am J Obstet Gynecol 145:882, 1983

37. O'Leary JA, Pollack NB: McRoberts maneuver for shoulder dystocia: a survey. Int J Gynaecol Obstet 35:129, 1991

38. Gonik B, Allen R, Sorab J: Objective evaluation of the shoulder dystocia phenomenon: effect of maternal pelvic orientation on force reduction. Obstet Gynecol 74:44, 1989

39. Allen R, Sorab J, Gonik B: Risk factors for shoulder dystocia: an engineering study of clinician-applied forces. Obstet Gynecol 77:352, 1991

40. Woods CE, Westbury NY: A principle of physics as

applicable to shoulder delivery. Am J Obstet Gynecol 45:796, 1943

41. Rubin A: Management of shoulder dystocia. JAMA 189:835, 1964

42. Barnum CG: Dystocia due to the shoulders. Am J Obstet Gynecol 50:439, 1945

43. Sandberg EC: The Zavanelli maneuver: a potentially revolutionary method for the resolution of shoulder dystocia. Am J Obstet Gynecol 152:479, 1985

44. Graham JM, Blanco JD, Wen T, Magee KP: The Zavanelli maneuver: a different perspective. Obstet Gynecol 79:883, 1992

45. Hibbard LT: Shoulder dystocia. Obstet Gynecol 34:424, 1969

46. Chavis WM: A new instrument for the management of shoulder dystocia. Int J Gynaecol Obstet 16:331, 1979

47. Shute WB: Management of shoulder dystocia with the Shute parallel forceps. Am J Obstet Gynecol 84:936, 1962

48. Schramm M: Impacted shoulder: a personal experience. Aust NZ J Obstet Gynaecol 23:28, 1986

49. Seedat EK, Crichton D: Symphysiotomy: technique, indications, and limitations. Lancet 1:554, 1962

50. van Roosmalen J: Safe motherhood: cesarean section or symphysiotomy? Am J Obstet Gynecol 163:1, 1990

51. Phelan JP: Medical-legal considerations in the post-date pregnancy. Clin Obstet Gynecol 32:294, 1989

52. Gross TL, Sokol RJ, Williams T, Thompson K: Shoulder dystocia: a fetal-physician risk. Am J Obstet Gynecol 156:1408, 1987

53. Acker DB: A shoulder dystocia intervention form. Obstet Gynecol 78:150, 1991

54. Steele KB, Javert CT: The mechanism of labor for transverse positions of the vertex. Surg Gynecol Obstet 75:477, 1942

55. Seeds JW: Malpresentations. p. 539. In Gabbe SG, Niebyl JR, Simpson JL (eds): Obstetrics: Normal and Problem Pregnancies. 2nd Ed. Churchill Livingstone, New York, 1991

56. Cunningham FG, MacDonald PC, Gant NF et al (eds): Williams' Obstetrics. 19th Ed. Appleton & Lange, E. Norwalk, CT, 1993

57. Crichton D, Seedat EK: The technique of symphysiotomy. S Afr Med J 37:277, 1963

Obstetric Hemorrhage

Stephen K. Hunter and Carl P. Weiner

MORTALITY

Obstetric hemorrhage remains a major and often preventable cause of maternal mortality. The Centers for Disease Control[1] (CDC) analyzed 2,067 nonabortive maternal deaths in the United States between 1974 and 1978 and concluded that hemorrhage was the direct cause of death in 13.4 percent. A separate report from the Maternal Mortality Collaborative[2] described hemorrhage as the direct cause of 11 percent of maternal deaths between 1980 and 1985. Any facility that delivers obstetric care should have the resources necessary to provide prompt blood replacement therapy.

Obstetric hemorrhage also poses a significant risk to the fetus. Pregnancies complicated by second- and third-trimester bleeding have preterm delivery and perinatal mortality rates that are at least quadruple[3] those not complicated by bleeding. In one series, antepartum hemorrhage precipitated 17 percent of deliveries associated with a very-low-birth weight infant.[4]

BLOOD LOSS DEFINITION AND ASSESSMENT

Blood loss exceeding 500 ml by completion of the third stage of labor is commonly used as the definition of postpartum hemorrhage. Approximately one-third of women undergoing vaginal delivery and almost all women undergoing cesarean section will lose this much blood or more if the loss is measured quantitatively.[5] In general, physicians tend to underestimate the actual blood loss. However, an accurate assessment of blood loss is the first step in providing appropriate and timely therapy.

The blood volume of a woman with a normal singleton pregnancy increases by 30 to 60 percent by term.[6] As a result, the woman will not manifest the normal physiologic responses to hemorrhage until she has lost more than the volume of blood added during pregnancy. Four classes of volume loss secondary to hemorrhage have been defined.[7] A loss of 15 percent or less of the total circulating volume is defined as a class 1 hemorrhage. Patients with such loss rarely exhibit signs or symptoms of volume deficit other than a mild tachycardia. Class 2 hemorrhage is defined as a blood loss of 15 to 25 percent of the patient's total volume. These patients have the usual signs and symptoms of hypovolemia: tachycardia, tachypnea, cold, clammy, pale skin, and orthostatic changes. In addition, these patients have decreased perfusion of the extremities as documented by a delayed capillary refilling time. Delayed filling is demonstrated by squeezing the hypothenar area of the hand to produce blanching and then releasing the pressure. The skin of a patient with normal volume status will return to a normal pink color within 1 to 2 seconds. A refilling time of more than 2 seconds represents a volume deficit of 15 to 25 percent. Another reliable response to volume deficit is narrowing of the patient's pulse pressure, usually secondary to diastolic hypertension. This results from vasoconstriction caused by stimulation of the sympathetic nervous system. Systolic pressure is usually affected only by larger volume deficits. Class 3 hemorrhage represents a blood loss of 25 to 35 percent. It is associated with a marked tachycardia (120 to 160 bpm), overt hypotension, tachypnea (respirations 30 to 50/min), and oliguria.

Urine output should be closely monitored in any patient with hemorrhage. During hypovolemia, blood flow is diverted away from nonvital organs (skin, kidneys, gut) to ensure perfusion of vital organs (heart, brain). Renal blood flow and renal output have a fairly good correlation. Often, a low urine output will be the first sign of hypovolemia. Any patient with significant blood loss, or the potential for hemorrhage, should have an indwelling bladder catheter in place. A normal urine output, in the absence of diuretic use, is a reassuring sign.

Class 4 hemorrhage represents a volume deficit of 40 percent or more. Patients with this degree of blood loss are usually in profound shock and often have no discernible peripheral blood pressure. They have either severe oliguria or anuria and are at very high risk of circulatory collapse if volume therapy is not initiated rapidly.

Although a hematocrit is useful in the assessment of blood loss, acute hemorrhage is not reflected in the hematocrit for at least 4 hours, and full equilibration may take 24 to 48 hours. Furthermore, fluid replacement will also affect the hematocrit. A hematocrit significantly lower than one obtained before the bleeding event usually indicates a significant hemorrhage. In addition to knowing the patient's hematocrit, it is important to be aware of any unusual blood type or the presence of antibodies that may delay the availability of cross-matched blood.

Pre-existing medical conditions or previously administered drugs may hide or alter the normal physiologic responses to volume loss. Patients with severe pre-eclampsia are already depleted of intravascular volume, and lack the usual protection provided by volume expansion during normal pregnancy. As a result, women with pre-eclampsia tend to become

hemodynamically unstable more rapidly, with blood losses usually classified as a class 1 hemorrhage. Moreover, blood pressure may be a misleading indicator of fluid status. A normal blood pressure in a previously hypertensive patient may indicate an already significant volume deficit. Serial blood pressure recordings are usually of more benefit than isolated readings, especially in patients with pre-existing hypertension.

Medications used for pain relief may also hinder a patient's ability to respond to volume loss. Epidural anesthesia and some narcotic medications can decrease blood pressure by diminishing or blocking the ability of the sympathetic nervous system to cause vasoconstriction of both the arterial and venous compartments. Drug- or anesthetic-induced hypotension may lead to an inaccurate assessment of volume status and consequently to inappropriate fluid-replacement therapy. Equally important is that the administration of these agents to a patient who already shows signs and symptoms of hypovolemia before appropriate therapy has been instituted may have severe consequences.

PATHOPHYSIOLOGY OF HYPOVOLEMIA AND SHOCK

Hypovolemia secondary to blood loss affects both the macrocirculatory and microcirculatory systems. Decreased blood volume leads to a decrease in cardiac return, which subsequently decreases cardiac output and finally arterial blood pressure. Compensatory mechanisms include increased sympathetic discharge causing tachycardia, increased myocardial contractility, and increased peripheral vascular resistance. A decrease in the hydrostatic pressure of the capillary bed causes fluid to be drawn from the interstitial space back into the capillaries, thus augmenting venous return. If the hemorrhage is severe and leads to shock, damage occurs to the endothelium of the capillary bed. This damage increases capillary permeability, which further exacerbates the intravascular volume deficit. Shock also alters electrolyte transport. There is an increase in the intracellular sodium and chloride concentrations, which tends to pull fluid from the interstitial space into the cell. Therefore, hemorrhagic shock is associated with a decrease in both intravascular and interstitial fluid volumes. Hence, the replacement of interstitial fluid and electrolytes in addition to restoration of intravascular volume is a primary goal of fluid resuscitation.

TREATMENT

Regardless of the cause, the treatment of hemorrhage is directed at maintaining intravascular volume so that perfusion and oxygenation are preserved while the cause of the blood loss is eliminated. Intravenous access with at least one and preferably two large-bore (18- or 16-gauge) catheters should be established early in the course of a bleeding episode. Whole blood can be infused eight times as rapidly through a 17-gauge needle as through a 21-gauge needle.[8] Urine output should be maintained at 30 ml/hr or more. Vital signs should be closely monitored, and when bleeding is severe, oxygen therapy providing 6 to 8 L/min of 100 percent oxygen by face mask should be initiated.

Fluid Resuscitation

Until blood or blood components are available, fluid resuscitation is initiated at a rapid infusion rate, usually 1 to 2 L over 30 to 60 minutes. Whether crystalloid or colloid fluids are initially preferable is controversial. When large volumes of crystalloid are given, the colloid osmotic pressure (COP) may be markedly reduced. This is usually of little concern in the healthy, nonpregnant patient. Lactated Ringer's solution or 0.9 percent sodium chloride (normal saline) are the crystalloid solutions of choice for the initial resuscitation. During pregnancy, the colloid osmotic pressure normally decreases, reaching its nadir in the peripartum period.[9] In hypovolemic shock, large volumes of crystalloid can reduce the COP to a level at which pulmonary edema occurs despite a normal pulmonary capillary wedge pressure. This is especially common in the pregnant patient who begins an episode of hypovolemic shock with a low COP. Colloid solutions have the advantage of maintaining the colloid osmotic pressure while expanding the plasma volume. On a volume-for-volume basis, colloids expand the plasma volume more than do crystalloids.[10] In one randomized clinical trial comparing 5 percent albumin, 6 percent hetastarch, and 0.9 percent saline for the resuscita-

tion of patients in hypovolemic or septic shock, from two to four times the volume of saline as of albumin or hetastarch solution was needed to reach the same hemodynamic endpoint.[11] Saline decreased the COP by 34 percent. Both albumin and hetastarch significantly raised the COP above baseline. Modest amounts of either crystalloid or colloid can be safely administered to previously healthy patients.

Blood Component Therapy

The decision to transfuse should be based on the clinical situation and the stability of the patient. In healthy patients, cardiac output does not dramatically increase until the hemoglobin decreases to below 7 g/ml.[12]

Whole Blood

Although whole blood would seem the ideal treatment for hypovolemia secondary to hemorrhage, it has some distinct disadvantages, and its use has been discouraged by blood bank centers in the United States. Storage of whole blood causes significant changes in some cellular elements and coagulation proteins. After 24 hours, white blood cells (WBCs) and platelets are either not present or are nonfunctional. After 14 days, factors V and VIII are decreased by 50 percent or more. Whole blood does provide red blood cells (RBCs) for oxygen delivery, and does contain most other coagulation factors at functional levels. In young, otherwise healthy obstetric patients in whom clotting is normal, the use of whole blood wastes many coagulation factors that could otherwise have been separated and used in a more appropriate situation. Packed RBCs, with crystalloid added for volume expansion, work as well as whole blood in most indications. However, massive hemorrhage remains an acceptable indication for the transfusion of whole blood.

Packed Red Blood Cells

The administration of packed RBCs is the most efficient way of restoring oxygen-carrying capacity to an anemic patient. Packed cells have an additional advantage should volume overload be a concern. Unless bleeding is massive, a combination of packed RBCs and crystalloid solution will suffice for most situations.[13] The administration of 1 U of packed

RBCs will, on average, increase the hematocrit 2 to 3 percent.

Fresh Frozen Plasma

Fresh frozen plasma (FFP) is prepared by the separation and freezing of plasma from whole blood within 6 hours of phlebotomy. It contains both labile and stable clotting factors. With the unavailability of whole blood, the prophylactic administration of FFP in conjunction with packed RBCs to provide clotting components has increased. However, in the absence of clotting abnormalities caused by decreased concentrations of soluble clotting factors as documented by abnormalities in the patient's prothrombin time (PT) and partial thromboplastin time (PTT), there are few data to support this practice. In fact, Martin and colleagues[14] showed that prophylactic FFP therapy did not efficiently restore coagulation activity. Microvascular bleeding is most commonly related to thrombocytopenia and hypofibrinogenemia; dilution of clotting factors is inconsequential and not the cause of the bleeding.[15] A consensus conference on the use of FFP also concluded that there is no justification for its use as a volume expander.[16] Indications as recommended by the National Institutes of Health (NIH) Consensus Conference for the use of FFP include replacement of isolated factor deficiencies, reversal of the effect of warfarin, massive blood transfusion (>1 blood volume within several hours), antithrombin III (AT III) deficiency, treatment of immunodeficiencies, and treatment of thrombotic thrombocytopenic purpura. Other volume expanding agents, such as crystalloid, colloid solutions containing albumin or plasma protein fractions, hydroxyethyl starch, or dextran should be used in place of FFP for all but the indications given above.

Platelet Concentrates

Platelet concentrates are indicated for the patient with an abnormality of platelet function, or who is thrombocytopenic and either actively bleeding or must undergo surgery. Patients who have platelet counts of 50,000/μl or more rarely bleed as a result of inadequate platelet numbers. One unit of platelets contains between 5,500 and 8,000 platelets, with 5,500 being the minimum allowed by the U.S. Food and Drug Administration (FDA).[17] Platelets are usually provided in 6- to 10-U packs. An NIH Consensus report dealing with platelet transfusion therapy counsels against the routine treatment of thrombocytopenia in the absence of clinically significant bleeding.[18] When necessary, type-specific platelets should be used, since RBC contamination of packed platelets is common and alloimmunization is possible.[13]

Cryoprecipitate

Cryoprecipitate contains significant amounts of factor VIII, von Willebrand's factor, and fibrinogen, and is therefore used to treat von Willebrand's disease, hemophilia A, and fibrinogen deficiencies or abnormalities. Each unit of cryoprecipitate will raise the serum fibrinogen concentration by approximately 10 mg/dl. Where fluid overload is a concern, cryoprecipitate will provide most of the coagulation factors in FFP plus factor VIII, but in only 15 percent of the volume. However, cryoprecipitate contains little AT III. In contrast to pooled plasma, cryoprecipitate may be collected from a single donor, thereby reducing the risk of infection. As with platelets, ABO- and Rh-compatible cryoprecipitate must be used.

Risks of Transfusion and Component Therapy

The transfusion of blood or blood products carries certain risks. The administration of incompatible blood, especially within the ABO system, usually causes an immediate transfusion reaction. Immunization to weak antigens whose antibodies are not detected by blood bank antigen panels may cause a delayed reaction characterized by fever, malaise, anemia, and jaundice 7 to 8 days after the transfusion. A delayed transfusion reaction, although usually not of immediate harm to the patient, could slow the future availability of cross-matched blood should the patient need it.

The greatest risk of transfusion therapy is the transmission of an infectious disease. Hepatitis B follows the transfusion of fewer than 1 in 2,000 U of blood; hepatitis C follows the use of approximately 1 in 1,000 U.[19] Human immunodeficiency virus (HIV) has had a major impact on blood banking practices. Routine screening of donor blood for HIV has been standard practice in the United States since 1985. The likelihood of HIV transmission in the transfusion of infected blood is extremely high (>95 percent).[20] The current risk of HIV infection from tested blood in the United States is estimated by the CDC to be 1 in 225,000 U.[21]

Risks of Blood and Component Transfusions

Whole blood and packed red blood cells
Hemolytic reaction
Febrile reaction
Allergic reactions
Fluid overload with noncardiogenic pulmonary edema
Infectious diseases
Adult respiratory distress syndrome

Fresh frozen plasma
Anaphylactoid reactions
Alloimmunization
Infectious disease transmission
Fluid overload

Platelets
Alloimmunization
Infectious diseases
Graft-versus-host disease (rare)

The current battery of screening tests performed in the United States on donor blood includes the rapid plasma reagin (RPR) test for syphilis, tests for hepatitis B surface antigen (HBsAg), anti-HBc antibody, hepatitis C virus, HIV-1 and HIV-2 antibodies, human T-cell leukemia viruses 1 and 2 (HTLV-1/ HTLV-2), and alanine aminotransferase (ALT). Transmission of other viral infections is also possible, these include cytomegalovirus (CMV), parvovirus, and Epstein-Barr virus infections. These viruses, and especially CMV, are primarily of concern in the immunocompromised patient. The use of leukocyte-poor filtered blood dramatically reduces the risks of infection by most of these agents.

Autologous Blood Donations

Recent years have seen renewed interest in the practice of autologous blood donation, owing to the concern of infection from homologous blood. The use of autologous blood in obstetrics has been more limited than in other disciplines. Kruskall and colleagues,[22] reporting on 48 women enrolled in a program of autologous blood donation in the third trimester of pregnancy, concluded that such donation was safe for both mother and fetus. Others have since confirmed its safety.[23–25]

However, the need for autologous donations in the obstetric population continues to be questioned. Less than 3 percent of patients who deliver vaginally require transfusion. One recent study reported that only 13 of 2,265 women (0.57 percent) required a transfusion.[26] Of these patients, 251 had risk factors prospectively necessitating transfusion, but only 4 (1.6 percent) required transfusion. The investigators questioned the need for routine autologous blood donation in view of the low frequency of use. However, they noted that 25 percent of patients with placenta previa receive a transfusion. In a cost-benefit analysis of autologous blood donation in pregnancy,[27] placenta previa was the only condition for which this procedure was justified. Another group that might benefit from autologous blood donation would be patients with rare antibodies that make difficult the provision of blood in emergency situations.

Disseminated Intravascular Coagulation

Hemorrhage associated with disseminated intravascular coagulation (DIC) may occur in several obstetric conditions, including placental abruption, amniotic fluid embolism, sepsis, pre-eclampsia, retained dead fetus syndrome, and uterine rupture. DIC is not a disease but rather the result of a pathologic condition that triggers the consumption of platelets and coagulation factors. The thrombus formed by platelets and fibrin includes plasminogen activated to plasmin, which then lyses fibrinogen and fibrin polymer to fibrin-fibrinogen degradation products (FDP). Marder[28] described three possible clinical consequences of DIC:

1. Hemorrhage due to the consumption of platelets and clotting factors and potentiated by the anticoagulant effects of FDP
2. Circulatory obstruction caused by fibrin plugs deposited in the microvasculature, producing tissue hypoxia and ischemic necrosis
3. Microangiopathic hemolysis due to the mechanical disruption of erythrocytes within small vessels in which fibrin has been deposited

The diagnosis of DIC is based on both clinical observation and laboratory findings. The patient with acute DIC typically bleeds from multiple sites. If the DIC is secondary to sepsis, the patient may have hypotension out of proportion to the amount of blood loss. The severe hypotension in these patients results from the activation of inducible nitric oxide synthase, with the constant release of nitric oxide by vascular smooth muscle.[29,30] Renal failure is also a common sequel to DIC.

Chronic DIC is more common than acute DIC in obstetric patients.[31] These patients are less likely to have severe hemorrhage, but may bruise easily or have minor mucosal or gingival bleeding. Laboratory documentation in patients with a chronic form of DIC is more reliable than clinical signs. The most sensitive laboratory test for DIC is the measurement of either AT III[31,32] or the AT III–thrombin complex. One-half of patients with acute DIC have a normal PT and PTT, and 15 percent have a normal FDP level.[33] Plasma AT III levels are essentially unchanged during normal pregnancy[34] but decline in women with a viral infection, bacterial pneumonia, pyelonephritis, or such pregnancy-specific conditions as pre-eclampsia.[35] This is in contrast to the nonpregnant patient, in whom AT III remains stable in the absence of overwhelming sepsis. This suggests that the "reserve" of AT III is reduced during pregnancy and that the sensitivity of AT III for excess clotting may be enhanced.[31]

The management of DIC, whether acute or chronic, is directed toward its underlying cause. Aggressive volume replacement may be necessary to minimize hypotension and hypoperfusion. Inotropic support may also be indicated. For patients in hypovolemic shock, intravascular volume must be restored (see the preceding section). In cases in which the vascular system is intact and the DIC is secondary to sepsis or dead fetus syndrome, low-dose heparin has been used as therapy. Heparin blocks the ongoing generation thrombin by interacting with AT III. Response to this therapy is followed both clinically and through laboratory parameters.[31,36]

ANTEPARTUM HEMORRHAGE
Placental Abruption

Placental abruption is the antenatal separation (complete or partial) of a normally implanted placenta. It results from bleeding into the decidua basalis, usu-

ally with retroplacental clot formation. The condition can be self-perpetuating, as further bleeding causes the clot to enlarge, lifting the placenta further away from the decidua. Although the reported incidence of placental abruption varies with the criteria used to make the diagnosis, it is estimated that 1 percent of all pregnancies are complicated by abruption; in about 10 percent of these the abruption is severe enough to kill the fetus. The CDC[37] reports that the incidence of abruption increased from 8.2 cases per 1,000 deliveries in 1979 to 11.5 per 1,000 deliveries in 1987. Placental abruption is classified as either mild (grade 1), moderate (grade 2), or severe (grade 3), depending on clinical and laboratory findings (Table 12-1).

Etiology

The exact etiology of placental abruption is unknown, but abnormalities of uterine blood vessels and the decidua have been postulated.[40] Unexplained increases in the maternal serum α-fetoprotein (AFP) concentration are associated with a severalfold increase in the incidence of abruption,[41] suggesting the possibility of a defect at the decidual–placental interface.

Several common obstetric complications are associated with abruption. The complication most strongly associated with the condition is maternal hypertension. Among patients with an abruption, as many as 44 percent have hypertension.[42] Over 50 percent of severe abruptions fatal to the fetus are associated with maternal hypertension. Both chronic hypertension and pregnancy-associated hypertension contribute to the incidence of abruption. A history of maternal trauma is noted in from 1.5 to 9.4 percent of abruptions.[43,44] Common causes of the trauma include falls, motor-vehicle accidents, and assault.

The use and abuse of various substances has been linked to placental abruption. According to a study by Voigt and colleagues,[45,46] cigarette smoking is associated with 40 percent of cases of abruption. However, Marbury et al[47] suggested that maternal ethanol consumption (≥14 drinks/wk), not smoking, was the predisposing factor for placental abruption. An association between placental abruption and cocaine abuse was first reported by Chasnoff et al[48] in

Table 12-1. Placental Abruption Classification

Grade of Abruption	Clinical/Laboratory Findings	Frequency (%)
Mild	Slight vaginal bleeding Minimal uterine irritability Normal maternal blood pressure and heart rate No evidence of coagulopathy Normal fetal heart rate pattern	40
Moderate	Mild to moderate vaginal bleeding Tetanic contractions are possible Maintenance of maternal blood pressure Maternal tachycardia Orthostatic changes in blood pressure and heart rate Hypofibrinogenemia (150–250 mg%) Fetal distress	45
Severe	Usually heavy vaginal bleeding, but may be concealed Tetanic, painful uterus Maternal hypotension Hypofibrinogenemia (<150 mg%) Other coagulation abnormalities Fetal death	15

1985. Since then, numerous studies have linked the use of cocaine with an increased risk of abruption.[49]

Other conditions that have been associated with placental abruption include preterm premature rupture of the membranes[50,51] and uterine leiomyoma,[52] especially if the leiomyoma is retroplacental.

Diagnosis

The diagnosis of placental abruption is usually based on the clinical presentation. The most commonly taught hallmark of placental abruption is vaginal bleeding with painful uterine contractions. There is, however, a wide range of presenting signs and symptoms associated with placental abruption. Approximately 80 percent of patients who eventually prove to have a placental abruption exhibit some degree of vaginal bleeding. The remaining 20 percent have a concealed abruption and are commonly diagnosed as having preterm labor.[38] Hurd observed that idiopathic preterm labor was the initial diagnosis in 22 percent of patients who subsequently developed other signs and symptoms, including fetal distress and fetal death, which made the diagnosis of placental abruption clear. Back pain was seen in 10 percent of the patients in a study by Sholl.[54]

The ultrasonographic diagnosis of placental abruption has in the past been disappointing. Hurd and colleagues[53] were able to recognize a retroplacental hematoma in only 1 of 59 patients. They concluded that ultrasound was useful only in excluding placenta previa. Sholl[54] was able to confirm abruption in 25 percent of his patients. It is likely that the increasing resolution capacity of diagnostic ultrasound has increased the sensitivity (Fig. 12-1). However, these studies stress that a negative ultrasound examination does not exclude the possibility of abruption. If all the blood lost in an abruption leaves the uterus through the cervical canal, there will be no sonographically detectable hematoma.[55]

In severe abruption, the patient may be in shock and the degree of shock may be out of proportion to the amount of external blood loss. Pritchard and Brekken[56] studied the blood loss associated with placental abruption severe enough to cause fetal death in 141 women. They found that the blood loss often amounted to at least one-half the blood volume of the pregnant patient. Much of the blood loss associated with placental abruption may remain retroplacental and become evident only at delivery.

In addition to shock, DIC is observed in approximately 30 percent of patients with placental abruption significant enough to cause fetal death. Fibrinogen will be decreased and the concentration of FDP will be increased (>100 μg/ml).[57] DIC in the absence

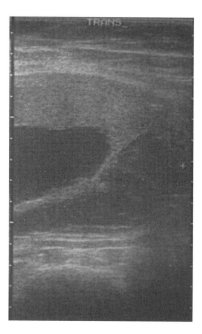

Fig. 12-1. Transverse view of placenta showing large blood collection in a retroplacental and retrochorionic position.

of fetal distress is most unusual. Delivery should be effected if the PTT is abnormal.

Acute renal failure is also seen with severe placental abruption. Incompletely treated hypotension and possibly fibrin deposition within the microvasculature of the kidney may be partially responsible. Grunfeld and Pertuiset[58] reported that 23 percent of 57 cases of acute renal failure were associated with placental abruption, most of them marked by reversible acute tubular necrosis. Of 19 women with acute cortical necrosis, 7 had placental abruption.

Although the diagnosis of severe placental abruption is usually obvious, the recognition of the more common, milder forms of the disorder may be very difficult, and the diagnosis may be one of exclusion.

The recurrence rate for placental abruption ranges from 5 to 17 percent.[51,59] There is a 25 percent chance of recurrence if the patient has had two prior abruptions.[38] Unfortunately, there is no way to predict who will have a recurrence, and therefore a prospective plan of management to reduce this risk has not been developed.

Management

The management of placental abruption is based on an assessment of the conditions of mother and fetus. If there is extensive hemorrhage with evidence of fetal distress, prompt delivery by cesarean section, with intensive fluid replacement therapy, is warranted. If there is evidence of DIC, FFP should be given. If the blood loss is not large and there is no evidence of fetal compromise, a more conservative approach may be taken. If the pregnancy is near or at term, steps for delivery are indicated. Vaginal delivery is not contraindicated as long as there is no evidence of fetal compromise. Continuous fetal monitoring as well as close observation of maternal vital signs and urine output are essential.

If the mother is hemodynamically stable, blood loss is minimal, there is no evidence of fetal distress, and the pregnancy is significantly preterm, careful expectant management with corticosteroids to accelerate fetal lung maturity can be considered. Sholl[54] observed that the fetuses in 50 percent of pregnancies between 26 and 37 weeks' gestation were delivered within 3 days of admission because of increased hemorrhage or fetal distress, or both. In a study by Bond and colleagues,[60] 43 women with placental abruption at less than 35 weeks' gestation were managed expectantly. The mean time to delivery was 12.4 days. There were no intrauterine deaths. The investigators concluded that in properly selected patients with preterm gestation and low-grade abruption, expectant management is reasonable. They advise antepartum fetal heart rate testing and serial hematologic and coagulation profiles if indicated.

The use of tocolytic agents in the setting of placental abruption is controversial. If true preterm labor is encountered, tocolytics of any kind are unlikely to prolong the pregnancy to any clinically significant extent. β-Adrenoreceptor agonists are usually not recommended because of their potential for dilating the vascular system in patients who may already have hypovolemia. However, the only animal study to examine this issue concluded that a β-adrenoceptor agonist is safer for both the fetus and the mother than is magnesium sulfate.[53] Although there is some evidence that the use of a β-adrenoceptor agonist may delay the diagnosis of placental abruption in some patients, especially when vaginal bleeding is not present,[54,62] other studies report improved outcomes with the use of tocolytic agents in a select group of hemodynamically stable patients with preterm contractions.[55,62]

Placenta Previa

Placenta previa is the implantation of the placenta over the cervical os. Three types of placenta previa are commonly described: total, partial, and marginal (Fig. 12-2). A total placenta previa is one that completely covers the cervical os; central complete previa is a total previa centrally located over the os. A total placenta previa is usually associated with a greater blood loss than either partial or marginal previas.[38] The type of placenta previa and the frequency with which each type is diagnosed will depend on the gestational age, degree of cervical dilatation at the time of the evaluation, and method of diagnosis (ultrasonographic versus digital).

The incidence of placenta previa is typically quoted at from 1 in 200 to 1 in 250 live births, and seems to vary with the population studied. The recurrence risk is reported to be from 3 to 3.5 percent.[64] Several factors associated with placenta previa include previous cesarean section,[65,66] multiparity, advanced maternal age,[67] and smoking.[68]

Diagnosis

The hallmark of placenta previa is painless vaginal bleeding. This is the presentation in 70 to 80 percent of cases.[69,70] In approximately 20 percent, bleeding is accompanied by uterine contractions. Typically, the first episode of bleeding is light. The lower uterine segment begins to form in the mid- to late second trimester, and the initial bleeding episode usually corresponds to this event. As the lower uterine segment develops, placental attachment is disrupted, causing bleeding from the exposed maternal vessels. The decreased ability of the lower uterine segment to contract accentuates the bleeding potential.

Placenta previa should be suspected in any pregnant women who presents with vaginal bleeding in the second or third trimester. Because of the potential for unexpected, profuse, life-threatening hemorrhage in these patients, steps to assure maternal vascular stability should be undertaken before ultrasonographic confirmation of the diagnosis. Ultrasonography is the diagnostic technique of choice, and digital examination of the cervix is absolutely contraindicated until placenta previa is ruled out. The accuracy of ultrasound examination is high, ranging up to 98 percent in some studies. Transabdominal, transvaginal, and transperineal methods have all been used with favorable results (Fig. 12-3).

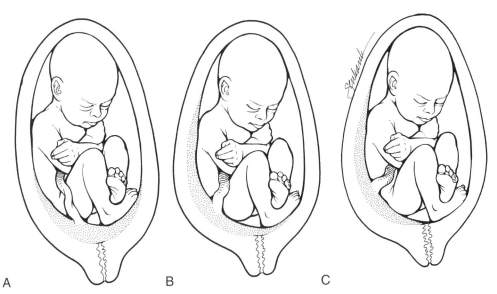

A   B   C

Fig. 12-2. Various types of placenta previa. **(A)** Total. **(B)** Partial. **(C)** Marginal.

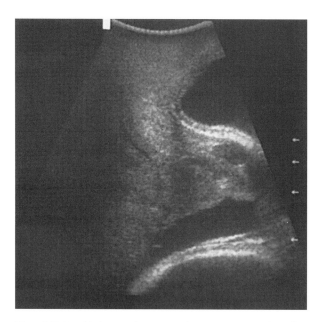

Fig. 12-3. Midsagittal view with a transvaginal probe demonstrating a complete placenta previa.

Management

Once the diagnosis of placenta previa is confirmed, management depends on such factors as gestational age, the amount of bleeding, maternal and fetal well-being, and fetal presentation. The previa diagnosed incidentally during an ultrasound examination done for other reasons does not require a change in pregnancy management, although abstinence from coitus seems prudent. Hospitalization cannot be justified.

If there is no clinically significant active bleeding when the patient is evaluated, and the fetus is preterm, expectant management is the treatment of choice. Cerclage has been recommended, but the experience with it is too small to permit endorsing it at this time. Expectant management consists of bed rest (preferably in a hospital setting) for at least the first several days after the diagnosis of placenta previa. If the patient remains without any bleeding for 1 week, bed rest at home may be considered. If the patient continues to bleed, even in small volumes, continued hospitalization is warranted. The patient should have a blood type and screen done to expedite the acquisition of blood products should they become necessary. The patient who has multi-

ple bleeding events not severe enough to warrant delivery but sufficient to cause a decrease in the hematocrit should receive blood replacement adequate to maintain the hematocrit above 30 percent. Placenta previa is one obstetric situation in which autologous blood donation is cost effective.[27]

Uterine contractions in patients with placenta previa may trigger hemorrhage. Tocolytic agents are safe[66,71] and cost effective[71] if contractions are present (see the section, *Placental Abruption*). Although in most cases of placenta previa, the hemorrhage observed is of maternal origin, there are case reports of fetal blood loss. Cotton et al[66] observed that 35 percent of infants born to mothers who required antepartum transfusions were also anemic and required transfusion. Unfortunately, it is unknown whether the fetal blood loss occurred before or during delivery, when the integrity of the placenta may have been interrupted. All Rh-negative women who are unsensitized should receive Rh immunoglobulin. The use of antenatal corticosteroids in this situation is appropriate.

The route of delivery in cases of placenta previa depends on the type of previa and the urgency for delivery. For women who are stable with a marginal previa, and either in labor or at term, a double set-up examination is indicated to both confirm the diagnosis and determine whether it is possible to rupture the membranes and attempt vaginal delivery. Although in most cases a cesarean section will be selected, a vaginal delivery is often possible, since the fetal head will tamponade the bleeding placental edge as it descends.

The double set-up examination is performed in an operating suite with the patient prepared and draped for cesarean section. The anesthesiologist and the rest of the operating staff should be in the room and ready to proceed immediately with a surgical delivery. A speculum examination is performed before the digital examination. If placental tissue cannot be seen, a careful digital examination of the vaginal fornices is performed. If a placenta previa is present, a fullness or a thrill in the fornix may be appreciated. The final step is a very careful and gentle digital examination through the cervical os. Even the most careful and gentle of digital examinations can result in profuse hemorrhage. If a vaginal delivery is deemed unsafe, then delivery should proceed via cesarean section. If the patient has a posterior previa, or a very low anterior previa, a low transverse hysterotomy incision can be safely made. If the placenta occupies most or all of the anterior lower uterine segment, the obstetrician has two options: a vertical incision above the placenta, or a transverse incision with rapid shearing of the placenta from the wall to reach a site in the membranes where the amniotomy can be performed. Delivery through the placenta should be avoided whenever possible.

There is an increased risk of placenta accreta, percreta, and increta with placenta previa (Fig. 12-4). The potential for blood loss is great if one of these conditions co-exists. Clark et al[72] reported that 5 percent of patients with a placenta previa also have placenta accreta. This incidence rises to 25 percent among patients who have had a prior cesarean section. The antepartum diagnosis of placenta accreta by ultrasound has been reported.[73] In those patients with a placenta previa and history of cesarean section, an ultrasound evaluation may be of value. Careful planning and anticipation may prove lifesaving. These patients should have at least 4 U of blood typed and cross-matched before proceeding with the cesarean delivery.

The bleeding associated with placenta accreta can

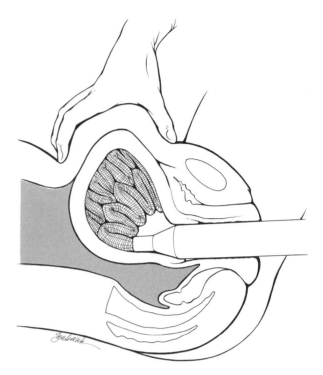

Fig. 12-5. Gauze packing of the uterine cavity.

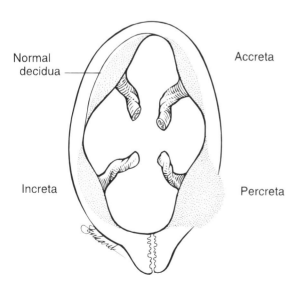

Fig. 12-4. Comparison of abnormal decidualization associated with placenta accreta, percreta, and increta and normal placentation.

be profuse and difficult to control. Ecbolic agents are often unsuccessful because of the decreased ability of the lower uterine segment to contract. If the patient does not desire future fertility, timely hysterectomy will decrease maternal morbidity and mortality. In patients who desire to preserve fertility, other conservative techniques include leaving the placenta in place (totally or in fragments),[74] localized resection and repair,[75] oversewing the defect,[76] blunt dissection and curettage,[77] packing of the uterus,[78–80] (Fig. 12-5) placement of a transvaginal pressure pack,[81,82] (Fig. 12-6) and ligation of uterine, ovarian or hypogastric vessels.[83] Cho and associates[84] describe the placement of interrupted 0-chromic sutures circumferentially around the lower uterine segment, above and below the transverse incision. They report success in all eight patients in whom this technique was employed.

Although retention of fertility is worthwhile, it is not without risk. Blood loss, infection rates, and overall morbidity rates are higher when conservative measures are tried without success, and only delay definitive treatment (i.e., hysterectomy).

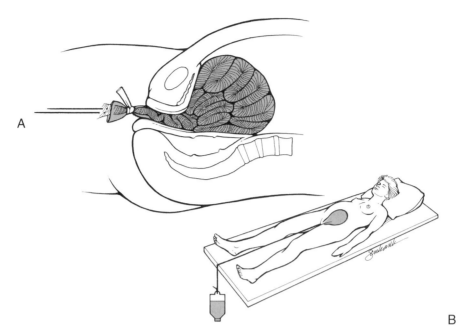

Fig. 12-6. (A & B) Transvaginal pressure pack with traction.

Vasa Previa

A rare cause of antepartum hemorrhage is fetal and not maternal in origin. Vasa previa is a condition in which the umbilical vessels present in advance of the fetal part during labor (Fig. 12-7). The condition is usually associated with a velamentous insertion of the umbilical cord into the placenta. The incidence of vasa previa is approximately 1 per 5,000 singleton deliveries.[85] Both a velamentous insertion of the cord and vasa previa are more common with multiple gestations. The fetal vessels are not protected by a surrounding Wharton's jelly, and are usually firmly attached to the fetal membranes. In both of these situations, the vessels are susceptible to rupture, especially at the time of membrane rupture (either spontaneous or artificial) and labor. Fetal mortality occurs in 75 to 100 percent of cases of rupture of these vessels.[86]

Diagnosis

Vessel rupture often occurs in association with ruptured membranes and results in painless vaginal bleeding with a rapid deterioration of the fetal heart rate pattern. If the vessels do not rupture but are compressed by the descending fetal part, variable fetal heart rate deceleration are typical. The diagnosis of this condition before rupture of the vessels or confirmation of a ruptured vasa previa requires a high index of suspicion. Occasionally, the fetal vessels can be palpated on vaginal examination as firm, usually pulseless, immobile cords. If digital examination raises suspicion of vasa previa, an examination with Doppler ultrasonography should be performed[87] (Fig. 12-8). If the patient presents with painless vaginal bleeding, and abruption and placenta previa have been ruled out, identification of fetal blood will quickly confirm the diagnosis. Often, however, the rapid deterioration of the fetal heart rate will not permit this prior to delivery.

Several laboratory tests are available to differentiate fetal from maternal blood. The Apt test[88] is rapid and inexpensive. Certain maternal hematologic conditions, such as sickle cell disease or thalassemia, may interfere with this test and give misleading results.[86] The Kleihauer–Betke test can both identify and quantitate fetal blood but is considerably more difficult to perform reproducibly, and takes longer than the Apt test.

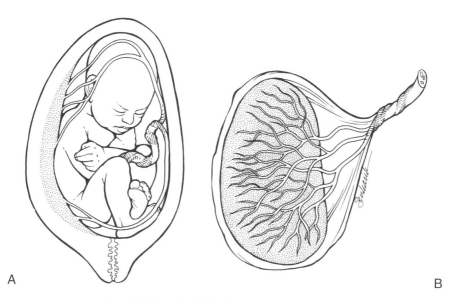

Fig. 12-7. (A & B) Schematic of vasa previa.

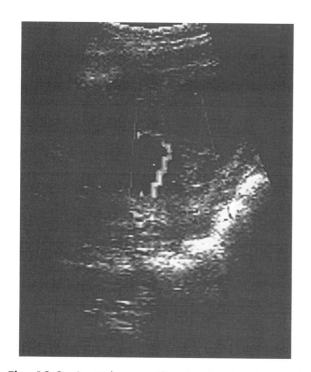

Fig. 12-8. Sagittal view with color Doppler ultrasound image showing vasa previa crossing the cervical os. (Color not shown.)

Management

If unruptured vasa previa is confirmed, amniotomy is absolutely contraindicated. Tocolytic therapy may prevent or delay spontaneous rupture of membranes in a laboring patient in cases of this diagnosis, and allow time for a controlled delivery by cesarean section. If rupture of the fetal vessels has occurred and the fetus is still alive and viable, delivery by rapid, emergent cesarean section may be lifesaving. The total blood volume of a term fetus is approximately 375 ml. Shock in the fetus will occur with the loss of only 72 ml of blood.[86] This amount of blood loss can occur within minutes of vascular rupture.

POSTPARTUM HEMORRHAGE

Postpartum hemorrhage (PPH), a relatively common and potentially lethal complication, is classified as early or late. Early postpartum hemorrhage occurs within 24 hours of delivery. Late postpartum hemorrhage occurs more than 24 hours but less than 6 weeks after delivery.

The most common cause of postpartum hemorrhage is uterine atony, which complicates approximately 1 in 20 deliveries. Twenty percent of women who develop uterine atony have no apparent risk factors for this condition.[89] Conditions that predis-

---

Causes of Postpartum Hemorrhage

Uterine atony

Genital tract lacerations

Uterine rupture

Uterine inversion

Placenta accreta or one of its variants

Retained products of conception

Coagulopathies

Common etiologies for late postpartum infection include

Endomyometritis

Subinvolution of the placental site

Retained products of conception

---

pose a patient to uterine atony include grand multiparity; uterine overdistension secondary to multiple gestations; hydramnios or a macrosomic fetus; prolonged labor, especially when associated with operative vaginal delivery or cesarean section; placental abruption; precipitous labor and delivery; chorioamnionitis; and myometrial relaxing medications, such as halogenated anesthetic agents and tocolytics. The recurrence rate for postpartum atony in a subsequent pregnancy is as high as 25 percent.[90]

Lower genital tract lacerations characteristically manifest immediately after delivery of the infant and before expulsion of the placenta. Lacerations of the upper genital tract may not be appreciated because of bleeding into an intra-abdominal potential space. Events associated with an increased risk of laceration of the genital tract include operative vaginal delivery, especially forceps delivery with rotation; precipitous labor and delivery; macrosomia with or without shoulder dystocia; and episiotomy.

Uterine rupture is a catastrophic event and is estimated to occur in approximately 1 in 2,000 deliveries. Spontaneous rupture of a nulliparous woman's intact uterus before the onset of labor is a reportable event. Conditions associated with uterine rupture include previous uterine surgery (cesarean section, myomectomy), operative vaginal delivery (midforceps, breech extraction, internal podalic version), high parity, abnormal fetal lies, and obstructed labor.

Uterine inversion occurs in approximately 1 in 2,500 deliveries.[91] Fundal implantation of the placenta and excessive cord traction may be contributing factors. Other factors reported to be associated with uterine inversion include macrosomia, use of oxytocin, and primiparity.[92] Conditions that produce uterine atony may predispose to this complication.

Failure of the placenta to separate is a common cause of PPH. Retained placenta can cause either early or late PPH, but is likely overdiagnosed. Conditions associated with early PPH include retention of a succenturiate lobe or placenta accreta. Placenta accreta occurs in approximately 1 in 2,000 deliveries. Factors predisposing to accreta include previous hysterotomy, previous puerperal curettage, placenta previa, and high parity.[82] Retention of placental fragments may also cause delayed PPH, which is usually associated with endomyometritis.

Congenital and acquired coagulopathies may either cause PPH or exacerbate a hemorrhagic condition. The most common congenital coagulopathy associated with hemorrhage in pregnancy is von Willebrand's disease, a common source of delayed postpartum hemorrhage.

The most common acquired coagulopathies are consumptive and include pre-eclampsia, abruption, sepsis, dead fetus syndrome, amniotic fluid embolism, and coagulopathy following massive blood loss. A dilutional coagulopathy may follow massive crystalloid fluid replacement. Rarely, autoimmune disorders such as idiopathic thrombocytopenic purpura are causes of PPH. Patients who are receiving anticoagulant medications are also at risk of PPH. Most hemorrhage secondary to coagulopathy is the result of soft tissue trauma or laceration, and is not secondary to uterine atony.

Management

Early recognition and acknowledgment of the diagnosis of PPH are crucial. If the patient has known risk factors for PPH, one or two large-bore intravenous catheters should be placed prior to delivery and arrangements made for the availability of blood products. If there are no known risk factors for PPH, intravenous access should be obtained as soon as the diagnosis is made. Initial laboratory studies should include a complete blood count (CBC), platelet count, and blood type and screen if not already done. A coagulation profile should be obtained when appropriate. Vital signs are monitored for evidence of severe hypovolemia (i.e., hypotension, tachycardia and oliguria). Hypovolemia is initially treated with crystalloid products, with the addition of blood as the situation dictates. Supplemental oxygen should be given by mask to increase oxygen delivery to the microvasculature.

Identification of the bleeding source is performed as the patient is stabilized. The timing of the onset of bleeding can provide important diagnostic clues. Bleeding that begins before delivery of the placenta is often due to a laceration of the lower genital tract or coagulopathy. Bleeding that occurs after delivery of the placenta suggests uterine atony, uterine inversion, or retained placental fragments (see above).

The placenta and lower genital tract should be carefully inspected in all patients. If the placenta is delivered in a piecemeal fashion, or if inspection of the placenta reveals missing cotyledons, then retained placental fragments should be suspected. Some obstetricians advocate a routine sweep of the uterine cavity after each delivery to guard against such surprises. If accessory vessels in the chorioamniotic membranes are seen, the presence of a retained succenturiate lobe should be considered. In addition to an inspection of the placenta, an examination should be done of the lower genital tract for cervical, vaginal, and perineal lacerations. It is important to have adequate exposure for this examination, even if a general anesthetic is required.

If the placenta appears normal and no lower genital tract lacerations are identified, a bimanual examination of the uterus is performed. An irregular or absent uterine fundus suggests some degree of uterine inversion. A soft, boggy uterus suggests uterine atony. Uterine rupture is identified by manual examination of the lower uterine segment following vaginal birth after cesarean section.

Lower Genital Tract Lacerations

When identified, specific sources of bleeding from lower genital tract lacerations should be ligated with absorbable suture. Any hematoma should be evacu-

ated and obvious bleeding sources ligated. If no specific source of bleeding is identified, placement of a vaginal pack may provide adequate hemostasis. The pack should be left in place for several hours before removal. Drains are placed if the laceration involves the deep pelvic tissues.

Uterine Inversion

Uterine inversion is best treated by rapid, manual replacement of the uterus into its anatomic position before the cervix has time to contract (Fig. 12-9). The placenta should not be removed if it is still attached. Following return of the uterus to its normal anatomic position, the placenta is manually removed and the uterine cavity explored. Manual massage of the uterus is performed and ecbolic agents administered to ensure uterine contraction. If the cervix has already contracted before the uterus can be restored, a uterine relaxant, such a halogenated anesthetic agent, may be necessary before replacement. In rare cases the uterus cannot be replaced manually and surgical intervention is required. Both transvaginal and transabdominal approaches have been described.[91] The abdominal approach is most often advocated.

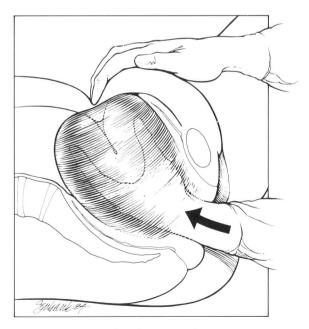

Fig. 12-9. Manual replacement of inverted uterus. (From Benedetti,[38] with permission.)

Uterine Rupture

Laparotomy is usually indicated if the uterus has ruptured. Conservative measures may be tried if the patient desires future fertility. The separated edges should be reapproximated after debridement of any nonviable tissue. If the bleeding cannot be controlled or the damage to the uterus is extensive, hysterectomy is necessary.

Uterine Atony: Medical Management

The initial management of PPH secondary to uterine atony consists of vigorous, bimanual fundal massage (Fig. 12-10), with the infusion of oxytocin. The typical dose of oxytocin is 10 to 40 U in 1,000 ml of normal saline or lactated Ringer's solution. Larger doses of oxytocin will not provide an additional effect. Moreover, there is also the potential for circulatory collapse if oxytocin is given as a rapid intravenous injection; therefore, this practice should be avoided. Oxytocin can be less effective after a prolonged augmentation of labor in which large doses of oxytocin have already been administered.

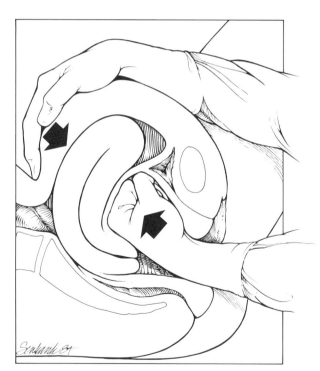

Fig. 12-10. Bimanual uterine compression and massage of the uterus to control hemorrhage from uterine artery. (From Benedetti,[38] with permission.)

If these measures fail to contract the uterus, other pharmacologic therapy is indicated. Methylergonovine (Methergine) 0.2 mg IM may be given every 6 hours, or 15-methyl prostaglandin-$F_{2\alpha}$ ($PGF_{2\alpha}$) (Hemabate) 0.25 mg IM may be given every 15 to 60 minutes. Hemabate has also been administered directly into the myometrium.[93] Both methylergonovine and 15-methyl-$PGF_{2\alpha}$ may exacerbate chronic and pre-eclamptic hypertension. Acute maternal oxygen desaturation has also been reported in some patients given $PGF_{2\alpha}$.[94] If pharmacologic therapy does not control hemorrhage and preservation of fertility is highly desired, uterine packing may be successful.[78,95] Concerns about infection and concealed hemorrhage with uterine packing are not supported by experience.[95] Angiographic arterial embolization has also been employed for the treatment PPH, but is more likely to be successful with bleeding from a discrete site rather than for uterine atony.[96,97]

Uterine Atony: Surgical Management

If medical management of uterine atony fails, aggressive surgical intervention is required. The choice of procedure depends on the patient's hemodynamic stability, her desire to preserve fertility, and the experience of the operator. If the patient desires preservation of fertility and is hemodynamically stable, ligation of the uterine and ovarian arteries or of the hypogastric artery may be performed. The goal in each procedure is to reduce the pulse pressure to the reproductive organs and thereby facilitate thrombus formation and hemostasis. Ligation of the uterine (Fig. 12-11) and ovarian arteries is a relatively simple procedure and reportedly reduces the pulse pressure by 60 to 70 percent. The bladder flap is dissected away from the cervix to displace the ureters laterally. The uterine arteries are ligated just above the bladder flap. The use of a large-diameter, delayed-absorption suture is recommended. The sutures should extend into the myometrium to avoid the ureters and ensure inclusion of enough tissue to maintain vascular compression. The vessels must not be cut. The ovarian arteries are then ligated near the utero-ovarian ligament.

Ligation of the anterior branch of the hypogastric artery (Fig. 12-12) is an alternative to ligation of the uterine and ovarian arteries. It is technically more difficult than ligation of the uterine arteries but will

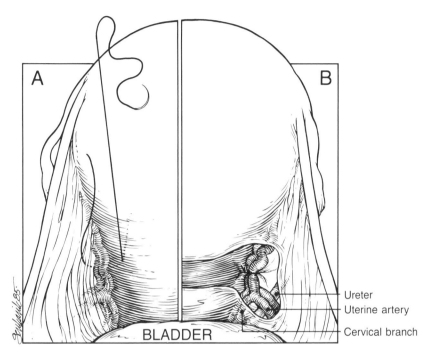

Fig. 12-11. Ligation of uterine artery. (From Benedetti,[38] with permission.)

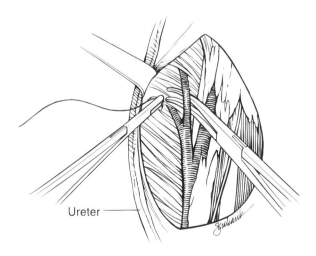

Fig. 12-12. Ligation of anterior branch of hypogastric artery.

include several pelvic anastomic sites missed by uterine/ovarian ligation. In patients with either a uterine rupture or a large broad-ligament hematoma, this procedure may be preferred to ligation of the uterine arteries. Correct anatomic identification is imperative before ligation. The posterior branch of the hypogastric artery provides blood to the gluteal muscles, and the external iliac artery is the sole supply of blood to the lower extremities. Mistaken ligation of these vessels would have severe consequences. Opening the lateral pelvic peritoneum at the level of the bifurcation of the common iliac artery provides access to the hypogastric artery. It is important to visualize the ureter on the medial leaf of the peritoneum to avoid its inadvertent ligation. The anterior and posterior branches of the hypogastric artery are then identified by careful dissection. Bilateral ligation of the hypogastric arteries reportedly decreases the mean arterial perfusion pressure by 25 percent, blood flow by 50 percent, and pulse pressure by 85 percent. Despite these reductions Clark and associates[98] found this procedure to be associated with the control of hemorrhage in only 42 percent of patients. In addition, ureteral injury and cardiac arrest were each reported. Attempting any or all of these procedures adds operative time and increases the total blood loss. They should be attempted only in patients who are hemodynamically stable.

In women who do not desire future fertility, are hemodynamically unstable, or continue to bleed after other procedures have been performed, hysterectomy is the procedure of choice. It is estimated that from the time the decision is made to proceed with hysterectomy to the time of its completion, an additional 2,000 ml of blood will be lost,[89] again emphasizing the importance of not delaying this decision. Because of the increased vascular size observed during pregnancy, all vascular pedicles should be doubly ligated.

REFERENCES

1. Kaunitz AM, Hughes JM, Grimes DA et al: Causes of maternal mortality in the United States. Obstet Gynecol 65:605, 1985
2. Rochat RW, Koonin LM, Atrash HK, Jewett JF: The Maternal Mortality Collaborative. Maternal mortality in the United States: report from the maternal mortality collaborative. Obstet Gynecol 72:91, 1988
3. Jouppilla P: Vaginal bleeding in the last two trimesters of pregnancy: a clinical and ultrasonic study. Acta Obstet Gynecol Scand 58:461, 1979
4. Hewitt BG, Newnham JP: A review of the obstetric and medical complications leading to the delivery of infants of very low birth weight. Obstet Gynecol Surv 45:369, 1988
5. Pritchard JA, Baldwin RM, Dickey JC, Wiggins KM: Blood volume changes in pregnancy and the puerperium. II. Red blood cell loss and changes in apparent blood volume during and following vaginal delivery, cesarean section, and cesarean section plus total hysterectomy. Am J Obstet Gynecol 84:1271, 1962
6. Pritchard JA, Baldwin RM, Dickey JC, Wiggins KM: Blood volume changes in pregnancy and the puerperium. Am J Obstet Gynecol 84:1271, 1962
7. Baker RJ: Evaluation and management of critically ill patients. Obstet Gynecol Ann 6:295, 1977
8. Walter CW, Bellamy D, Murphy WP: The mechanical factors responsible for rapid infusion of blood. Surg Gynecol Obstet 101:115, 1955
9. Moise KJ, Cotton DB: The use of colloid osmotic pressure in pregnancy. Clin Perinatol 13:827, 1986
10. Hayashi RH: Hemorrhagic shock in obstetrics. Clin Perinatol 13:755, 1986
11. Rackow EC, Falk JL, Fein IA: Fluid resuscitation in circulatory shock: a comparison of the cardiorespiratory effects of albumin, hetastarch, and saline solutions in patients with hypovolemic and septic shock. Crit Care Med 11:839, 1983
12. Consensus Development Panel: Perioperative red blood cell transfusion. JAMA 260:2700, 1988
13. Blood Component Therapy. ACOG Technical Bulletin No 78.: American College of Obstetricians and Gynecologists, Washington, DC, July, 1984
14. Martin DJ, Lucas CE, Ledgerwood AM et al: Fresh frozen plasma supplement to massive red blood cell transfusion. Ann Surg 202:505, 1985
15. Ciavarella D, Reed RL, Counts RB et al: Clotting factor levels and the risk of diffuse microvascular bleeding in the massively transfused patient. Br J Haematol 67:365, 1987
16. Consensus Development Panel: Fresh-frozen plasma: indictions and risks. JAMA 253:551, 1985
17. Nolan TE, Gallup DG: Massive transfusion: a current review. Obstet Gynecol Surv 46:289, 1991
18. Consensus Development Panel: Platelet transfusion therapy. Conn Med 51:105, 1987
19. Berkman SA: Infectious complications of blood transfusions. Blood Rev 2:206, 1988
20. Perkins HA, Samson S, Garner J et al: Risk of AIDS for receipients of blood components from donors who subsequently developed AIDS. Blood 5:1604, 1987
21. Ness PM: The safety of blood transfusions in obstetric patients. Postgrad Obstet Gynecol 13:1, 1993
22. Kruskall MS, Leonard S, Klapholz H: Autologous blood donation during pregnancy: Analysis of safety and blood use. Obstet Gynecol 70:938, 1987
23. Druzin ML, Wolf CFW, Edersheim TG et al: Donation of blood by the pregnant patient for autologous transfusion. Am J Obstet Gynecol 159:1023, 1988
24. Herbert WNP, Owen HG, Collins ML: Autologous blood storage in obstetrics. Obstet Gynecol 72:166, 1988
25. Droste S, Sorensen T, Price T et al: Maternal and fetal hemodynamic effects of autologous blood donation during pregnancy. Am J Obstet Gynecol 167:89, 1992
26. Andres RL, Piacquadio KM, Resnik R: A reappraisal of the need for autologous blood donation in the obstetric patient. Am J Obstet Gynecol 163:1551, 1990
27. Combs CA, Murphy EL, Laros RK: Cost-benefit analysis of autologous blood donation in obstetrics. Obstet Gynecol 80:621, 1992
28. Marder VJ: Consumptive thrombohemorrhagic disorders. p. 1523. In Williams WJ, Beutler E, Erslev AJ,

Lichtman MA (eds): Hematology. 4th Ed. McGraw-Hill, New York, 1990

29. Moncada S, Palmer RMJ, Higgs EA: Nitric oxide: physiology, pathophysiology, and pharmacology. Pharmacol Rev 43:109, 1991

30. Kilbourn RG, Gross SS, Jubran A et al: N^G-methyl-L-Arginine inhibits tumor necrosis factor-induced hypotension: implications for the involvement of nitric oxide. Proc Natl Acad Sci USA 87:3629, 1990

31. Weiner CP: The obstetric patient and disseminated intravascular coagulation. Clin Perinatol 13:705, 1986

32. Bick RK, Dukes ML, Wilson WL et al: Antithrombin III as a diagnostic aid in disseminated intravascular coagulation. Thromb Res 10:721, 1977

33. Bick RK: Disseminated intravascular coagulation and related syndromes: etiology, pathophysiology, diagnosis, and management. Am J Hematol 5:265, 1978

34. Weiner CP, Brandt J: Plasma antithrombin III activity in normal pregnancy. Obstet Gynecol 56:601, 1980

35. Weiner CP, Brandt J: Plasma antithrombin III activity: an aid in the diagnosis of preeclampsia-eclampsia. Am J Obstet Gynecol 142:275, 1982

36. Brandjes DPM, Schenk BE, Büller HR, ten Cate JW: Management of disseminated intravascular coagulation in obstetrics. Eur J Obstet Gynecol Reprod Biol 42:S87, 1991

37. Saftlas AF, Olson DR, Atrash HK et al: National trends in the incidence of abruptio placentae, 1979–1987. Obstet Gynecol 78:1081, 1991

38. Benedetti TJ: Obstetric hemorrhage. p. 573. In Gabbe SG, Niebyl JR, Simpson JL (eds): Obstetrics: Normal and Problem Pregnancies. 2nd Ed. Churchill Livingstone, New York, 1991

39. Fleming AD: Abruptio placentae. Crit Care Clin 7:865, 1991

40. Green JR: Placenta previa and abruptio placentae. p. 592. In Creasy RK, Resnik R (eds): Maternal-Fetal Medicine: Principles and Practice. 2nd Ed. WB Saunders, Philadelphia, 1989

41. Katz VL, Chescheir NC, Cefalo RC: Unexplained elevations of maternal serum alpha-fetoprotein. Obstet Gynecol Surv 45:719, 1990

42. Pritchard JA, Mason R, Corley M, Pritchard S: Genesis of severe placental abruption. Am J Obstet Gynecol 108:22, 1970

43. Williams JK, McClain L, Rosemurgy AS, Colorado NM: Evaluation of blunt abdominal trauma in the third trimester of pregnancy. maternal and fetal considerations. Obstet Gynecol 75:33, 1990

44. Pearlman MD, Tintinalli JE, Lorenz RP: A prospective controlled study of outcome after trauma during pregnancy. Am J Obstet Gynecol 162:1502, 1990

45. Naeye RL: Abruptio placentae and placenta previa: frequency, perinatal mortality, and cigarette smoking. Obstet Gynecol 55:701, 1980

46. Voigt LF, Hollenbach KA, Krohn MA, et al: The relationship of abruptio placentae with maternal smoking and small for gestational age infants. Obstet Gynecol 75:771, 1990

47. Marbury MC, Linn S, Monson R et al: The association of alcohol consumption with outcome of pregnancy. Am J Public Health 73:1165, 1983

48. Chasnoff I, Burns W, Schnoll S, Burns K: Cocaine use in pregnancy. N Engl J Med 313:666, 1985

49. Slutsker L: Risks associated with cocaine using during pregnancy. Obstet Gynecol 79:778, 1992

50. Gonen R, Hannah ME, Milligan JE: Does prolonged preterm premature rupture of the membranes predispose to abruptio placenta? Obstet Gynecol 74:347, 1989

51. Pritchard JA, Cunningham FG, Pritchard SA, Mason RA: On reducing the frequency of severe abruptio placaentae. Am J Obstet Gynecol 165:1345, 1991

52. Rice JP, Kay HH, Mahony BS: The clinical significance of uterine leiomyomas in pregnancy. Am J Obstet Gynecol 160:1212, 1989

53. Chestnut DH, Thompson CS, McLaughlin GL, Weiner CP: Dose the intravenous infusion of ritodrine or magnesium sulfate alter the hemodynamic response to hemorrhage in gravid ewes? Am J Obstet Gynecol 159:1467, 1988

54. Hurd WW, Miodovnik M, Hertzberg V, Lavin JP: Selective management of abruptio placentae: a prospective study. Obstet Gynecol 61:467, 1983

55. Sholl JS: Abruptio placentae: clinical management in nonacute cases. Am J Obstet Gynecol 156:40, 1987

56. Sprit BA, Kagan EH, Rozanski RM: Abruptio placentae: sonographic and pathologic correlation. AJR 133:877, 1979

57. Pritchard JA, Brekken AL: Clinical and laboratory studies on severe abruptio placentae. Am J Obstet Gynecol 97:681, 1967

58. Cunningham FG, MacDonald PC, Gant NF et al (eds): Obstetrical hemorrhage. p. 819. In: William's Obstetrics. 19th Ed. Appleton & Lange, E. Norwalk CT, 1993

59. Grünfeld JP, Pertuiset N: Acute renal failure in pregnancy: 1987. Am J Kidney Dis 9:359, 1987

60. Hibbard B, Jeffcoate T: Abruptio placentae. Obstet Gynecol 27:155, 1966

61. Bond AL, Edersheim TG, Curry L et al: Expectant management of abruptio placentae before 35 weeks gestation. Am J Perinatol 6:121, 1989

62. Astedt B: Risk of β-receptor agonists delaying diagno-

sis of abruptio placentae. Acta Obstet Gynecol Scand, suppl. 108:35, 1982

63. Combs CA, Nyberg DA, Mack LA et al: Expectant management after sonographic diagnosis of placental abruption. Am J Perinatol 9:170, 1992

64. Thomas RL: How to manage third-trimester bleeding. Fem Patient 15:17, 1990

65. Brenner W, Edelman D, Hendricks C: Characteristics of patients with placenta previa and results of "expectant management." Am J Obstet Gynecol 132:180, 1978

66. Cotton D, Ead J, Paul R, Quilligan EJ: The conservative aggressive management of placenta previa. Am J Obstet Gynecol 17:687, 1980

67. Cunningham FG, Leveno KJ: Pregnancy after thirty-five. In William's Obstetrics. 18th Ed, (Suppl. 2). Appleton & Lange, E. Norwalk, CT, 1989

68. Williams MA, Mittendorf R, Lieberman E et al: Cigarette smoking during pregnancy in relation to placenta previa. Am J Obstet Gynecol 165:28, 1991

69. Silver R, Depp R, Sabbbagha RE et al: Placenta previa: aggressive expectant management. Am J Obstet Gynecol 150:15, 1984

70. Cotton DB, Read JA, Paul RH et al: The conservative aggressive management of placenta previa. Am J Obstet Gynecol 137:687, 1980

71. Tomich PG: Prolonged use of tocolytic agents in the expectant management of placenta previa. J Reprod Med 30:745, 1985

72. Clark SL, Koonings PP, Phelan JP: Placenta previa/accreta and prior cesarean section. Obstet Gynecol 66:89, 1985

73. Tabsch KMA, Brinkman CR, King W: Ultrasound diagnosis of placenta increta. J Clin Ultrasound 10:288, 1982

74. Arulkumaran S, Ratnam SS: Medical treatment of placenta accreta with methotrexate. Acta Obstet Gynecol Scand 65:285, 1986

75. McGuinness TB, Jackson JR, Schnapf DJ: Conservative surgical management of placental implantation site hemorrhage. Obstet Gynecol 81:830, 1993

76. Cox SM, Carpenter RJ, Cotton DB: Placenta percreta: ultrasound diagnosis and conservative management. Obstet Gynecol 71:454, 1988

77. Zahn CM, Yeomans ER: Postpartum hemorrhage: placenta accreta, uterine inversion, and puerperal hematomas. Clin Obstet Gynecol 33:422, 1990

78. Maier RC: Control of postpartum hemorrhage with uterine packing. Am J Obstet Gynecol 169:317, 1993

79. Hester JD: Postpartum hemorrhage and reevaluation of uterine packing. Obstet Gynecol 45:501, 1975

80. Druzin ML: Packing of lower uterine segment for control of postcesarean bleeding in instances of placenta previa. Surg Gynecol Obstet 169:543, 1989

81. Hallak M, Dildy GA, Hurley TJ, Moise KJ: Transvaginal pressure pack for life-threatening pelvic hemorrhage secondary to placenta accreta. Obstet Gynecol 78:938, 1991

82. Dildy GA, Clark SL: Postpartum hemorrhage. Contemp Obstet Gynecol 38:21, 1993

83. Thavarasah AS, Sivalingam N, Almohdzar SA: Internal iliac and ovarian artery ligation in the control of pelvic haemorrhage. Aust NZ J Obstet Gynaecol 29:22, 1989

84. Cho JY, Kim SJ, Cha KY et al: Interrupted circular suture: bleeding control during cesarean delivery in placenta previa accreta. Obstet Gynecol 78:876, 1991

85. Quek SP, Tan KL: Vasa previa. Aust NZ J Obstet Gynaecol 12:206, 1972

86. Carlan SJ, Knuppel RA: Vasa previa: approaches to detection. Fem Patient 15:37, 1990

87. Gianapoulos J, Carver T, Tomich P et al: Diagnosis of vasa previa with ultrasonography. Obstet Gynecol 69:488, 1987

88. Apt L, Downy W: Melena neonatorum: the swallowed blood syndrome: a simple test for differentiation of adult and fetal Hgb in blood stool. J Pediatr 47:6, 1955

89. Varner M: Postpartum hemorrhage. Crit Care Clin 7:883, 1991

90. Dewhurst CJ, Dutton WAW: Recurrent abnormalities of the third stage of labor. Lancet 2:764, 1957

91. Didley GA, Clark SL: Acute puerperal uterine inversion. Contemp Ob/Gyn 37:13, 1993

92. Brar HS, Greenspoon JS, Platt LD et al: Acute puerperal uterine inversion. New approaches to management. J Reprod Med 34:173, 1989

93. Bruce SL, Paul RH, Van Dorsten JP: Control of postpartum uterine atony by intramyometrial prostaglandin. Obstet Gynecol 59:47S, 1982

94. Hankins GDV, Berryman GK, Scott RT, Hood D: Maternal arterial desaturation with 15-methyl prostaglandin F_2 alpha for uterine atony. Obstet Gynecol 72:367, 1988

95. Maier RC: Control of postpartum hemorrhage with uterine packing. Am J Obstet Gynecol 169:317, 1993

96. Duggan PM, Jamieson MG, Wattie WJ: Intractable postpartum haemorrhage managed by angiographic embolization: case report and review. Aust NZ J Obstet Gynaecol 31:229, 1991

97. Mitty HA, Sterling KM, Alvarez M, Gendler R: Obstetric hemorrhage: prophylactic and emergency arterial catheterization and embolotherapy. Radiology 188:183, 1993

98. Clark SL, Phelan JP, Yeh SY et al: Hypogastric artery ligation for obstetric hemorrhage. Obstet Gynecol 66:353, 1985

Chapter 13

Operative Obstetrics, Vaginal Birth After Cesarean Section, and Puerperal Hysterectomy

Carolyn M. Zelop and Leonard E. Safon

OPERATIVE OBSTETRICS

According to the Centers for Disease Control's National Hospital Discharge Survey for 1991, 966,000 (23.5 percent) of the 4,111,000 live births in the United States during that year were by cesarean section. Of these, an estimated 338,000 (35 percent) births were by repeat cesarean section and 628,000 (65 percent) were by primary cesarean section. Of all cesarean sections performed in 1991 on a national basis, 35 percent were associated with previous cesarean sections, 30.4 percent with dystocia, 11.7 percent with breech presentation, and 9.2 percent with fetal distress, and 13.7 percent were done for all other specified indications. These statistics demonstrate the rising trend in the cesarean section rate beginning in 1965, and prevailing into the 1990s.[1] Because from a public health and economic viewpoint there is little evidence that maternal- and child-health status have continued to improve dramatically during this period, debate continues about the legitimacy of the current cesarean section rate.

Indications

Indications for cesarean section are divided into two major categories: maternal and fetal. Maternal indications include failed medical induction; obstetric hemorrhage, including placenta previa; and cephalopelvic disproportion (CPD) secondary to a contracted pelvis. CPD and/or failure to progress (FTP) may result from abnormal uterine labor or relative fetal dystocia. Fetal indications for cesarean section include fetal distress; fetal anomalies leading to relative dystocia; fetal malpresentation, including multiple gestations; and vasa previa. Whatever the indication for it, it is important that the decision to perform cesarean section be based on logical and concrete factors that are acceptable to both the patient and physician. Many areas of controversy remain about the absolute need for cesarean section. The following clinical situations deserve special mention here. However, they are extensive topics for discussion in and of themselves.

Class R Diabetes Mellitus

Cesarean section at our institution has traditionally been recommended as the preferred route of delivery for patients with class R diabetes mellitus who show evidence of active neovasculization and have a history of recent laser therapy. More recently, however, patients with class R diabetes with quiescent retinal disease who have undergone frequent ocular antepartum examinations have been considered candidates for vaginal delivery with an assisted second stage of labor.

Immune Thrombocytopenia

Immune thrombocytopenia (ITP) poses potential risks for the mother and fetus that are in direct opposition to one another. Thrombocytopenia may, for

---

Indications for Cesarean Section

Maternal

Hemorrhage secondary to previa or abruption

CPD/failure to progress

Skeletal dysplasia leading to contracted pelvis

Active genital herpes (lesions present)

Failed medical induction

Previous classical hysterotomy

Previous cornual resection

Previous myomectomy involving uterine cavity violation

Fetal

Fetal distress

Fetal malpresentation, including unfavorable breech presentation

Multiple gestations:

a. nonvertex-presenting fetus

b. triplet gestations

c. non-vertex nonpresenting fetus can be offered trial of labor, a relative indication

Vasa previa

Macrosomia of 4,500 or more in the nondiabetic population, and of 4,000 g or more in the diabetic population

Fetal anomalies leading to relative dystocia

Cord prolapse

---

example, cause maternal bleeding at the time of a cesarean section designed to protect the fetus from intracranial hemorrhage. Although controversies continue, the consensus advocates cesarean section for cases of alloimmune thrombocytopenia.[2] Platelets collected from the fetal scalp during the intrapartum period can be used for testing in cases of maternal ITP, with recognition of the 14 percent risk of falsely decreased fetal platelet values low enough

to incorrectly alter obstetric management.[3] By contrast, Cook et al[4] have suggested that the route of delivery does not affect the rate of intracranial hemorrhage in thrombocytopenic newborns.

Fetal Anomalies

Controversy also continues over the correct route of delivery for fetuses with congenital anomalies. For example, the literature supports the delivery of fetuses with neural tube defects by cesarean section to protect the fetus from infection. In cases of fetal hernial defects such as gastroschisis and omphalocele, the support for cesarean delivery is less clear, since increased survival has not been found with respect to the route of delivery. However, the size of the defect as well as concern that extracorporeal viscera are at risk of avulsion or tear injuries (or both) during a vaginal delivery may tip the balance toward delivery by elective cesarean section.[5] A biparietal diameter (BPD) of 11.0 cm or more in the setting of macrosomia or fetal intracranial anomaly usually necessitates delivery by cesarean section.

Maternal Intracranial Vascular Lesions

Maternal aneurysms and AV malformations, particularly when newly diagnosed in the antepartum period in the setting of intracranial hemorrhage, traditionally mandate cesarean section delivery. However, patients who have undergone successful surgical repair of such lesions remote from the time of delivery may be potential candidates for vaginal delivery with assisted second stages.[6]

Choice of Skin and Uterine Incisions

Identification of the indication for cesarean delivery can influence the choice of skin and uterine incisions. However, most situations can be adequately handled with the use of the Pfannenstiel skin incision and the Kerr or lower-uterine-segment transverse hysterotomy. In the morbidly obese patient the Pfannenstiel incision, made several centimeters cephalad to the usual landmarks, provides the ideal approach to this most challenging surgical situation. Bilateral support of the pannus may be required, using temporary skin sutures or tape attached to a secured divider anteriorly. The incision, however, should not be made within a deep skin fold. Cases of fetal distress or hemostatic difficulties may lend themselves to a vertical skin incision, since this expedites entry into the abdomen and reduces bleeding in the midline.

The lower transverse uterine incision is also extremely versatile and can be used in most clinical situations. Exceptions to this include malpresentation of a premature infant, a transverse lie at any gestational age, multiple gestations, and fetal macrosomia when the lower uterine segment is thickened and undeveloped. If necessary, a Kerr incision can be extended by creating a J extension, which may be preferable to performing a uterine hysterotomy with a T incision. However, care must be taken to avoid extension into the uterine vessels. A low vertical incision, defined as an incision kept below the superior insertion of the round ligament, can be extended if necessary to a classical hysterotomy.

Surgical Technique and Choice of Suture

The Bovie cautery used widely in other surgical subspecialities can be used to facilitate hemostasis during cesarean section. The surgeon should always document that the patient has been properly grounded prior to its use. The Bovie technique should not be used to incise the uterus when performing a hysterotomy.

Following entrance into the abdominal peritoneal cavity, a bladder flap is created by incising the visceral peritoneum in the midline and extending the incision bilaterally, using suture forceps and Metzenbaum scissors. The bladder flap is then developed through gentle blunt dissection. Following this, a Doyen bladder retractor is placed under the bladder flap for retraction. Inability to create a bladder flap because of previous scar tissue or severe varicosities will necessitate a vertical hysterotomy. Alternatively, a higher transverse hysterotomy can be performed. Following placement of the Doyen retractor, the lower uterine segment is examined and a choice of incision is made as discussed above. The Kerr incision can be extended bluntly using a finger technique once the midline of the uterus is incised. Alternatively, the incision can be extended using bandage scissors. The goal of both techniques is to avoid laceration of the ascending branch of the uterine artery in the broad ligament. Following delivery of the fetus and placenta, the margins of the uterine incision are reapproximated. Exteriorization of the uterus to facilitate its exposure has mainly been a matter of the operator's personal preference. Typically, an absorbable suture such as chromic catgut is employed to minimize tearing through the "buttery" peripartum uterine texture. The short duration of suture tensile strength (approximately 7 days) is adequate for the rapidly healing uterus with its tremendous blood supply. A two-layer approach is utilized in closing the hysterotomy wound, with the first layer primarily used to secure hemostasis. The second layer is used to imbricate the endopelvic fascia. However, single-layer closures incorporating both of the layers can be used, and is not associated with an increased risk of dehiscence.[7]

A Kronig (low vertical) or classical hysterotomy may require an additional interrupted layer to facilitate reapproximation of the margins of the incision and decrease tension along the incision border. The Irving suture technique is performed by dividing the tissue on either side of the hysterotomy into halves (Fig. 13-1). The suture is begun from the outer half, brought over the other side in a backhanded fashion and inserted in the two inner halves. Finally, the suture is made to join the outer half on the proximal side, to complete the interrupted suture.

Reperitonealization of the visceral and parietal peritoneum occurs spontaneously within 48 hours.

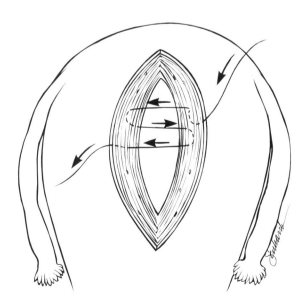

Fig. 13-1. Irving suture technique.

Thus, the need for suture reapproximation is unclear. Allowing spontaneous reperitonealization may decrease bladder adhesion as well as operative time.[8] Closure of the fascia is again dictated by the type of incision used. The transverse incision can be closed with a running suture divided in half. The vertical fascial incision is traditionally closed with interrupted figures of eight made with a delayed-absorption suture (i.e., vicryl). No randomized controlled studies have examined the occurrence of peripartum dehiscence following the closure of vertical fascial incisions, with the interrupted as opposed to running suture technique with delayed-absorption sutures such as vicryl, Maxon, or PDS. The surgeon may elect to use a running closure with the incision divided in half if the patient has no risk factors for poor healing, such as obesity, infection, steroid dependence, or diabetes. In this case, a longer lasting delayed-absorption suture such as maxon should be used.

Postoperative Morbidity and Mortality

The appropriate use of cesarean section may decrease perinatal morbidity and mortality, but is accompanied by an increase in maternal morbidity. Although complication rates may vary with the demographic characteristics of the cohort and with such risk factors as emergency cesarean section and the duration of rupture of membranes, infection is by far the most frequent complication of cesarean section. In a prospective 3-year study[9] in Sweden involving 1,319 women undergoing cesarean section, an overall complication rate of 14.5 percent was observed. Morbidity resulting from cesarean section included wound abscess, hematoma, endometritis, urogenital tract injury, venous thromboembolism, and ileus (Table 13-1). Mortality related to cesarean section is somewhat difficult to quantify due because of its rarity. Sachs and colleagues[10] demonstrated the relative safety of cesarean section by examining the morbidity and mortality related to the procedure in Massachusetts from 1954 to 1985. Despite the quadrupling of the cesarean section rate over this period, the number of related deaths per 100,000 live births did not change. Between 1976 and 1984 there were 649,375 births and 121,217 cesarean sections in the state of Massachusetts. Seven deaths were directly related to cesarean section, giving a rate of 5.8 deaths per 100,000 cesarean sections performed. Surprisingly, the death rate for vaginal deliveries was 10.8 per 100,000.

Strategies For Prevention of Perioperative Complications

Antibiotic Prophylaxis

The most common complication of cesarean section is endometritis. There is substantial clinical evidence that a short course of perioperative antibiotic ther-

Table 13-1. Morbidity of Cesarean Section

Complication	Prevalence (%)
Minor (N = 1,319)	
Paralytic ileus	0.2 (3/1,319)
Endometritis	6.6 (87/1,319)
Urinary tract infection	3.1 (41/1,319)
Superficial wound infection	1.6 (21/1,319)
Major (N = 1,319)	
Reoperation secondary to intra-abdominal hemorrhage	0.3 (4/1,319)
Reoperation secondary to pelvic abscess	0.6 (8/1,319)
Paraendometritis	0.9 (12/1,319)
Pneumonia	0.5 (6/1,319)
Bladder paresis and urethral catheter $\geq$5 days	0.2 (2/1,319)
Severe paralytic ileus >5 days	0.2 (2/1,319)
Thrombosis	0.1 (1/1,319)
Pneumothorax	0.1 (1/1,319)
Sepsis	0.1 (1/1,319)
Hysterectomy secondary to increased bleeding in the uterine scar	0.1 (1/1,319)

apy significantly reduces the frequency of endometritis in patients undergoing nonelective cesarean section.[11] From both an economic and clinical standpoint, limited spectrum antibiotics such as first-generation cephalosporins (i.e., cefazolin) appear to be as effective as broader spectrum agents. A single dose after cord clamping is adequate for prophylaxis.[12]

Autologous Blood Donation

Depending on the study and patient cohort, the transfusion frequency related to cesarean section can range from 2.2 to 7.3 percent.[13] Risk factors suggesting the possible need for transfusion include a previous history of transfusion, placenta previa, multiple gestation, pregnancy-induced hypertension, and repeat cesarean section. However, the risk factors may vary in their ability to predict the need for transfusion.[14] Donor-directed blood banking is an option in the high-risk patient unable to donate blood because of anemia. Nonetheless, autologous blood donation appears to be safe for both the mother and fetus.

Deep Vein Thrombosis Prophylaxis

The incidence of venous thrombosis in pregnancy ranges from 0.13 to 1.1 percent in the antepartum period to 0.61 to 1.2 percent in the postpartum patient. Post cesarean section, the risk may be as high as 1.8 to 3.0 percent.[15] Therefore, patients with increased risk factors, including prolonged bed rest, obesity, diabetes, and sickle cell disease, may benefit from prophylaxis before a cesarean section. Prolonged surgeries, such as for patients with multiple laparotomies or cesarean sections for placenta previa, should also prompt consideration of prophylaxis against deep vein thrombosis (DVT). Thigh-high pneumatic boots can be used for such prophylaxis, but no randomized, controlled studies have been done to document their efficacy in the peripartum period, particularly when a pelvic condition is the most likely source of a thrombotic event. In addition to providing a local mechanical effect, the pneumatic device stimulates the fibrinolytic system as a consequence of recurrent cycles of deflation and inflation. Alternatives to pneumatic devices include subcutaneous heparin at a dose of 5,000 U subcutaneously, with the first dose given 2 hours before surgery and

further dosing continuing postoperatively every 8 hours until the patient is ambulatory. Heparin has not been associated with an increased risk of surgical bleeding complications.

Perimortem Cesarean Section

A carefully timed perimortem cesarean section has the potential to be lifesaving to both the mother and fetus. Cesarean section is an important component of successful maternal resuscitation in the event of maternal cardiac arrest. Ideally, every obstetrician should know when to initiate this procedure in order to facilitate the resuscitation process. Causes of arrest in pregnancy include pre-existing heart disease, peripartum cardiomyopathy, severe pregnancy-induced hypertension, laryngeal edema/anaphylaxis, aspiration pneumonia, pulmonary embolism, sepsis, trauma, hypoalbuminemia/hemorrhage, drug poisoning with overdose, and electrolyte abnormalities, including elevated concentrations of magnesium or potassium.

The unique changes in maternal and fetal physiology that occur with normal pregnancy help explain the increased susceptibility to hemodynamic instability during this period. Oxygen deprivation is not well tolerated, owing to the increased basal metabolic rate, increased oxygen consumption, and decreased functional residual capacity (FRC). The gravid uterus, causing aortocaval compression, compromises the ability to generate sufficient cardiac output through cardiopulmonary resuscitation (CPR). Lateral uterine displacement, the hallmark of maternal resuscitation, will not totally correct this problem, and will in addition prevent adequate thoracic compression.[16,17] Therefore, in the setting of cardiac arrest, if the mother is not improving by 4 minutes after the beginning of CPR, cesarean section should be initiated, with delivery by 5 minutes. The 5-minute limit until delivery is derived from knowledge of the effect of anoxia on the mother. Without adequate cerebral perfusion, irreversible brain damage occurs within 4 to 6 minutes.[18,19]

VAGINAL BIRTH AFTER CESAREAN SECTION

Vaginal birth after cesarean section (VBAC) was introduced in 1982 to combat the rising trend in the rate of cesarean section. This was because repeat cesarean section had become a major factor compounding the growing rate of cesarean section delivery.[20]

Candidates

Eligible candidates for VBAC include those with two or fewer prior Kerr hysterotomies or one prior low-vertical hysterotomy. Contraindications include known T-shaped hysterotomy scars and known classical hysterotomy.[21] More controversial with regard to risk are a trial of labor in a patient with an unknown uterine scar[22] and VBAC with a previous Kerr hysterotomy in the setting of twin gestation.[23] Both of these latter two clinical situations are examples of settings in which cesarean section is best individualized rather than mandated. However, both are acceptable for VBAC. The patient with an unknown uterine scar can be offered VBAC. According to Pruett and colleagues,[22] the rate of VBAC success in and of maternal and fetal morbidity after the procedure were no different in patients with an unknown prior uterine incision than in those with a known prior low-transverse incision.[22] With regard to VBAC in patients with a greater number of previous scars (i.e., >2), the number of cases is too small to permit the ascertainment of specific guidelines.[24]

Success Indicators

Ideally, a previous cesarean section should become an infrequent indication for cesarean section. However, not every candidate for VBAC may be suitable for the procedure. Pickhardt and colleagues were unsuccessful in an attempt to develop a reliable linear-regression model to predict the likelihood of success in VBAC regardless of past obstetric history or clinical parameters,[25] and with other investigators concluded that VBAC should be strongly encouraged. Review of the various multi-center trials of VBAC demonstrates a range of success rates varying from 50 to 85 percent. A meta-analysis of several pre-existing indicators for VBAC was done by Rosen and Dickinson.[26] According to their composite success rates, the average success rate for a patient previously sectioned for CPD/FTP is 67 percent and that for a patient with a previous breech delivery was 85 percent. Patients who had at least one prior vaginal delivery had an 84 percent average success rate with VBAC, and patients with more than one previous

cesarean section had an average success rate of 75 percent. Should estimated fetal weight factor into the equation? The meta-analysis data showed no statistically significant association between higher birth weight and higher failure rates for VBAC.

The use of oxytocin in the patient undergoing VBAC deserves special consideration. Again, the meta-analysis done by Rosen and Dickinson demonstrated an average VBAC success rate of 63 percent in patients receiving oxytocin.[26] However, the success rate of the procedure was clearly lower in trials in which oxytocin was used than in those in which it was not employed. Although the literature[27,28] supports the use of oxytocin in the setting of VBAC, attesting to its safety, caution in its use is still required. In our unit, 20 mU/min of oxytocin is the maximum allowable dose for multiparous patients with or without a prior uterine scar. Intrauterine pressure catheters are not routinely used, but should be used if uterine contractions cannot be recorded with an external tocometer.

The guidelines of the American College of Obstetricians and Gynecologists (ACOG) contain a precautionary statement about an estimated fetal weight of more than 4,000 g in VBAC. The success of VBAC in trials of the procedure is biased toward a lower threshold for performing surgery in the previous cesarean section group. Moreover, the ability to reliably estimate macrosomia by ultrasonography declines as fetal weight increases beyond 4,000 g. According to Flam and Goings,[29] an increased risk of uterine rupture was not observed in a trial of VBAC in 301 patients having infants with birth weights of 4,000 g or more as compared with 1,475 trials of labor in patients having fetuses with estimated weights of less than 4,000 g. Although no statistically significant difference in maternal and neonatal morbidity was found in a comparison of the outcomes of 301 trials of labor involving macrosomic infants with those of 301 consecutive control patients with no previous uterine surgery delivering infants of 4,000 g or more, shoulder dystocia occurred in 6 of 165 (3.6 percent) of cases and 7 of 269 (2.6 percent) of cases in the control group.

Morbidity and Mortality

The intent to reduce the cesarean section rate must be balanced against potential complications of VBAC. Many studies with small numbers of subjects lack the statistical power to provide reliable data on rare outcome events. A meta-analysis by Rosen and colleagues[30] included 31 studies with a total of 11,417 trials of labor in an attempt to evaluate the association between the route of delivery after cesarean section and the morbidity and mortality for the mother and fetus.

Maternal mortality rates were 2.8 in 10,000 for patients undergoing a trial of labor, versus 2.4 in 10,000 for patients undergoing elective repeat cesarean section. Febrile morbidity was lowest in the successful trials of labor and highest in the failed trials (P <0.001). Rupture or dehiscence complicated about 2 percent of 6,000 deliveries in 11 studies. Meta-analysis revealed no statistically significant difference in the rate of dehiscence or uterine rupture after VBAC versus elective repeat cesarean section ($P = 0.3$). However, the rate of uterine rupture after a failed trial of labor was 2.8 times that following a repeat cesarean section (P <0.01). The use of oxytocin during a trial of labor did not appear to influence the risk of uterine dehiscence or uterine rupture ($P = 0.7$). After excluding fetal deaths occurring before labor, cases involving very-low-birth-weight infants (less than 750 g), and infants with congenital anomalies, an association between an increased perinatal mortality rate and trial of labor appeared unsupported.

Uterine Rupture

The true incidence of uterine rupture during VBAC is hampered by the incomplete identification of such cases, since dehiscence may be a silent event. The incidence of clinically significant uterine dehiscence in patients undergoing VBAC is less than 1 percent.[31] Leung and colleagues[32] quoted an incidence of 0.82 percent in a case control study of 8,513 trials of labor and 70 cases of uterine rupture. Results of this same study illustrated an increased risk of uterine rupture in patients who received excessive amounts of oxytocin. Dysfunctional labor patterns, particularly active-phase arrest disorders, were associated with an increased risk of uterine rupture. A history of two or more prior cesarean sections is another risk factor. Epidural anesthesia, macrosomia, an unknown uterine scar, and a history of cesarean section for CPD are not associated with uterine rupture per se. Successful VBAC after cesarean section

does not appear to protect against uterine rupture.[33,34]

Should the type of uterine scar affect the decision to allow VBAC? A known classical uterine incision is a contraindication to VBAC. Most of the literature concentrates on the lower transverse uterine incision (i.e., Kerr hysterotomy), and studies involving unknown scars assume that more than 90 to 95 percent of prior incisions would be of the lower transverse variety. Consequently, studies of the outcome in cases of past low vertical incisions are lacking. At the Brigham and Women's Hospital, patients with low vertical uterine incisions are permitted the option of VBAC.

SURGICAL MANAGEMENT OF POSTPARTUM HEMORRHAGE

Vascular Ligation

The management of postpartum hemorrhage begins with the assessment of its etiology and the implementation of conservative procedures, including the mechanical and pharmacologic interventions discussed in Chapter 12. When these are unsuccessful, the next step in the algorithm is vascular ligation, including uterine artery ligation, also known as the O'Leary[35] suture, and hypogastric artery ligation (Fig. 13-2).

Candidates for vascular ligation must be carefully selected. According to Evans and McShane,[36] hypogastric artery ligation appears effective for controlling hemorrhage secondary to uterine atony and midline perforation. Patients with suspected abnormal placentation (i.e., placenta accreta) will usually require total abdominal hysterectomy for complete management of hemorrhage, as discussed in the next section. Candidates for vascular ligation should be of low parity and should be hemodynamically stable before being considered for ligation.

Burchell, during the 1960s,[36] investigated the hemodynamic effects of hypogastric artery ligation on pelvic blood flow. Ipsilateral arterial ligation decreased pulse pressure by 77 percent, blood flow by 49 percent, and mean pressure by 22 percent. Bilateral ligation decreased pulse pressure by 85 percent, mean pressure by 24 percent, and blood flow by 48 percent. The rich collateral blood supply of the pel-

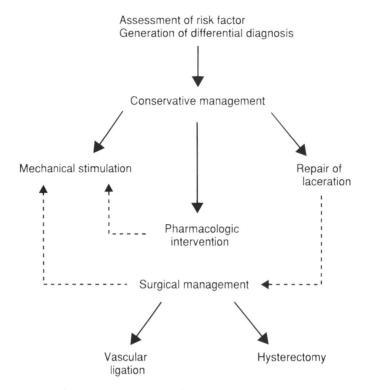

Fig. 13-2. Treatment of postpartum hemorrhage.

vis insures postprocedural blood flow so that tissue integrity is not compromised. However, it is this rich collateral circulation that also limits the overall effectiveness of hypogastric artery ligation. Successful pregnancies have been documented in patients who have previously undergone hypogastric artery ligation. Blood flow is maintained through three major specific collateral arterial anastomoses: lumbar–iliolumbar, middle sacral–lateral sacral, and superior hemorrhoidal–middle hemorrhoidal arteries.

PUERPERAL HYSTERECTOMY

Indications

Emergency peripartum hysterectomy is generally performed in the setting of life-threatening hemorrhage. The frequency of this procedure ranges from 1.3 to 1.55 per 1,000 births, depending on the series studied. Two large series reported in 1993, one from the East and the other from the West Coast, both demonstrated the emergence of abnormal adherent placentation as the leading clinical indication for

hysterectomy in the gravid state.[37,38] According to Zelop and associates,[37] among 117 cases of puerperal hysterectomy performed at the Brigham and Women's Hospital, the clinical indication for the procedure was classified as abnormal placentation in 75 (64 percent) of the cases, uterine atony in 25 (24.1 percent), uterine rupture in 10 (8.5 percent), sepsis in 3 (2.6%), fibroids in 2 (1.7%), and extension of a uterine scar in 2 (1.7%). Increases in the cesarean section rate coupled with advances in pharmacologic modalities for the treatment of uterine atony (i.e., prostaglandin-$F_{2\alpha}$ [Hemabate][39]) may be responsible for the predominance of abnormal adherent placentation leading to gravid hysterectomy.

Prenatal Diagnosis of Abnormal Adherent Placentation

Three types of abnormal adherent placentation are identified, according to the severity of placental invasion: placenta accreta, in which placental villi are attached to the myometrium, placenta increta, in which placental villi invade the myometrium, and

Uterine Artery Ligation/O'Leary Suture[35]

1. Advance the vesicouterine peritoneum off the lower uterine segment to expose the contents of the broad ligament
2. Identify the ascending branch of the uterine artery by palpation
3. Using #1 chromic suture, pass the needle in and through the myometrium from anterior to posterior, from 2 to 3 cm medial to the uterine vessels, then bring it forward through the avascular area of the broad ligament lateral to the artery and vein
4. Secure the ligature
5. Do not divide the vessels (Fig. 13-3).

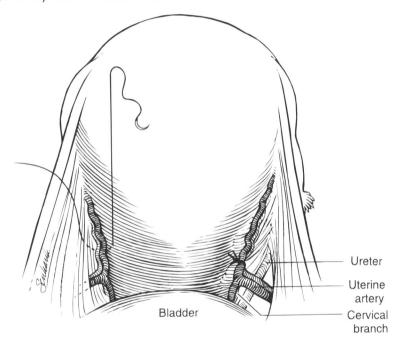

Ureter

Uterine artery

Cervical branch

Bladder

Fig. 13-3. Uterine artery ligation. Demonstration of the placement of a suture around the ascending branch of the uterine artery and vein as described by O'Leary and O'Leary.[35] Note that 2 to 3 cm of myometrium medial to the vessels has been included.

placenta percreta, in which placental villi penetrate through the myometrium into other tissue (Fig. 13-5). All three types of adherent placentation result from the partial or total absence of the decidua basalis and imperfect development of the fibrinoid layer, known as Nitabuch's layer.

Case control studies have identified patients at increased risk of abnormal adherent placentation. The risk is increased with increasing parity, and is strongly influenced by placenta previa and a history of cesarean section. Clark and associates[40] quoted a 5 percent risk of placenta accreta in patients presenting with an unscarred uterus and placenta previa. With placenta previa and one previous cesarean section, the risk of accreta was 24 percent. With two prior cesarean sections the risk increased to 47 percent. One can extrapolate from this to conclude that other procedures or conditions causing uterine scarring might predispose to accreta by similar mechanisms. These include prior dilatation and curettage, myomectomy, Asherman's syndrome, and submucous fibroids. Bleeding occurs because the involved

Hypogastric Artery Ligation Resection

1. Pack the bowel and gain good exposure
2. Ligate the round ligament doubly in the midportion, leaving approximately 1 to 2 cm between each tie
3. Divide the round ligament
4. Develop the retroperitoneal space through gentle traction
5. Incise the peritoneum of the pelvic side-wall, working toward the infundibulopelvic ligament until the retroperitoneum is adequately exposed
6. Using a peanut as a dissector, identify the external iliac artery and its bifurcation
7. Carefully identify the ureters. The ureters run along the common iliac artery and then cross over the iliac vessels as they enter the pelvis. The right and left ureters vary slightly from one another. The right ureter crosses at the bifurcation of the iliac artery, while the left ureter crosses 1 to 2 cm above the bifurcation. The ureters then travel medially as they continue toward the bladder in the retroperitoneum. Each ureter can be found peristalsing on the medial leaf of the parietal peritoneum of the broad ligament
8. Identify the hypogastric artery for a distance of 3 to 4 cm below the bifurcation of the common iliac artery. This will allow ligation of the anterior division of the hypogastric artery, which is the branch of interest. A right-angle clamp is then passed around the lateral and posterior aspect of the anterior division of the hypogastric artery. The jaws of the clamp are opened and two silk ties are inserted into the jaws. The clamp is gently withdrawn, leaving the free ties in place for double ligation
9. Avoid injury to the hypogastric vein, which lies posterior and medial to the hypogastric artery
10. Palpate distal pulses to insure against inadvertent ligation of the external iliac artery (Fig. 13-4).

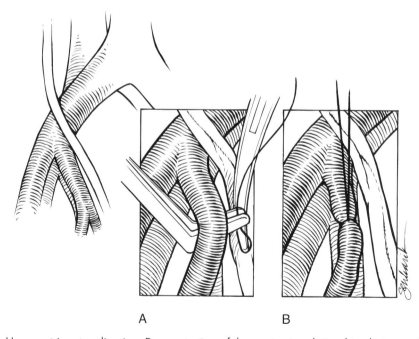

A   B

Fig. 13-4. Hypogastric artery ligation. Demonstration of the anatomic relationships between the ureter and the hypogastric vessels in the retroperitoneum. Placement of the suture ligation around the anterior division of the hypogastric artery must avoid injury to the hypogastric vein, which lies posterior and medial to the hypogastric artery.

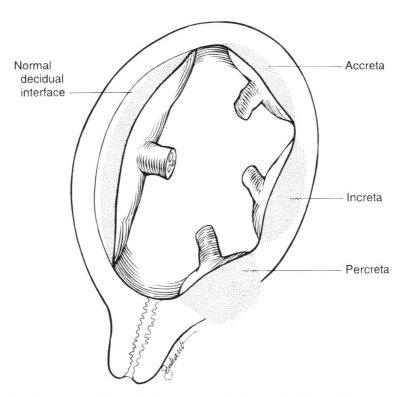

Fig. 13-5. Uteroplacental relationships with abnormal adherent placentation.

cotyledon is either pulled off the myometrium, with somewhat excessive bleeding from the implantation site, or because the cotyledon is torn from the placenta and adheres to the implantation site with increased bleeding.

α-Fetoprotein (AFP) screening in maternal serum is now used routinely to detect fetuses at risk of structural defects and chromosomal abnormalities. Women who have increased maternal serum AFP concentrations are also at increased risk of adverse pregnancy outcome in the third trimester, including preterm delivery, premature rupture of membranes, intrauterine growth retardation, and placental abnormalities. Placental abnormalities such as hydropic changes, subchorionic hemorrhage, and intraplacental hemorrhage are known to be associated with increased maternal serum AFP concentrations. A comparison of patients with simple placenta previa and those with concurrent placenta previa and adherent placentation demonstrated a significant association between an unexplained increase in the ma-

ternal serum AFP concentration and placenta accreta, increta, and percreta. Patients with unexplained elevations of maternal serum AFP as well as placenta previa or a low-lying placenta may therefore be at increased risk of abnormal placental adherence.[41]

The implications of a prospective sonographic diagnosis of placenta accreta are that the patient can be carefully counseled and that surgical management can be planned in advance in detail. Finberg and Williams[42] performed a prospective evaluation for possible placenta accreta in 34 patients with placenta previa and a history of one or more cesarean sections. The sonographic criteria used included the following: (1) loss of the normal hypoechoic retroplacental myometrial zone; (2) thinning or disruption of the hyperechoic uterine serosa–bladder interface; and (3) the presence of a local exophytic mass protruding from the uterus. Using these criteria, Finberg and Williams correctly diagnosed placenta accreta in 14 of 18 cases with positive sono-

---

Ultrasound Characteristics and Probability of Adherent Placentation

High-probability characteristics

Attenuation or interruption of the hyperechoic uterine serosa

Placental nodularity extending beyond the uterine margin

Presence of marked intraparenchymal placental vascular spaces

Intermediate-probability characteristics

Loss of hypoechoic myometrial zone

Low-probability characteristics

Preservation of a normal hypoechoic myometrial zone

---

graphic findings. There were 4 false-positive diagnoses and 1 false-negative diagnosis in a cohort of 34 patients. In light of their commentary, transabdominal and transvaginal ultrasound can be used to generate a probability of the likelihood of accreta rather than a "yes-no" diagnosis (Fig. 13-6). Mag-

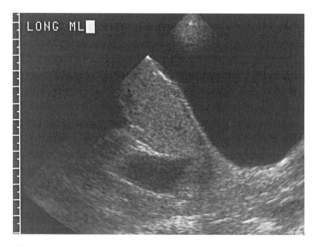

Fig. 13-6. Antenatal ultrasonogram demonstrating placenta previa and placenta increta. Pathology examination following delivery confirmed placenta increta.

netic resonance imaging (MRI) potentially offers two major advantages over ultrasonography that make it particularly suitable for third-trimester bleeding.[43] These advantages include potentially better tissue differentiation and an ability to highlight blood. However, the exact role of MRI in the diagnosis of abnormal adherent placentation has yet to be established. To date, only case reports[44] involving the use of this modality to diagnose abnormal adherent placentation have appeared in the literature. Currently, MRI may be used to clarify inconclusive ultrasonographic findings. A positive diagnosis will enhance the preparation of definitive surgical management. However, a negative diagnosis should not instill a false sense of security, especially in a patient with multiple clinical risk factors for abnormal adherent placentation (Fig. 13-7).

Preoperative Preparation and Operative Management

Early planning and patient counseling are the cornerstones of the management of the patient with suspected placenta accreta, increta, or percreta. Collaboration of the obstetric and anesthesia teams is essential. The blood bank should be notified and prepared for a potentially high transfusion requirement. Thigh-high pneumatic boots should be applied before beginning the cesarean section for DVT prophylaxis. Puerperal hysterectomy with minimal placental disruption can be considered for high-risk patients, particularly in the setting of suspected placenta percreta. Individual patient input about future fertility can and should influence an obstetric plan to proceed with a cesarean hysterectomy. In cases of suspected placenta percreta involving the bladder, preoperative placement of stents and cystoscopy to determine the extent of placental invasion are recommended. Conservative therapy for a placenta accreta involving a limited area of the placenta has been reported. The decision to leave the entire placenta in situ, with a good outcome has also been recently reported.[45] These procedures involve a combination of oversewing of the placental bed and the use of utero-tonic agents. Uterine packing and the postoperative use of methotrexate have also been described. However, significant hemorrhage can usually be controlled only by hysterectomy.

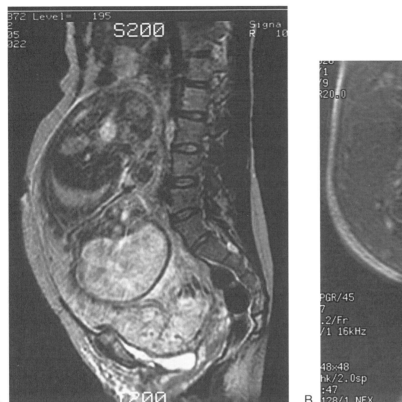

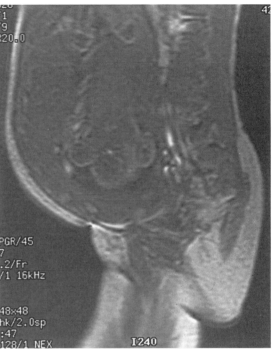

A   B

Fig. 13-7. **(A)** MRI performed in the third trimester on patient with placenta previa and pathologic confirmation of placenta increta following delivery. Although the thinness of intervening myometrium is apparent, it represents only a subtle difference from the normal thinness of the third-trimester myometrium. **(B)** Third-trimester MRI performed for clarification of adnexal pathology. Note thinness of the myometrium, which is a normal characteristic in the third trimester.

Operative Approach

The operative approach to hysterectomy may vary according to the suspected pathologic entity. Supracervical hysterectomy can be appropriate for the management of atony that is unresponsive to pharmacologic therapy, unless the lower uterine segment is also involved. Total abdominal hysterectomy is recommended in the setting of abnormal adherent placentation, since the subtotal approach leaves the cervical branch of the uterine artery intact, which may predispose to hematoma formation. In cases of anterior placenta previa and concurrent suspected abnormal adherent placentation, a vertical uterine hysterotomy can be made to decrease placental manipulation leading to hemorrhage. A vertical hyster-

otomy can be performed without raising a bladder flap, which can be avoided until the degree of placental invasion can be assessed. Technical performance of a hysterectomy is aided by the maintenance of a dry surgical field. A tourniquet of 0.5-in. Penrose drain material can be placed around the lower uterine segment. Bilateral hypogastric artery ligation can be considered to decrease the rate of hemorrhage. These steps, however, will not obviate the need for proceeding with puerperal hysterectomy. Aggressive maintenance of intravenous crystalloid and the titration of blood products are necessary to avoid dilutional coagulopathy.

Although the execution of a gravid hysterectomy closely resembles the standard approach used to perform any hysterectomy, the surgeon should keep several caveats in mind. The tissue in the gravid peripartum state is highly vascular and easily torn. Therefore, a noncutting suture, such as a Q1 chromic suture, is preferable. Vascular pedicles can be secured with triple ties if necessary. Bovie cautery can be used to achieve hemostasis. Prophylactic antibiotics providing aerobic and anaerobic coverage should be administered. Several surgical drains should be placed to assess hemostasis and the integrity of any urologic anastomoses.

When placenta percreta involves the urinary bladder, separation of the lower uterine segment becomes more difficult. Two approaches are suggested.[46] The dome of the bladder can be incised and opened so that dissection between the lower uterine segment and bladder can be performed under direct visualization of the ureteral orifices (Fig. 13-8). Alternatively, the hysterectomy can be executed through a posterior approach. With the latter technique, the uterus is mobilized first by dividing the uterosacral ligaments and then entering the vagina posteriorly. The ureter is then retracted laterally while the medial parametria are serially isolated and divided, moving in a cephalad to caudal direction. Once the uterus is mobilized, the portion of the bladder adherent to the placenta is resected, along with the surgical specimen. Genitourinary reconstruction can then be addressed. This may involve a two-layer closure of the dome of the bladder or more extensive repair if the trigone and ureters were involved. Ideally, a graft of omentum should be placed between the bladder suture and vaginal cuff to prevent fistula formation or adhesions. If the distal ureter or trigone (or both) has been resected, ureteroneocystostomy accompanied by bladder repair is performed. Ureteral injury distal to the bladder may involve ureteroureterostomy, transureteroureterostomy, or cutaneous ureterostomy. Points of anastomosis and suture lines should be tension-free and water-tight.

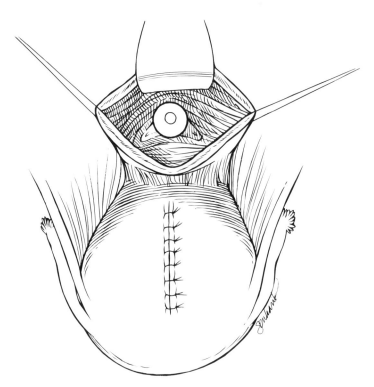

Fig. 13-8. When placenta percreta involves the urinary bladder, separation of the lower uterine segment can be accomplished under direct visualization of the ureteral orifices after incising the dome of the bladder.

Intraoperative and Perioperative Complications

The patient undergoing puerperal hysterectomy is at risk of significant morbidity. The degree of hemorrhage exposes the patient to coagulopathy and the need for multiple blood products. Re-exploration in the setting of hematoma formation or continued bleeding is another potential complication. In our recent series[37] of 117 emergency peripartum hysterectomy patients, 50 of 117, or nearly 50 percent, sustained infectious complications, including wound infection in 4 patients and sepsis in 4 patients. Respiratory complications such as acute respiratory distress syndrome (ARDS), prolonged intubation, pulmonary edema, atelectasis, or chest, tube placement occurred in 21 percent of cases. Intraoperative urologic complications can involve both the bladder and ureter. In our series,[37] 9 percent of the patients sustained urologic injuries, including cystotomies in 9 patients and ureteral injuries requiring stent placement in 3. Because of the severity and variety of intraoperative and postoperative complications, the patient is best co-managed by her obstetrician in conjunction with anesthesiologists and physicians trained in critical care medicine.

REFERENCES

1. Office of Vital and Health Statistics Systems, National Center for Health Statistics, Centers for Disease Control: Rates of cesarean delivery—United States, 1991. JAMA 18:2360, 1993

2. Burrows RF, Kelton JG: Fetal thrombocytopenia and its relation to maternal thrombocytopenia. N Engl J Med 11:1463, 1993

3. Christiaens GCML, Helmerhorst FM: Validity of intrapartum diagnosis of fetal thrombocytopenia. Am J Obstet Gynecol 157:864, 1987

4. Cook RL, Miller RC, Katz VL, Cefalo RC: Immune thrombocytopenic purpura in pregnancy: a reappraisal of management. Obstet Gynecol 78:578, 1991

5. Sakala EP, Erhard LN, White JJ: Elective cesarean section improves outcomes of neonates with gastroschisis. Am J Obstet Gynecol 169:1050, 1993

6. Dias MS, Sekhar LN: Intracranial hemorrhage from aneurysms and arteriovenous malformations during pregnancy and the puerperium. Neurosurgery 27:855, 1990

7. Hauth JC, Owen J, Davis RO: Transverse uterine incision closure: one versus two layers. Am J Obstet Gynecol 167:1108, 1992

8. Hull DB, Varner MW: A randomized study of closure of the peritoneum at cesarean delivery. Obstet Gynecol 77:818, 1991

9. Nielson TF, Hokegard KH: Postoperative cesarean section morbidity: A prospective study. Am J Obstet Gynecol 146:911, 1983

10. Sachs BP, Yeh J, Acker D et al: Cesarean section related maternal mortality in Massachusetts, 1954–1985. Obstet Gynecol 71:385, 1988

11. Duff P: Prophylactic antibiotics for cesarean delivery: a simple cost-effective strategy for prevention of postoperative morbidity. Am J Obstet Gynecol 157:794, 1987

12. Carlson C, Duff P: Antibiotic prophylaxis for cesarean delivery: is an extended-spectrum agent necessary? Obstet Gynecol 76:343, 1990

13. Kruskall MS, Leonard S, Klapholz H: Autologous blood donation during pregnancy: analysis of safety and blood use. Obstet Gynecol 70:938, 1987

14. Combs CA, Murphy EL, Laros RK: Cost-benefit analysis of autologous blood donation in obstetrics. Obstet Gynecol 80:621, 1992

15. Mercer BM, Garner P: Thrombophlebitis. Principles and practice of medical therapy. p. 1284. In Gleicher N (ed): Pregnancy. Appleton & Lange, E. Norwalk, CT, 1992

16. Lee RV, Rodgers BD, White LM, Harvey RC: Cardiopulmonary resuscitation of pregnant women. Am J Med 81:311, 1986

17. Troiano NH: Cardiopulmonary resuscitation of the pregnant woman. Perinat Neonat Nurs 3:1, 1989

18. Katz VL, Dotters DJ, Droegemueller W: Perimortem cesarean delivery. Obstet Gynecol 68:571, 1986

19. Lindsay SL, Hanson GC: Cardiac arrest in near-term pregnancy. Anesth 42:1074, 1987

20. Pridjian G, Hibbard JU, Moawad AH: Cesarean: changing the trends. Obstet Gynecol 77:195, 1991

21. Pridjian G: Labor after prior cesarean section. Clin Obstet Gynecol 35:445, 1992

22. Pruett KM, Kirshon B, Cotton DB: Unknown uterine scar and trial of labor. Am J Obstet Gynecol 159:807, 1988

23. Strong TH, Phelan JP, Ahn MO, Sarno AP: Vaginal birth after cesarean delivery in the twin gestation. Am J Obstet Gynecol 161:29, 1989

24. Novas J, Myers SA, Gleicher N: Obstetric outcome of patients with more than one previous cesarean section. Am J Obstet Gynecol 160:364, 1989

25. Pickhardt MG, Martin JN, Meydrech EF et al: Vaginal birth after cesarean delivery: are there useful and valid predictors of success or failure? Am J Obstet Gynecol 166:1811, 1992

26. Rosen MG, Dickinson JC: Vaginal birth after cesarean: a meta-analysis of indicators for success. Obstet Gynecol 76:865, 1990

27. Flamm BL, Goings JR, Fuelberth NJ et al: Oxytocin during labor after previous cesarean section: results of a multicenter study. Obstet Gynecol 70:709, 1987

28. Silver R, Gibbs RS: Predictors of vaginal delivery in patients with a previous cesarean section who require oxytocin. Am J Obstet Gynecol 156:57, 1987

29. Flamm BL, Goings JR: Vaginal birth after cesarean section: is suspected fetal mascrosomia a contraindication? Obstet Gynecol 74:694, 1989

30. Rosen MG, Dickinson JC, Westhoff CL: Vaginal birth after cesarean: a meta-analysis of morbidity and mortality. Obstet Gynecol 77:465, 1991

31. Jones RO, Nagashima AW, Hartnett-Goodman MM, Goodlin RC: Rupture of low transverse cesarean scars during trial of labor. Obstet Gynecol 77:815, 1991

32. Leung AS, Farmer RM, Leung EK et al: Risk factors associated with uterine rupture during trial of labor after cesarean delivery: a case-control study. Am J Obstet Gynecol 168:1358, 1993

33. Nielsen TF, Ljungblad U, Hagberg H: Rupture and dehiscence of cesarean section scar during pregnancy and delivery. Am J Obstet Gynecol 160:569, 1989

34. Eden RD, Parker RT, Gall SA: Rupture of the pregnant uterus: a 52-year review. Obstet Gynecol 68:671, 1986

35. O'Leary JL, O'Leary JA: Uterine artery ligation for control of postcesarean section hemorrhage. Obstet Gynecol 43:849, 1974

36. Evans S, McShane P: The efficacy of internal iliac artery ligation in obstetric hemorrhage. Surg Gynecol Obstet 160:250, 1985

37. Zelop CM, Harlow BL, Frigoletto FD et al: Emergency peripartum hysterectomy. Am J Obstet Gynecol 168:1443, 1993

38. Stanco LM, Schrimmer DB, Paul RH, Mishell DR: Emergency peripartum hysterectomy and associated risk factors. Am J Obstet Gynecol 168:879, 1993

39. Hayashi RH, Castillo MS, Noah ML: Management of severe postpartum hemorrhage due to uterine atony using an analogue of prostaglandin $F_{2\alpha}$. Obstet Gynecol 58:426, 1981

40. Clark SL, Koonings PP, Phelan JP: Placenta previa/accreta and prior cesarean section. Obstet Gynecol 66:89, 1985

41. Zelop C, Nadel A, Frigoletto FD et al: Placenta accreta/percreta/increta: a cause of elevated maternal serum alpha-fetoprotein. Obstet Gynecol 80:693, 1992

42. Finberg H, Williams JW: Placenta accreta: prospective sonographic diagnosis in patients with placenta previa and prior cesarean section. J Ultrasound Med 11:333, 1992

43. Kay H, Spritzer CE: Preliminary experience with magnetic resonance imaging in patients with third-trimester bleeding. Obstet Gynecol 78:424, 1991

44. Thorp JM, Councell RB, Sandridge DA, Wiest HH: Antepartum diagnosis: placenta previa percreta by magnetic resonance imaging. Obstet Gynecol 80:506, 1992

45. Legro RS, Price FV, Hill LM, Carites SN: Nonsurgical management of placenta previa a case report. Obstet Gynecol 83:847, 1994

46. Price FV, Resnik E, Heller KA, Christopherson WA: Placenta previa percreta involving the urinary bladder: a report of two cases and review of the literature. Obstet Gynecol 78:508, 1991

Chapter 14

Creation and Use of a Labor-and-Delivery Intensive Care Unit

William C. Mabie

The intensive care unit (ICU) had its origin in the postoperative recovery room. In 1863, Florence Nightingale wrote that it was not uncommon to have a room set aside near the operating rooms for patients recovering from the immediate effects of surgery. In 1923, Walter Dandy started the first postoperative neurosurgical unit at the Johns Hopkins Hospital in Baltimore. Dwight Harkin established the first cardiac surgery ICU in Boston in 1951. During the Scandinavian polio epidemic of 1952, Blegdam Hospital in Copenhagen opened a 105-bed respiratory care unit for endotracheal intubation and positive pressure ventilation of polio victims. The first coronary care unit was established by Hughes Day in Kansas City in 1962. Today, in addition to these ICUs, it is not uncommon for large tertiary care centers to have burn, trauma, medical, surgical, pediatric, and neonatal ICUs. The philosophy behind the operation of all ICUs is the same: place the sickest patients in a room with the best nurses in a 1:1 or 2:1 patient/nurse ratio. Within the past decade, several large obstetric services have created ICUs in their labor and delivery units or contiguous areas. The purpose of these units is intensive maternal and fetal surveillance and supportive care during the antepartum and immediate postpartum periods.

The obstetric ICU is an outgrowth of the subspecialty of maternal-fetal medicine. Although in utero diagnosis and fetal therapy are the primary concerns of current research in maternal-fetal medicine, a major clinical role of the subspecialist in maternal-fetal medicine continues to be that of an "internist for pregnant women." Other factors contributing to the development of the obstetric ICU are regionalization of care, new knowledge, new equipment, a more liberal attitude among physicians in allowing pregnancy in patients with major organ or multisystem disease, and better treatment for chronic diseases (e.g., kidney, liver, and heart transplantation, surgical correction of congenital heart disease, and cancer chemotherapy).[1]

Regionalization of care expands the availability of technology through more efficient utilization at high-volume centers, enhances the experience base of the staff, facilitates education and research because of the expanded patient pool, saves money by reducing duplication of services, and improves recruitment and retention of personnel. Examples of new knowledge put into practice in the ICU include concepts of preload and afterload augmentation and reduction, oxygen delivery and consumption, and pharmacologic support with antiarrhythmic, inotropic, vasopressor, vasodilator, and β-blocking drugs. Examples of new equipment are intra-arterial blood pressure monitors, pulse oximeters, pulmonary artery catheters, continuous mixed venous oxygen saturation monitors, intracranial pressure monitors, ventilators, computed tomographic (CT) scanners, ultrasound machines, echocardiography machines, bronchoscopes, and other endoscopy equipment. On large obstetric services that are sometimes overwhelmed by the number of patients in labor, simply identifying the sick patient and placing her in an ICU, even if it is not elaborately equipped, improves the patient's chances of having a favorable outcome, because she is singled out as someone who requires extraordinary and meticulous care.

Although improvement in patient care and patient outcome are the driving forces for such technologic developments as the obstetric ICU, the benefits of intensive care are difficult to prove. The only study of the efficacy of obstetric intensive care compared maternal mortality during the 3 years after establishment of an obstetric ICU to that during the prior 3 years when patients were transferred to a medical ICU. Maternal mortality was essentially the same (approximately 22 per 100,000 deliveries). The authors concluded that an obstetric ICU staffed by maternal-fetal medicine specialists and anesthesiologists can provide the same level of care for critically ill obstetric patients as that provided by medical intensive care specialists.[2]

The following discussion of obstetric intensive care is influenced by my own past 8 years' experience as director of the obstetric ICU at the University of Tennessee in Memphis. The aim of our ICU is to treat all critically ill pregnant women, except women having major trauma (who are treated in our institution's trauma center), neurosurgical disorders, or the need for mechanical ventilation for more than 5 days.

NEED FOR AN OBSTETRIC ICU

As seen from a Medline literature review for the years 1987 to 1994 and summarized in Table 14-1, the percentage of obstetric patients requiring intensive care is small, ranging from 0.1 to 0.9 percent.[1-8] For all practical purposes, unless one has a large number of deliveries (>6,000/yr) or a large number of critically ill maternal transfer patients, it makes more sense to manage these patients in a medical or surgical ICU. The patient's ICU care could be under the guidance of both the obstetric and the ICU teams, as outlined by Kilpatrick and Matthay.[5]

In our particular situation, the hospital has approximately 7,500 deliveries per year and serves as the referral center for a five-state region. The referral area has approximately 40,000 deliveries per year, and there are no towns with a population of more than 100,000 within a 100-mile radius of Memphis. We have found the benefits of an obstetric ICU to be: (1) intensive observation and organization al-

Table 14-1. Use of the Intensive Care Unit by Obstetric Services

Author	Year	Location	Time Period	Deliveries	Patients Admitted to ICU		Nonsurvivors (% of Admissions)
					N	%	
Graham et al[4]	1989	Nottingham, England (Medical-Surgical ICU)	1982–1986	21,983	23	0.1	8.7
Mabie et al[1]	1990	Memphis (Obstetric ICU)	1986–1989	22,651	200	0.9	3.5
Kirshon et al[2]	1990	Houston (Obstetric ICU)	1984–1987	49,700	141	0.3	7.8
Stephens[8]	1991	Brisbane, Australia (Medical-Surgical ICU)	1979–1989	61,435	126	0.2	
Kilpatrick et al[5]	1992	San Francisco (Medical-Surgical ICU)	1985–1990	8,000[a]	32	0.4	12.5
Ng et al[7]	1992	Singapore (Surgical ICU)	1985–1990	16,264	37	0.2	5.4
Collop et al[3]	1993	Charleston (Medical ICU)	1988–1991	6,667[a]	20	0.3	20.0
Monaco et al[6]	1993	Chapel Hill (various ICUs)	1983–1990	15,323	38	0.3	18.0

[a] Number of deliveries estimated from data in article.

lows for prevention or early recognition and treatment of complications; (2) familiarity with invasive monitoring permits personnel to exert prompt, rational treatment of hemodynamically unstable patients; (3) continuity of care is improved before and after delivery; and (4) residents and fellows learn a great deal about intensive care and the management of rare medical complications of pregnancy.[1]

FACILITIES

The size of the obstetric ICU depends on the volume of deliveries. In most cases, a one- or two-bed unit will suffice. The ICU should have the capability of isolating infected patients (wound infections, varicella, tuberculosis). Handwashing facilities should be available inside the room. There should be enough space around the bed for maneuvering portable radiography equipment and for several caretakers to be present at the bedside. A view box for reviewing chest radiographs, wall suction, and oxygen (including setup for a ventilator) should be available.

Our obstetric ICU consists of one large room (approximately 700 ft²), which is located next to the recovery room. Major equipment includes one six-channel and two three-channel Hewlett-Packard hemodynamic monitors, two Hewlett-Packard cardiac output computers, a strip chart recorder and printer, a Nellcor pulse oximeter, a Wescor colloid oncometer, two electric hospital beds, and one birthing bed that can be used for vaginal delivery for patients in the ICU. Emergency equipment includes a "crash" cart, defibrillator, suction machine, and electrocardiograph machine. Portable fetal monitors are brought in as needed.

DIRECTOR OF THE ICU

In addition to routine obstetrics, certain specialized clinical skills are frequently needed in the ICU, such as the ability to insert radial and pulmonary artery catheters, perform endotracheal intubation, manage a ventilator, read an electrocardiogram (ECG), direct cardiopulmonary resuscitation (CPR), and perform a cesarean hysterectomy or bilateral hypogastric artery ligation.

We have repeatedly observed the following emergencies: pulmonary edema, massive hemorrhage,

disseminated intravascular coagulation (DIC), septic shock, adult respiratory distress syndrome (ARDS), acute renal failure, hypertensive crisis, cardiac arrhythmias, status asthmaticus, status epilepticus, stroke, pulmonary embolism, diabetic ketoacidosis, and thyroid storm. Training to manage these emergencies must be given if an ICU is to exist. Training can be provided in several ways, including a critical care fellowship, a medicine residency, or a maternal-fetal medicine fellowship involving interaction with the subspecialists.

I completed residencies in internal medicine and obstetrics and gynecology, and a fellowship in maternal-fetal medicine. I am board-certified in these specialties, as well as in critical care medicine. Other obstetric ICU directors have completed obstetric and gynecology residencies and fellowships in critical care medicine, and work part-time as attending physicians in medical or surgical ICUs to maintain their skills. They have joint appointments in both departments.

Because of the limited number of critically ill obstetric patients, the obstetric ICU director will be a part-time staff member. The ICU director must also be available 24 hours per day because the need is unpredictable. On the bright side, some of the administrative hassles of a multidisciplinary combined medical-surgical unit are absent in the obstetric ICU. These include: (1) making triage decisions during periods of high census, (2) managing diverse patient populations and diverse physician specialties, (3) caring for the chronically critically ill who are deteriorating with time, and (4) establishing consensus on futile care.

NURSES

It is relatively easy to obtain equipment for an ICU, but quite another matter to recruit experienced, well-trained nurses. Some centers use a labor-and-delivery nurse for the obstetric care and a medical ICU nurse for managing hemodynamic monitoring. This is expensive and less than ideal in terms of merging the two disciplines for optimal patient management (i.e., one nurse who can put the whole picture together). We find that regular obstetric nurses can function well in the ICU setting. Indeed, the unit attracts bright, enthusiastic, energetic nurses, but they often "move up" into nursing administration or transfer to other areas. Therefore, one constantly trains new nurses. Some of the reasons for this are long hours in a high-stress environment, inadequate reimbursement, and the situation at many institutions in which 75 percent of the ICU nurse's time is spent in charting, developing care plans, giving reports, obtaining laboratory data, and performing various secretarial duties.

Our unit is staffed by 10 obstetric nurses who control their own work schedule and ensure that at least one of them is available 24 hours per day, 7 days per week. All the nurses have had at least 2 years of labor floor experience; previous medical or surgical intensive care experience is desirable although not essential. All the nurses are given a 4-week course in high-risk obstetric nursing, a 1-week course in obstetric intensive care, a 1-week course in medical intensive care, a 2-day course in hemodynamic monitoring, and a 1-day course in mechanical ventilation. They are encouraged to become certified in advanced cardiac life support (ACLS). Nurses also gain clinical experience by working in the medical ICU, and refresh their knowledge by working there 1 day per month.

ADMISSION CRITERIA

Patients in the ICU may be divided into three categories: (1) a low-risk monitoring group, (2) patients requiring intensive conventional therapy, and (3) patients requiring ICU therapy. Patients in the first group require frequent monitoring of their vital signs, neurologic evaluation, ECG monitoring, or pulse oximetry monitoring (e.g., for suspected myocardial infarction or drug overdose). Intensive conventional therapy is designed primarily for the prevention of complications (e.g., abdominal surgery in a massively obese patient) or for active medical therapy (e.g., for asthma or pneumonia, to prevent intubation). Specific ICU therapy includes hemodynamic monitoring with the Swan–Ganz catheter, mechanical ventilation, and titration of vasoactive drugs (e.g., for septic shock or ARDS). In one series of 2,693 admissions to a medical ICU, the need for noninvasive monitoring, rather than immediate major intervention, was responsible for 77 percent of the admissions. Among those admitted for moni-

---

Obstetric ICU Admission Criteria

1. Intubated patient requiring mechanical ventilation or airway protection
2. Impending respiratory failure (e.g., status asthmaticus, varicella pneumonia)
3. Titration of intravenous vasoactive drugs (e.g., dopamine, sodium nitroprusside)
4. Shock or impending shock (e.g., hypovolemic, cardiogenic, obstructive, or distributive)
5. Invasive hemodynamic monitoring (e.g., Swan–Ganz catheter)
6. Patients requiring plasmapheresis
7. Patients requiring hemodialysis
8. Specialized patients (e.g., high spinal or epidural anesthesia, traumatic intubation, drug overdose)

---

toring, only 10 percent ultimately required active interventions that justified admission to the ICU. These low-risk monitoring patients could have been monitored outside the ICU.[9]

Although we do not have good data on monitoring in obstetric patients, the low admission rate of obstetric patients suggests that few are admitted for monitoring only. Because the nurse/patient ratio in a labor-and-delivery suite is roughly 1:2, noninvasive monitoring and intra-arterial blood pressure monitoring can usually be accomplished in the labor rooms and does not require transfer to an ICU. Of my own first 200 ICU patients, 76 percent had radial artery lines, 37 percent had pulmonary artery catheterization, 12 percent required mechanical ventilation, and 4 percent underwent dialysis.[1] In the study by Kilpatrick and Matthay,[5] an arterial line was used in 88 percent of patients, a pulmonary artery catheter in 34 percent, and a ventilator in 59 percent.[5] The criteria for admission to our obstetric ICU are summarized in the box above.

CONSULTATIONS

The knowledge base used for treatment in the ICU is changing constantly. In such a dynamic environment it is necessary to use consultants. Our primary consultants are specialists in pulmonary medicine and cardiology; however, other consultants have included specialists in hematology, gastroenterology, hepatology, infectious disease, nephrology, neurology, general surgery, plastic surgery, hyperalimentation, ear-nose-and throat medicine, ophthalmology, and psychiatry.

TRANSFERS

Of the first 200 cases admitted to our obstetric ICU, 9 patients (4.5 percent) required transfer to another ICU. The main indication for transfer was prolonged mechanical ventilation for ARDS. Although residents and faculty members in anesthesiology are readily available to help in the obstetric ICU, we have found that adverse occurrences are fairly frequent in mechanically ventilated patients (e.g., self extubation, accidental intubation of the right main-stem bronchus, sinusitis, and pneumothorax). If a patient clearly has ARDS or has another condition that will most likely require mechanical ventilation for 5 days or longer, we arrange transfer to the medical or surgical ICU. However, with a rapidly progressive illness such as influenza or varicella pneumonia, the patient may be too unstable to transfer for several days.

COSTS

The monitoring and other ICU equipment cost several thousand dollars, but the main expenses of an ICU are supplies (intravenous fluids, blood products, medications) and personnel. Our nurses do not receive extra pay for working in the ICU. The benefits to them are restricted to intellectual stimulation, variation from routine obstetrics, and the satisfaction of helping a critically ill patient to recover. When there are no patients in the ICU, nurses work in the labor-and-delivery area. Such variety prevents burn-out and raises the general level of nursing care in labor and delivery. Similarly, other personnel, such as respiratory therapists, ECG, electroencephalography (EEG), and radiology technicians, and phlebotomists are used on an as-needed basis when there is a patient in the unit. The average length of stay in our ICU is 2.5 ± 2.0 days.[1]

Whether an obstetric ICU will be financially viable depends on the money actually spent by the hospital in treating a patient in the ICU compared to the reimbursement for such treatment. In areas of the United States with heavy penetration by managed care organizations, this is a difficult calculation. Several managed care organizations may send patients to a particular hospital, and reimbursement schemes for these patients' care may vary from 80 percent of charges to a capitated rate for prenatal care and delivery no matter how complicated the case.

QUALITY ASSURANCE

Since our obstetric ICU has a smaller census than that of a typical ICU, our quality assessment is performed by the quality assurance coordinator for our labor and delivery division. The Joint Commission on the Accreditation of Healthcare Organizations requires that there be written nursing protocols and standards of practice in all special care units. This serves as the template against which the adequacy of patient care is judged. The quality assurance coordinator reviews the chart of each patient discharged from the ICU to see that the standards were met, that nursing notes are completed, and that all orders were executed. All maternal deaths are reviewed by the chief of the division of maternal-fetal medicine and by the chairman of the OB/GYN department. The quality assurance coordinator also tries to identify and correct any problems or conflicts with the services involved in patient care in the ICU (e.g., radiology, laboratory, respiratory therapy, pharmacy, dietetics, bioengineering, and the various consultants to the ICU). Incident reports are also filed to identify problems, their cause, and their solution.

MOST COMMON DISORDERS

About 40 percent of admissions to our obstetric ICU are for pre-eclampsia-eclampsia and its complications, 10 percent are for massive hemorrhage, and 50 percent are for various medical problems of pregnancy listed by organ system. Since true intensive care involves invasive hemodynamic monitoring, mechanical ventilation, and titration of vasoactive drugs, each of these is considered in some detail.

**Main Indications for Admission to the
Obstetric ICU**

Hypertensive disorders
  Severe pre-eclampsia with pulmonary edema
  or oliguria
  Eclampsia
  HELLP (hemolysis, elevated liver enzymes, and
  low platelet count) syndrome
  Liver rupture
  Refractory hypertension
Massive hemorrhage
  Abruption
  Previa
  Accreta
  Uterine atony
  Uterine rupture
  Postoperative bleeding
Medical problems of pregnancy
  Cardiac problems
    Pulmonary edema
    Cardiomyopathy
    Congenital heart disease
    Arrhythmias
    Myocardial infarction
  Pulmonary problems
    Pneumonia
    Asthma
    Pulmonary embolism
  Renal problems
    Acute tubular necrosis
    Chronic renal failure
  Gastrointestinal problems
    Acute fatty liver of pregnancy
    Ruptured appendix
    Sickle hepatopathy
  Sepsis
    Pyelonephritis
    Septic shock
    Septic pelvic thrombophlebitis
  Endocrine problems
    Diabetic ketoacidosis
    Thyroid storm
  Central nervous system problems
    Stroke
    Status epilepticus
    Meningitis

INVASIVE HEMODYNAMIC MONITORING

The Swan–Ganz pulmonary artery catheter was introduced into clinical practice in 1970 for the evaluation of patients with cardiac disease.[10] The first publications on its use in obstetrics appeared in 1980.[11,12] Swan–Ganz monitoring should be considered in any critically ill patient whose volume status the physician needs to know. The standards and criteria for invasive monitoring should be the same for pregnant as for nonpregnant patients.

The Swan–Ganz catheter is useful in differentiating cardiogenic from noncardiogenic forms of pulmonary edema. It may also be used to guide diuretic therapy and manipulations of cardiac output, such as preload and afterload reduction or inotropic therapy. In patients with oliguria, the catheter may be used to assess volume status. In pre-eclampsia it has been shown that central venous pressure is not adequate for assessing volume status. The changes in wedge pressure and cardiac output in response to a fluid challenge are the most important guides to intravascular volume. Although invasive hemodynamic monitoring is not necessary for acute resuscitation from hemorrhagic shock, it is useful in the

---

**Indications for Invasive Hemodynamic
Monitoring in Obstetrics**

Refractory or unexplained pulmonary edema

Refractory or unexplained oliguria

Massive hemorrhage

Septic shock

Adult respiratory distress syndrome

New York Heart Association class III and IV cardiac disease

Intraoperative or intrapartum cardiovascular decompensation

Respiratory distress of unknown cause

Invasive monitoring is not necessary in every patient with one of these conditions, nor is this an all-inclusive list.[13]

subsequent 24 to 72 hours to guide fluid therapy in complex cases in which it is not clear whether internal bleeding is continuing or whether oliguria, pulmonary edema, liver dysfunction, or severe coagulopathy are present. In septic shock, invasive monitoring allows manipulation of cardiovascular parameters with fluid and inotropic therapy, as well as assessment of the response to therapy through such parameters as oxygen delivery and consumption. In ARDS, the Swan–Ganz catheter is used to exclude cardiogenic pulmonary edema and to guide supportive therapy with mechanical ventilation, positive end-expiratory pressure, intravenous fluids, diuretics, and inotropic agents. Cardiac patients in New York Heart Association Classes III and IV require invasive monitoring for fluid therapy, drug therapy, and anesthetic management during labor and delivery. The cause of sudden intraoperative or intrapartum cardiovascular decompensation may be clarified by obtaining the wedge pressure and cardiac output. The final indication for use of the Swan–Ganz catheter is for patients in whom the contribution of cardiac or pulmonary disease to respiratory distress is unclear by clinical examination. The pulmonary artery catheter can help to differentiate heart failure, pneumonia, pulmonary emboli, ARDS, and chronic pulmonary disorders.

The risks and benefits of bedside catheterization were reviewed by Matthay and Chatterjee.[14] These authors considered four areas: (1) complications, (2) obtaining reliable data, (3) clinical versus invasive assessment of hemodynamic status, and (4) the effect of monitoring on outcome.

Complications of bedside catheterization have decreased over the years, at least partially through better physician and nurse awareness. The incidence of pneumothorax has decreased from 6 to 1 percent in the early literature to less than 0.1 percent now. Pulmonary infarction has decreased from 7.2 percent in 1974 to 0 to 1.3 percent in recent studies. Pulmonary artery rupture has fallen from 0.1 to 0.2 percent to almost 0 percent. Local vascular thrombosis has decreased with the use of heparin-bonded catheters. Septicemia has decreased from 2 to 0.5 percent. However, complications of catheterization have not been eliminated.

There are multiple causes for interpretive error in catheter readings, including improper calibra-

tion, air or blood in the lines, the use of digital readout rather than a hard copy printout, and failure to measure wedge pressure at end-expiration when pleural pressure is zero. Pulmonary capillary wedge pressure may not reflect left ventricular end-diastolic pressure in the setting of aortic insufficiency, mitral stenosis, or mitral insufficiency. In addition, the relation between left ventricular end-diastolic pressure and left ventricular end-diastolic volume may vary with changes in left ventricular compliance, such as during myocardial ischemia.

Two studies have shown that prediction of cardiac output and wedge pressure based on history, physical examination and chest radiography are about 75 percent accurate in coronary care unit patients.[15,16] However, three studies have shown that clinical criteria may accurately predict wedge pressure and cardiac output only about 50 percent of the time in a more heterogeneous group of general ICU patients.[17–19] Information from invasive monitoring also made a difference in treatment (fluids, diuretics, vasopressors, or vasodilators) about 50 percent of the time.[17–19]

Does use of the Swan–Ganz catheter improve outcome? No hard data exist to prove this, and a large, prospective, randomized trial would be needed. The authors emphasize that the Swan–Ganz catheter is only a diagnostic device. It will improve outcome only if it permits the diagnosis of conditions for which treatment exists. For example, it may improve outcome in acute myocardial infarction with heart failure, because afterload reduction, inotropic agents, and intra-aortic balloon counterpulsation may be applied. By contrast, patients with septic shock are unlikely to benefit from the catheter because no new therapeutic option exists for this condition. However, invasive monitoring may make management of the hemodynamically unstable septic patient more rational.[14]

The normal hemodynamic values for healthy nonpregnant women compared with healthy primiparous women at 36 to 38 weeks' gestation and 11 to 13 weeks' postpartum are summarized in Table 14-2.[13] Central venous pressure and pulmonary capillary wedge pressure are unchanged in pregnancy. Cardiac output is increased as the result of an increase in both heart rate and stroke volume. Sys-

Table 14-2. Hemodynamic Values in Healthy Nonpregnant, Pregnant, and Postpartum Subjects

Parameter	Hemodynamic Values in Subjects[a]		
	Nonpregnant	36–38 Weeks of Gestation[b]	Postpartum
Heart Rate (beats/min)	60–100	83 ± 10	71 ± 10
Central venous pressure (mm Hg)	5–10	3.6 ± 2.5	3.7 ± 2.6
Mean pulmonary artery pressure (mm Hg)	15–20	—[c]	—[c]
Pulmonary capillary wedge pressure (mm Hg)	6–12	7.5 ± 1.8	6.3 ± 2.1
Mean arterial pressure (mm Hg)	90–110	90.3 ± 5.8	86.4 ± 7.5
Cardiac output (L/min)	4.3–6.0	6.2 ± 1.0	4.3 ± 0.9
Stroke volume (ml/beat)	57–71	74.7	60.6
Systemic vascular resistance (dyne·cm·sec^{-5})	900–1,400	1,210 ± 266	1,530 ± 520
Pulmonary vascular resistance (dyne·cm·sec^{-5})	<250	78 ± 22	119 ± 47

[a] Where available, data are given as mean ± standard deviation.
[b] Values in pregnant patients were determined with patient in left lateral decubitis position.
[c] Not reported.
(Adapted from ACOG Technical Buletin No. 175,[13] with permission.)

temic and pulmonary vascular resistances are decreased during pregnancy.

MECHANICAL VENTILATION

Managing a pregnant woman on a mechanical ventilator is a big step above managing a pregnant woman through invasive hemodynamic monitoring. There are several types of ventilators, including negative-pressure ventilators (e.g., the iron lung) and positive-pressure ventilators (e.g., pressure-cycled, volume-cycled, time-cycled, and flow-cycled). The standard ventilator is a volume-cycled ventilator because it delivers a constant tidal volume despite changes in the patient's lung compliance and airway resistance. There are also several modes of mechanical ventilation, but the most commonly used are controlled mandatory ventilation, assisted/controlled ventilation, and synchronized intermittent mandatory ventilation. The disease processes complicating pregnancy that may require intubation and mechanical ventilation are listed in the box.

The arterial blood gas criteria for acute respiratory failure are an arterial oxygen partial pressure (PaO$_2$) below 50 mm Hg or an arterial carbon dioxide partial pressure (PaCO$_2$) above 50 mm Hg on room air. The blood gas analysis reveals what the patient is accomplishing. It does not reveal how hard

Maternal Diseases That May Require Mechanical Ventilation

Bacterial pneumonia

Viral pneumonia

Aspiration pneumonia

Asthma

Pulmonary edema

Status epilepticus

Septic shock

Adult respiratory distress syndrome

Postoperative pseudocholinesterase deficiency

Postoperative hemodynamic instability

High spinal or epidural anesthesia

Difficult intubation

Laryngeal edema

Drug overdose

Cardiac arrest

Hypoxic encephalopathy

she is working to do it. If the patient is severely dyspneic, restless, confused, or fatigued, it may be wise to intubate her prophylactically. Mechanical ventilation is performed for (1) oxygenation failure, (2) ventilatory failure, or (3) to decrease the work of breathing to allow oxygen delivery to other organ systems during systemic illness. Oxygenation failure occurs with ventilation–perfusion mismatch (e.g., atelectasis, ARDS) or low-perfusion states (e.g., pulmonary embolism, cardiogenic shock). Ventilatory failure results from a depressed ventilatory drive (e.g., from drugs or spinal cord injury) or from overloaded re-

spiratory muscles (e.g., stiff lungs, neuromuscular disease, or electrolyte imbalance).

The period during initiation of ventilatory support can be a time of patient instability. Positive pressure ventilation interferes with venous return to the heart, reducing cardiac output and blood pressure. The patient's breathing is often uncoordinated with the ventilator. It is useful to begin with the patient breathing 100 percent oxygen in the conditioned gas provided by the ventilator. Once the patient's initial blood gas data are available, the inhaled oxygen fraction can be decreased to a more appropriate

---

Complications of Mechanical Ventilation

Pulmonary complications
  Barotrauma
    Pulmonary interstitial emphysema
    Pneumothorax
    Pneumomediastinum
    Subcutaneous emphysema
    Pneumoperitoneum
    Air embolism
  Pulmonary embolism
  Pulmonary fibrosis
Complications related to airway management
  Right main-stem bronchus intubation
  Self extubation
  Laryngeal edema, ulceration, hemorrhage
  Stridor
  Hoarseness
  Paranasal sinusitis
  Aspiration
  Tracheal stenosis
Complications associated with tracheostomy
  Tracheoinnominate fistula
  Tracheoesophageal fistula
  Tracheal stenosis
Cardiovascular complications
  Myocardial ischemia
  Arrhythmias
Gastrointestinal complications
  Hemorrhage
  Altered motility
  Malnutrition

Complications of enteral nutrition
  Vomiting
  Abdominal distension
  Diarrhea
  Electrolyte abnormalities
  Hypercapnea
Complications of total parenteral nutrition
  Hyperchloremic acidosis
  Hyperglycemia
  Hypophosphatemia
  Liver function abnormalities
  Hypercapnia
Infection
  Line sepsis
  Endocarditis
  Septic thrombophlebitis
  Acalculous cholecystitis
  Nosocomial pneumonia
  Decubitus ulcer
  Sinusitis
  Meningitis
Renal complications
  Positive fluid balance
  Acute renal failure

level for the patient's needs. The respiratory rate may be set at 8 to 16 breaths per minute. Tidal volume is set at about 10 ml/kg of body weight. The peak flow rate is set at about 45 L/min. The inspiratory time/expiratory time ratio should be about 1 : 2. Peak inspiratory pressure should be maintained below 60 cm H_2O to reduce the risk of barotrauma. Positive end-expiratory pressure (PEEP) may be used in patients with diffuse lung injury (e.g., noncardiogenic pulmonary edema) who require high oxygen settings. PEEP helps to prevent airway and alveolar collapse and recruits partially collapsed alveoli. It should not be used in lobar pneumonia or other localized lung disease because it will overdistend the compliant, normal alveoli, decreasing their perfusion. The resulting ventilation–perfusion mismatch may actually worsen oxygenation.[20]

While the patient is maintained on mechanical ventilation, a number of parameters may be followed. Arterial blood gas data should be obtained about 20 minutes after each ventilator change to make sure oxygenation, ventilation, and acid–base status are normal. Other parameters that may be followed include vital signs; ECG, chest-radiographic, and pulse oximetry data; alveolar–arterial oxygen gradient; static and dynamic compliance of the lung; and end-tidal carbon dioxide concentration. When mixed venous blood gas data are obtained from blood drawn from the distal port of the Swan-Ganz catheter, and cardiac output and hemoglobin are known, oxygen delivery and consumption and the intrapulmonary shunt fraction can be calculated.

Trained and experienced personnel are required for monitoring ventilated patients. Adverse occurrences (e.g., self extubation, right main-stem bronchus intubation, pneumothorax, ventilator malfunction) are fairly frequent.[21]

Weaning from mechanical ventilation in previously healthy patients with acute lung injury can occur as soon as the acute pulmonary process has resolved. In patients with pre-existing lung disease, weaning can be very difficult. Numerous weaning parameters (e.g., minute ventilation <10 L/min, negative inspiratory force of >−20 cm H_2O) can be used to support the clinical decision to stop mechanical ventilation. The mnemonic "weans now" is useful for recalling the factors that optimize weaning potential.[22]

TITRATION OF VASOACTIVE DRUGS

In this section I discuss the five vasoactive agents most commonly titrated by intravenous infusion in the obstetric ICU (Table 14-3). In treating patients with shock, the first line of therapy, even in cardiogenic shock, is intravenous fluid administration. Inotropes and vasopressors should be withheld until intravascular volume is optimized. An appropriate approach to fluid resuscitation of a patient in shock is to place a pulmonary artery catheter and measure the wedge pressure and cardiac output serially as increments of fluid are given. In obstetrics, the most common type of shock is hypovolemic shock due to hemorrhage. In the young, previously healthy woman, rapid fluid resuscitation may be accomplished by monitoring urine output, mental status, heart rate, blood pressure, respiratory rate, and temperature. Invasive monitoring may be reserved for women who remain in shock after initial resuscitation, those who deteriorate after an initial response, or those who have poor physiologic reserve and are unlikely to tolerate errors in the resuscitation attempt. In the 1960s, Weil and Shubin[23] developed a method of fluid challenge involving the administration of 200-ml boluses over periods of 10 minutes while observing the change in central venous pressure or pulmonary capillary wedge pressure. This is

---

Optimizing Weaning Potential

W   Check *Weaning* parameters

E   Use the largest possible *Endotracheal* tube to minimize airway resistance

A   Optimize *Arterial* blood gases

N   Maintain adequate *Nutrition*

S   Clear *Secretions* from endotracheal or tracheostomy tube

N   Ascertain that *Neuromuscular* blocking agents have worn off

O   Reverse airway *Obstruction* with bronchodilators or corticosteroids

W   Wean when the patient is *Wakeful*

Table 14-3. Vasoactive Drug Dose Chart

Agent	Dopamine	Dobutamine	Norpinephrine	Nitroprusside	Nitroglycerin
Mix in 250 ml D_5W (mg)	400	250	8	50	50
Concentration (μg/ml)	1,600	1,000	32	200	200
Usual dose (μg/kg/min)	5	10	0.1	1	1
Dose range (μg/kg/min)	1–20	5–20	0.1–1	0.25–5	0.25–3

a useful protocol for avoiding overzealous treatment in patients with poor physiologic reserve. For 30 years there has been a controversy over whether to use crystalloid or colloid solutions for fluid resuscitation. Numerous clinical studies and meta-analyses of these studies have failed to demonstrate a clear advantage of colloid administration that would justify its cost.[24,25]

Dopamine

Dopamine is an inotropic vasoconstrictor. It has both α- and β-adrenergic effects, depending on the dose employed. At doses of 0.5 to 3 μg/kg/min the dopaminergic effects predominate, causing selective renal, splanchnic, and cerebral vasodilation. At 3 to 10 μg/kg/min, the β_1 and β_2 effects predominate, resulting in a positive inotropic and chronotropic effect on the heart. At doses of 10 to 20 μg/kg/min, the α-adrenergic effect predominates, resulting in vasoconstriction. Dopamine is the most widely used drug for treating hypotension, and is particularly indicated in cardiogenic shock, septic shock, and during the first few hours of oliguric renal failure. Its adverse effects include tachyarrhythmias, myocardial ischemia, and renal and splanchnic ischemia (a flow rate of >15 mg/kg/min). In practice, if 20 μg/kg/min does not satisfactorily raise blood pressure, the dopamine infusion rate is reduced to a nephrotonic dose of 3 μg/kg/min, and another agent, such as norepinephrine, is begun.[26]

Dobutamine

Dobutamine is an inotropic vasodilator. At low doses, the β_1 effects predominate (cardiac stimulation), while at higher doses, the β_2 effects increase (peripheral vasodilation). The peripheral vasodilator effect of dobutamine distinguishes it from dopamine. Cardiac output increases and peripheral resistance falls, leaving the blood pressure more or less unchanged. Dobutamine also causes less tachycardia

than dopamine, and is less arrhythmogenic. It is the inotropic agent of choice for acute management of heart failure, providing simultaneous inotropic support and afterload reduction. Its side effects include tachyarrhythmias and hypotension in hypovolemic patients.[26]

Norepinephrine

Norepinephrine has 60 percent α- and 40 percent β-agonist effects. Its propensity to cause profound vasoconstriction, especially in the splanchnic beds, limits the use of this drug. Norepinephrine increases blood pressure by increasing systemic vascular resistance. Cardiac output may not rise despite increased contractility, because of the elevated systemic vascular resistance. Myocardial oxygen consumption increases markedly. Norepinephrine is used for life-threatening hypotension caused by acute blood loss (while providing aggressive fluid resuscitation), for septic shock, and during surgery for pheochromotoma. Its adverse effects are myocardial ischemia, lactic acidosis, splanchnic ischemia, and skin necrosis from extravasation.[26]

Sodium Nitroprusside

Nitroprusside is an equal arteriolar and venular vasodilator, acting directly on the vessel wall. It enhances myocardial function, causing an increase in stroke volume by reducing afterload. The pulmonary capillary wedge pressure falls partly because of venodilation. Nitroprusside also reduces pulmonary vascular resistance. Nitroprusside crosses the placenta; it has no effect on uterine contractility.[27] Uterine blood flow has been reported to increase,[28] to decrease,[29] and to remain unchanged[30] with nitroprusside therapy. The rapid onset and disappearance of activity (15 to 30 seconds) of nitroprusside make it the best drug available for the control of acute hypertensive emergencies. Other indications include acute left ventricular failure in the absence of hypotension, and intraoperative control of blood pressure. Adverse effects of the drug are overshoot hypotension, undesired vasodilation in some vascular beds (increased intracranial pressure and intrapulmonary shunting), and cyanide and thiocyanate toxicity. The cyanide toxicity appears to be dose-related. Infusion rates should be limited to less than 5 μg/kg/min if possible. Antidotes include amyl nitrite, sodium nitrite, sodium thiosulfate, and hydroxycobalamin.[26] It has been recommended that sodium nitroprusside not be used during pregnancy for longer than 30 minutes because of the risk of fetal cyanide toxicity,[31] although some reports have described its longer use.[27,32] Monitoring with an indwelling arterial catheter is mandatory during nitroprusside therapy. Additionally, nitroprusside must be shielded from light.

Nitroglycerin

Nitroglycerin is a direct-acting vasodilator. It is distinguished from nitroprusside in that at low dosage (<50 μg/min) it is predominantly a venodilator. At higher doses (>200 μg/min), its predominant effect is arterial dilatation. It dilates coronary arteries and reverses myocardial ischemia.[26] Nitroglycerin is rarely used in obstetrics. It can be used as an antihypertensive agent for minute-to-minute titration of blood pressure. It may also be used to reduce preload in patients with cardiogenic pulmonary edema.[33] Nitroglycerin can be used acutely to reduce the mean arterial pressure by 10 percent to decrease infarct size in the rare patient with acute myocardial infarction in pregnancy. With a molecular weight of 227 daltons and not being ionized, nitroglycerin crosses the placenta to the fetus; however, hypotension and serious fetal side effects are rare.[34] Nitroglycerin increases uterine blood flow in hypertensive gravid ewes.[35,36] The main concern with this drug is that it increases intracranial pressure in animal studies, raising the possibility that it might be detrimental in pre-eclampsia.[37] Other side effects of nitroglycerin include headache, tachyphylaxis, and methemoglobinemia. Nitroglycerin binds to polyvinylchloride tubing, necessitating the use of pretreated tubing for intravenous administration.[26]

REFERENCES

1. Mabie WC, Sibai BM: Treatment in an obstetric intensive care unit. Am J Obstet Gynecol 162:1, 1990
2. Kirshon B, Hinkley CM, Cotton DB, Miller J: Maternal mortality in a maternal-fetal medicine intensive care unit. J Reprod Med 35:25, 1990
3. Collop NA, Sahn SA: Critical illness in pregnancy. Chest 103:1548, 1993
4. Graham SG, Luxton MC: The requirement for intensive care support for the pregnant population. Anesthesia 44:581, 1989
5. Kilpatrick SJ, Matthay MA: Obstetric patients requiring critical care: a five-year review. Chest 101:1407, 1992
6. Monaco TJ, Spielman FJ, Katz VL: Pregnant patients in the intensive care unit: a descriptive analysis. South Med J 86:414, 1993
7. Ng TI, Lim E, Tweed WA, Arulkumaran S: Obstetric admissions to the intensive care unit—a retrospective review. Ann Acad Med 21:804, 1992
8. Stephens ID: Occasional survey: ICU admissions from an obstetrical hospital. Can J Anaesth 38:677, 1991
9. Thibault G, Mulley A, Barnett et al: Medical intensive care: indications, interventions, and outcomes. N Engl J Med 302:939, 1980
10. Forrester JS, Diamond G, McHugh TH, Swan HJC: Filling pressures in the right and left sides of the heart in acute myocardial infarction. N Engl J Med 283:190, 1970
11. Berkowitz RL, Rafferty TD: Pulmonary artery flow-directed catheter use in the obstetric patient. Obstet Gynecol 55:507, 1980
12. Cotton DB, Benedetti TJ: Use of the Swan–Ganz catheter in obstetrics and gynecology. Obstet Gynecol 56:641, 1980
13. Invasive hemodynamic monitoring in obstetrics and gynecology. ACOG Technical Bulletin No. 175. American College of Obstetricians and Gynecologists, Washington, DC, December, 1992
14. Matthay MA, Chatterjee K: Bedside catheterization of the pulmonary artery: risks compared with benefits. Ann Intern Med 109:826, 1988
15. Forrester JC, Diamond G, Swan HJC: Correlative classification of clinical and hemodynamic function after acute myocardial infarction. Am J Cardiol 39:137, 1977
16. Bayliss J, Norell M, Ryan A et al: Bedside hemodynamic monitoring: experience in a general hospital. BMJ 287:187, 1983
17. Connor AF Jr, McCaffree DR, Gray BA: Evaluation of right heart catheterization in the critically ill patient

without acute myocardial infarction. N Engl J Med 308:263, 1983

18. Eisenberg PR, Jaffe AS, Schuster DR: Clinical evaluation compared to pulmonary artery catheterization in the hemodynamic assessment of critically ill patients. Crit Care Med 12:549, 1984

19. Fein AM, Goldberg SK, Wahlenstein MD et al: Is pulmonary artery catheterization necessary for the diagnosis of pulmonary edema? Am Rev Respir Dis 129: 1006, 1984

20. Balk RA: Mechanical ventilation. p. 24. In Parillo JE (ed): Current Therapy in Critical Care Medicine. 2nd Ed. BC Decker, Philadelphia, 1991

21. Pingleton SK: Complications of acute respiratory failure. Am Rev Respir Dis 137:1463, 1988

22. Beaton N, Bone RC: Criteria for weaning your patients from respirators. J Respir Dis 6:80, 1985

23. Weil MH, Shubin H: The VIP approach to the bedside management of shock. JAMA 207:337, 1969

24. Gould SA, Sehgal LR, Sehgal HL, Moss GS: Hypovolemic shock. Crit Care Clin 9:239, 1993

25. Imm A, Carlson RW: Fluid resuscitation in circulatory shock. Crit Care Clin 9:313, 1993

26. Marino PL: Hemodynamic drugs. p. 241. In: The ICU Book. Lea & Febiger, Malvern, PA, 1991

27. Stempel JE, O'Grady JP, Morton MJ, Johnson KA: Use of sodium nitroprusside in complications of gestational hypertension. Obstet Gynecol 60:533, 1982

28. Ellis SC, Wheeler AS, James III FM et al: Fetal and maternal effects of sodium nitroprusside used to counteract hypertension in gravid ewes. Am J Obstet Gynecol 143:766, 1982

29. Lieb SM, Zugaib M, Nuwayhid B et al: Nitroprusside-induced hemodynamic alteration in normotensive and hypertensive pregnant sheep. Am J Obstet Gynecol 139:925, 1981

30. Ring G, Kranes E, Shnider SM et al: Comparison of nitroprusside and hydralazine in hypertensive pregnant ewes. Obstet Gynecol 50:598, 1977

31. Naulty J, Cefalo RC, Lewis PE: Fetal toxicity of nitroprusside in the pregnant ewe. Am J Obstet Gynecol 139:708, 1981

32. Shoemaker CT, Meyers M: Sodium nitroprusside for control of severe hypertensive disease of pregnancy: a case report and discussion of potential toxicity. Am J Obstet Gynecol 149:171, 1984

33. Cotton DB, Jones MM, Longmire S et al: Role of intravenous nitroglycerin in the treatment of severe pregnancy-induced hypertension complicated by pulmonary edema. Am J Obstet Gynecol 154:91, 1986

34. Snyder SW, Wheeler AS, James III FM: The use of nitroglycerin to control severe hypertension of pregnancy during cesarean section. Anesthesiology 51:563, 1979

35. Wheeler AS, James III FM, Meis PJ et al: Effects of nitroglycerin and nitroprusside on the uterine vasculature of gravid ewes. Anesthesiology 52:390, 1980

36. Craft JB Jr, Co EG, Yonekura ML, Gilman RM: Nitroglycerin effect in the hypertensive pregnant ewe. Anesthesiology 51:S308, 1979

37. Writer WDR, James III FM, Stullken EH Jr, Koontz FA: Intracranial effects of nitroglycerin—an obstetrical hazard? Anesthesiology 52:S309, 1980

Chapter 15

Pre-eclampsia and Hypertension

John T. Repke

Pre-eclampsia and hypertension are terms frequently interchanged in the setting of pregnancy. As research in these areas continues, the controversy grows. Pre-eclampsia has been categorized as pregnancy-induced hypertension with proteinuria, but variants include pregnancy-induced hypertension without proteinuria. In addition, pregnancy may be complicated by pre-existing chronic hypertension, or what has been currently termed transient hypertension of pregnancy. For the practicing clinician, chronic hypertension and pre-eclampsia are the two most important conditions in terms of intrapartum management. The definitions of the hypertensive disorders of pregnancy as determined by the Committee on Terminology of the American College of Obstetricians and Gynecologists are summarized in box below.

PRE-ECLAMPSIA

Pre-eclampsia is an idiopathic disorder of pregnancy characterized by hypertension, proteinuria, and edema that resolves on delivery of the fetus and placenta. A variety of terms have been used to describe this disorder, including toxemia, edema-proteinuria, hypertension-gestosis, hypertension with proteinuria, and pregnancy-induced hypertension. The overwhelming majority of cases of pre-eclampsia culminate in successful outcomes for mother and fetus,

but in the most severe cases the condition may result in severe multisystem decompensation, cardiovascular collapse, and death of the mother or fetus, or both. Pre-eclampsia remains a major cause of maternal mortality worldwide, and continues to be one of the leading causes of maternal and perinatal morbidity and mortality in the United States. Despite aggressive research efforts, there remains a limited understanding of the etiology of this disease. Epidemiologically, patients who are young, nulliparous, and from lower socioeconomic groups seem to be at greatest risk of the development of pre-eclampsia.

Etiology

Over the years, multiple etiologies have been proposed for pre-eclampsia (Table 15-1). To date, no satisfactory, single unifying explanation has been advanced for the origin of the protean manifestations of this disorder. Given the incomplete understanding of the pathogenesis of pre-eclampsia, the development of rational treatment and prevention programs for it has been quite difficult.[1,2] Recent observations have increasingly shown that although blood pressure elevation is an important component of pre-eclampsia, numerous other pathophysiologic events contribute to its evolution. Increased vascular reactivity to pressor substances, reduction in maternal intravascular volume, alterations in prostanoid metabolism, and abnormalities of the coagulation

Hypertensive Disorders of Pregnancy

Hypertension: Systolic blood pressure above 140 mm Hg, diastolic blood pressure above 90 mm Hg; or a systolic increase of 30 mm Hg, diastolic increase of 15 mm Hg

Proteinuria: Protein levels above 300 mg in 24 hours or above 1 g/L on dipstick testing in at least two random urine specimens collected 6 or more hours apart

Pre-eclampsia: The development of hypertension with proteinuria or edema, or both, after 20 weeks' gestation

Eclampsia: The occurrence of convulsions in a pre-eclamptic patient in the absence of coincidental neurologic disease

Chronic hypertension: The presence of persistent hypertension of whatever cause before 20 weeks' gestation in the absence of neoplastic trophoblastic disease

Superimposed pre-eclampsia or eclampsia: The development of pre-eclampsia or eclampsia in a woman with pre-existing hypertensive vascular or renal disease

Gestational hypertension: Hypertension developing in the latter half of pregnancy without other evidence of pre-eclampsia or chronic hypertensive vascular disease

Severe pre-eclampsia: A blood pressure above 160/110 mm Hg, proteinuria (>5 g in 24 hours), rising serum creatinine, persistent visual disturbances, epigastric or right upper quadrant pain, pulmonary edema or right upper quadrant pain, pulmonary edema or cyanosis, thrombocytopenia or overt hemolysis, hepatocellular damage, and intrauterine growth retardation

Table 15-1. Theories of Etiology of Pre-eclampsia

Theory	Evidence
Excessive placental mass	Increased incidence in twins, molar gestation
Immunologic	Increased incidence in first pregnancy
Placental ischemia	Increased incidence of fetal growth retardation
Genetic	Familial inheritance pattern
Imbalance of prostaglandins	Aspirin therapy is somewhat protective
Endothelial injury	Renal hepatic dysfunction, coagulopathy

injury. When endothelial cell injury occurs, it sets the stage for a variety of pathologic events that are manifested as the typical clinical signs and symptoms of pre-eclampsia.[3] These include increased vascular tone, alterations in prostanoid metabolism, activation of the coagulation cascade, and capillary leak syndrome (Table 15-2).

Although this view may be an oversimplification, it serves to highlight the need for an effective means of primary prevention. Preventive efforts have focused primarily on minimizing vascular sensitivity to pressor substances, altering prostaglandin synthesis, and finally, averting the endothelial cell damage leading to the pathologic cascade ultimately recognized as clinical pre-eclampsia. As with chronic hypertension, and discussed later in this chapter, schemes for preventing pre-eclampsia include both nonpharmacologic and pharmacologic approaches.

Prevention

By the time pre-eclampsia is clinically evident, the disease process is quite advanced and therapeutic options available to the clinician are limited. For this reason, primary prevention of this disease would be ideal. To develop an approach for primary prevention, a reasonable screening test that can predict susceptibility to pre-eclampsia must be established. Thus far, an easily applied, safe, noninvasive, and reliable screening test does not exist. Nevertheless, populations of patients who are at high risk of pre-eclampsia have been identified. Examples of such high-risk groups include adolescents, nulliparous

mechanism have all been observed in pre-eclampsia. Viewed in a more global context, pre-eclampsia may be described as a failure of the normal adaptive mechanisms of pregnancy. Currently, the most favored paradigm of the pathogenesis of pre-eclampsia emphasizes the critical role of endothelial cell

Table 15-2. Manifestations of Pre-eclampsia

Finding	Pathology	Putative Mechanism

Hypertension	Increased cardiac contractility
	Increased sensitivity to endogenous
	  angiotensin
	? Vasospasm
		Excess of thromboxane, decreased
		  prostacyclin

Proteinuria	Glomerular endotheliosis	Endothelial cell damage
Peripheral edema	Capillary leak	Endothelial cell damage
Decreased intravascular volume	? Capillary leak	Endothelial cell damage
Pulmonary edema	Capillary leak	Endothelial cell damage
Visual disturbances	? Vasospasm	Excess of thromboxane, decreased prostacyclin
Hepatic dysfunction	Platelet/fibrin plugging of sinusoids	Excess of thromboxane, decreased prostacyclin

Thrombocytopenia, hemolysis	Platelet activation, microvascular
	  thrombosis
		Excess of thromboxane, decreased
		  prostacyclin

Seizures, altered consciousness	? Cerebral vasospasm	Excess of thromboxane, decreased prostacyclin

patients, patients of lower socioeconomic status, and patients with chronic hypertension, insulin-dependent diabetes, or multifetal gestations. Women with a previous history of pre-eclampsia are also at increased risk. Provocative tests (e.g., angiotensin challenge tests)[4] to screen for increased maternal vascular reactivity have been proposed, but are expensive, time-consuming, and not applicable to the general population.

Nonpharmacologic Prevention

A number of nonpharmacologic approaches have been proposed to reduce the incidence of pre-eclampsia. In an effort to alter vascular sensitivity and possibly affect prostaglandin ratios, strict sodium restriction and alteration of medium-chain triglycerides in the diet have been attempted. Other nutritional approaches have included supplementation with zinc, magnesium, and calcium. While there is evidence that relative zinc deficiency may be associated with an increased incidence of pre-eclampsia, zinc deficiency is a very rare complication in the American diet.

Dietary magnesium supplementation has enjoyed an intuitive popularity, based on the use of magnesium sulfate in the intrapartum clinical management of pre-eclampsia. While several studies have suggested that magnesium supplementation may effectively reduce the incidence of pre-eclampsia,[5,6] a randomized clinical trial completed in 1989 failed to support that association.[7] Calcium supplementation has also been proposed as a means of reducing the incidence of pre-eclampsia.[8] There is a well-described relationship between calcium and blood pressure. increased dietary calcium has been associated with reduced blood pressure in both pregnant and nonpregnant populations. Additionally, several randomized clinical trials have shown that calcium supplementation may reduce vascular sensitivity to angiotensin II and thus lower the clinical incidence of pre-eclampsia.[1] Larger, multicenter clinical trials are currently in progress to investigate this issue more definitively.

The precise mechanism whereby calcium supplementation lowers blood pressure and possibly reduces the incidence of pre-eclampsia is an intriguing one that is undergoing rapid investigation.[9,10]

Pharmacologic Prevention

Currently, the principal pharmacologic approach to preventing pre-eclampsia remains the use of low-dose aspirin (40 to 100 mg/day). The theory behind this approach involves the ability of low-dose aspirin to inhibit platelet thromboxane synthesis while minimally affecting prostacyclin synthesis by the endothelial cell.[11,12] Presumably, favorably altering the prostacyclin/thromboxane ratio protects the endothelial cell from damage and prevents the initiation of a cascade of intravascular events, subsequently leading to clinically evident pre-eclampsia.

To date, multiple small clinical trials have successfully shown that low-dose aspirin markedly reduces the incidence of pre-eclampsia, but definitive studies of the appropriate population sample size for this are still pending. The most recent large-scale investigation of the role of low-dose aspirin for the prevention of pre-eclampsia in healthy nulliparous women concluded that while low-dose aspirin decreased the incidence of pre-eclampsia, there was no decrease in perinatal morbidity, and a suggestion of an increase in the risk of placental abruption.[13] This led the investigator to conclude that routine use of low-dose aspirin in healthy nulliparous women could not be recommended. These findings do not necessarily preclude the use of low-dose aspirin in high-risk clinical settings. Although criteria for identifying those patients who would qualify for low-dose aspirin treatment are not universally agreed on, present criteria may include such therapy for patients with a history of severe pre-eclampsia, a previous pregnancy with unexplained severe intrauterine growth restriction (IUGR), or a positive serology result for the lupus anticoagulant or anticardiolipin antibodies. Other, less well-established indications include multiple gestation, type I diabetes, and moderate chronic hypertension.

When informing the patient of the possible benefits of low-dose aspirin therapy, it is also necessary to review its potential risks. Several studies have suggested that early first-trimester exposure to aspirin could have teratogenic effects,[14,15] specifically comprising an increased risk of various congenital cardiac anomalies. Although no definitive studies have been done in this area, these concerns have led clinicians to avoid aspirin therapy until after the first trimester unless the benefit of its use clearly outweighs any theoretical risks. Other potential risks include fetal pulmonary hypertension, delay of onset of labor, and coagulation disorders in the mother or fetus (or both). It has also been suggested that aspirin use during pregnancy may be associated with reduced intelligence quotient (IQ) scores for the children born in such cases.[16] Data from the collaborative perinatal project have, however, failed

Diagnosis of Pre-eclampsia

Mild
  Blood pressure
    Above 140/90 mm Hg, two measurements 6 or more hours apart or an increase of 30 mm Hg systolic/15 mm Hg diastolic from first-trimester values
  Proteinuria
    Above 300 mg/24 hr
      OR
    Above 1 + on two consecutive specimens
  Significant nondependent edema

Severe
  Central nervous system dysfunction
    Blurry vision, scotomata, severe headaches, altered sensorium
  Pulmonary edema/cyanosis
    Rales, chest radiograph evidence of pulmonary edema, hypoxia on blood gas analysis
  Eclampsia
    Seizures or postictal state
  Blood pressure
    Persistently above 160/110 mm Hg
  Proteinuria
    Above 5 g/24 hr
  Oliguria
    Below 30 ml/hr, <400 ml/24 hr
  Right upper quadrant or epigastric pain
    Suggests liver capsule distension
  HELLP syndrome
    Hemolysis, elevated transaminases ($>2\times$ normal) low platelets ($<100,000$ mm^3)
  Significant fetal growth retardation
    Tapering or cessation of growth, growth at or below the 10th percentile

Other useful parameters
  24-Hour urinary calcium
    Below 12 mg/dl
  Uric Acid
    Above 6.0 mg/dl
  Rising blood urea nitrogen creatinine

to substantiate this concern. When the aspirin dose is limited to less than 100 mg/day, existing data do not suggest that any of these latter events should be anything more than a theoretical concern. Definitive studies of this, however, are not available.

Until the issue of low-dose aspirin therapy for preventing pre-eclampsia is clarified, such therapy should be undertaken only after informed consent is obtained from the patient and only under the supervision of a knowledgeable physician. When indicated, aspirin therapy is usually begun at 16 to 20 weeks' gestation in doses of 60 to 80 mg/day PO and continued until delivery occurs.

Treatment

In the absence of primary prevention of pre-eclampsia, its complete prevention remains an unachieved goal. Consequently, the obstetrician is often faced with the dilemma of managing the patient who presents with well-advanced pre-eclampsia. Clinicians must be rigorous in their application of the criteria for making the diagnosis of pre-eclampsia. As noted earlier, the disease is defined as the presence of hypertension with proteinuria or edema, or both. Once the diagnosis of pre-eclampsia is made with relative certainty, decisions about its management and the timing of delivery become critical.

Antepartum Management

The management of pre-eclampsia depends on the severity of its symptoms and the gestational age at diagnosis. An algorithm for triage management of these patients is presented in Figure 15-1. Once the diagnosis of pre-eclampsia is ascertained, a complete evaluation for hypertension should be initiated. Initial management of mild pre-eclampsia usually requires little more than close and frequent observation. In stable, compliant patients with mild disease, strict bed rest at home, with close fetal and maternal surveillance, is reasonable. For the motivated patient, this may include dipstick urinalysis for proteinuria and blood pressure measurement at home. Semiweekly fetal biophysical testing in either the home or clinic is also recommended. In general, mild pre-eclampsia at term may be managed expectantly until the spontaneous onset of labor, or until a Bishop cervical score favorable for a safe induction of labor is obtained. Any suggestion of worsening pre-

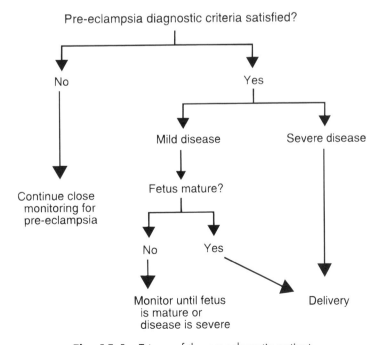

Fig. 15-1. Triage of the pre-eclamptic patient.

Laboratory Evaluation of the Pre-eclamptic Patient

Complete blood count (with platelets)

Chemistry panel

    Electrolytes

    Blood urea nitrogen

    Creatinine

    Uric acid

    Transaminases

    Total protein, albumin

    Calcium, magnesium

24-Hour urine for protein

    Creatinine

    Calcium

Electrocardiogram (optional)

Prothrombin time, partial thromboplastin time, fibrinogen (optional)

---

eclampsia or fetal compromise should prompt immediate hospitalization and further evaluation.

Once the patient is hospitalized, the goals are to minimize maternal morbidity and optimize perinatal outcome. These are best accomplished through close monitoring for signs of severe disease or fetal maturity (Fig. 15-2). Traditionally, the notion of continued observation of the preterm patient with severe pre-eclampsia, while attractive, has been frowned on. A recent report of 95 patients, however, suggests that expectant management of severe pre-eclampsia up to 32 weeks' gestation may in fact reduce neonatal complications and the neonatal stay in the newborn intensive care unit.[17] A review of this topic by the same group of investigators has recently been published,[18] with guidelines summarized in Tables 15-3 and 15-4.

Basically, any patient with mild pre-eclampsia and a mature fetus, or any patient with severe disease, should be evaluated for delivery. An exception to this is extreme fetal immaturity. Furthermore, with the availability of the data mentioned previously, expectant management of severe pre-eclampsia may be a consideration in gestations of up to 34 weeks, provided that such management is meticulous and takes place in a tertiary care center (Fig. 15-3). When patients are hospitalized and undergoing monitoring for signs of severe pre-eclampsia, prudent clinical judgment is essential. In a premature fetus, more than one sign of severe disease may be desirable before initiating delivery. In the patient at 34 to 36 weeks' gestation who has mild pre-eclampsia, the potential morbidity of amniocentesis to demonstrate fetal maturity and failed induction of labor should be weighed against the perceived benefits of delivery.

Intrapartum Management

Once pre-eclampsia has progressed to the point at which delivery is required (Fig. 15-1), the next priority is to prevent the progression of disease to eclampsia. The optimal management in such cases is again not without controversy. Magnesium sulfate remains the drug most commonly used in the United States for prevention of eclampsia. Although the need for intrapartum magnesium sulfate therapy for mild pre-eclampsia is not universally accepted, it is common practice to use such therapy during the intrapartum period for the prevention of eclampsia, and to continue it for a minimum of 24 hours after delivery. Because eclampsia is a potentially life-threatening event, and because statistically, most seizures occur during the antepartum or intrapartum periods or within the first 24 hours postpartum, most authorities advise concentrating prophylactic efforts within these time frames.

There is also a continuing controversy about whether magnesium sulfate should be used at all for the prevention of seizures. The details of this controversy have been presented elsewhere in the literature, and the issue remains unresolved.[19,20] In brief, animal and basic science data do not demonstrate a convincing effect of magnesium sulfate in preventing or ameliorating experimentally induced seizures. Indeed, the mechanism for the clinically observed benefit of magnesium sulfate treatment in pre-eclampsia or eclampsia is not clear. However, accumulated clinical experience with this agent suggests its superiority over a number of other single and polypharmaceutical regimens.[21] For this rea-

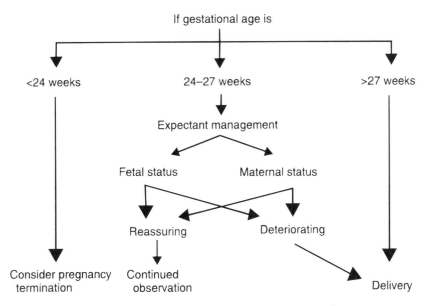

Fig. 15-2. Conservative management of severe pre-eclampsia.

Table 15-3. Maternal Guidelines for Expedited Delivery and Conservative Management of Severe Pre-eclampsia Remote From Term

Management	Clinical Findings

Expedited delivery (within 72 hours)	One or more of the following
	    Uncontrolled severe hypertension[a]
	    Eclampsia
	    Platelet count <100,000/μl
	    AST or ALT >2 × upper limit of normal with epigastric pain or right upper quadrant tenderness
	    Pulmonary edema
	    Compromised renal function[b]
	    Persistent severe headache or visual changes

Conservative management	One or more of the following
	    Controlled hypertension
	    Urinary protein >5,000 mg/24 hr
	    Oliguira (<0.5 mL/kg/hr) that resolves with routine fluid or food intake
	    AST or ALT >2 × upper limit of normal without epigastric pain or right upper quadrant tenderness

AST, aspartate aminotransferase; ALT, alamine aminotransferase.

[a] Blood pressure persistently ≥160 mm Hg systolic or ≥110 mmHg diastolic despite maximum recommended doses of two antihypertensive medications.

[b] Persistent oliguria (<0.5 ml/kg/hr) or a rise in serum creatinine of 1 mg/dl over baseline levels.

Table 15-4. Fetal Guidelines for Expedited Delivery and Conservative Management of Severe Pre-eclampsia Remote From Term

Management	Clinical Findings
Expedited delivery (within 72 hours)	One or more of the following Fetal distress by fetal heart rate tracing or biophysical profile Amniotic fluid index ≤ 2 Ultrasonographically estimated fetal weight $\leq$5th percentile Reverse umbilical artery diastolic flow
Conservative management	One or more of the following Biophysical profile ≥ 6 Amniotic fluid index >2 Ultrasonographically estimated fetal weight $>$5th percentile

son, magnesium sulfate continues to be the drug of choice in the management of pre-eclampsia.

Administration regimens for magnesium sulfate in preventing seizures are summarized in Table 15-5. When magnesium sulfate is administered for the prevention of seizures, an intramuscular or intravenous route is employed. Since the pathogenesis of eclamptic seizures is not completely understood, and since the mechanism of action of magnesium sulfate is likewise incompletely understood, proper use of this agent has been largely based on empirical obser-

vation. It is known that magnesium competes with calcium for specific ion channels, and may therefore minimize cellular excitability. Clinically, magnesium also exerts a peripheral effect at the neuromuscular junction. Abolition of patellar reflexes is an early sign of magnesium toxicity and may be noted at serum magnesium levels as low as 4 to 6 mEq/L. High levels of magnesium sulfate may also produce respiratory depression and cardiotoxicity. These signs must be carefully monitored in the patient receiving parenteral magnesium sulfate therapy. Also,

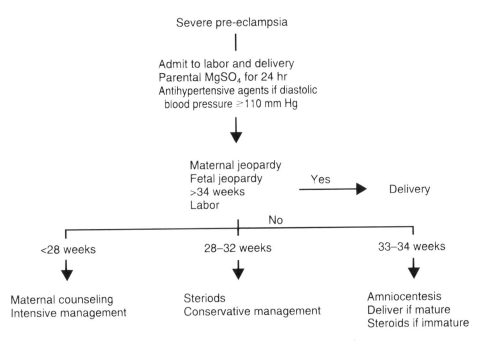

Fig. 15-3. Alternative management of severe pre-eclampsia.

Table 15-5. Magnesium Sulfate Administration for Seizure Prophylaxis

Intramuscular	Intravenous
10 g (5 IM deep in each buttock)[a]	6 g bolus over 15 minutes
5 g IM deep q4h, alternating sides	1–3 g/hr by continuous infusion pump[a]
	May be mixed in 100 ml crystalloid; if given by intravenous push, make up as 20% solution; push at maximum rate of 1 g/min
	40 g $MgSO_4 \cdot 7H_2O$ in 1,000 ml Ringers lactate; run at 25–75 ml/hr (1–3 g/hr)[a]

[a] Made up as 50% solution.

magnesium sulfate has been reported to be an effective tocolytic agent, and patients receiving magnesium sulfate therapy may require oxytocin augmentation for continuation of labor.

While magnesium sulfate has a wide margin of safety, serious complications have been associated with its use. Consequently, it has become increasingly common to monitor serum magnesium levels in patients being treated with this agent. Levels between 4 and 8 mEq/L have generally been accepted as therapeutic, although there is no indisputable

clinical basis for choosing these levels. Levels above 6 mEq/L are associated with lethargy and loss of patellar reflexes. Respiratory depression is seen at levels of 8 to 10 mEq/L, and cardiorespiratory arrest can occur when the serum magnesium level rises above 12 mEq/L. Suffice it to say that although serum magnesium levels may be useful in helping to establish a rate of magnesium infusion to achieve a steady state, these levels should not serve as a substitute for frequent clinical assessment of the patient. Guidelines for monitoring the patient on magnesium sulfate are summarized in the box titled *Monitoring the Patient on Magnesium Sulfate.*

Monitoring the Patient on Magnesium Sulfate

Assess patient's vital signs, urine output, and reflexes every 2 to 4 hours
  Patellar reflexes above 1+
  Respiratory rate above 12/min
  Monitor pulse for arrythmia
  Watch for oxygen desaturation
  Watch for widening QRS or prolonged Q-T interval on ECG
  If urine output below 30 ml/hr, check level, adjust infusion
Laboratory values
  Therapeutic levels accepted as 4 to 8 mEq/L
  Toxicities
    Absence of deep tendon reflexes (>4 to 6 mEq/L)
    Somnolence (>8 mEq/L)
    Respiratory depression (>8 mEq/L)
    Cardiotoxicity (>15 mEq/L)

Alternative Pharmacotherapy

Interest has recently grown in alternative pharmacotherapy for the management of pre-eclampsia and for the prevention of eclampsia. As stated previously, magnesium sulfate remains the most widely used drug for the prevention of eclampsia in the United States. Worldwide, however, a number of other agents have been employed for this purpose, including phenytoin and diazepam.[22,23] Both of these drugs have a fairly long history in neurologic practice for the management of acute seizures, but their potential roles in the management of pre-eclampsia and eclampsia are not as clear. Diazepam has been shown to have negative effects on the fetus, including reduced tone, hypothermia, and respiratory depression, and for this reason is not widely used in pregnancy. Phenytoin, by control, does not have these effects, and may ultimately prove to have a role in the prevention or management of eclampsia. Multiple regimens for phenytoin administration have been proposed. The regimen I have developed and employed is summarized in Table 15-6.

Table 15-6. Protocol for Administering Intravenous Phenytoin

Initial dosage based on patient weight[a]

Weight Patient	Dosage
<50 kg	1,000 mg
50–70 kg	1,250 mg
>70 kg	1,500 mg

Further dosing based on serum phenytoin levels

Serum Level	Additional Dose
<10 mg/L	500 mg
10–12 mg/L	250 mg
>12 mg/L	None

[a] First 750 mg of phenytoin administered at 25 mg/min; remainder of dose administered at 12.5 mg/min; ECG tracing (lead II) obtained for 1 minute of every 10 minutes during the first 750 mg of phenytoin.
(From Repke et al,[19] with permission.)

ECLAMPSIA

Eclampsia is defined as the occurrence of a grand mal tonic clonic seizure in a patient exhibiting symptoms of pre-eclampsia in the absence of underlying neurologic disease. Although eclampsia is a relatively rare event, it occurs frequently enough (1 per 1,000 deliveries) that most clinicians will personally encounter one or more cases in their professional careers. Although the pathophysiology of eclamptic seizures is not well understood, the maternal and fetal consequences of eclampsia have been recognized and feared for centuries. Until the introduc-

---

Initiation of Magnesium Sulfate

Eclampsia
  50 percent antepartum
  20 percent intrapartum
  30 percent postpartum
Poor prediction of who will have seizures

---

tion of magnesium sulfate therapy in the 1930s, maternal mortality in cases of eclamptic seizures approached 30 percent.

Initial Management

The best management for eclamptic seizures is prevention. Awareness of the categories of pre-eclamptic patients at greatest risk of convulsions would be helpful, but unfortunately, eclampsia, the Greek word for lightning, often has few warning signs and frequently occurs in the patient with previously mild disease. Predicting the timing of eclampsia is just as difficult as predicting its occurrence. A study of 186 cases at the University of Tennessee[24] found that seizures occurred postpartum in 28 percent of patients, and one-half of these occurred more than 48 hours after delivery. Indeed, only approximately one-third of eclamptic events occurred during labor, with almost one-half of all patients suffering convulsions before admission to the delivery unit (Table 15-7).

The initial management of the patient who develops an eclamptic seizure is extremely important. An approach to the management of eclampsia is sum-

---

Morbid Sequelae of Eclampsia

Maternal apnea, fetal asphyxia

Cerebral edema, coma

Intracerebral hemorrhage

Aspiration of gastric contents

Placental abruption

Maternal death

Fetal death

Table 15-7. Patient Symptoms Preceding Eclampsia

Symptoms	Patients (%)
Headache	83
Hyperreflexia	80
Clonus	46
Proteinuria	80
Visual signs	45
Epigastric pain	20

Management of Eclampsia

Protect maternal airway; prevent patient injury

Wait for convulsion to abate

Maternal resuscitation
 Maximum oxygenation (mask or endotracheal oxygen)
 Intravenous access and judicious hydration

Fetal resuscitation
 Maternal oxygen, left lateral positioning
 Continuous fetal heart rate monitoring

Maternal postictal assessment
 Complete blood count, platelets, electrolytes, glucose, calcium, magnesium, toxin screen, blood type and antibody screen
 Careful neurologic examination
 Cervical examination

Magnesium sulfate$_4$ prophylaxis for subsequent seizures

Formulate delivery strategy

---

marized in the boxes titled *Management of Eclampsia* and *Delivery of the Eclamptic Patient*. Most eclamptic seizures are self-limited, and if appropriate maternal protection is afforded, are resolved without significant sequelae. However, seizures may recur and result in intracerebral hemorrhage, placental abrup-

---

Delivery of the Eclamptic Patient

Avoid emergent (STAT) cesarean section

Stabilize maternal and fetal oxygenation, hemodynamics

Start or reassess magnesium sulfate therapy

Assess cervix and maternal and fetal reserve

Vaginal delivery usually yields the best outcome overall

Normalize coagulation prior to cesarean section

---

tion, fetal asphyxia, or maternal cardiovascular collapse. As with most grand mal seizures, the seizure event is characterized by maternal apnea and transient hypoxia. This is accompanied almost routinely by transient fetal bradycardia. Protection of the maternal airway and administration of oxygen postictally will usually result in eventual in utero resuscitation of the fetus. The initial resolution of the fetal bradycardia is followed by a compensatory tachycardia, usually with some loss of baseline variability. As the patient recovers, and with supportive management, the fetal heart rate will usually return to its preseizure state within 20 to 30 minutes.

In patients who are brought to the hospital after an eclamptic seizure and in those already hospitalized who suffer a seizure while not receiving magnesium sulfate, treatment with magnesium sulfate should be instituted. Patients who suffer an eclamptic seizure while being treated with magnesium sulfate or who are otherwise atypical in their presentation should have their magnesium level determined immediately, and consideration should be given to adding a standard anticonvulsant such as phenytoin until a neurologic evaluation is completed. This recommendation is based on reports that pathologic central nervous system (CNS) abnormalities are more common in patients who experience seizures while receiving magnesium sulfate than might otherwise be expected.

If phenytoin therapy is instituted, close monitoring of the patient is essential. Potentially, the most life-threatened complication of phenytoin administration is cardiotoxicity, although this is extremely uncommon in young, healthy patients receiving intravenous phenytoin at continuous infusion rates of less than 50 mg/min. As discussed earlier, when phenytoin therapy is begun, a serum level measurement of the drug should be obtained 30 to 60 minutes after the infusion is completed. Subsequent serum levels may be measured every 12 hours, and additional phenytoin can be administered as needed in the manner summarized in Table 15-6.

Delivery

Once the eclamptic patient has been stabilized, the timing and route of delivery must be determined. In general, the occurrence of eclampsia in an antepartum patient is an indication for delivery. These patients should be managed identically to patients categorized as having severe pre-eclampsia. Ideally, delivery procedures should await stabilization of the mother and fetus. Emergency delivery, especially by cesarean section immediately after an eclamptic seizure, puts the mother and the fetus at a substantially greater risk of morbidity. As stated above, in utero resuscitation of the fetus should be the primary goal in the management of eclampsia, provided no other catastrophe has occurred during the eclamptic seizure, such as maternal stroke or placental abruption. When delivery is safe, both the vaginal and cesarean routes should be considered. When cesarean section is necessary, epidural anesthesia is usually the anesthetic technique of choice, since it produces the fewest acute physiologic alterations.[25] However, if epidural anesthesia is used in the eclamptic or severely pre-eclamptic patient, certain requirements must be met, including adequate intravenous access, an accurate method for blood pressure determination, and ample time for stepwise, preblock maternal intravascular volume expansion. The patient's coagulation profile should be within acceptable limits, and an anesthesiology team skilled in the administration of epidural anesthesia should be present. If these requirements cannot be fulfilled, balanced general anesthesia is preferred, with careful attention given to blood pressure control at the time of induction of anesthesia, to avoid the exaggerated hypertensive response that may occur with the induction of anesthesia in these patients.

Postpartum Management

Once the patient with severe pre-eclampsia or eclampsia has delivered, postpartum management should consist of close monitoring of blood pressure, intravascular volume, and urinary output. Seizure prophylaxis should continue for at least 24 hours postpartum; in some cases, continuation of magnesium sulfate therapy beyond 24 hours postpartum is indicated if there is evidence of continuing or worsening vasospasm or renal, hepatic, or pulmonary dysfunction. Generally, resolution of the disease will be characterized by a gradual reduction in blood pressure and proteinuria, accompanied by a brisk, profound diuresis. Transient thrombocytopenia, observed in many patients with severe pre-eclampsia, can usually be managed expectantly. The platelet count typically reaches a nadir on postpartum day 2 or 3 and then gradually returns to normal levels. Platelet transfusion may be useful if surgery is contemplated for the patient with a markedly abnormal bleeding time, or if venous oozing from intravenous sites is noted. In severe cases of thrombocytopenia, normalization of the platelet count may take up to 7 days.[26]

Invasive Hemodynamic Monitoring

Both severe pre-eclampsia and eclampsia can represent a significant risk to the patient and her fetus. Such cases should always be managed at a tertiary care center. At such centers the availability of expertise and technology will allow for management of even the most severely ill patients. The use of invasive hemodynamic monitoring in these patients may provide a sensitive and useful method for assessing maternal volume status and guiding volume replacement therapy. The actual role of such monitoring in pre-eclampsia and eclampsia remains controversial. Many investigators have argued for utilization of a pulmonary artery catheter in cases of severe pre-eclampsia, claiming that central venous pressure may not accurately reflect left ventricular function. In most obstetric patients, the absence of pre-existing cardiovascular disease usually allows for management without invasive hemodynamic monitoring of any kind, and in cases in which invasive hemodynamic monitoring is thought to be necessary, an arterial line and central venous pressure line are usually sufficient. The indications for use of a pulmonary artery catheter will vary from one institution to another. Clinical circumstances that might suggest the utility of such an approach include refractory pulmonary edema, uncontrollable hypertension, or pre-existing cardiac disease in a patient with severe pre-eclampsia. At our institution it is rarely necessary to employ pulmonary artery catheters for the management of pre-eclamptic patients except in the extreme circumstances described above.

HELLP SYNDROME

The HELLP syndrome, named in 1982 by Weinstein,[27] is characterized by *h*emolytic anemia, *el*evated *l*iver enzymes, and thrombocytopenia (*low* *p*latelet count). It deserves separate presentation because of its unique features. Although frequently managed and interpreted as a variant of severe pre-eclampsia, the HELLP syndrome may appear without associated hypertension or proteinuria. Although many clinicians consider the syndrome an indication of severe pre-eclampsia, most insist on at least one additional criterion for the disorder to qualify as severe. The management scheme for patients with HELLP syndrome is similar to that presented in Figure 15-1 for the management of patients with pre-eclampsia. The primary objective is to stabilize the mother and fetus and to make appropriate decisions about the timing and route of delivery.

As many as 30 percent of cases of HELLP syndrome will occur after delivery. Of patients in whom the HELLP syndrome develops before delivery, the overwhelming majority will describe flu-like symptoms consisting of fatigue and malaise for the few days preceding their clinical presentation. Epigastric and right upper quadrant pain in this setting are pathognomonic for the disease. Nausea and vomiting may occur in such cases, and because of the multiple constitutional symptoms accompanying the HELLP syndrome, differential diagnosis can be extensive. Not infrequently, the first diagnosis will usually pertain to the specialty of the consultant called. For this reason it is important to remember that obstetricians are the specialists most suited to make the diagnosis of HELLP syndrome and to manage the patient with it. A few of the diagnoses that can be confused with HELLP syndrome include viral hepatitis, gastroenteritis, gallbladder disease, immune thrombocytopenia, appendicitis, and acute fatty liver of pregnancy. The laboratory valves in the differential diagnosis of HELLP syndrome and acute fatty liver of pregnancy are presented in Table 15-8. Although the HELLP syndrome is not an indication for immediate cesarean section, management decisions should be guided by the patient's stability, according to the suggestions made for the management of severe pre-eclampsia. Our policy for managing patients with HELLP syndrome has been to assess the severity of disease, stabilize the patient, and proceed with delivery. While vaginal delivery is preferred, cesarean section is not contraindicated, provided that blood products are available to deal with

Table 15-8. Laboratory Differentiation of AFLP and the HELLP Syndrome

	AFLP	HELLP Syndrome
Hematologic		
Platelet count	Low or	Low
Fibrinogen	normal	Normal to
Prothrombin time	Low	increased
Partial thromboplastin	Prolonged	Normal
time	Prolonged	Normal
Serum chemistries	Low	Normal
Glucose	High	High
Uric acid	High	High
Creatinine	High	Normal
Ammonia		

AFLP, acute fatty liver of pregnancy; HELLP, hemolytic anemia, elevated liver enzymes, low platelets.
(From Barton and Sibai,[28] with permission.)

any complications of bleeding that may be encountered in such patients. Again, for this reason, among others, these severely ill patients are best managed in a tertiary care center, where both medical expertise and sufficient laboratory and blood bank facilities are available for their management. The general policy at Brigham and Women's Hospital is to withhold platelet transfusions for symptomatic bleeding, without any absolute platelet count mandating platelet transfusion. In cases of significant hepatic dysfunction, the availability of fresh frozen plasma (FFP) and cryoprecipitate may also be necessary to assist in the correction of coagulation factor deficiencies until there is spontaneous reversal of the disease process. Patients with HELLP syndrome, even in the absence of hypertension and proteinuria, should be considered at risk of eclamptic seizures, just as in the case of patients with severe pre-eclampsia. For those reasons, magnesium sulfate should be administered to these patients and continued until there is evidence of resolution of their disease process. One general policy has been to entirely close the abdominal incision when cesarean section is performed, to limit bleeding. Others have reported success with delayed closure of the abdomen to minimize the risk of hematoma formation.[28]

CHRONIC HYPERTENSION

Chronic hypertension will occur in up to 4 percent of pregnancies, and presents a unique challenge to the practicing obstetrician. Patients with this condition will generally present to the obstetrician in one of four ways. Patients with previously diagnosed chronic hypertension controlled with medication may present to the obstetrician for prenatal care after having discontinued their therapy when pregnancy was suspected. Other patients presenting for prenatal care may never have been diagnosed as hypertensive, but are markedly hypertensive at the time of their first visit. In the third situation a patient may present in whom hypertension is well controlled but who is taking medication not suitable for use during pregnancy. The fourth situation, which is probably the least common but the most desirable, is that of the patient with chronic hypertension who seeks out the obstetrician for counseling before attempting pregnancy, so that the risks of pregnancy may be fully understood and appropriate pharmacotherapeutic changes made before conception.

Diagnosis

Although hypertension may arise from renal disease and from adrenal tumors or other endocrinopathies, the average practitioner predominantly encounters essential hypertension in pregnant patients. By definition, essential hypertension is hypertension of uncertain etiology despite a thorough laboratory and physical evaluation. Pregnant patients with essential hypertension should have previously had a complete hypertensive evaluation. If they have not, this should be completed by the obstetrician as soon as possible after the first prenatal visit, so that appropriate intervention and counseling can be initiated. Establishing the diagnosis of essential hypertension is quite difficult in the patient who presents in the later stages of pregnancy. In general, blood pressure before the 20th week of gestation must be consistently above 140/90 mm/Hg to satisfy the definition of chronic hypertension. Other etiologies of hypertension should be excluded by a comprehensive laboratory work-up and physical examination.

The key component in the diagnosis of hypertension is the accurate recording of blood pressure. The optimal method of making this measurement remains a source of considerable controversy. The most important aspects of blood pressure measurement are its accuracy, consistency, and standardization. Lack of standardization introduces significant error into the clinical data and leads to both over- and underdiagnosis of hypertension.[29] Standardization of the techniques of blood pressure measurement used by clinic personnel is also important, in order to teach the patient consistent methods of home blood pressure monitoring, an effective method for reducing hospital stay without compromising outcome.[30] The use of an appropriately sized sphygmomanometer cuff is essential. Measurements should be obtained in the clinic or at home after the patient has been allowed to rest quietly for at least 5 to 10 minutes. Blood pressure may then be recorded in the sitting position, with the patient's arm well supported and the blood pressure cuff approximately at the level of the patient's heart.

Counseling

The patient who presents with chronic hypertension in early pregnancy should be appropriately counseled about the risks that her pregnancy poses to her medical condition and the risks that her hypertension poses to her pregnancy. She should also understand the additional prenatal testing of both mother and fetus required in this disease. In general, patients without evidence of significant renal impairment who have undergone a prior hypertensive evaluation and who are well controlled at the initial visit should expect a reasonably good pregnancy outcome. Although there is disagreement about the magnitude of the risk, patients with underlying hypertensive disease are at increased risk of superimposed pre-eclampsia. Interestingly, this risk does not seem to be affected by antihypertensive therapy. A number of risk factors may effect pregnancy outcome in chronic hypertension. Additionally, certain complications of pregnancy have been directly attributed to chronic hypertension. It is noteworthy that most of these complications are not altered by the administration of antihypertensive medication. It is generally agreed that antihypertensive therapy for chronic hypertension in pregnancy will decrease the incidence of cardiovascular complications and the risk of stroke, but will have little or no effect on perinatal morbidity and mortality. There are limited data on the outcome of pregnancy in patients with severe hypertension at the time of their initial presentation. The data that do exist, however, suggest that these patients are at very high risk of an adverse pregnancy outcome ranging from miscarriage to second- or third-trimester pregnancy loss. For this reason, the importance of preconceptional counseling and management cannot be overemphasized.

The use of antihypertensive medications during pregnancy prompts most of the questions that patients raise in prenatal visits. Many experienced clinicians reserve medical therapy for the patient with blood pressures consistently above 160/100 mm/Hg. Others initiate antihypertensive medication whenever blood pressures consistently exceed 140/90 mm/Hg. However, patients with modest or borderline blood pressure elevations during the first trimester have not been conclusively shown to benefit from antihypertensive medication during pregnancy. A randomized clinical trial reported in 1990 failed to demonstrate a significant improvement in perinatal outcome among patients with mild to moderate chronic hypertension treated with placebo or with agents such as labetolol or α-methyldopa.[31] Thus, it is not currently clear whether mild to moderate chronic hypertension should be treated, although the long-term end-organ effects of untreated moderate chronic hypertension may be significant. The issue here, however, is whether pharmacotherapy over the short course of pregnancy is beneficial to pregnancy outcome. Additionally, decisions about pharmacotherapy should consider other factors in addition to blood pressure, including the patient's lifestyle, child-care responsibilities, and career obligations.

Management

The clinician faces several important management decisions regarding treatment of the pregnant, chronically hypertensive patient. Uncontrolled severe maternal hypertension may lead to stroke, placental abruption, and maternal or fetal death. Injudicious medical therapy, however, may provoke unpleasant maternal symptoms and compromise fetal well-being and growth. The typical first step in the management of increased blood pressure is limitation of physical activity. Research has shown that bed rest or sedentary positioning reduces blood pressure in susceptible pregnant individuals.[4] It is not always possible, however, for women to remain sedentary or on a limited activity schedule for the greater part of their pregnancy. In this circumstance, pharmacologic therapy or some of the nonpharmacologic alternatives may be attempted.

The use of antihypertensive therapy is often based on blood pressure levels in the first or second trimester. Patients with marked hypertension (>160/100 mm/Hg) before 12 weeks' gestation are more likely to experience precipitous increases in blood pressure in the third trimester, necessitating premature delivery. Initiation of antihypertensive therapy early in pregnancy may facilitate smoother control of this third-trimester increase in blood pressure, helping to prolong pregnancy closer to term. Also of great concern is the patient who experiences significant blood pressure elevation within the second trimester. Normally, mean arterial pressure and vascular resistance fall during the second trimester, then rise modestly as term approaches.[32] An increase in blood pressure in the second trimester may lead to an upswing to dangerous levels in the third trimester, creating a potentially critical clinical situation. By contrast, overly aggressive pharmacologic reduction of maternal blood pressure may reduce uteroplacental perfusion and compromise fetal growth and oxygenation. Because of these conflicting effects, and because reliable scientific studies are lacking, indications for initiating and modulating antihypertensive medications during pregnancy remain highly controversial. In any event, the decision of whether to use pharmacotherapy is an important one, and the risks and benefits of this decision must be fully discussed with the patient.

Nonpharmacologic Approaches

Several nonpharmacologic interventions have been suggested for the management of chronic hypertension. These have included limitation of physical activity, dietary manipulation, biofeedback, and other modalities. Limited physical activity may be the approach with the fewest side effects, but is also often the least practical. Another approach to chronic hypertension is nutritional alteration. The classic example of this approach in the nonpregnant population has been sodium restriction.[33] In hypertensive gravid women, sodium restriction is generally not recommended unless there is clear evidence of excessive sodium intake, as convincing studies of this issue in pregnant patients are lacking. I find that sodium restriction has no place in my clinical practice for the management of hypertensive gravid women.

Alternative nutritional approaches have included the use of various supplements, including zinc, magnesium, and calcium. Many of the studies exploring these compounds have focused on their ability to reduce blood pressure and prevent pre-eclampsia.[34] There is considerable literature indicating that populations with a lower calcium intake have higher blood pressures. Recent evidence further suggests that calcium supplementation may be associated with mild to moderate blood pressure reductions in both pregnant and nonpregnant populations.[35] In general, the extent of calcium supplementation has been on the order of 2,000 mg/day of elemental calcium.[36]

The close association of calcium with blood pressure has a rational explanation.[37] A recent review of this topic has been presented elsewhere.[10] Since numerous studies have now confirmed this moderate blood pressure-lowering effect, and because it lacks adverse side effects, calcium supplementation is a reasonable first option for the patient with mild to moderate chronic hypertension.[38] Since the demands for calcium in pregnancy are increased over those in the nonpregnant state, this approach may also have additional nutritional benefits. Dietary calcium supplementation generally requires approximately 4 to 5 weeks for its blood pressure-lowering effect to be observed. Therefore, it may not be effective when instituted late in the third trimester, and its use at this time should be viewed as a purely prophylactic measure rather than a treatment approach to the management of pre-eclampsia.

Pharmacologic Treatment

When pharmacotherapy is indicated for the management of chronic hypertension during pregnancy, the obstetrician has several medications available for use. The most commonly used drugs are α-methyldopa, β-blocking agents, hydralazine, thiazide diuretics, and calcium-channel blockers, the last of which are being used with increasing frequency.[39]

α-Methyldopa

α-Methyl dopa remains the drug of first choice in the United States, primarily because of the extensive accumulated experience with this drug in pregnancy, and its apparently wide margin of safety. Long experience with α-methyldopa has failed to show significant adverse maternal, fetal, or neonatal side effects. Administration of the drug is summarized in Table 15-9. While α-methyldopa is generally well tolerated, a small percentage of patients receiving it will experience a drug-induced hepatitis evidenced by rising liver enzyme values. This complication is completely reversible on discontinuation of the drug. Some patients also experience a positive direct Coomb's test in response to α-methyldopa, but this does not require discontinuation of the drug.

β-Adrenergic Blocking Agents

Other drugs, such as the β-adrenergic blocking agents, have become increasingly popular for the management of chronic hypertension in pregnancy in the United States since the early 1980s. The prototype drug of this class of drugs is propranolol, although the most commonly used agents in pregnant patients are atenolol and labetolol. Initial concerns about β-adrenergic blocking agents included teratogenesis, IUGR, and fetal distress. To date there is no evidence that β-adrenergic blocking agents are teratogenic. Early reports suggesting that these drugs might be associated with IUGR were primarily based on retrospective analyses, although more recent evidence has strengthened this association with respect to atenolol. Further evaluation of these data suggest that the observed IUGR was more likely due to the underlying condition (hypertension) than to the β-blocking agent itself. With regard to fetal distress, it is important to note that fetal heart rate reactivity and cardioacceleration are mediated by the sympathetic nervous system of the fetus. Thus, β-blocking agents that freely cross the placenta make it possible for the maternal administration of these drugs to reduce fetal heart rate reactivity and decrease the fetal capability for compensatory tachycardia in the face of uteroplacental insufficiency or hypoxia. None of these facts contraindicates the use of β-blocking agents, but clinicians should be aware of them when interpreting fetal biophysical information.

Table 15-9. Medical Treatment of the Pregnant Hypertensive Woman

Drug	Usual Dose	Disadvantages
First-line agents		
α-methyldopa	250 mg tid to 500 mg qid	Rare: drug-induced hepatitis, positive Coombs' test
β-blockers: labetalol	100 mg bid to 300 mg qid	Possible: decreased fetal growth, fetal bradycardia
Second-line agents		
Hydralazine	50 mg qd to 100 mg tid	Postural hypotension, edema, lupus-like syndrome
Calcium-channel blockers: nifedipine		Maternal hypotension, uteroplacental insufficiency, IUGR
Diuretics: furosemide		Maternal hypovolemia, decreased placental perfusion
ACE inhibitors: enalapril		Fetal oliguria, renal failure, death

ACE, angiotensin-converting enzyme; IUGR, intrauterine growth restriction.

Although there has been increasing concern about the association of atenolol with IUGR, this drug is still used in my clinical practice and by many obstetricians in the management of chronic hypertension. The usual initial dose of atenolol is 50 mg once daily, with a maximum dose of 50 mg bid or 100 mg once daily. An occasional patient may be managed with up to 200 mg/day. Labetolol has also become popular since its approval by the U.S. Food and Drug Administration (FDA) in the mid-1980s. Labetolol has the advantage of being both an α- and β-adrenergic blocking agent, which allows for many of the benefits of β-blockade without some of the annoying side effects. Labetolol may be started at 100 mg PO bid, and increased to a maximum dose of 300 mg bid or qid. Other β-blocking agents, such as metaprolol and acebutalol, have been used during pregnancy, but since experience with these agents is limited, atenolol and labetolol remain the most commonly used members of the class. The clinician should remember that β-blockers have never been conclusively shown to be superior to α-methyldopa for the management of chronic hypertension. There may be selected circumstances (e.g., documented high-renin hypertension) in which β-blocker therapy may offer an advantage over α-methyldopa, but these cases must be evaluated individually. Moreover, neither β-blocking agents nor α-methyldopa have been conclusively demonstrated to be superior to placebo in preventing pre-eclampsia or improving perinatal outcome. The main benefit of pharmacotherapy is maternal. Also, the clinician must remember that at the doses required to treat hypertension, even the so-called cardioselective β-blocking agents have constrictive effects on the bronchial tree. Therefore, β-blocking agents should be avoided in patients with asthma. Additionally, since β-blocking agents can mask the effects of hypoglycemia, they should be avoided or used with great caution in patients with insulin-dependent diabetes. Finally, another concern frequently raised by clinicians is whether use of β-blockers increases the risk of preterm labor. There are no data to suggest that β-blocker therapy increases the risk of preterm labor, and in fact some data suggest that the nonpregnant uterus is more susceptible to the effects of β-blockade than is the pregnant uterus.[40]

Hydralazine

Another drug that may be used for the management of chronic hypertension during pregnancy is hydralazine, although it is not widely used in my clinic for this purpose. Hydralazine is a peripheral vasodilator with a long history of use during pregnancy. It is generally given orally in divided doses to a total dose of 50 to 300 mg/day. The most common adverse side effect of hydralazine reported by patients is postural hypotension, which is frequently a first dose phenomenon.

Long-term side effects of hydralazine include sodium and water retention. A lupus-like syndrome has been reported, but this has generally occurred in patients receiving very high doses for longer than 6 months. This syndrome is also reversible on discontinuation of the drug.

Other Agents

Although α-methyldopa, β-blocking agents, and hydralazine are the drugs primarily used for managing the pregnant patient with chronic hypertension, other agents, including calcium-channel blockers, diuretics, and angiotensin-converting enzyme (ACE) inhibitors have also been used.

Calcium-channel blockers are very useful in the treatment of hypertension in nonpregnant patients. However, because of potentially adverse effects on uteroplacental blood flow and on the fetal cardiac conduction system, these drugs should be avoided during pregnancy unless the benefit of their use clearly outweighs the risks to the fetus.[41]

The use of diuretics has also been the subject of decades-long controversy in obstetrics. Because of reports of thrombocytopenia in the fetus and hemorrhagic pancreatitis in the mother, diuretic use has not been popular for pregnant patients in the United States. Adverse effects on serum glucose, uric acid, and potassium have also made diuretics less attractive for use in pregnancy, and additional concerns have been raised about the possible negative effects of diuretics on maternal intravascular volume expansion during pregnancy.[42] Since diuretics are generally used only in patients with mild hypertension, it is not recommended that they be used or continued during pregnancy. Of course, as with many medications, there may be an occasional patient in whom diuretics are helpful, but as a general rule they should be avoided or discontinued in pregnant patients.

ACE inhibitors are very effective antihypertensive agents and are frequently employed as first-line agents in nonpregnant women. They have the advantage of producing very few systemic side effects such as hypotension or lethargy, which makes them particularly suitable for more physically active individuals. Since pregnancy is a state of increased plasma renin activity, increased aldosterone, and increased angiotensin II, these agents would seem to be ideally suited for use in pregnancy. However, recent reports have documented adverse effects of ACE inhibitors on the fetal urinary tract, and specifically on fetal nephron development.[43] In addition to the concerns about congenital malformations and fetal urinary dysfunction, ACE inhibitors may also

have adverse effects on prostaglandin synthesis and uteroplacental perfusion.[44] Therefore, these agents should be discontinued or avoided in pregnancy.

Postpartum Care

The management of the patient with chronic hypertension is somewhat simplified after the delivery of the fetus. The management is even more straightforward for patients who are not breast-feeding, since their treatment may immediately be converted to generally accepted first-line agents for nonpregnant patients. In the breast-feeding mother, however, the same antihypertensive regimen that was used antepartum is usually maintained. It is advisable to discuss this regimen with the infant's pediatrician. Perhaps one notable finding with regard to management of the postpartum patient is that because of abrupt decreases in plasma renin activity following parturition, ACE inhibitors seem to be less effective than other antihypertensive agents.

When postpartum patients with chronic hypertension are discharged from the hospital, it is essential that close follow-up of their hypertension be arranged. Frequently, this is initially provided by the obstetrician or perinatologist. When an internist is consulted, it is important to remember that resolution of the anatomic and physiologic changes of pregnancy and a return to prepregnancy status may take up to 12 weeks.

MANAGEMENT OF HYPERTENSIVE CRISIS

Whether the underlying disorder is chronic hypertension, pre-eclampsia, eclampsia, or some combination thereof, some patients require intensive intervention for control of blood pressure and acute management of other physiologic problems. While all severely pre-eclamptic and eclamptic patients should be considered critically ill, many may be managed with standard equipment, including routine peripheral intravenous lines and Foley catheterization for urinary output determinations. In some cases of labile, blood pressure, arterial line placement may be useful for more meticulous management of blood pressure. Additionally, as stated previously, some patients may require more aggressive and invasive hemodynamic monitoring, such as through the placement of a central venous pressure catheter or pulmonary artery catheter. The indications for invasive hemodynamic monitoring include refractory oliguria, pulmonary edema, and severe hypertension that is difficult to control. It is estimated that the average labor-and-delivery service would require full critical care intervention in about 1 per 2,000 deliveries. Because many centers cannot maintain this level of nursing or physician skill, transfer of the patient to the intensive care unit of a tertiary care center, where critical obstetric care is available, may be necessary.

By contrast, hypertensive crisis (blood pressure >200/115 mm Hg) is not an uncommon event in obstetrics. Because patients with pre-eclampsia have enhanced vascular reactivity, they may be at particular risk of labile hypertension. The pre-eclamptic patient with uncontrolled blood pressure is at risk of a cerebral vascular accident and placental abruption. A number of pharmacologic agents are available for the management of patients in hypertensive crisis. Because of long experience with it and its safety, hydralazine remains the drug most commonly used for the acute management of blood pressure emergencies in the antepartum period. Intravenous hydralazine may be given as an initial 5-mg bolus, followed by an additional 5 mg after 10 minutes. If significant hypotension does not occur, 10-mg intravenous boluses may be administered at 20-minute intervals until blood pressure control is achieved. The goal of such therapy is maintenance of blood pressure in the range of 140 to 150/90 to 100 mm Hg to avoid uterine hypoperfusion. (Table 15-10).

Because one of the side effects of hydralazine may be tachycardia, and because hypertension in some pre-eclamptic patients is the result of increased cardiac output, alternative methods of blood pressure management are worth considering. Sodium nitroprusside has been used successfully, and may be started at a rate of 0.5 μg/kg/min and increased by 0.5 μg/kg/min every 5 to 10 minutes until blood pressure control is achieved. A similar intravenous infusion method may be employed for hydralazine, using the same dosage schedule. Intravenous hydralazine has a relatively longer half-life than nitroprusside, and is therefore less easily titrated. Gradual reduction of blood pressure with these agents may also benefit uteroplacental perfusion. Although with nitroprusside selective concentration of cyanide and thiocyanate in the fetus can theoretically cause poisoning of the electron transport chain and subsequent asphyxia, brief use of this agent to control arterial pressure before and during cesarean section has not been associated with any adverse fetal effects. Likewise, intermittent administration of nitroglycerine, usually in 50-μg boluses, can be employed for a similar purpose.

Intravenous labetalol (Table 15-10) may also be used for the antepartum management of acute hypertension. The use of labetolol may have several advantages, not the least of which is avoidance of the adverse side effect of tachycardia frequently encountered with the peripheral vasodilators such as hydralazine. Since obstetricians are generally less familiar with its parenteral administration, labetalol is a less popular drug, and hydralazine frequently takes first preference. Other agents have been successfully used in the treatment of hypertensive crises in nonpregnant populations. These agents have included

Table 15-10. Pharmacologic Management of Acute Hypertension

Hydralazine	5 mg IV; repeat in 10 minutes; then 10 mg IV every 20 minutes until stable blood pressure (140–150/90–100 mm Hg) achieved
Labetalol	5–15 mg IV push; repeat every 10–20 minutes by doubling dose to a maximum of 300 mg total
Sodium nitroprusside[a,b] (best used for refractory hypertension)	Controlled infusion, 0.5–3 μ/kg/min not to exceed 800 μg/min
Nifedipine[b]	10 mg sublingual, repeat in 30 minutes; then 10–20 mg PO 4–6 h
Nitroglycerin[a]	Should be used only by practitioners thoroughly familiar with its use in obstetrics

[a] Requires an arterial line for continuous blood pressure monitoring.
[b] Avoid use in antepartum patients; profound hypotension may result.

calcium-channel blockers, ACE inhibitors, sodium nitroprusside, and diazoxide. Any of these agents may be appropriate for use in the postpartum patient having a hypertensive crisis, but all should be used with great caution in the antepartum patient because of the risk of uncontrolled maternal hypotension and subsequent fetal distress.

The importance of prompt recognition and management of the hypertensive crisis in the pregnant patient cannot be overemphasized. Hypertension remains a leading cause of maternal mortality, with cerebrovascular accident the most common direct cause of death in hypertensive patients. For these reasons, patients with significant hypertensive disease, be it chronic hypertension or severe preeclampsia, are best managed in tertiary care centers where a multidisciplinary approach by physicians skilled in the management of such patients can serve to optimize the outcomes for both the mother and fetus.

SUMMARY

The hypertensive disorders in pregnancy present a significant challenge for clinician and patient. Close maternal observation, control of blood pressure, and prolongation of pregnancy to term are the goals of intervention for these disorders. Clinical trials of new pharmacologic agents may lead to better control of hypertension in the pregnant patient without compromising fetal oxygenation. Continued research into the etiology and pathophysiology of preeclampsia may allow for better control of this disease, or, ideally, to better ways of preventing its occurrence. As research in this area continues to yield benefits, so will the ability to more effectively manage all pregnant patients with hypertensive disorders.

REFERENCES

1. Repke JT: Prevention of preeclampsia. Clin Perinatol 18:779, 1991
2. Roberts JM, Taylor RN, Musci TJ, Rodgers GM: Serum from preeclamptic women contains a factor which damages human endothelial cells. Clin Exp Hypertens 8:119, 1989
3. Friedman SA, Taylor RN, Roberts JM: Pathophysiology or pre-eclampsia. Clin Perinatol 18:661, 1991
4. Gant NF, Dailey GL, Chand S et al: A study of angiotensin II pressor response throughout primigravida pregnancy. J Clin Invest 52:2682, 1973
5. Conradt A, Weidinger H, Algayer H: On the role of magnesium in fetal hypotrophy, pregnancy-induced hypertension, and preeclampsia. Magnesium Bull 6:68, 1984
6. Spatling L, Spatling G: Magnesium supplementation in pregnancy: a double blind study. Br J Obstet Gynaecol 95:120, 1988
7. Sibai BM, Villar MA, Bray E: Magnesium supplementation during pregnancy: a double blind randomized controlled clinical trial. Am J Obstet Gynecol 161:115, 1989
8. Repke JT: Prevention and treatment of pregnancy-induced hypertension. Comp Ther 17:25, 1991
9. Szal SE, Repke JT, Seely EW et al: Calcium signaling in pregnant human myometrium. Am J Physiol (Endocrinol Metab) 267:E77, 1994
10. Repke JT: Calcium and vitamin D. Clin Obstet Gynecol 37:550, 1994
11. Schiff E, Peleg E, Goldenberg M et al: The use of aspirin to prevent pregnancy-induced hypertension and lower the ratio of thromboxane A_2 to prostacyclin in relatively high risk pregnancies. N Engl J Med 321:351, 1989
12. Benigni A, Gregorini G, Frusca T et al: Effective low dose aspirin on fetal and maternal generation of thromboxane by platelets in women at risk for pregnancy-induced hypertension. N Engl J Med 321:357, 1989
13. Sibai BM, Caritis SN, Thom E et al: Prevention of preeclampsia with low dose aspirin in healthy, nulliparous pregnant women. N Engl J Med 329:1213, 1993
14. McNeil J: The possible teratogenic effect of salicylates on the developing fetus: brief summaries of eight suggestive cases. Clin Pediatr 12:347, 1973
15. Sloan D, Heinonen OP, Kaufman DW et al: Aspirin and congenital malformations. Lancet 1:1373, 1976
16. Streissguth AP, Treder RP, Barr HM et al: Aspirin and acetaminophen use by pregnant women and subsequent child IQ and attention decrements. Teratology 35:211, 1987
17. Sibai BM, Mercer BM, Schiff E, Friedman SA: Aggressive versus expectant management of severe preeclampsia at 28–32 weeks gestation: a randomized controlled trial. Am J Obstet Gynecol 171:818, 1994
18. Schiff E, Friedman SA, Sibai BM: Conservative management of severe preeclampsia remote from term. Obstet Gynecol 84:626, 1994
19. Repke JT, Friedman SA, Kaplan PW: Prophylaxis of

eclamptic seizures: current controversies. Clin Obstet Gynecol 35:365, 1992

20. Kaplan P, Repke JT: Complications of pregnancy-eclampsia. Neurol Clin 12:565, 1994
21. Pritchard JA, Cunningham FG, Pritchard SA: Parkland Memorial Hospital protocol for treatment of eclampsia. Evaluation of 245 cases. Am J Obstet Gynecol 148:951, 1984
22. Domisse J: Phenytoin, sodium and magnesium sulfate in the management of eclampsia. Br J Obstet Gynaecol 7:104, 1990
23. Crowther C: Magnesium sulfate versus diazepam in the management of eclampsia: a randomized controlled trial. Br J Obstet Gynaecol 97:110, 1990
24. Sibai BM, Schneider JM, Morrison JC: The late postpartum eclampsia controversy. Obstet Gynecol 55:75, 1980
25. Ramanathan J, coleman P, Sibai B: Anesthetic modification of hemodynamic and neuroendocrine stress responses to cesarean delivery in women with severe pre-eclampsia. Anesth Analg 73:772, 1991
26. Martin JN, Blake PG, Lowry SL et al: Pregnancy complicated by preeclampsia/eclampsia with the syndrome of hemolysis, elevated liver enzymes, and low platelet count: how rapid is postpartum recovery? Obstet Gynecol 76:737, 1990
27. Weinstein L: Syndrome of hemolysis, elevated liver enzymes and low platelet count: a severe consequence of hypertension in pregnancy. Am J Obstet Gynecol 142:159, 1982
28. Barton JR, Sibai BM: Care of the pregnancy complicated by HELLP syndrome. Obstet Gynecol Clin North Am 18:165, 1991
29. Villar J, Repke JT, Markush L et al: The measuring of blood pressure during pregnancy. Am J Obstet Gynecol 161:1019, 1989
30. Zuspan FP, Rayburn WF: Blood pressure self monitoring during pregnancy: practical considerations. Am J Obstet Gynecol 164:2, 1991
31. Sibai BM, Mabie WC, Shamsa F et al: A comparison of no medication versus methyldopa or labetolol in chronic hypertension during pregnancy. Am J Obstet Gynecol 162:960, 1990
32. Sibai BM, Abdella TN, Anderson GD: Pregnancy outcome in 211 patients with mild chronic hypertension. Obstet Gynecol 61:571, 1983
33. Genest J, Nowaczynski W, Bousche R, Kuchel O: Role of the adrenal cortex and sodium in the pathogenesis of human hypertension. Can Med Assoc J 118:538, 1978
34. Repke JT: The role of calcium, magnesium, and zinc supplementation and perinatal outcome. Clin Obstet Gynecol 34:262, 1991
35. Belizan J, Villar J, Repke J: The relationship between calcium intake and pregnancy-induced hypertension: up to date evidence. Am J Obstet Gynecol 158:898, 1988
36. Villar J, Repke JT: Calcium supplementation during pregnancy may reduce preterm delivery in high-risk populations. Am J Obstet Gynecol 163:1124, 1990
37. Repke JT, Villar J, Anderson C et al: Biochemical changes associated with calcium supplementation induced blood pressure reduction during pregnancy. Am J Obstet Gynecol 160:684, 1989
38. Belizan J, Villar J, Gonzalez L et al: Calcium supplementation to prevent hypertensive disorders of pregnancy. N Engl J Med 325:1399, 1992
39. Maden RP, Redman CWG: Antihypertensive drugs in pregnancy. Clin Perinatol 12:521, 1985
40. Wansbrough H, Nakanishi H, Wood C: The effect of adrenogenic receptor blocking drugs on the human uterus. Br J Obstet Gynaecol 75:189, 1968
41. Fenakel K, Lorie S: The use of calcium channel blockers in obstetrics and gynecology: a review. Eur J Obstet Gynaecol Reprod Biol 37:199, 1990
42. Sibai BM, Grossman RA, Grossman HE: Effects of diuretics on plasma volume in pregnancies with long-term hypertension. Am J Obstet Gynecol 150:831, 1984
43. Rosa FW, Bosco LA, Graham CF et al: Neonatal anuria with maternal angiotensin converting enzyme inhibitor. Obstet Gynecol 74:371, 1989
44. Ferris TF, Weir EK: Effect of captopril on uterine blood flow and prostaglandin E synthesis in the pregnant rabbit. J Clin Invest 71:809, 1983

Chapter 16

Preterm Labor

James E. Ferguson II and Richard E. Besinger

Preterm labor and delivery is the most important problem in modern obstetrics. It is disappointing to recognize that the incidence of preterm birth in the United States is not only not decreasing, but actually seems to be increasing. In 1981, the incidence of births ending before 37 weeks of gestation was 9.4 percent, whereas in 1989 it was reported to be 10.6 percent.[1] A recently reported multicenter trial revealed that the incidence of preterm delivery between 20 and 36 completed weeks of gestation was 9.6 percent.[2] In the study by Copper et al,[2] two-thirds of all neonatal deaths followed pregnancies ending before 29 completed weeks of gestation. These investigators demonstrated that neonatal survival exceeds 90 percent by 30 completed weeks of gestation, and that 90 percent of otherwise uncomplicated preterm births occur between 30 and 36 weeks of gestation.[2] It is thus apparent that we cannot look at reductions in perinatal mortality alone to substantiate tocolytic therapy, but must also look to improvements in preventing neonatal morbidity.[2,3] It is known that the incidence of respiratory morbidity, patent ductus arteriosus, necrotizing enterocolitis, intraventricular hemorrhage, and nursery stay decreases with advancing gestational age.[3] Figure 16-1 shows the dramatic reduction in neonatal morbidity associated with prolonged gestation. Aside from the marked increase in perinatal morbidity and mortality associated with preterm delivery,

such deliveries have many other adverse long-term consequences. Morrison[4] has noted a marked increase in neonatal death and hospital readmission for preterm infants, and that neurodevelopmental handicaps such as cerebral palsy, seizure disorders, and mental retardation are 22 times more common among infants weighing less than 1,500 g at birth than among those weighing 2,500 g or more. He further noted that 5-million hospital days per year are devoted to the care of preterm offspring, and that neonatal intensive-care costs exceed $5 billion per year.[4]

Additionally, the widespread use of tocolytic agents has not significantly reduced the incidence of low birth weight among infants born in the United States.[5] It is estimated that 60 to 80 percent of low-birth-weight deliveries are attributable to preterm labor or preterm premature rupture of membranes, and that the remainder are iatrogenic preterm deliveries for maternal or fetal compromise.[6] Controversy exists about the use of tocolytic agents in patients with preterm premature rupture of membranes, and there exist a variety of different therapeutic approaches to this problem.[7] In general, only 10 to 20 percent of women presenting with preterm labor are considered routine candidates for tocolysis.[8] While some have questioned the role of tocolytic agents in the treatment of preterm labor,[9] we remain convinced that in appropriate circumstances

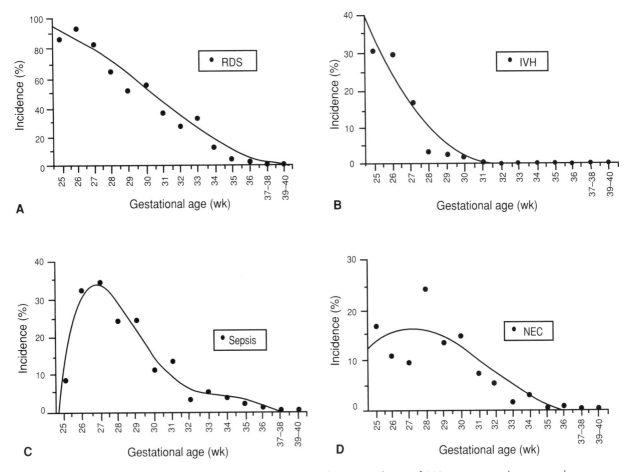

Fig. 16-1. Neonatal morbidity according to gestational age. Incidence of **(A)** respiratory distress syndrome (RDS), **(B)** intravenous hemorrhage (IVH) grades III and IV, **(C)** sepsis, **(D)** necrotizing enterocolitis (NEC). *(Figure continues.)*

the benefits to be gained in perinatal morbidity and mortality by delaying delivery are great, particularly in pregnancies between 24 and 30 weeks.[10] The purpose of this chapter is to present clinically relevant information about preterm labor and to provide pertinent guidelines for the use of tocolytic agents.

DEFINITION

There currently is no universal definition of preterm labor. Studies report differing criteria related to the important signs of cervical effacement and dilatation, and the frequency of uterine contractions. A recent survey study[7] found that cervical dilatation or effacement, or both, were required as diagnostic

criteria by only 60 percent of the respondents. For other respondents, the maternal perception of contractions was a sufficient indicator. Aside from discrepancies in establishing the diagnosis of preterm labor, not all practitioners agree on the gestational ages that define the limits of preterm gestation.[7] The World Health Organization defines a preterm infant as one born before 37 completed weeks of gestation (259 days). Since the delivery of a fetus before 20 completed weeks of gestation (140 days) is defined as an abortion, it seems apparent that a preterm birth is one in which delivery occurs between 20 and 37 weeks. Clearly, birth weight alone is inappropriate as a criterion for preterm birth. In previous studies, we have used a rigid set of criteria to diagnose pre-

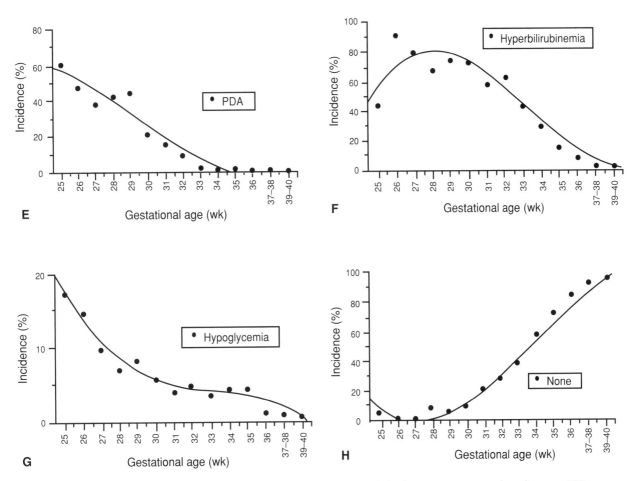

Fig. 16-1 *(Continued).* **(E)** patient ductus arteriosus (PDA), **(F)** hyperbilirubinemia requiring phototherapy, **(G)** hypoglycemia, and **(H)** no specific neonatal morbidities displayed by gestational age at birth.

term labor; these criteria include regular uterine contractions at a frequency of eight or more per hour, in association with progressive cervical dilatation or effacement or both.[11] Another common definition of preterm labor and delivery that Creasy and Heron[12] proposed is outlined in Figure 16-2. While we favor the upper limit of 37 weeks to define preterm labor, we generally do not treat preterm labor beyond 35 to 36 weeks' gestation. It is obvious that patient care must be individualized and that the risk of neonatal morbidity and mortality at specific gestational ages needs to be weighed against the maternal and fetal risks of tocolysis at each specific institution. Finally, there is the issue of definition of tocolytic "success." A variety of parameters have been utilized for this, including temporary arrest of uterine contractions; delay of delivery for 24, 48, or rarely 72 hours; delay of delivery for 1 week; and delay of delivery until the birth weight reaches 2,500 g or the gestational age reaches 36 or 37 weeks. It is important to keep these issues in mind when evaluating the reported efficacy of any tocolytic agent.

ETIOLOGY

Preterm labor and delivery can either be planned or unplanned. Planned preterm deliveries can occur through carelessness, as in the case of a lack of accurate knowledge of the gestational age when performing a repeat cesarean section, but are usually due to

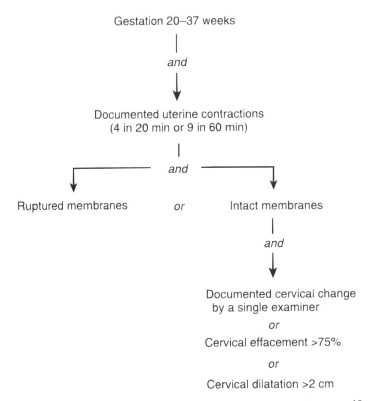

Gestation 20–37 weeks

and

Documented uterine contractions
(4 in 20 min or 9 in 60 min)

and

Ruptured membranes   *or*   Intact membranes

and

Documented cervical change
by a single examiner

or

Cervical effacement >75%

or

Cervical dilatation >2 cm

Fig. 16-2. Criteria for diagnosis of preterm labor. (Adapted from Creasy and Herron,[12] with permission.)

maternal or fetal indications. In the latter circumstance, the practitioner determines that it is in either the mother's or fetus's best interest to effect early delivery. Well-known indications for early delivery include severe pre-eclampsia, in which the well-being of the mother is compromised, and such fetal indications as severe intrauterine growth retardation (IUGR) coupled with oligohydramnios and fetal monitoring tests that indicate a compromised fetus at risk of demise in utero. Unplanned preterm labor and delivery account for more than 95 percent of early deliveries. The cause of unplanned preterm labor is generally unknown, although its association with obstetric factors such as placental abruption, multiple gestation, hydramnios, fetal anomaly, uterine malformation, and preterm premature rupture of membranes is well known. Probably because of a lack of awareness of the mechanism underlying preterm labor, a substantial number of cases remain characterized as idiopathic. In addition to the factors described above, compelling evidence is accumulat-

ing for a role in preterm labor of a subclinical or clinical infection in a mother's lower genital tract, fetal membranes, decidua, or amniotic fluid. A number of clinical studies have implicated vaginal and endocervical colonization with microorganisms such as group B streptococci, *Chlamydia trachomatis*, and mycoplasmas in the initiation of preterm labor.[13] Additionally, a significantly increased risk of preterm labor (relative risk of 3.8) has been reported among patients with bacterial vaginosis.[14] Many microorganisms (e.g., *Gardneralla vaginalis* and anaerobes, as seen in bacterial vaginosis) are known to produce phospholipase A_2 activity. Phospholipase A_2 causes the release of arachidonic-acid precursors, and may therefore initiate the local production of prostaglandins, with the associated potential for premature cervical ripening and preterm labor. Proteases, collagenases, and mucinases are also produced by the microorganisms and may facilitate the passage of additional microorganisms through the cervical mucus to the amnion, chorion, and decidua, which these organisms may colonize, thus compromising the integrity of the fetal membranes and possibly allowing the development of an intra-amniotic infection or preterm premature rupture of the membranes. In a recent study[15] of 264 pregnant women in preterm labor, involving amniocentesis and the evaluation of amniotic fluid for the presence of intra-amniotic infection, 9 percent of the patients undergoing amniocentesis were noted to have intra-amniotic infections. *Ureaplasma urealyticum, Fusobacterium* species, and *Mycoplasma hominis* were noted to be important agents, in addition to other well-known microorganisms.

DIAGNOSIS AND GENERAL TREATMENT CONSIDERATIONS

The clinical diagnosis of preterm labor remains extremely problematic. The identification of preterm labor requires that the physician have a high index of suspicion for its existence. The most common signs and symptoms of women presenting with preterm labor include uterine contractions, abdominal pain, backache, watery vaginal discharge, bloody vaginal discharge, vaginal bleeding, suprapubic pressure, vaginal pressure, change in vaginal discharge, and thigh aches. While these complaints should be seriously considered in any pregnant woman, they are especially important in women who have a high a priori risk of preterm labor, such as those who have had a prior preterm delivery and those with a multiple gestation, or known uterine anomaly. The presence of uterine contractions and clinical examination of the cervix are critical factors to consider in making the diagnosis of preterm labor. These factors must be considered in relationship to the gestational age at the time of patient presentation. If a patient has presented with possible preterm labor yet has not met such diagnostic criteria as those outlined earlier, further evaluation should be undertaken for a period of 1 to 2 hours to document cervical dilatation or effacement. This period of observation probably does not adversely affect the success of subsequent tocolysis.[16] Despite the best clinical efforts, it is clear that the diagnostic ability needed for accurately predicting preterm labor is less than desirable. Keirse and colleagues,[17] in their meta-analysis of 15 placebo-controlled trials

of tocolysis, reported that 60 percent (range, 27 to 89 percent) of patients had delivery delayed by placebo for 48 hours or more, and that 37 percent (range, 0 to 73 percent) reached term following placebo. Oncofetal fibronectin has been reported to have a positive predictive value of 83.1 percent for preterm delivery when present in the cervical vaginal secretions of patients with preterm uterine contractions.[18] Testing for oncofetal fibronectin in conjunction with cervical evaluation may improve the positive predictive value and sensitivity of the diagnosis of preterm labor.[19] Because of the lack of accuracy in diagnosing preterm labor and the high incidence of false preterm labor, some women who do not have progressive preterm labor are unnecessarily treated with potentially dangerous tocolytic agents.

The patient who is determined to be in preterm labor, becomes a candidate for tocolysis. It is generally accepted that tocolytic agents do prolong gestation when preterm labor is present,[20] but any and all of these agents clearly pose risks to the mother and fetus. The physician must therefore individualize patient care and formulate a risk/benefit assessment for each patient. Preterm labor in association with overt chorioamnionitis, frank placental abruption, fetal distress, a fetal anomaly incompatible with life, or fetal demise probably represents an absolute contraindication to tocolysis. Relative contraindications include significant vaginal bleeding and maternal medical conditions in which prolongation of gestation may be detrimental to the mother, such as peripartal cardiomyopathy or other significant cardiovascular disease and severe pre-eclampsia. Controversy surrounds the role of tocolysis in patients with preterm labor associated with preterm premature rupture of membranes. Although tocolysis in this setting may increase the risk of fetal and maternal infection, an argument can be made for short-term tocolysis in an effort to allow the administration of glucocorticoids.

After the risk/benefit assessment has been made by the physician, it should be presented to the patient in a direct and understandable manner, with treatment alternatives outlined and a treatment plan suggested. Such an approach helps to relieve patient anxiety and allows the patient an opportunity to be part of the decision-making process. At times it is useful to obtain a neonatal/pediatric consultation to discuss with the parents the issues related to perinatal mortality and morbidity. A complete history and physical examination would already have been performed at this point to identify any underlying maternal or fetal risks. Baseline laboratory evaluations should be obtained, including complete blood counts with differential counts, and serum chemistries. A baseline electrocardiogram (ECG) is indicated, and a pulse oximetry determination may reveal unsuspected abnormalities. A coagulation profile should be obtained for patients at risk of subclinical abruption, and consideration should be given to performing a toxicology screen on all patients in preterm labor. Cervical cultures should be obtained for gonorrhea and chlamydia, and vaginal cultures for group B streptococcal infection. We favor the approach of initiating antibiotic treatment with ampicillin or, in the face of penicillin allergy, clindamicin on an empiric basis until culture results are available. If the cervical and vaginal cultures are negative, the antibiotic is discontinued. If the results are positive, the antibiotic is continued for an appropriate period and repeat cultures are performed. Fetal assessment is required and should include fetal heart rate monitoring and sonography. Ultrasonographic information that should be specifically sought includes a confirmation of the gestational age, evaluation of fetal growth, detailed evaluation of fetal anatomy, assessment of amniotic fluid volume, and evaluation for retroplacental clots, uterine malformations, and myomas.

Consideration is often given to the usefulness of long-term antibiotic prophylaxis in patients with intact membranes, the value of amniocentesis and preterm labor, and the advisability of glucocorticoid administration. Because subclinical infection is noted in association with preterm labor and delivery, several investigators have added adjunctive antibiotic treatment for 5 days or more to standard tocolytic therapy in an effort to improve perinatal outcome. Morales et al[21] found a prolongation of pregnancy in an antibiotic-treated group, whereas Newton and colleagues[22] did not. A recent multicenter collaborative trial reported by Romero et al[23] evaluated 277 patients in preterm labor with intact membranes. In this double-blind, placebo-controlled trial, no significant difference between the antibiotic group and

the placebo group was found in relationship to maternal outcomes, including duration of the interval between randomization and delivery, frequency of preterm delivery, frequency of preterm premature rupture of membranes, clinical infection, or number of subsequent admissions for preterm labor. There was also no significant difference in severe neonatal morbidity when the groups were compared. While the overall data remain unclear as to whether antibiotic administration improves latency, all studies are consistent in reporting that adjunctive antibiotic administration does not have an effect on perinatal morbidity or mortality. We believe that the data taken in aggregate do not support the routine use of prolonged antibiotic administration in women in preterm labor, but continue to recommend the empiric use of antibiotics on a short-term basis until cervical/vaginal culture results are available (generally 24 to 48 hours).

Controversy also exists about whether all patients in preterm labor require an amniocentesis, either to rule out intra-amniotic infection or to determine fetal lung maturity. We believe the use of amniocentesis should be individualized, but generally support its use in earlier gestations when the likelihood of intrauterine infection is greatest. The amniotic fluid should be subjected to a Gram stain, culture, cell count, glucose assay, and interleukin-6 assay.[24] Intra-amniotic infection mandates discontinuation of tocolysis and the initiation of antibiotics and maneuvers to effect delivery.

Another area of clinical uncertainty surrounds the use of glucocorticoid administration. The two most commonly used steroids are betamethasone (12.5 mg IM with doses given 24 hours apart) and dexamethasone (6.0 mg IM given in four doses at 12-hour intervals). In general, the enhancing effect of glucocorticoids on fetal lung maturity is thought to last for 1 week. Recently, a National Institutes of Health (NIH) consensus panel[25] reached the conclusions and recommendations reported in the box below.

Once the clinician has considered all the above issues and initiated a treatment plan, a prolonged period of clinical observation begins. Knowledge about specific pharmacologic agents for tocolysis (as outlined in the remainder of this chapter and in Ch. 17) is of paramount importance in administering

NIH Consensus Panel Conclusions and Recommendations

The benefits of antenatal administration of corticosteroids to fetuses at risk of preterm delivery vastly outweigh the potential risks. The benefits include not only a reduction in the risk of respiratory distress syndrome (RDS), but also a substantial reduction in mortality and interventricular hemorrhage (IVH).

All fetuses between 24 and 34 weeks' gestation and at risk of preterm delivery should be considered candidates for antenatal treatment with corticosteroids

The decision to use antenatal corticosteroids should not be altered by fetal race or gender or by the availability of surfactant replacement therapy

Patients eligible for therapy with tocolytic agents should also be eligible for treatment with antenatal corticosteroids

Because treatment with corticosteroids for less than 24 hours is still associated with significant reductions in neonatal mortality, RDS, and IVH, antenatal corticosteroids should be given unless immediate delivery is anticipated

In preterm premature rupture of membranes at 30 to 32 weeks' gestation in the absence of clinical chorioamnionitis, antenatal corticosteroid use is recommended

In complicated pregnancies in which delivery before 34 weeks' gestation is likely, antenatal corticosteroid use is recommended unless there is evidence that corticosteroids will have an adverse effect on the mother or delivery is imminent

these medications in a safe manner and decreasing the risk of maternal-fetal-neonatal complications. If signs of maternal or fetal compromise occur during the course of tocolysis, it is necessary to re-evaluate the entire clinical situation. If maternal cardiac compromise, pulmonary edema, respiratory depression, persistent hypotension, or uncorrectable fetal distress develop, it may be necessary to change tocolytic agents or perhaps discontinue tocolysis. The patient should be evaluated frequently to ensure that clinical signs of chorioamnionitis have not developed. If chorioamnionitis is suspected, amniocentesis, as outlined previously, is invaluable. Amniocentesis should also be considered in cases of refractory preterm labor. It is reasonable to treat patients with progressive preterm labor sequentially with different tocolytic agents, since there will often be a response in this situation.[11] Except in pregnancies of the very earliest gestational age, it is probably reasonable to discontinue tocolysis if progressive cervical dilatation exceeds 4 cm.

If acute tocolysis is successful, the clinician must determine the need for oral tocolysis at discharge. We believe it is reasonable to provide oral tocolysis if it has been well tolerated in the hospital setting, yet the consensus for the advisability of this practice is waning. A recent study[26] failed to demonstrate any benefit of oral terbutaline as compared with placebo. If an oral agent is well tolerated in long-term therapy it should be given through 36 to 37 completed weeks of gestation.

PHARMACOLOGIC THERAPY

In 1961, the first β-mimetic tocolytic agent, isoxsuprine, was proposed for the treatment of preterm contractions.[27] The clinical use of isoxsuprine was subsequently limited by its nonselective β-adrenergic side effects. Over the next 15 years, a wide variety of selective β-mimetic medications were proposed for tocolytic therapy. Some gained popularity with clinicians around the world, and the U.S. Food and Drug Administration (FDA) approved the use of ritodrine hydrochloride for clinical use in 1980.[28] The need to develop safe and effective alternatives to β-mimetic agents led to a re-evaluation of the tocolytic effects of magnesium sulfate during the early 1980s.[29] More recently, other tocolytic agents, such as prostaglandin synthetase inhibitors, calcium-channel blockers, and oxytocin antagonists have undergone critical clinical evaluation.

β-Adrenergic Tocolytic Agents
Mechanisms of Action

β-Mimetic stimulation had one of the earliest recognized inhibitory effects on uterine contractility. β-Mimetic agents act on intramembranous β-receptors that activate the enzyme adenylate cyclase and cause an increase in the intracellular concentration of cyclic adenosine monophosphate (cAMP).[30,31] This latter intracellular messenger initiates a series of reactions that reduce intracellular calcium levels and decrease the sensitivity of the myosin–actin contractile unit of muscle to the effects of calcium and prostaglandins.[30] The resulting inhibition of uterine contractility occurs even if oxytocin is given simultaneously.[30]

Clinical Efficacy

Ritodrine hydrochloride (Yutopar) remains the clinical standard against which all subsequent tocolytic agents have been judged. The certification of its safety and efficacy by the FDA came after more than 10 years of clinical investigation with ritodrine. The approval for its clinical use in the United States was supported by data supplied by a number of independent investigators studying small numbers of subjects in different treatment protocols. The β_2-selective nature of ritodrine led to hope that it would exhibit an efficacy similar to that of previously developed β-mimetic tocolytics, with fewer side effects.

A large number of placebo-controlled clinical trials have evaluated the efficacy of ritodrine for the inhibition of preterm labor. Initial randomized clinical trials at multiple sites in Europe and the United States showed a significant prolongation of pregnancy with an increase in birth weight associated ritodrine tocolysis.[32,33] The Phase III FDA clinical trial of ritodrine compared it with either placebo or ethanol in 313 singleton gestations.[33,34] Despite the reported success of the drug, however, many valid criticisms of this study have been voiced, including its lack of standardized enrollment criteria, the varying treatment protocols at the different participating centers, the small subject numbers at individual institutions, and the inclusion of a small number of patients with preterm premature rupture of membranes. Results from one of the five study centers that were published separately failed to demonstrate any beneficial effect of ritodrine.[35] Even more disconcerting was that no serious maternal complications or significant patient intolerance were reported in the large study population.[34]

More recent and better-designed clinical trials raise serious doubts about the long-term efficacy of ritodrine in the inhibition of preterm labor.[36–39] Most of these trials failed to demonstrate a significant long-term delay of delivery, increased birth weight, or decreased neonatal mortality associated with ritodrine tocolysis. Several of the trials did, however, suggest a realistic short-term gain in delaying delivery for more than 24 to 48 hours.[37,38]

The largest multicenter clinical trial evaluating the efficacy of ritodrine was performed and reported by the Canadian Preterm Labor Investigators Group.[39] This placebo-controlled trial involved 708 women and failed to demonstrate any long-term delay of delivery change in the frequency of low-birth-weight infants, or differences in perinatal mortality statistics with ritodrine. Nevertheless, the study did confirm that β-mimetic tocolysis was effective in delaying preterm delivery for 48 hours, despite its apparent minimal impact perinatal survival.

A recent meta-analysis of 16 methodologically acceptable trials of β-mimetic agents supports the overview that ritodrine is, at most, effective in postponing a preterm delivery for only 24 to 48 hours.[40] Utilizing a data base of 890 women (the Canadian study data were not included) the analysis showed that β-mimetic tocolysis reduced the frequency of preterm birth and low birth weight without an accompanying reduction in perinatal mortality or the incidence of severe neonatal respiratory problems. Despite these findings, ritodrine remains the gold standard of modern tocolytic therapy and has a definite role in the treatment of prematurity. A recent FDA report to a meeting of tocolytic experts supports this consensus.[41]

Several small, placebo-controlled trials have produced conflicting results regarding the tocolytic effect of another selective β_2-agonist, terbutaline (Brethine/Bricanyl), in the treatment of preterm labor. Although the initial study showed a significant prolongation of pregnancy with terbutaline tocolysis,[42] more recent studies failed to demonstrate either short- or long-term effects.[43,44] By contrast, subsequent comparative clinical trials with ritodrine[45–47] have shown it to have a similar short-term efficacy in the treatment of preterm labor.

Limited attention has been given to the efficacy of maintenance β-mimetic tocolysis after successful parenteral therapy. Most clinical studies have by design used oral therapy once the initial contractions had been arrested. An initial single study had shown that maintenance therapy with oral β-mimetic agents was successful in preventing recurrent preterm labor, with fewer relapses, longer intervals to first relapse, and an overall increase in the delay of delivery.[48] However, a more recent randomized, placebo-controlled trial involving 55 patients failed to demonstrate any beneficial clinical effect.[26] Further complicating the issue of maintenance tocolysis is that several comparative trials of oral ritodrine and oral terbutaline have shown as much as a 2-week difference between these agents in the long-term delay of preterm delivery.[45–46]

Serum ritodrine or terbutaline concentrations vary widely during oral maintenance therapy, and are significantly lower than with intravenous dosing.[49–51] Oral administration of ritodrine produces a peak serum concentration within approximately 30 minutes, with a bioavailability approaching only 20 to 30 percent.[50–52] Experts speculate that the observed failure of β-mimetic tocolysis to provide a long-term delay of delivery may be directly attributable to these pharmacologic shortcomings.[41]

Tolerance to the metabolic and cardiovascular effects of long-term therapy with β-mimetic agents is well documented.[53] In humans, chronic administration of β-mimetic agents results in the development of tolerance to uterine smooth muscle relaxation.[54,55] This phenomenon probably follows from down regulation and cellular internalization of membranous β-receptors, with subsequent loss of myometrial relaxation in response to additional β-mimetics.[56,57] The existence of this biologic phenomenon also suggests that chronic β-mimetic tocolysis may have only a transitory ability to arrest preterm labor, lasting on the order of 1 to 2 weeks.[58]

In animal models, the pulsatile administration of β-mimetic agents decreases the degree of receptor down regulation and preserves a chronic physiologic response.[56,59] A continuous low-level infusion of terbutaline, with intermittently scheduled boluses administered by a computerized, subcutaneous infusion pump system, has been developed to address this provocative finding in the clinical setting.[60] Unfortunately, published scientific support for the intriguing laboratory observations is scant. An original report of an uncontrolled study of nine women with recurrent preterm labor treated with subcutaneous terbutaline delivered by a pump documents a mean prolongation of 9.2 weeks to delivery after the initiation of therapy.[61] Patients typically receive 3 to 4 mg/day of terbutaline, receiving continuous infusion therapy, compared with 40 to 50 mg/day with oral administration. No published clinical trials have addressed this provocative tocolytic issue. Pending its further scientific evaluation, subcutaneous terbutaline pump therapy is perhaps best restricted to cases of recurrent or refractile preterm labor. The metabolic and physiologic effects of this method of terbutaline administration during acute treatment of preterm labor are also not well defined.

Recommended Clinical Use

Tocolysis with ritodrine is begun with intravenous dosing at an initial rate of 50 to 100 μg/min, and is increased every 15 to 30 minutes until uterine activity is controlled, unacceptable side effects develop, or a maximum dose of 350 μg/min is reached (Table 16-1). When infused intravenously for tocolysis, ritodrine reaches therapeutic levels rapidly, with an initial half-life of 6 to 9 minutes followed by an elimination phase with a half-life of approximately 2 to 3 hours.[52,62] Steady-state concentrations at constant infusion rates are reached within 8 to 12 hours.[62,63] Ritodrine can be administered intramuscularly, but the intravenous route is preferred because it avoids the fluctuating serum concentrations observed with the former technique.[52] However, some investigators believe that intramuscular administration of the drug (5 to 10 mg every 2 to 4 hours) produces superior results, has fewer side effects, and requires less intravenous hydration than with the intravenous route.[36,64,65]

Infusion protocols for ritodrine based on pharmacologic data recommend that its infusion be started at a rate of 50 μg/min, increased by 50 μg/min every 20 minutes until tocolysis is achieved, and maintained at this dose for only 60 minutes before decreasing the infusion rate by 50 μg/min every 30 minutes until the lowest effective infusion rate is achieved.[66] Maintenance intravenous therapy should be discontinued after 12 to 24 hours of uterine quiescence. This infusion regimen reduces average and peak ritodrine concentrations and minimizes the total amount of drug administered, in accord with sound pharmacologic principles.[66]

Table 16-1. Tocolytic Agents

Drug	Initial Dose	Maximum Dose	Maintenance Dose
Ritodrine	0.05–0.10 mg/min IV	0.35 mg/min IV	10–20 mg PO q3–4h
Terbutaline	0.01–0.015 mg/min IV	0.025 mg/min IV	2.5–5.0 mg PO q3–4h
Magnesium sulfate	4–6 g in 10% solution over 15–30 minutes	2–4 g/hr	1 g PO q2–4h (magnesium oxide)
Indomethacin	50 mg PO 100 mg PRO	50 mg PO q4h	25 mg PO q4–6h
Nifedipine	10 mg PO or SL (may repeat at 20-minute intervals)	40 mg during a 1-hour period	10–20 mg PO q4–6h

Transplacental transfer of intravenously administered ritodrine and terbutaline is rapid and appreciable.[62] After maternal administration of ritodrine has been discontinued, levels of the drug in umbilical cord blood at delivery remain significant for up to 5 hours.[52] Because of this, if tocolysis fails and delivery is deemed inevitable, intravenous β-mimetic therapy should be discontinued in order to decrease neonatal levels of the drug.

Because the elimination half-life of oral ritodrine is approximately 1.3 to 2 hours, frequent oral administration is required to maintain therapeutic serum levels.[41,52] The usually recommended dosing interval of 10 to 20 mg every 3 to 4 hours may not provide the sustained serum concentrations necessary for adequate maintenance tocolysis.

Terbutaline can also be given intravenously, at an initial rate of 10 μg/min that is increased every 15 to 30 minutes until contractions have ceased, unacceptable side effects develop, or a maximum dosage of 25 μg/min has been achieved (Table 16-1). The intravenous infusion of terbutaline produces therapeutic levels rapidly, with a mean elimination half-life of 3.7 hours.[51] Limited pharmacologic data make it difficult to determine a therapeutic plasma level for terbutaline in tocolysis.

Several groups of investigators advocate the subcutaneous administration of terbutaline as an alternative to its intravenous administration[67,68] When given subcutaneously, terbutaline is absorbed rapidly, with a half-life of 7 minutes.[69] The common subcutaneous dose is 0.25 mg every 20 to 60 minutes until contractions have subsided. Intermittent subcutaneous dosing can then be maintained at a 2 to 4 hour interval. The ease of subcutaneous administra-tion of terbutaline and its avoidance of excessive intravenous hydration make it clinically attractive. Toxic effects of terbutaline have, however, been described with its continuous subcutaneous administration.[70]

The nature and degree of subjective maternal side effects of parenteral β-mimetic therapy have tended to limit its widespread clinical use. These effects are extensively discussed in Chapter 17. Worrisome symptoms include palpitations, tremor, nausea, vomiting, headache, nervousness, and restlessness. Chest discomfort, shortness of breath, and excessive maternal/fetal tachycardia are also common. Many troublesome symptoms require the discontinuation of infusion or diminution of infusion rates. Infusions of β-mimetic agents should be titrated to minimize side effects on an individual basis, while ensuring adequate tocolysis. Severe side effects are most commonly observed when the infusion rate and concentration of ritodrine are increasing.[62] Thus, slower increases in infusion rates and maintenance of the lowest effective infusion rate may allow the continued administration of ritodrine even in individuals experiencing minimal side effects. The maternal side effects of terbutaline are similar to those of ritodrine. Most randomized comparison studies have not shown any difference in the incidence of tachycardia, hypotension, chest pain, arrhythmia, hypokalemia, or jitteriness with intravenous infusions.[45–47] One single-center comparative study noted an unacceptable level of cardiac side effects with intravenous doses of terbutaline, and discontinued its use by this route.[47] Comparative trials of the oral forms of terbutaline and ritodrine likewise suggest no significant difference in the incidence of maternal side effects.[71] The clinical experience with ritodrine infusion suggests that it may be possible to reduce worrisome effects by minimizing infusion rates and subsequently reducing overall plasma concentrations.

Magnesium Sulfate

Magnesium has long been known to decrease uterine contractility.[72] The infusion of magnesium sulfate for seizure prophylaxis during pre-eclamptic labor is commonly associated with decreased uterine activity,[72] although the apparent reduction in uterine activity is generally transitory.[73] Magnesium sulfate has been used as a tocolytic agent for some time; however, renewed interest in its use arose in the 1980s from concern about complications of cardiac stimulation and pulmonary edema induced by β-mimetic agents.[7] While its use has gained popularity in the United States over the past decade, many potential complications of tocolysis with magnesium sulfate have also come to light with its expanded clinical use (Table 16-2).

Mechanism of Action

The basis of the tocolytic action of magnesium sulfate remains unknown. Because magnesium decreases the frequency of depolarization of the smooth muscle cell and uncouples the adenosine triphosphate (ATP)-linked activation of the actin–myosin unit during in vitro studies, it has been suggested that magnesium competes with calcium for entry into the muscle cell through voltage-operated calcium channels.[74] More recently, it has been proposed that magnesium competitively binds with calcium storage sites in the myometrial endoplasmic

Table 16-2. Adverse Effects of Magnesium Sulfate Tocolytic Therapy in 355 Patients

Side Effect	%
Pulmonary edema	1.1
Chest pain	1.1
Severe nausea or flushing	3.6
Drowsiness or blurred vision	0.8
Total	6.6

(From Elliott,[133] with permission.)

reticulum.[30] Magnesium concentrations approximating 4 to 8 mEq/L appear to be necessary for the in vitro contraction inhibition human myometrium.[30,74]

Clinical Efficacy

Placebo-controlled studies[44,47,75,76] of the efficacy of magnesium sulfate in inhibiting preterm labor have been limited. Several randomized trials showed that intravenous magnesium sulfate at 2 to 3 g/hr produced no significant short-term delay of delivery, increase in birth weight, or difference in perinatal mortality.[47,76] On the basis of these limited results and the observation that tocolytic success is inversely related to the degree of cervical dilatation,[75] the documented tocolytic effect of magnesium sulfate remains in question.

Randomized, comparative clinical trials with ritodrine[47,77,78] and terbutaline[44,47,79] have also been used to evaluate the clinical effectiveness of magnesium sulfate tocolysis. These relatively large clinical trials show no significant difference in delay of delivery for more than 48 hours with magnesium sulfate as compared with intravenous β-mimetic agents. The trial data suggest that magnesium sulfate may be comparable to β-mimetic drugs as a short-term tocolytic agent.

By contrast, evaluation of the long-term efficacy of magnesium tocolysis was initially difficult because of the lack of an oral dosage form. Most long-term studies substituted an oral β-mimetic agent for maintenance tocolysis following successful intravenous magnesium sulfate therapy.[44,77,78] Recently, several oral magnesium preparations have been evaluated.[80–82] Baseline serum magnesium levels increase modestly after the oral administration of 1 g of magnesium sulfate every 4 hours.[80] Several randomized trials comparing oral magnesium gluconate or magnesium oxide with oral β-mimetic agents have shown a similar efficacy in the prolongation of pregnancy.[81,82]

With regard to the overall efficacy of magnesium sulfate as a tocolytic agent, the clinical studies so far reported are difficult to compare because of the small numbers of patients, differing rates and durations of administration, and possible inclusion of a high percentage of patients with false preterm labor. Similarly, the relationship between specific magnesium sulfate concentrations and its tocolytic effect need to be better defined.[83] Although the apparent lack of a tocolytic effect in placebo-controlled trials represents a significant concern, the comparable success rate of β-mimetic and magnesium sulfate therapies has made magnesium tocolysis popular in clinical practice.[7] Some clinicians strongly believe that magnesium sulfate should be a first-line agent for preterm labor inhibition in the United States.

Other authors advocate the use of sequential regimens of tocolytic therapy, with magnesium sulfate being offered to patients for whom initial therapy with a β-mimetic agent proves unsuccessful.[84,85] Uncontrolled reports of overall success rates ranging from 40 to 90 percent with sequential treatment suggest that magnesium sulfate may be beneficial in prolonging selected pregnancies.[84–86] Even in cases marked by a significant progression of cervical dilatation before magnesium sulfate therapy is initiated, the sequential use of more than one tocolytic agent does not decrease the probability of successful therapy.[85,86] However, because no clinical trials have been reported in which patients in whom ritodrine proves unsuccessful have been randomized to magnesium sulfate or placebo, the true efficacy of sequential magnesium sulfate therapy to treat first-line tocolytic failure remains unproved.

Recommended Clinical Use

Current therapeutic recommendations for magnesium sulfate are an initial loading dose of 4–6 g in 10% solution, given intravenously over 15 to 30 minutes and followed by a continuous infusion at a rate of 2 to 4 g/hr (Table 16-1). A serum magnesium concentration of 5 to 6 mEq/L can be achieved with an infusion rate of 3 g/hr.[29,87] An increase in the infusion rate can be made relatively rapidly, with the realization that toxic levels will be reached more rapidly. Magnesium is eliminated almost entirely by renal excretion.[29] With intravenous infusion, 75 percent of the administered dose is excreted during a bolus infusion, and 90 percent within 24 hours after treatment.[87] Under these circumstances, high infusion rates are required to maintain therapeutic serum concentrations. All patients receiving high-dose magnesium tocolytic therapy should have their urine outputs and deep tendon reflexes monitored frequently. Pulse oximetry is also a helpful adjunct

for the early detection of magnesium toxicity. In patients with impaired renal function, serum magnesium levels must be monitored frequently to prevent toxicity at levels above 8 mEq/L. In order to reduce maternal symptoms, patients should be maintained with the lowest possible rate of magnesium infusion necessary to control contractility. Under circumstances of failed tocolysis and inevitable delivery, intravenous magnesium tocolysis should be discontinued to decrease neonatal levels of the drug.

Once uterine activity has been well controlled for a 12- to 24-hour period with intravenous magnesium sulfate, patients can generally be converted to oral maintenance therapy with a β-mimetic agent. One can give an initial oral dose of a β-mimetic drug and discontinue the magnesium infusion approximately 20 to 30 minutes later. Some centers choose to administer oral magnesium oxide at doses of 1 g every 2 to 4 hours as an alternative maintenance tocolytic agent.

Prostaglandin Synthetase Inhibitors

Indirect clinical observations have suggested that prostaglandin synthetase inhibitors suppress the process of labor. Pregnant patients taking high-dose salicylate for rheumatoid diseases were found to have significant increases in the mean length of gestation, frequency of postdate pregnancy, and mean duration of spontaneous labor.[88,89] The administration of indomethacin to patients in active term labor results in complete cessation of labor or prolongation of the active phase.[90]

Mechanisms of Action

Prostaglandins are important modulators of uterine contractility during preterm labor. Increased concentrations of prostaglandin metabolites have been measured in patients experiencing preterm labor.[91,92] Prostaglandins activate the calcium channels within the myometrial cell membrane, in addition to functioning as secondary messengers to modulate calcium release from the sarcoplasmic reticulum.[30] All currently available prostaglandin synthetase inhibitors act on cyclooxygenase to prevent the cascade of prostaglandins from their precursor, arachidonic acid.[93,94] Indomethacin (Indocin), naproxen (Naprosyn, Anaprox), and fenoprofen (Nalfon) are more effective inhibitors of prostaglandin synthesis than is aspirin.[93,94] These prostaglandin synthetase inhibitors decrease the contractility of excised uterine muscle strips.[95,96] Administration of indomethacin[97–99] or ritodrine[100,101] during labor in humans results in a significant reduction in plasma prostaglandin levels. Indomethacin is the most widely used prostaglandin synthetase inhibitor for the treatment of preterm labor.

Clinical Efficacy

Initial clinical experience with prostaglandin synthetase inhibitors in patients in whom other tocolytic agents proved unsuccessful was encouraging.[102] The largest clinical experience with indomethacin as a first-line tocolytic agent involved 252 patients, of whom 88 percent had a prolongation for more than 1 week.[103]

Placebo-controlled clinical trials have documented the efficacy of indomethacin in the inhibition of preterm labor.[99,104] These short-term studies demonstrated that indomethacin was more effective than placebo in delaying preterm delivery during a 24-hour course of therapy.

Several randomized comparative trials with ritodrine have demonstrated the efficacy of indomethacin in arresting preterm labor. In a short-term study in which patients were randomized to intravenous ritodrine or oral indomethacin for 48 hours, similar rates of successful tocolysis were reported.[105] A small study of the long-term efficacy of intravenous or oral ritodrine and oral indomethacin showed comparable prolongation rates of approximately 3 weeks.[106] A recent, small comparative study with oral terbutaline suggests an efficacy similar to indomethacin tocolysis.[107]

Several randomized clinical trials of combination tocolytic therapy have also demonstrated a positive additive tocolytic effect with indomethacin. A combination of ethanol and indomethacin was more effective than either salbutamol or ethanol alone in arresting preterm labor.[108] Two studies comparing treatment regimens of ritodrine alone versus combined ritodrine/indomethacin showed an improved tocolytic effect of the combination regimen.[109,110]

These prospective, controlled clinical trials suggest that indomethacin is one of the most effective tocolytic agents for the treatment of preterm labor. Few tocolytic agents to date have demonstrated such consistently salutory effects in placebo-controlled and comparative trials.

Recommended Clinical Use

Indomethacin is usually administered initially as a 50-mg oral loading dose, followed by 25 mg every 4 to 6 hours (Table 16-1). Indomethacin can also be administered initially in the form of a 100-mg rectal suppository. The drug is rapidly absorbed after oral ingestion, reaching peak plasma concentrations within 1 to 2 hours.[111] In women in labor, the peak serum concentration of indomethacin following its oral administration is reached later, but still within 1.5 to 2.0 hours.[111] The half-life of excretion of indomethacin in the nonpregnant adult is approximately 2.2 hours.[94] The drug is readily transferred across the placental unit to the fetus, and appears in the fetal blood within 15 minutes.[112,113] Fetal concentrations of indomethacin equilibrate with maternal levels within 5 to 6 hours.[113] Placental transfer of the drug does not appear to vary with gestational age.[113] The half-life excretion of indomethacin in the term neonate ranges from 11 to 15 hours,[94,111] and is prolonged to 19 hours in neonates born before 32 weeks.[112] As a precaution, indomethacin tocolysis should be discontinued once it is apparent that a preterm birth is inevitable, in order to minimize neonatal drug levels.

Potential fetal-neonatal complications of indomethacin therapy can be minimized by selective and limited use of this tocolytic agent. Indomethacin should not be considered as a first-line agent unless β-mimetic or magnesium sulfate tocolysis is absolutely contraindicated. Its clinical use in the treatment of first-line tocolytic failures may be justified when the risk of prematurity is greater than the perceived risk of the medication. It seems appropriate to limit the use of indomethacin in most modern perinatal centers to gestations of less than 32 weeks, on the basis of the nearly universal neonatal survival in gestations exceeding 32 to 34 weeks. Limiting the use of indomethacin to short-term therapy (24 to 48 hours) may also prove to be an effective strategy for avoiding potential fetal-neonatal complications. Attempting to discontinue indomethacin at 24 hours before delivery would also be helpful in reducing neonatal complications, but is probably difficult to achieve in an unpredictable clinical setting. Maternal, fetal, and neonatal effects of indomethacin are discussed in Chapter 17.

All pregnant women undergoing chronic tocolytic therapy with indomethacin should have periodic ultrasound examinations for drug-induced oligohydramnios. Intermittent examination of blood flow through the fetal ductus arteriosus should be undertaken, if available in the local medical community. Indomethacin therapy should be discontinued if significant oligohydramnios or ductal constriction is documented. These conservative recommendations are prudent until additional knowledge permits minimizing the potential neonatal complications of indomethacin tocolysis.

Calcium-Channel Blockers

Background and Mechanism of Action

Although magnesium sulfate, β-adrenergic agents, and prostaglandin synthetase inhibitors are available as tocolytic agents, each is associated with drawbacks that have led to a continuing search for alternative therapies. Interest has increased in the calcium-channel blockers, such as nifedipine, nicardipine, diltiazem, and verapamil, as possible tocolytic agents, but only nifedipine has been used regularly in the treatment of preterm labor. This section provides details of the current understanding of the role of nifedipine in the treatment of preterm labor, and focuses on clinically relevant data derived from its human use. Information about maternal physiologic effects and fetal-neonatal side effects of nifedipine is discussed in Chapter 17, and has recently been reviewed.[114]

The cytoplasmic concentration of free calcium directly affects the degree of myometrial contraction or relaxation. It is well known that increases in cytoplasmic free calcium cause myometrial contraction, whereas decreases are usually associated with relaxation. The predominant portion of intracellular free calcium results from passage of the calcium ion through voltage-dependent calcium channels in the cell membrane. Nifedipine, a dihydropyridine-type calcium-channel blocker, effectively inhibits myometrial activity by blocking the transmembrane influx of calcium through these voltage-dependent calcium channels.[115] In vitro studies have shown the effectiveness of nifedipine in inhibiting spontaneous uterine contractions and those elicited by vasopressors or potassium deplorization in isolated strips of human myometrium.[116] Furthermore, in vivo studies using microtransducer techniques[117] have shown nifedipine to be effective in inhibiting uterine contractions during menstruation,[118] those caused by intraamniotic prostaglandin F_{2a} (PGF_{2a}),[119] and those seen in the immediate postpartum period.[120] Recent work by Young[121] has shed further light on the mechanism of action of nifedipine. Using freshly dispersed human uterine myocytes from pregnant patients he identified T-type and L-type voltage-activated calcium currents in these cells. Nifedipine at 10^{-6} mol/L blocked the L-type but not the T-type currents, suggesting that the primary tocolytic effect of nifedipine may result from a decrease in the strength of contractions rather than in their frequency.

Clinical Efficacy

The initial experience with nifedipine as a tocolytic agent was reported in the 1980s by Ulmsten and colleagues.[112,123] In their first study, 10 patients were treated with the drug and all had uterine activity abolished for 3 days or more.[122] In 1984, Ulmsten[123] reported on 28 patients who were in preterm labor (8 of whom were also hypertensive). To be included in the study, the patients were required to have two or more uterine contractions within 10 minutes and to have an effaced cervix that was not dilated beyond 4 cm. In 80 percent of the patients, tocolysis was reported to be successful for 72 hours or longer. All 8 patients who had hypertension in addition to preterm labor became normotensive and were delivered beyond 38 weeks of gestation.

Read and Welby,[124] describing a nonrandomized group of patients who received nifedipine, ritodrine, or no tocolytic treatment, reported a significantly greater percentage of "postponement of delivery" (48 to 72 hours) in patients treated with nifedipine (15 of 20, 75 percent) as compared to those treated with ritodrine (9 of 20, 45 percent) or those who were untreated (7 of 20, 35 percent). In this study, patients were included for the treatment of preterm labor if they had contractions at a frequency of at least once every 10 minutes, their membranes were intact, and their cervix was not dilated beyond 4 cm. Three more recent studies have compared nifedipine to ritodrine or magnesium sulfate in a prospective randomized format.[11,125,126] Ferguson et al[11] prospectively randomized 64 patients at 20 to 36 weeks' gestation to receive either sublingual followed by oral nifedipine or intravenous followed by oral ritodrine. Preterm labor was defined as consisting of regular uterine contractions occurring at a frequency of eight or more per hour, with a documented change in cervical dilatation or effacement, before 36 weeks' gestational age. Patients receiving nifedipine for tocolysis were given a 10-mg capsule sublingually. If uterine contractions persisted after 20 minutes, a similar dose was repeated at intervals of 20 minutes to a maximal dose of 40 mg during the first hour of treatment. If sublingual nifedipine stopped uterine activity, oral therapy with 10 to 20 mg of nifedipine was initiated 6 hours after the last sublingual capsule. This dose was repeated at 4- to 6-hour intervals or, if needed to continue tocolysis, occasionally at more frequent intervals. Ritodrine was initiated at 50 μg/min and increased by 50 μg every 15 to 30 minutes, as previously reported.[127] Oral therapy (10 to 20 mg every 4 to 6 hours) was started 30 minutes before the discontinuation of intravenous ritodrine. Patients who had recurrent preterm labor while receiving oral nifedipine or ritodrine were treated sublingually or intravenously, respectively, with the same drug to which they had been randomized. If their uterine contractions stopped, the patients were again given their assigned oral tocolytic agents. Additionally, in 10 cases, patients who had persistent uterine contractions with progressive cervical dilatation or a maternal side effect requiring discontinuation of the tocolytic agent were switched to the other drug in an attempt to prevent delivery.

The goal of therapy was to delay delivery for 48 hours in patients with ruptured membranes, and to complete 36 weeks of gestation in patients whose membranes were intact. Therapy was considered successful in each respective group when delivery was delayed for these intervals. In patients with intact membranes, the ability of tocolysis to delay delivery for 1 week was also evaluated. Treatment failure was said to occur if uterine quiescence could not be achieved and delivery occurred despite maximal dosages of nifedipine or ritodrine, or if continued uterine contractions and cervical dilatation necessi-

tated the switching of a patient to the alternative therapy before the prescribed interval of tocolysis had been achieved. If the patient experienced a significant side effect that the attending obstetrician judged necessitated the discontinuation of the medication or a change to alternative therapy, or the patient experienced a spontaneous rupture of membranes, a treatment failure was said to have occurred.

Overall, there was no significant difference in the ability of nifedipine or ritodrine to delay delivery at 48 hours, 7 days, or 36 weeks. Nifedipine successfully delayed delivery in 27 of 32 patients (84 percent) for 48 hours, whereas ritodrine delayed delivery for the same period in 23 of 32 (72 percent) of patients (P = NS). At 7 days and 36 weeks, nifedipine was successful in delaying delivery in 16 of 23 (70 percent) and 9 of 22 (41 percent) of patients, respectively, compared with 17 of 27 (63 percent) and 14 of 27 (52 percent) in the ritodrine group (P = NS). Treatment failure occurred in 15 patients in the nifedipine group. In 5 instances, crossover therapy with intravenous and oral ritodrine was attempted, and further tocolysis was accomplished in 3 cases, but failed in the other 2. In the remaining 10 cases, no alternative agent was used, and delivery occurred in all 10 within 12 hours. There were 16 treatment failures in the ritodrine group. Crossover treatment with sublingual followed by oral nifedipine was attempted in 5 cases, and delivery was delayed in 3 of these cases for 50, 68, and 84 days, respectively. In the remaining 11 patients in whom no alternative agent was used, delivery occurred within 12 hours. Overall, the probability of delaying delivery beyond 48 hours was significantly greater in patients in whom crossover therapy with the alternative agent was attempted (P < 0.001) than in those in whom it was not used.

Meyer et al[125] treated 58 women in preterm labor (diagnosed as having either progressive cervical changes or regular uterine contractions numbering 6 within 30 minutes). The patients were randomly assigned to receive either ritodrine or nifedipine. Women treated with nifedipine received an initial oral dose of 30 mg followed by 20 mg PO every 6 hours during the first 24 hours, and 20 mg PO every 8 hours on the second day. On the third day, the dosage was reduced to 10 mg PO every 8 hours. Ritodrine was initiated at 50 μg/min and given according to standard protocols.[127] Among the 34 women assigned to receive nifedipine, tocolysis was successful (delay of delivery >48 hours) in 19 (56 percent), as compared with 10 (42 percent) of the 24 women who received ritodrine. These differences were not statistically significant. Tocolytic failures in each group were subsequently treated with magnesium sulfate, with an equal percentage (67 percent) of success. A recent study by Glock and Morales[126] compared the efficacy and safety of nifedipine versus magnesium sulfate in arresting preterm labor, and the efficacy of nifedipine versus terbutaline in preventing recurrent preterm labor. Thirty-nine patients were randomized to the nifedipine group and 41 to the magnesium sulfate group. The patients were generally comparable in terms of clinically significant entry variables. Those in the nifedipine group were initially treated as outlined previously by Ferguson and colleagues.[11] If sublingual tocolysis stopped uterine activity, 20 mg of nifedipine was initiated 4 hours after the last sublingual capsule and repeated every 4 hours for 48 hours. Patients were then treated with 10 mg of nifedipine orally every 8 hours until 34 weeks of pregnancy were completed. Patients randomized to receive magnesium sulfate were given a loading dose of 6 g IV over 30 minutes, followed by an infusion of 2 g/hr, increasing to a maximum of 4 g/hr as needed to arrest labor for 24 hours. Patients were weaned from the drugs after contractions had been arrested for 24 hours. When the rate of magnesium sulfate infusion was at 0.5 g/hr, 5 mg of oral terbutaline was administered and repeated every 6 hours until 34 weeks of pregnancy had been completed. In the nifedipine group, delivery was delayed for 2 or more days in 36 of 39 patients, for 34 weeks or more in 24 of 39 (62 percent) and for 37 weeks or more in 16 of 39 (41 percent). These differences were nonsignificant when similar comparisons were made with the group receiving ritodrine: 38 of 41 (93 percent), 28 of 41 (68 percent) and 17 of 41 (41 percent), respectively.

The studies described above verify the tocolytic efficacy of nifedipine. Overall, the ability of nifedipine to delay delivery appears to be comparable with, but not superior to, that of ritodrine and magnesium sulfate for acute tocolysis and ritodrine and terbutaline for long-term tocolysis. Additionally,

nifedipine can be used to delay delivery in patients with spontaneous rupture of membranes.

Recommended Protocol/Clinical Use

Different dosing regimens of nifedipine were used in the studies described above; there is no unanimity in the dose or timing of administration. Furthermore, no studies have compared differences in these factors in terms of efficacy or associated physiologic alterations or side effects.

Once the diagnosis of preterm labor has been made, the patient should receive a continuous intravenous infusion of crystalloid after a 200 to 500-ml fluid bolus. We favor the initiation of nifedipine tocolysis with a 10-mg capsule given sublingually (Table 16-1). The capsule can either be bitten into and held for buccal absorption or bitten and swallowed. If uterine contractions persist after 20 minutes, similar doses are repeated at intervals of 20 minutes to a maximum dose of 40 mg during the first hour of treatment. If sublingual treatment with nifedipine is successful in stopping uterine activity, oral therapy with 20 mg of nifedipine should be initiated 6 hours after the last sublingual capsule. This dose is repeated at 4 to 6 hour intervals or if needed to continue tocolysis, occasionally at more frequent intervals. If a patient has recurrent preterm labor while receiving oral nifedipine, it is reasonable to treat with a repeat sublingual dose. If that approach is ineffective, it is probably reasonable to employ sequential tocolysis with an alternative tocolytic agent. β-Adenergic agents are good choices for this, although one must be careful if magnesium sulfate is chosen, since profound hypotension has been documented when this agent and nifedipine are used concurrently.[128] Pharmacokinetic data have been obtained from patients receiving nifedipine, as previously described. Patients receiving sublingual nifedipine generally demonstrate increasing plasma concentrations after each successive dose of the drug.[129] The mean half-life (mean ± SD) of nifedipine, calculated from plasma concentrations obtained hourly after the last sublingual dose before the first oral dose, was 81 ± 26 minutes (range, 49 to 137 minutes). Following oral administration, mean serum concentrations were 7.2 ± 5.5 ng/ml. The plasma levels of the drug generally ranged from 1.5 to 21 ng/ml. If nifedipine is given more often than every 6 hours, some drug accumulation can occur. It can thus be appreciated that substantial interpatient variability exists in nifedipine levels, and that all therapies must be individualized.

Oxytocin Antagonists

Recently, a new class of polypeptide oxytocin antagonists has been under development in Europe and the United States as potential tocolytic agents.[130] These experimental agents represent a selective pharmacologic strategy for reducing preterm uterine contractility while limiting multiorgan side effects. Their potential specificity and lack of serious side effects make these agents attractive alternatives to currently available tocolytic agents. Phase III clinical trials of the first of these oxytocin antagonist agents, Atosiban (1-deamino-2-D-tyr-(OET)-4-thr-8-orn-vasotocin/oxytocin), have recently been initiated in the United States.

Oxytocin receptors significantly increase in numbers during the propagation of preterm labor,[30] and probably act as a common pathway in uterine activation. Administration of oxytocin antagonists in animal studies clearly demonstrates a decrease in the frequency and magnitude of uterine contractile activity.[131]

Preliminary human studies with atosiban have shown promising results in cases of early preterm labor.[132] Short-term administration of this oxytocin antagonist produced a significant decrease in uterine contraction frequency during a 2-hour infusion period. More exciting was the readily apparent lack of maternal symptomatology associated with this polypeptide infusion.

This class of tocolytic agents must be administered intravenously or subcutaneously because of the polypeptide nature.[130] No demonstrable changes in maternal heart rate, blood pressure, or urinary output are produced. Rare cases of nausea and hypersensitivity represent the only observed maternal side effects of these drugs to date. Transplacental transfer appears to be minimal, and the fetal/neonatal risks are thought to be minuscule.[130] This new class of high-specificity tocolytic agents offers great promise, although expanded clinical experimentation seems quite reasonable before promoting oxytocin antagonists as safe and effective tocolytic agents.

REFERENCES

1. National Center for Health Statistics: Vital Statistics of the United States, 1989, Vol. I, Natality. U.S. Department of Health and Human Services Publication No. (PHS)93-1100. U.S. Government Printing Office, Washington, DC, 1993
2. Copper RL, Goldenberg RL, Creasy RK et al: A multicenter study of preterm birth weight and gestational age-specific neonatal mortality. Am J Obstet Gynecol 168:78, 1993
3. Robertson PA, Sniderman SH, Laros RK et al: Neonatal morbidity according to gestational age and birth weight from five tertiary care centers in the United States, 1983 through 1986. Am J Obstet Gynecol 166:1629, 1992
4. Morrison JC: Preterm birth: a puzzle worth solving. Obstet Gynecol 76:5S, 1990
5. Leveno KJ, Little BB, Cunningham FG: The national impact of ritodrine hydrochloride for inhibition of preterm labor. Obstet Gynecol 76:12, 1990
6. Meis PJ, Ernest JM, Moore ML: Causes of low birthweight in public and private patients. Am J Obstet Gynecol 156:1165, 1987
7. Taslimi MM, Sibai BM, Amon E et al: A national survey on preterm labor. Am J Obstet Gynecol 160:1352, 1989
8. Zlatnik FJ: The applicability of labor inhibition to the problem of prematurity. Am J Obstet Gynecol 113:704, 1973
9. Higby K, Xenakis MJ, Pauerstein CJ: Do tocolytic agents stop preterm labor? A critical and comprehensive review of efficacy and safety. Am J Obstet Gynecol 168:1247, 1993
10. Besinger RE, Repke JT, Ferguson II JE: Preterm labor and intrauterine growth retardation: complex obstetrical problems with low birth weight infants. In Stevenson DK, Sunshine P (eds): Fetal and Neonatal Brain Injury: Mechanisms, Management and the Risks of Practice. B.C. Decker, Toronto, 1989
11. Ferguson JE, Dyson DC, Schutz T et al: A comparison of tocolysis with nifedipine or ritodrine: analysis of efficacy and maternal, fetal, and neonatal outcome. Am J Obstet Gynecol 163:105, 1990
12. Creasy RK, Herron MA: Prevention of preterm birth. Semin Perinatol 5:295, 1981
13. Armer TL, Duff P: Intraamniotic infection of patients with intact membranes and preterm labor. Obstet Gynecol Surv 46:589, 1991
14. Gravett MG, Hummel D, Eschenbach DA et al: Preterm labor associated with subclinical amniotic fluid infection with bacterial vaginosis. Obstet Gynecol 67:229, 1986

15. Romero R, Sirtori M, Oyarzun E et al: Infection and labor. V. Prevalence, microbiology, and clinical significance of intraamniotic infection in women with preterm labor and intact membranes. Am J Obstet Gynecol 161:817, 1989

16. Utter GO, Dooley SL, Tamura RK et al: Awaiting cervical change for the diagnosis of preterm labor does not compromise the efficacy of ritodrine tocolysis. Am J Obstet Gynecol 163:882, 1990

17. Keirse MJNC, Grant A, King JF: Preterm labour. p. 694 In Chalmers I, Enkin M, Keirse MJNC (eds): Effective Care in Pregnancy and Childbirth. Oxford University Press, New York, 1989

18. Lockwood CJ, Senyel AE, Dische MR et al: Fetal fibronectin in cervical and vaginal secretions as a predictor or preterm delivery. N Engl J Med 325:669, 1991

19. Creasy RK: Preterm birth prevention: where are we? Am J Obstet Gynecol 168:1223, 1993

20. King JF, Grant A, Keirse MJ, Chalmers I: Beta-mimetics in preterm labour: an overview of the randomized controlled trials. Br J Obstet Gynaecol 95:211, 1988

21. Morales WJ, Angel JL, O'Brien WF et al: A randomized study of antibiotic therapy in idiopathic preterm labor. Obstet Gynecol 72:829, 1988

22. Newton ER, Dinsmoor MJ, Gibbs RS: A randomized, blinded, placebo-controlled trial of antibiotics in idiopathic preterm labor. Obstet Gynecol 74:562, 1989

23. Romero R, Sibai B, Caritis S et al: Antibiotic treatment of preterm labor with intact membranes: a multicenter, randomized, double-blinded, placebo-controlled trial. Am J Obstet Gynecol 169:764, 1993

24. Romero R, Yoon BH, Kenney JS et al: Amniotic fluid interleukin-6 determinations are of diagnostic and prognostic value in preterm labor. Am J Reprod Immunol 30:167, 1993

25. NIH Consensus Development Panel: The effect of corticosteroids for fetal maturation on perinatal outcomes. JAMA 273:413, 1995

26. Parilla BV, Dooley SL, Minogue JP et al: The efficacy of oral terbutaline after intravenous tocolysis. Am J Obstet Gynecol 169:965, 1993

27. Bishop EH, Wouterxz TB: Isoxsuprine, a myometrial relaxant. Obstet Gynecol 17:442, 1961

28. Ritodrine approved for premature labor. FDA Bulletin 10:22, 1980

29. Petrie RH: Tocolysis using magnesium sulfate. Semin Perinatol 5:266, 1981

30. Carsten ME, Miller JD: A new look at uterine muscle contraction. Am J Obstet Gynecol 157:1303, 1987

31. Scheid CR, Honeyman TW, Fay FS: Mechanism of β-adrenergic relaxation of smooth muscle. Nature 277:32, 1979

32. Wesselius-de Casparis A, Thiery M, Sian A et al: Results of double-blind, multicentre study with ritodrine in premature labor. BMJ 3:144, 1971

33. Merkatz IR, Peter JB, Barden TP: Ritodrine hydrochloride: a betamimetic agent for use in preterm labor. II. Evidence of efficacy. Obstet Gynecol 56:7, 1980

34. Barden TP, Peter JB, Merkatz IR: Ritodrine hydrochloride: a betamimetic agent for use in preterm labor. Pharmacology, clinical history, administration, side-effects and safety. Obstet Gynecol 56:1, 1980

35. Spellacy WN, Cruz AC, Birk SA et al: Treatment of premature labor with ritodrine: a randomized controlled study. Obstet Gynecol 54:220, 1979

36. Larsen JF, Hansen MK, Hesseldahl H et al: Ritodrine in the treatment of preterm labor. A clinical trial to compare a standard treatment with three regimens involving the use of ritodrine. Br J Obstet Gynaecol 87:949, 1980

37. Larsen JF, Eldon K, Lange AP et al: Ritodrine in the treatment of preterm labor: second Danish multicenter study. Obstet Gynecol 67:607, 1986

38. Leveno KJ, Guzick DS, Hankins GD et al: Single-center randomized trial of ritodrine hydrochloride for preterm labor. Lancet 1:1293, 1986

39. Canadian Preterm Labor Investigation Group: Treatment of preterm labor with the beta-adrenergic agonist ritodrine. N Engl J Med 327:308, 1992

40. King JA, Grant A, Keirse MJNC: Betamimetics in preterm labor: an overview of randomized controlled trials. Br J Obstet Gynaecol 95:211, 1988

41. Price PH: Review of betamimetic drugs for tocolysis. Special report to FDA public meeting on re-evaluation of ritodrine labelling. October 28, 1992

42. Ingemarsson I: Effect of terbutaline on premature labor. A double-blind placebo-controlled study. Am J Obstet Gynecol 125:520, 1975

43. Howard TE Jr, Killam AP, Penney LL et al: A double blind randomized study of terbutaline in premature labor. Mil Med 147:305, 1982

44. Cotton DB, Strassner HT, Hill LM et al: Comparison of magnesium sulfate, terbutaline and a placebo for inhibition of preterm labor. A randomized study. J Reprod Med 29:92, 1984

45. Caritis SN, Toig G, Heddinger LS et al: A double-blind study comparing ritodrine and terbutaline in the treatment of preterm labor. Am J Obstet Gynecol 150:7, 1984

46. Kosasa TS, Nakayama RT, Hale RW et al: Ritodrine

and terbutaline compared for the treatment of preterm labor. Acta Obstet Gynecol Scand 64:421, 1985

47. Beall MH, Edgar BW, Paul RH et al: A comparison of ritodrine, terbutaline, and magnesium sulfate for the suppression of preterm labor. Am J Obstet Gynecol 153:854, 1985

48. Creasy RD, Golbus MS, Laros RD Jr: Oral ritodrine maintenance in the treatment of preterm labor. Am J Obstet Gynecol 137:212, 1980

49. Caritis SN, Lin LS, Venkataramanan R et al: Effect of pregnancy on ritodrine pharmacokinetics. Am J Obstet Gynecol 159:328, 1988

50. Smit DA, Essed GGM, deHaan J: Serum levels of ritodrine during oral maintenance therapy. Gynecol Obstet Invest 18:10, 1984

51. Lyrenas S, Grahnen A, Lindberg B et al: Pharmacokinetics of terbutaline during pregnancy. Eur J Clin Pharmacol 29:619, 1986

52. Gandar R, deZoeten LW, van der Schoot JB: Serum level of ritodrine in man. Eur J Clin Pharmacol 17:117, 1980

53. Bredholm B, Lunell NO, Persson B et al: Development of tolerance to the metabolic actions beta$_2$-adrenoceptor stimulating drugs. Acta Obstet Gynecol Scand Suppl 108:53, 1982

54. Berg G, Andersson RGG, Ryden G: Beta-adrenergic receptors in human myometrium during pregnancy: changes in the number of receptors after beta-mimetic treatment. Am J Obstet Gynecol 151:392, 1985

55. Berg G, Andersson RGG, Ryden G: Effects of selective beta-adrenergic agonists on spontaneous contraction, cAMP levels and phosphodiesterase activity in myometrial strips from pregnant women treated with terbutaline. Gynecol Obstet Invest 14:56, 1982

56. Caritis SN, Chiao JP, Kridgen P: Comparison of pulsatile and continuous ritodrine administration: effect on uterine contractility and beta-adrenergic receptor cascade. Am J Obstet Gynecol 164:1005, 1991

57. Benoy CJ, El-Fellah MS, Schneider R et al: Tolerance to sympathomimetic bronchodilators in guinea-pig isolated lungs following chronic administration in vivo. Br J Pharmacol 55:547, 1975

58. Ryden G, Anderson RGG, Berg G: Is the relaxing effect of beta-adrenergic agonists on the human myometrium only transitory? Acta Obstet Gynecol Scand Suppl 108:47, 1982

59. Casper RF, Lye SJ: Myometrial desensitization to continuous but not to intermittent beta-adrenergic agonist infusion in the sheep. Am J Obstet Gynecol 154:301, 1986

60. Fischer JR, Kaatz BL: Continuous subcutaneous infusion of terbutaline for suppression of preterm labor. Clin Pharm 10:292, 1991

61. Lam F, Gill P, Smith M et al: Use of subcutaneous terbutaline pump for long-term tocolysis. Obstet Gynecol 72:810, 1988

62. Caritis SN, Lin LS, Toig G et al: Pharmacodynamics of ritodrine in pregnant women during preterm labor. Am J Obstet Gynecol 147:752, 1983

63. Gross TL, Kuhnert BR, Kuhnert PM et al: Maternal and fetal plasma concentrations of ritodrine. Obstet Gynecol 65:793, 1985

64. Schreyer P, Caspi E, Snir E: Metabolic effects of intramuscular and oral administration of ritodrine during pregnancy. Obstet Gynecol 57:730, 1981

65. Gonik B, Benedetti T, Creasy RK et al: Intramuscular versus intravenous ritodrine hydrochloride for preterm labor management. Am J Obstet Gynecol 159:323, 1988

66. Caritis SN: A pharmacologic approach to the infusion of ritodrine. Am J Obstet Gynecol 158:380, 1988

67. Stubblefield PG, Heyl PS: Treatment of premature labor with subcutaneous terbutaline. Obstet Gynecol 59:457, 1982

68. Haspedis L: Terbutaline in the treatment of preterm labor: a comparison of intravenous and subcutaneous administration. J Am Osteopath Assoc 88:489, 1988

69. Leferink JG, Lamont H, Giebel R et al: Pharmacokinetics of terbutaline after subcutaneous administration. Int J Clin Pharmacol Biopharm 17:189, 1979

70. Hill WC: Overdosage of subcutaneous terbutaline in the treatment of preterm labor. Nebr Med J 71:242, 1986

71. Kopelman JN, Duff P, Read JA: Randomized comparison of oral terbutaline and ritodrine in preventing recurrent preterm labor. J Reprod Med 34:225, 1989

72. Hall DG, McGaughery HS, Corey EL et al: The effect of magnesium therapy on the duration of labor. Am J Obstet Gynecol 78:27, 1959

73. Stallworth JC, Yeh SY, Petrie AH: Effect of magnesium sulfate on fetal heart rate variability and uterine activity. Am J Obstet Gynecol 140:702, 1981

74. Guiet-Bara A, Bara M, Durlach J: Comparative study of the effect of two tocolytic agents (magnesium sulfate and alcohol) on the ionic transfer through the isolated human amnion. Eur J Obstet Gynecol Reprod Biol 20:297, 1985

75. Steer CM, Petrie RH: A comparison of magnesium sulfate and alcohol for the prevention of premature labor. Am J Obstet Gynecol 129:1, 1977

76. Cox SM, Sherman ML, Leveno KJ: Randomized in-

vestigation of magnesium sulfate for prevention of preterm birth. Am J Obstet Gynecol 163:767, 1990

77. Tchilinguirian MG, Majem R, Sullivan GB et al: The use of ritodrine and magnesium sulfate in the arrest of premature labor. Int J Gynaecol Obstet 22:117, 1984

78. Hollander DI, Nagey DA, Pupkin MJ: Magnesium sulfate and ritodrine hydrochloride: A randomized comparison. Am J Obstet Gynecol 156:631, 1987

79. Miller JM Jr, Keane MWD, Horger EO III: A comparison of magnesium sulfate and terbutaline for the arrest of premature labor. A preliminary report. J Reprod Med 27:348, 1982

80. Martin RW, Gaddy DK, Martin JN Jr et al: Tocolysis with oral magnesium. Am J Obstet Gynecol 156:433, 1987

81. Martin RW, Martin JN Jr, Pryor JA et al: Comparison of oral ritodrine and magnesium gluconate for ambulatory tocolysis. Am J Obstet Gynecol 158:1440, 1988

82. Ridgeway LE, Muise K, Wright JW et al: A prospective randomized comparison of oral terbutaline and magnesium oxide for the maintenance of tocolysis. Am J Obstet Gynecol 163:879, 1990

83. Madden C, Owens J, Hauth JC: Magnesium tocolysis: serum levels versus success. Am J Obstet Gynecol 162: 1177, 1990

84. Ogburn PJ, Hansen CA, Williams PP et al: Magnesium sulfate and beta-mimetic dual-agent tocolysis in preterm labor after single-agent therapy. J Reprod Med 30:583, 1985

85. Valenzuela G, Cline S: Use of magnesium sulfate in premature labor that fails to respond to beta-mimetic drugs. Am J Obstet Gynecol 143:718, 1982

86. Hatjis CG, Swain M, Nelson LH et al: Efficacy of combined administration of magnesium sulfate and ritodrine in the treatment of premature labor. Obstet Gynecol 69:317, 1987

87. Cruikshank DP, Pitkins RM, Donnelly E et al: Urinary magnesium, calcium and phosphate excretion during magnesium sulfate infusion. Obstet Gynecol 58: 430, 1981

88. Lewis RB, Schulman JD: Influence of acetylsalicylic acid, an inhibitor of prostaglandin synthesis on the duration of human gestation and labor. Lancet 2: 1159, 1973

89. Collins E, Turner GF: Salicylates and pregnancy. Lancet 2:1494, 1973

90. Reiss U, Atad J, Rubinstein I et al: The effect of indomethacin in labor at term. Int J Gynaecol Obstet 14: 369, 1976

91. Weitz CM, Ghondgaonkar RB, Dubin NH et al: Pros-

taglandin F metabolite concentration as a prognostic factor in preterm labor. Obstet Gynecol 67:496, 1986

92. Dubin NH, Johnson JWC, Calhoun S et al: Plasma prostaglandin in pregnant women with term and preterm deliveries. Obstet Gynecol 57:203, 1981

93. Niebyl JR: Prostaglandin synthetase inhibitors, Semin Perinatol 5:274, 1981

94. Repke JT, Neibyl JR: Role of prostaglandin synthetase inhibitors in the treatment of preterm labor. Semin Reprod Endocrinol 3:259, 1985

95. Johnson WC, Harbert GM Jr, Martin CB: Pharmacologic control of uterine contractility. Am J Obstet Gynecol 123:364, 1975

96. Garrioch DB: The effect of indomethacin on spontaneous activity in the isolated human myometrium and on the response to oxytocin and prostaglandin. Br J Obstet Gynaecol 85:47, 1978

97. Zuckerman JH, Reiss U, Atad J et al: The effect of indomethacin on plasma levels of prostaglandin F_{2a} in women in labor. Br J Obstet Gynaecol 84:339, 1977

98. Wiqvist N, Lundstrom V, Green K: Premature labor and indomethacin. Prostaglandins 10:515, 1975

99. Niebyl JR, Blake DA, White RD et al: The inhibition of premature labor with indomethacin. Am J Obstet Gynecol 136:1014, 1980

100. Karin SMM, Devlin J: Prostaglandin content of amniotic fluid during pregnancy and labor. J Obstet Gynaecol Br Commonw 74:230, 1967

101. Fuchs AR, Husslein R, Sumulong L et al: Plasma levels of oxytocin and 13, 14-dihydro-15-keto prostaglandin F_{2a} in preterm labor and the effect of ethanol and ritodrine. Am J Obstet Gynecol 144:753, 1982

102. Zuckerman H, Reiss U, Rubinstein I: Inhibition of human premature labor by indomethacin. Obstet Gynecol 44:787, 1974

103. Zuckerman H, Shalev E, Gilad G et al: Further study of the inhibition of premature labor by indomethacin. Part I. Clinical experience. J Perinat Med 12:19, 1984

104. Zuckerman H, Shalev E, Gilad G et al: Further study of the inhibition of premature labor by indomethacin. Part II. Double-blind study. J Perinat Med 12: 25, 1984

105. Morales WJ, Smith SG, Angel JL et al: Efficacy and safety of indomethacin versus ritodrine in the management of preterm labor: a randomized study. Obstet Gynecol 74:567, 1989

106. Besinger RE, Niebyl JR, Keyes WG et al: Randomized comparative trial of indomethacin and ritodrine for the long-term treatment of preterm labor. Am J Obstet Gynecol 164:981, 1991

107. Bivins HA, Newman RB, Fyfe DA et al: Randomized

trial of oral indomethacin and terbutaline sulfate for the long-term suppression of preterm labor. Am J Obstet Gynecol 169:1065, 1993

108. Spearing G: Alcohol, indomethacin, and salbutamol. Obstet Gynecol 53:171, 1979

109. Gamissans O, Canas E, Cararach V et al: A study of indomethacin combined with ritodrine in threatened preterm labor. Eur J Obstet Gynecol Reprod Biol 8: 123, 1978

110. Katz Z, Lancet M, Yemini M et al: Treatment of premature labor contractions with combined ritodrine and indomethacin. Int J Gynaecol Obstet 21:337, 1983

111. Alvan G, Orme M, Bertilsson L et al: Pharmacokinetics of indomethacin. Clin Pharm Ther 18:364, 1975

112. Bhat R, Vidyasagar D, Vadapalli MD et al: Disposition of indomethacin in preterm infants. J Pediatr 95:313, 1976

113. Moise KJ, Ching-Nan O, Kirshon B et al: Placental transfer of indomethacin in the human pregnancy. Am J Obstet Gynecol 162:549, 1990

114. Ferguson II, Bruns ME, Bruns DE: Calcium channel blockers: role in preterm labor tocolysis. p. 241. In Parsons MT (ed): Clinical Consultations in Obstetrics and Gynecology. Vol. 3 WB Saunders, Philadelphia, 1991

115. Batra SC, Popper LD: Characterization of membrane calcium channels in nonpregnant and pregnant human uterus. Gynecol Obstet Invest 27:57, 1989

116. Forman A, Andersson KE, Persson CGA et al: Relaxant effects of nifedipine of isolated, human myometrium. Acta Pharmacol Toxicol 45:81, 1979

117. Ulmsten U, Andersson KE: Multichannel intrauterine pressure recording by means of microtransducers. Acta Obstet Gynecol Scand 58:115, 1979

118. Ulmsten U, Andersson KE, Forman A: Relaxing effects of nifedipine on the nonpregnant human uterus in vitro and in vivo. Obstet Gynecol 52:436, 1978

119. Andersson KE, Ingemarrson I, Ulmsten U et al: Inhibition of prostaglandin-induced uterine activity by nifedipine. Br J Obstet Gynaecol 86:175, 1979

120. Forman A, Gandrup P, Andersson KE et al: Effects of nifedipine on oxytocin- and prostaglandin F_2 alpha-induced activity in the postpartum uterus. Am J Obstet Gynecol 144:665, 1982

121. Young RC, Smith LH, McLaren MD: T-type and L-type calcium currents in freshly dispersed human uterine smooth muscle cells. Am J Obstet Gynecol 169:785, 1993

122. Ulmsten U, Andersson KE, Wingerup L: Treatment of premature labor with the calcium antagonist nifedipine. Arch Gynecol 229:1, 1980

123. Ulmsten U: Treatment of normotensive and hypertensive patients with preterm labor using oral nifedipine, a calcium antagonist. Arch Gynecol 236:69, 1984

124. Read MD, Welby DE: The use of a calcium antagonist (nifedipine) to suppress preterm labor. Br J Obstet Gynaecol 98:933, 1986

125. Meyer WR, Randall HW, Graves WL: Nifedipine versus ritodrine for suppressing preterm labor. J Reprod Med 35:649, 1990

126. Glock JL, Morales WJ: Efficacy and safety of nifedipine versus magnesium sulfate in the management of preterm labor: a randomized study. Am J Obstet Gynecol 169:960, 1993

127. Ferguson JE II, Hensleigh PA, Kredenster D: Adjunctive use of magnesium sulfate with ritodrine for preterm labor tocolysis. Am J Obstet Gynecol 148:166, 1984

128. Snyder SW, Cardwell MS: Neuromuscular blockade with magnesium sulfate and nifedipine. Am J Obstet Gynecol 161:35, 1989

129. Ferguson JE II, Schutz T, Pershe R et al: Nifedipine pharmacokinetics during preterm labor tocolysis. Am J Obstet Gynecol 161:1485, 1989

130. Melin P: Oxytocin antagonist in preterm labor and delivery, review. Baillieres Clin Obstet Gynecol 7: 577, 1993

131. Wilson L, Parsons MT, Ouano L et al: A new tocolytic agent: Development of an oxytocin antagonist for inhibiting uterine contractions. Am J Obstet Gynecol 163:195, 1990

132. Goodwin TM, Paul R, Silver H et al: The effect of oxytocin antagonist atosiban on preterm uterine activity in the human. Am J Obstet Gynecol 170:474, 1994

133. Elliott J: Magnesium sulfate as a tocolytic agent. Am J Obstet Gynecol 147:277, 1983

Consequences of Tocolysis: Maternal, Fetal, and Neonatal Effects

Richard E. Besinger and James E. Ferguson II

Modern tocolytic therapy presents a pharmacologic dilemma to the practicing obstetrician. Current scientific evidence suggests that aggressive tocolysis has some degree of measurable success and clinical utility in the treatment of preterm labor. Varying classes of tocolytic agents have been evaluated and accepted for contemporary clinical use. Chapter 16 outlines the varying mechanisms of action of these drugs and provides safe clinical protocols for their administration. However, expanded clinical experience with these powerful pharmacologic agents has raised new issues of maternal-fetal-neonatal safety.

Most modern tocolytic agents carry inherent risks of undesirable side effects through their nonselective pharmacologic action on other maternal or fetal organs. Any perceived risks to the mother or fetus from these interventions must be balanced against the potential for improved perinatal outcome in the face of a possible preterm birth. It is critical that the prescribing physician be aware of the potential risks and benefits of the tocolytic agents if they are to be used effectively and safely in the clinical setting. The purpose of this chapter is to review the potential adverse consequences of tocolytic therapy and to promote vigilance for tocolytic-induced complications on the part of the obstetric practioner. The application of the concept of primum non nocere to this important clinical problem seems prudent and humane.

β-ADRENERGIC TOCOLYTIC AGENTS

Maternal Physiologic Effects

Intravenous β-mimetic agents stimulate β-receptors in multiple organ systems and can produce a wide range of clinically significant side effects.[1,2] Under most clinical conditions, even selective β-mimetic agents activate both β_1 and β_2 receptors. This produces marked physiologic changes in the maternal cardiovascular system, including hypotension, tachycardia, and arrhythmia. Therefore, the use of β-mimetic tocolytic agents in patients with intravascular depletion secondary to hemorrhage or dehydration can produce profound maternal and fetal effects.

The activation of vascular β_2-adrenergic receptors leads to generalized vasodilation resulting in diastolic hypotension.[3] Physiologic consequences of β-mimetic administration include a compensatory increase in heart rate, stroke volume, cardiac output, and systolic blood pressure.[4] Maternal cardiac output during β-mimetic therapy can be increased 40 to 60 percent over basal levels.[4,5] β-mimetic tocolysis produces a marked increase in left ventricular contraction velocity with no significant evidence of cardiac failure or change in cardiac chamber dimensions.[4-6] Direct inotropic and chronotropic cardiac effects can also be attributed to the β-mimetic agents.[6] Given these pronounced alterations in cardiac function, β-mimetic tocolysis should not even be considered for patients with inherent cardiac compromise. Clinical use of these powerful cardiac stimulants may unmask asymptomatic cardiac disease in the pregnant patient.[1,7–12]

The β-mimetic agents also affect the minute-to-minute function of the peripheral vascular system. Use of selective $β_2$-adrenergic agents should lessen the degree of peripheral vasodilation and resultant hypotension. Notwithstanding this, tocolysis with intravenous ritodrine or terbutaline produces a significant decrease in diastolic blood pressure and peripheral vascular resistance.[13,14] Mean arterial pressures remain relatively unchanged because of increased systolic pressures attributable to increased cardiac output.[14] With intravenous infusions of terbutaline in late pregnancy, decreases in serum aldosterone levels are observed, with corresponding increases in serum renin and angiotensin II levels.[14,15]

The other major category of physiologic alterations produced by β-mimetic tocolytic agents are fluctuations in glucose, insulin, potassium, and lactic acid metabolism. Parenteral administration results in an acute increase in the plasma glucose concentration.[16] This phenomenon is mediated by direct β-adrenergic stimulation of the maternal pancreas to secrete glucagon, which in turn results in gluconeogenesis and glycogenolysis.[16] An initial insulin release from the maternal pancreas apparently precedes the onset of tocolytic-induced hyperglycemia.[17] Thereafter, serum insulin levels parallel the level of maternal hyperglycemia. Profound hypoglycemia following discontinuation of high-dose ritodrine has been described in fasting individuals.[18] These dramatic metabolic alterations are commonly seen with intravenous, intramuscular, and subcutaneous administration of these tocolytic agents.

The effects of orally administered β-mimetic agents on blood glucose levels is less clear. Oral administration of maintenance doses does not appear to cause overt hyperglycemia.[19] However, chronic administration of β-mimetic agents has been associated with maternal glucose intolerance. This effect is probably mediated by glucagon release and diminished insulin sensitivity during pregnancy.[20] Terbutaline produces the most obvious alteration in glucose tolerance.[20,21] However, this is not necessarily

the case with chronic oral ritodrine therapy.[22] The glucose intolerance associated with terbutaline is transient and generally resolves with discontinuation of oral therapy.[21] It therefore seems prudent that patients receiving chronic oral β-mimetic therapy be screened for the presence of existing or new-onset gestational diabetes.

The haphazard administration of β-mimetic tocolytic agents to insulin-dependent diabetic patients can precipitate diabetic ketoacidosis.[23] Diabetic patients receiving β-mimetic tocolytic agents have a significantly greater increase in serum glucose, lactate, and free fatty acids than do nondiabetic patients.[24] The degree of metabolic alteration in the insulin-dependent patient seems to parallel the severity of insulin deficiency.[24] This potentially hazardous situation can be controlled with concurrent intravenous insulin administration.[24–26] The greatest potential risk in administering β-mimetic tocolytic agents probably occurs in the unrecognized insulin-dependent diabetic patient.[27] Consequently, it is prudent to follow serum glucose and urinary ketone levels serially in patients receiving intravenous β-mimetic therapy. Intravenous insulin therapy should be instituted in those individuals with evidence of significant hyperglycemia (>200 mg%).

β-Mimetic stimulation also leads to significant increases in glycogenolysis and lipolysis. These changes result in enhanced lactate production, which parallels the alterations in blood glucose levels and produces a dramatic increase in serum lactate levels.[28–30] In the absence of glucose intolerance, significant changes in maternal serum pH do not occur.[28] However, β-mimetic-induced acidosis has been reported in nondiabetic pregnancies.[30] Whereas serial determinations of maternal serum pH are probably not warranted during tocolysis, closer evaluation of normoglycemia and ketosis during tocolysis may be indicated.

Significant and rapid shifts in serum potassium concentrations occur in patients receiving β-mimetic agents parenterally for tocolysis.[17,31,32] A maximal decline in serum potassium of 0.6 to 1.5 mEq below preinfusion values occurs approximately 2 to 3 hours after initiation of therapy.[31,32] After 10 to 20 hours of continuous infusion, the serum potassium concentration tends to normalize.[17,32] Parenteral administration of β-mimetic agents does not significantly increase the urinary excretion of potassium[33] or alter aldosterone-mediated potassium urinary losses.[34] The observed shifts in serum potassium parallel the alterations in glucose homeostasis. It appears that extracellular potassium is actually transported into an intracellular location during glucose and insulin translocation.[32,35] Although this mechanism of potassium transport clearly exists, direct β-adrenergic receptor stimulation resulting in transport of potassium across cellular membranes may also be important.[31] Orally administered β-mimetic agents do not significantly alter potassium metabolism.[19]

Because total body potassium is apparently not decreased with β-mimetic tocolysis, potassium replacement is rarely necessary during treatment with these drugs. However, intravenous potassium replacement should be considered when serum potassium levels drop below 2.0 mEq/L, a cardiac arrhythmia is present, or furosemide is administered. Reduced serum levels of calcium and magnesium have also been noted with parenteral β-mimetic tocolysis,[36] although the clinical significance of this remains unclear.

Central nervous system stimulation, manifesting as tremors, is a common physiologic occurrence during β-mimetic tocolysis.[37] In general, the tremors are benign and their severity decreases with continued physiologic adaptation.

Maternal Side Effects

Cardiac arrhythmias have been commonly reported with β-adrenergic tocolytic therapy. The most commonly observed electrocardiographic (ECG) abnormality is supraventricular tachycardia.[38–43] Other common β-mimetic-induced cardiac arrhythmias include atrial fibrillation,[41] atrial premature contractions,[41] ventricular ectopy,[41] and ventricular tachyarrhythmias.[44–48] Cases of potentiation of these adverse cardiac effects by general anesthesia[44] and antiarrythmic agents[45] have been anecdotally described. Maternal sinus bradycardia following discontinuation of chronic ritodrine therapy, presumably as a result of β-receptor downregulation, has also been described.[47] In general, palpitations or chest pain (or both) are not temporally associated with these rhythm abnormalities. The electrocardiac alterations seen during β-mimetic tocolysis are frequently missed with routine monitoring meth-

---

Maternal Risks of Potential β-Mimetic-Specific Complications

Cardiovascular
  Cardiac stimulation
  Tachycardia
  Peripheral vasodilation
  Hypotension
  Cardiac arrhythmia
  Myocardial ischemia
  Pulmonary edema
  Sodium/water retention

Metabolic
  Hyperglycemia
  Hyperinsulinemia
  Hypoglycemia
  Glucosee intolerance
  Hyperlactacidemia
  Hypokalemia
  Hypocalcemia
  Hypomagnesemia
  Diabetic ketoacidosis
  Euglycemic acidosis

Neuromuscular
  Central nervous system stimulation
  Tremor
  Cerebral vasospasm/ischemia
  Neuromuscular alterations

Other
  Altered thyroid function
  Elevated transaminase levels
  Agranulocytosis
  Bone marrow suppression
  Salivary gland enlargement
  Erythema multiforme
  Hemolytic anemia
  Cutaneous vasculitis

Multifactorial maternal death
  Pulmonary edema
  Unrecognized cardiac disease
  Underlying cardiac arrhythmia
  Hyperthyroid crisis

ods.[41,43] Continuous ECG monitoring of the symptomatic patient receiving intravenous β-mimetic therapy may be required to identify significant cardiac arrhythmias. A maternal death clearly attributable to the precipitation of an unrecognized malignant cardiac arrythmia has been reported.[48]

The degree of cardiac stimulation produced by the β-mimetic class of tocolytics may ultimately unmask asymptomatic cardiopulmonary disease. β-mimetic-induced increases in cardiac work may lead to cardiac decompensation manifesting as pulmonary edema, decreased systemic perfusion, or hypoxia. Multiple cases of unrecognized cardiomyopathy,[7-10] atrial myoma,[11] valvular disease,[1,7,12] and pulmonary hypertension[7] have been recognized during tocolysis with these cardiac stimulating agents.

Clinical suspicion of myocardial ischemia has also been reported in association with intravenous β-mimetic tocolysis. However, although chest pain is a relatively common maternal symptom during β-mimetic therapy, relatively few authors have reported ECG changes indicative of myocardial ischemia.[38,49-52] Transient ST-segment depression appears most commonly,[38,53-57] appears to be dose related,[50,54,55] and usually resolves with discontinuation of therapy. Because ST-segment depression has been reversed in some patients with the administration of sublingual nitroglycerin, it has been suggested that inadequate coronary blood flow may be responsible.[49] Subclinical myocardial damage, as evidenced by elevated levels of cardiac enzymes or cardiac-specific myoglobin, has not been described in these patients.[51-53] Similarly, the apparent lack of correlation between the timing of patients' symptoms and electrophysiologic alterations suggests an alternative explanation.[54,55] Closer analysis of these ECG alterations in patients receiving intravenous ritodrine, using paired serial ECGs and serum electrolyte measurements, suggests that most of the electrophysiologic findings can be attributed to ritodrine-induced hypokalemia and tachycardia.[55] Other investigators have discounted this supposition.[56] A more intriguing hypothesis is that β-mimetic-induced ST-segment depression represents only a physiologic adaptation to a high prevalence of pretreatment ECG alterations in patients treated with these drugs.[57] In all probability, the ECG criteria for discontinuation of β-mimetic tocolytic therapy need to be reassessed. Nonetheless, ST-segment depression associated with chest pain is an indication to reduce or discontinue the β-mimetic therapy.

Pulmonary edema represents the most common maternal cardiovascular complication attributable to intravenous β-mimetic therapy for tocolysis. A significant controversy exists about the actual incidence of this complication, with estimates ranging from 0.01 to 9.0 percent.[58,59] In 1981, an original estimate of 5 percent of such edema with intravenous terbutaline was reported in twin pregnancies.[38] Reputable authors have recently published incidences as high as 3 to 9 percent[60] on the basis of a limited number of clinical references.[38,61,62] These alarming estimates, one would lead one to expect approximately 3,000 to 9,000 cases of tocolytic-induced pulmonary edema in the United States each year.[58] A recent survey of practicing perinatologists suggests that this complication is common, with 68 percent of respondents stating that they had encountered this particular complication.[63] Approximately 120 documented cases of β-mimetic-induced pulmonary edema have been reported in the literature to date.[2] Despite the inherent difficulties in establishing a definite rate of this life-threatening complication, a more realistic estimate of 1 case per 350 to 400 treated patients can be derived from the existing obstetric literature.[59,64] This estimate seems to parallel the incidence of only one case of pulmonary edema in 352 patients treated with β-mimetic agents in the largest clinical trial of these agents to date.[65]

Pulmonary edema can occur at any time during β-mimetic tocolytic therapy, but has occurred during antepartum treatment in most cases. Pulmonary edema induced by β-mimetic agents has occurred with and without concurrent glucocorticoid therapy for accelerated fetal lung maturation, suggesting that the contribution of steroids with low mineralocorticoid activity is minimal. The presence of a positive fluid balance in excess of 3 to 5 L is almost universal in reported cases. Multiple gestation, anemia, hypertension, renal disease, saline infusions, unrecognized pre-eclampsia, prolonged therapy, need for a blood transfusion, and multiple-drug regimens all appear to be clinical risk factors for the development of pulmonary edema during β-mimetic tocolysis.[7]

The pathophysiology of β-mimetic-induced pulmonary edema has still not been well delineated. Initially, this complication was thought to be secondary to cardiac dysfunction and to result from excessive myocardial stimulation. However, neither noninvasive nor invasive studies of cardiac function have been able to document myocardial failure in patients with a normal cardiac history.[5,6] Possible noncardiogenic causes of β-mimetic-induced pulmonary edema include increased pulmonary capillary permeability or hydrostatic pressures (or both) from fluid overload. An antidiuretic effect of β-mimetic agents, with sodium and water retention mediated by activation of the renin-aldosterone system during tocolysis, has been described in humans.[15,66–68] A combination of fluid retention,[15,66,67] decreased colloid pressures,[68,69] and increased capillary pressures[13,62,69] associated with intravenous β-mimetic tocolysis appears to be the major factor in development of this dangerous pulmonary complication. A provocative association between maternal infections during tocolysis and subsequent pulmonary edema resulting from altered capillary permeability deserves further investigation.[62] Regardless of its etiology, the liberal use of saline infusions during tocolysis may predispose a patient to this complication.[70] To confuse issues further, a case of pulmonary edema during oral tocolysis only has been described.[71]

Irrespective of the pathophysiology of this life-threatening complication, initial treatment for edema occurring during β-mimetic tocolytic therapy should include discontinuation of tocolytic therapy, oxygen administration, upright positioning of the patient, and attempted diuresis with furosemide. The presence of persistent hypoxia should prompt the initiation of invasive hemodynamic monitoring and preparations to provide ventilatory support with continuous positive airway pressure. Based on the supposition that tocolytic-induced pulmonary edema is noncardiogenic, it is doubtful that the use of cardiac glycosides would be helpful in the management of affected patients.

It seems most appropriate to avoid pulmonary edema in patients undergoing β-mimetic tocolysis, particularly in cases in which aggressive and prolonged treatment may be in progress. Recommendations for this include limiting intravenous fluid to 2 L of 5 percent dextrose in water or quarter-normal saline solution over each 24-hour period, minimizing the total time during which the patient receives intravenous β-mimetic tocolytic therapy, avoidance of transfusions during intravenous tocolysis, and choosing alternative tocolytic agents in patients with severe anemia, twin gestation, or hypertension. Careful monitoring of fluid intake and output, frequent chest examinations, and pulse oximetry may help to identify those individuals destined to develop this life-threatening complication.

Approximately 25 maternal deaths have been reported following the administration of β-mimetic therapy over the past two decades.[2,7] More disconcerting is that 5.1 percent of perinatologists responding to a national survey have encountered maternal mortality attributable to β-mimetic tocolytic therapy.[63] Most of the reported maternal deaths resulted from intractable pulmonary edema. Pre-existing medical conditions, such as cardiomyopathy, pulmonary hypertension, fatal arrythmia, uncontrolled hypertension, sickle cell crisis, and cardiac aneurysm have also contributed to these mortalities. Other maternal deaths have been associated with Gram-negative sepsis, pulmonary embolism, and hyperkalemia. These tragic cases point to the importance of pretreatment screening of pregnant patients for cardiopulmonary disease, minimizing iatrogenic β-mimetic-induced pulmonary edema, and careful observation for complications during β-mimetic tocolytic therapy.

The possibility of β-mimetic-induced cerebral vasospasm has recently been raised. Initially, this side effect was reported in patients with pre-existing migraine syndrome.[72] More recently, reports of this reversible phenomenon have been documented in normal patients without antecedent histories of migraine headaches.[73] Exacerbation of pre-existing neuromuscular disease by β-mimetic tocolysis has also been described in patients with myasthenia gravis[74] and myotonic dystrophy.[75]

Altered thyroid function has also been described with β-mimetic tocolysis.[76] Significant increases in circulating triiodothyronine (T_3) concentrations have been observed without changes in free thyroxine or thyroid-stimulating hormone. While there are no reports to date of an exacerbation of unrecognized hyperthyroidism by β-mimetic tocolysis, the theoretical concern for this possibility still exists.

Other significant maternal side effects described

with the use of β-mimetic agents for tocolysis include transient increases in maternal serum transaminase,[77] paralytic ileus,[78] drug-induced agranulocytosis,[79] hemolytic anemia,[80] and drug-induced vasculitis.[80,81]

Fetal-Neonatal Side Effects

Placental transfer of β-mimetic tocolytic agents produces a stimulated β-adrenergic state in the exposed fetus. Development of fetal tachycardia is readily apparent with β-mimetic therapy[82,83] and is presumably due to direct β-adrenergic stimulation of the fetal myocardium. Originally, no pathologic arrhythmias were noted in short-term fetal ECGs recorded during β-mimetic infusion.[82,83] However, several cases of fetal tachyarrhythmias in utero have recently been described in association with β-mimetic tocolysis.[84,85]

Fetal-Neonatal Risks of Potential β-Mimetic-Specific Complications

Cardiac
  Cardiac stimulation
  Tachycardia
  Bradycardia
  Cardiac arrhythima
  Peripheral vasodilation
  Myocardial ischemia
  Septal hypertrophy
  Myocardial necrosis
  Cardiovascular decompensation
  Altered uteroplacental blood flow
  Exacerbation of fetal hypoxia

Metabolic
  Hyperglycemia
  Hypoglycemia
  Hyperinsulinemia
  Hypocalcemia
  Hyperbilirubinemia
  Hyercholesterolemia

Other
  Intraventricular hemorrhage
  Renal insufficiency
  Leukemoid reaction

Recent noninvasive evaluations of human fetal hemodynamics during β-mimetic tocolysis suggest that drug-induced increases in heart rate and contractility serve to augment cardiac output and increase peripheral blood flow.[86,87] No significant changes in other functional cardiac parameters or chamber size occur as a result of β-mimetic therapy.[87] Blood flow through the fetal aorta increases as a result of increased cardiac output without significant central vasodilation, while cerebral and renal vessels exhibit peripheral vasodilation.[87]

Initial concerns for fetal cardiac toxicity were raised with reports of myocardial lipid necrosis based on isolated clinical cases[88–90] and in vitro animal models.[88,90] This complication has been observed by some investigators[89] but not by others[90,91] at the time of neonatal autopsy in infants exposed to β-mimetic agents in utero. The controversy has resurfaced with the recent report of a case involving similar histologic findings associated with long-term subcutaneous terbutaline pump therapy.[92] The isolated cases of fetal hydrops, cardiac failure, and myocardial infarction in fetuses of mothers given β-mimetic tocolytic therapy may represent β-mimetic cardiac toxicity caused by catecholamine overload, myocardial ischemia, and altered myocardial calcium regulation.[93] Other authors believe that these worrisome cases are isolated, and that β-mimetic stimulation of the fetal myocardium is minimal owing to the relative immaturity of fetal-neonatal sympathetic innervation.[94]

Cardiac stimulation may also be responsible for the observation of ventricular septal hypertrophy in chronically exposed fetuses.[95] This morphometric effect correlated with the duration of maternal therapy and resolved approximately 3 months after birth.[95] This provocative finding has been attributable to direct myocardial stimulation[93] or fetal hyperinsulinemia,[96] both of which have been observed in offspring of diabetic mothers treated with β-mimetic agents.[97]

In general, uteroplacental blood flow is increased with β-mimetic tocolysis.[98–100] The waveforms of umbilical Doppler ultrasonograms show varying degrees of decreased uteroplacental resistance during such therapy.[99,100] Ritodrine infusion stimulates the production of vasodilatory prostacyclin,[99] which is a major modulator of uteroplacental circulation.[101] While this has been shown to have a beneficial fetal effect in cases of intrauterine growth retardation (IUGR) and chronic hypertension,[98] recent experimental data in a hypoxic animal model suggests a significant risk of fetal decompensation or death with β-mimetic infusions.[102]

Clinical evidence supports the use of acute β-mimetic tocolysis for fetal resuscitation during intrapartum fetal distress.[103,104] A significant improvement in fetal pH following subcutaneous administration of terbutaline has been reported in controlled studies.[103,104] Administration of low-dose ritodrine during the second stage of labor results in the abolishment of progressive fetal respiratory acidosis.[105] The exact mechanisms responsible for these beneficial effects are unknown, but it is hypothesized that increased uteroplacental blood flow, enhanced glucose transfer, and improved gas exchange may all be important.

The antepartum administration of β-mimetic agents has also been associated with a decreased incidence of hyaline membrane disease in the preterm infant.[106–109] An increased rate of surfactant release, as opposed to increased production of surfactant, is probably responsible for this phenomenon.[107–109]

Clinical observations in neonates during the immediate transition period of life have been reassuring following β-mimetic tocolysis. Depression of neonatal central nervous function has not been described.[110–114] Likewise, no significant adverse fetal acid-base effects have been described.[111,112]

As stated previously, the literature has carried isolated reports of altered neonatal cardiac electrophysiology during β-mimetic tocolysis. Transient neonatal tachycardia has been commonly described in preterm neonates exposed to these agents until the time of birth.[110] As stated previously, isolated cases of tachyarrhythmia have been observed before birth and continued to be a management problem after birth.[84,85,93] Digitalization, direct current cardioversion, and spontaneous resolution have resulted in favorable outcomes in these selected cases. Transient ST-segment changes have recently been described in neonates exposed to β-mimetic agents.[115] This suggests the possibility of fetal-neonatal myocardial ischemia in association with β-mimetic therapy, although all these infants had normal creatine phosphokinase (CPK) levels. Another provocative report described severe cardiac decompensation in three of four neonates from an exposed quadruplet

pregnancy.[116] Downregulation of β-adrenergic receptors was hypothesized in this pregnancy exposed to 9 weeks of subcutaneous terbutaline pump therapy. The affected infants demonstrated poor cardiac output, increased peripheral resistance, and impaired myocardial function that responded only to dobutamine infusion.

Hypoglycemia is a common observation in the preterm infant, but β-mimetic tocolysis has also been associated with altered glucose homeostasis in the neonate.[110,114,117–119] This phenomenon may be related to hyperinsulinemia and elevated growth hormone levels induced by β-mimetic stimulation of the fetal pancreas before birth.[117–119] Continuous β-mimetic tocolysis for more than 6 weeks is associated with an increased risk of reactive hypoglycemia after birth.[114] Significant shifts in neonatal potassium levels have not been described in neonates exposed to β-mimetic agents.[111] While severe neonatal hypocalcemia has been associated with isoxsuprine tocolysis,[110] this phenomenon has not been observed with ritodrine.[111] Neonatal thyroid function does not appear to be altered by β-mimetic tocolysis.[120]

Neonatal bilirubin metabolism does appear to be affected by β-mimetic tocolysis.[114,121,122] Animal studies show no significant increase in total bilirubin production, and suggest a binding-site displacement phenomenon for the hyperbilirubinemic effects of these drugs.[123] The clinical significance of tocolytic-induced neonatal hyperbilirubinemia seems minimal. A case of tocolytic-induced hypercholesterolemia in a neonate has been reported.[124]

An association between β-mimetic tocolysis and an increased incidence of intraventricular hemorrhage (IVH) has lately been suggested.[125,126] These retrospective comparisons demonstrate a fourfold increase in IVH rates in infants exposed to β-mimetic agents over that in untreated or magnesium-treated controls.[125] The concept that tocolytic-induced alterations in cerebrovascular blood flow are responsible for this finding is unproved, but these preliminary observations may parallel the pathologic effects of β-mimetic agents in the maternal cerebrovascular system. By contrast, other investigators have specifically failed to demonstrate an increased rate of fetal IVH under similar conditions.[127]

There is no evidence of β-mimetic-induced alterations in neonatal renal function, such as have been observed in mothers undergoing parenteral tocolysis.[128] Exposed infants exhibit normal urinary electrolyte excretion and osmolalities, but demonstrate lower inulin clearance and higher renin activity on the first day of life only. A transient fetal leukemoid reaction has been described in association with maternal ritodrine administration.[129]

Long-term follow-up studies of infant and child development after β-mimetic tocolysis has been reassuring. The developmental outcomes assessed after 1 to 9 years do not differ significantly from those of preterm controls.[91,130,131] No significant alterations in growth, head circumference, or neurologic, psychomotor, or social developmental milestones have been associated with any of the β-mimetic tocolytic agents.

Tocolysis with β-mimetic agents remains the mainstay of pharmacologic management of preterm labor. The extensive clinical use of these agents over the past three decades has fostered both familiarity and trepidation among clinicians. Although the potential for significant maternal-fetal-neonatal complications has become more evident over the years, these powerful tocolytic agents can be safely used by the vigilant practitioner.

MAGNESIUM SULFATE

Maternal Physiologic Effects

When intravenous magnesium sulfate therapy is maintained within a nontoxic range, maternal physiologic changes are minimal. Maternal tachycardia is not associated with the administration of magnesium sulfate, and cardiac output remains essentially unchanged.[132] Transient hypotension has been described after the initial loading dose, but hemodynamic alterations appear minimal.[132] The minimal impact of magnesium sulfate on maternal hemodynamics makes it a potentially useful medication in patients at risk of antepartum hemorrhage.

The major potential adverse effect of intravenous magnesium sulfate occurs when toxic serum concentrations are reached. The loss of deep tendon reflexes occurs with serum magnesium levels of 4 to 8 mEq/L; respiratory depression can occur at 12 to 15 mEq/L.[133] At higher concentrations than these, cardiac conduction abnormalities and cardiac arrest may occur. On the basis of these data, serum concentrations above 8 mEq/L should be avoided, and all patients receiving magnesium sulfate for tocolysis should be monitored closely for the loss of deep tendon reflexes, elevated serum levels of magnesium and respiratory depression.

Maternal Side Effects

The clinical popularity of magnesium sulfate tocolysis can be directly attributed to the perceived paucity of maternal side effects compared with intravenous β-mimetic therapy, and to most obstetricians' familiarity with this agent for seizure prophylaxis. The absence of identifiable physiologic alterations in

---

Maternal Risks of Potential Magnesium Sulfate-Specific Complications

Cardiopulmonary
   Respiratory depression
   Respiratory arrest
   Altered cardiac conduction
   Subendocardial ischemia
   Pulmonary edema
   Water retention
   Osmotic diuresis
   Chest tightness

Neurologic
   Altered sensorium/lethargy
   Ophthalmologic alterations
   Generalized muscle weakness
   Neuromuscular blockade
   Dysphagia/aspiration

Metabolic
   Hypocalcemia
   Hyperkalemia
   Cutaneous vasodilation
   Hypothermia

Gastrointestinal
   Nausea/vomiting
   Paralytic Ileus
   Constipation

Other
   Hypersensitivity

the maternal cardiovascular system is a particularly appealing aspect of magnesium sulfate tocolysis to clinicians searching for an alternative to β-mimetic therapy.

In a large, randomized comparative trial, significant side effects necessitating discontinuation of intravenous therapy were observed in only 2 percent of patients receiving magnesium sulfate, as compared with 38 percent of patients receiving ritodrine and 60 percent of patients receiving terbutaline.[134] Clinical data from other medical centers indicate maternal complaints in 22 percent of patients receiving ritodrine and 14 percent of those exposed to magnesium sulfate.[135] Significant maternal side effects are usually observed during the loading bolus of this agent. The most common complaint is an initial sensation of generalized heat and flushing. Nausea, chest tightness, generalized muscle weakness, and lethargy are other observed side effects during infusion, and are also associated with high serum magnesium concentrations during aggressive and prolonged administration.

Intravenous magnesium sulfate tocolysis appears to have a less dramatic impact on maternal fluid balance than does β-mimetic tocolysis. Maternal fluid dynamics during therapy suggest a positive fluid balance, with a reduction in colloid pressures despite increased sodium excretion and osmotic diuresis.[136] A major etiology for any detrimental fluid balance is iatrogenic overhydration. Despite the generally reassuring safety profile of magnesium sulfate, several cases of magnesium-induced pulmonary edema have recently raised clinical suspicions about the safety of this medication.[137,138]

The cardiovascular safety of magnesium sulfate tocolysis has also been challenged. A case of symptomatic subendocardial ischemia during such therapy has been well documented[139] and raises questions about its producing unrecognized myocardial alterations. A case of neuromuscular blockade at magnesium sulfate doses within therapeutic limits, attributable to concurrent magnesium and nifedipine tocolysis, has also been described.[140]

Neuro-ophthalmologic alterations have been well documented in patients undergoing magnesium sulfate tocolysis.[141] Transient patient complaints of blurred vision and diplopia are common. Common physical findings include ptosis, accommodative and convergence insufficiency, and abnormal pupillary responses to light. All these alterations resolve shortly after the discontinuation of therapy.

Treatment compliance is another issue that must be raised with regard to patients receiving high-dose magnesium sulfate tocolysis. The generalized flushing, nausea, vomiting, constipation, chest tightness, generalized muscle weakness, lethargy, and altered sensorium tend to correlate directly with higher serum magnesium concentrations, and also appear to be related to the duration of therapy. Although these symptoms may seem like manageable side effects to health care providers, they render many patients reluctant to consent to repetitive courses of this uncomfortable therapy.

Significant alterations in maternal calcium homeostasis have also been observed with magnesium sulfate tocolysis.[142,143] Serum concentrations of ionized and unionized calcium decrease dramatically during the infusion period. This is due in part to increased renal excretion of calcium, with substantial urinary losses of 800 to 900 mg/day being recorded.[143] Magnesium-induced changes in maternal levels of parathyroid hormone have also been implicated in this pathologic process.[142-144] Maternal mineralization studies clearly demonstrate a significant degree of decreased bone density with prolonged magnesium sulfate tocolysis.[143] Other maternal complications attributable to the profound hypocalcemia induced by magnesium sulfate remain uncharacterized. Two cases of profound hyperkalemia represent another example of a potential metabolic alteration associated with magnesium tocolysis.[145]

Besides these effects, a decrease in maternal temperature has been described with magnesium sulfate tocolysis.[146] This is most likely caused by cutaneous vasodilation and resultant heat loss with magnesium infusion. In addition to this, paralytic ileus has been described in association with magnesium sulfate tocolysis.[147] Altered gastrointestinal motility seems a reasonable but unexplored complication of this smooth muscle relaxant therapy. A case of hypersensitivity manifesting as a systemic urticarial reaction has also been described.[148]

Fetal-Neonatal Side Effects

Magnesium sulfate tocolysis does not appear to alter uteroplacental blood flow under routine clinical conditions.[100] Despite this, some investigators have re-

---

Fetal-Neonatal Risks of Potentional Magnesium Sulfate-Specific Complications

Altered heart rate variability

Altered biophysical activities

Amniotic accumulation

Hyermagnesium

Respiratory depression

Hypotonia

Meconium Ileus

Neonatal rickets

---

ported a decreased fetal heart rate variability with such therapy,[149] while others report no such effect.[150] At maternal serum magnesium concentrations above 6 mEq/L, the biophysical activity of fetal breathing and movement is suppressed.[151] The observed alterations in biophysical parameters are probably a direct effect of fetal hypermagnesemia rather than uteroplacental insufficiency. Significant accumulations of magnesium have been reported in fetal serum and amniotic fluid.[152,153]

Serum magnesium concentrations associated with tocolysis are rarely toxic in the newborn,[154–156] but neonatal hypotonia and respiratory depression due to hypermagnesemia have been described.[156] Neonatal hypermagnesemia is usually associated with magnesium sulfate infusions lasting longer than 24 hours, intramuscular administration of the drug, and birth during its infusion.[154,155] The newborn requires up to 48 to 72 hours to satisfactorily excrete the resulting magnesium load.[155] Two cases of decreased bowel peristalsis mimicking meconium ileus have been described during neonatal hypermagnesemia.[157] It seems prudent to discontinue maternal tocolysis as soon as delivery seems inevitable, in order to reduce the risks of these effects.

Recent evidence of maternal calcium losses has raised new concerns of neonatal rickets with prolonged magnesium sulfate tocolysis. Several cases of unexplained demineralization in the neonate have been described,[158] and a controlled analysis of neonatal radiographs suggests a significant calcium-

depleting effect in cases of prolonged maternal tocolysis with magnesium sulfate.[159] Further investigation of this provocative finding seems warranted.

In summary, substantial clinical evidence suggests that magnesium sulfate is a safe and effective tocolytic agent for the inhibition of preterm labor. While the scientific evidence to substantiate this claim is developing, magnesium sulfate can be considered an appropriate clinical alternative to intravenous β-mimetic therapy for tocolysis.

PROSTAGLANDIN SYNTHETASE INHIBITORS
Maternal Physiologic Effects

Alterations in maternal physiology attributable to indomethacin appear to be minimal. This medication does not alter maternal heart rate or blood pressure.[160] Fluid management during indomethacin tocolysis is generally simplified by oral or rectal administration. However, several independent reports of transient, indomethacin-induced renal insufficiency have been described.[161,162] Women exposed to the drug appear to be at risk of oliguria and azotemia, which resolve after the discontinuation of therapy.

Ingestion of aspirin before delivery has been associated with an increased incidence of maternal antepartum and postpartum hemorrhage.[163,164] By contrast, the effect of indomethacin on maternal platelet function is reversible[165] and does not lead to increased maternal hemorrhage during preterm parturition.[166] Postpartum hemorrhage did occur in 3 of 16 term patients who had received a single 100-mg suppository of indomethacin.[167] The clinical risk of severe indomethacin-induced antepartum/intrapartum bleeding during premature labor is still undefined.

Antipyretic effects of indomethacin are theoretically possible, and may potentially mask occult chorioamnionitis. Chronic maternal ingestion of indomethacin has been associated with altered T-suppressor lymphocyte activity in both the mother and neonate.[168]

Maternal Side Effects

The most common maternal side effects associated with oral to colytic therapy is nausea, heartburn, and gastric upset. Repeated rectal administration may produce proctitis and hematochezia. However, most

---

Maternal Risks of Potential Prostaglandin Synthetase Inhibitor-Specific Complications

Gastrointestinal irritation

Platelet dysfunction

Altered immune response

Antipyretic effect

Transient oliguria

---

mothers have few complaints during oral therapy. These tocolytic agents are best avoided in patients with a history of peptic ulceration, gastrointestinal bleeding, or a bleeding diasthesis.

Fetal-Neonatal Side Effects

Indomethacin therapy during preterm labor does not appear to significantly alter uteroplacental blood flow. Tocolysis with indomethacin in animal models

---

Fetal-Neonatal Risks of Potential Prostaglandin Synthetase Inhibitor-Specific Complications

Oligohydramnios

Constriction of ductus arteriosus

Fetal hydrops

Altered cerebral blood flow

Exacerbation of congenital heart disease

Persistent pulmonary hypertension

Oliguria

Renal dysfunction

Necrotizing enterocolitis

Cystic brain lesions

Intraventricular hemorrhage

Patent ductus arteriosus

Altered immune response

Hyperbilirubinemia

---

produces either transient vasoconstriction or no significant change in maternal-fetal blood flow.[169] Doppler maternal uterine artery and fetal umbilical artery waveforms remain unchanged with indomethacin tocolysis.[170] Likewise, Apgar scores remain unaffected by this particular class of tocolytic agents.[160]

One of the first recognized potential fetal complications of indomethacin tocolysis was oligohydramnios.[171,172] Additional cases of fetal oligohydramnios were reported with expanded clinical use of indomethacin tocolysis,[173,174] with an incidence in large clinical studies varying from 10 to 30 percent.[175,176] Significant decreases in hourly urine output in exposed fetuses have been reported with both short- and long-term indomethacin therapy.[177,178] An absence of changes in fetal renal blood flow with therapy suggests that the responsible mechanism is an alteration in prostaglandin-mediated tubular function.[179] This phenomenon appears to be dose dependent[180] and reversed in utero with discontinuation of indomethacin tocolysis.

Several isolated cases of subsequent renal failure in neonates exposed to prostaglandin synthetase inhibitors suggest a continuing pathologic situation after birth.[171–173,180] These cases of renal dysfunction are usually reversible over time, but several cases have culminated in neonatal death.[171,172,180] However, when the results of specific renal function tests in exposed fetuses were compared with those in age-adjusted controls, no significant tocolytic-induced alterations in neonatal renal function were noted.[161]

A significant alteration in fetal ductus arteriosus physiology has repeatedly been described in humans exposed to prostaglandin synthetase inhibitors.[181] This vasoconstrictive effect is observed in 20 to 50 percent of exposed fetuses, lasts for up to 2 hours after a dose, and completely resolves on re-examination 24 hours after discontinuation.[181] The phenomenon appears to be related to gestational age, with dramatic constriction of the ductus arteriosus being limited to fetuses of gestational ages above 32 weeks.[182] Cases of unexplained fetal hydrops[183] and tricuspid insufficiency[184] have been associated with indomethacin therapy. Recently, the dangers of indomethacin use have been illustrated in mothers of fetuses with ductus-dependent congenital cardiac disease.[185]

Unexplained cases of persistent fetal circulation

in premature neonates exposed to indomethacin tocolysis are commonly reported. Initial clinical cases appeared to be limited to near-term exposures,[183,186] but long-term exposure to indomethacin in a preterm population has also been associated with this life-threatening complication.[187] Chronic constriction of the fetal ductus arteriosus may result in hypertrophy of the fetal pulmonary vasculature and may ultimately be responsible for this troublesome neonatal event.[186,188] The risk of persistent fetal circulation increases with fetal exposure for to indomethacin for more than 48 hours and in populations at more than 32 weeks gestation. Currently, a preliminary estimate of a 5 percent incidence of indomethacin-induced persistent pulmonary hypertension seems reasonable.

Hypothetically, other blood flow alterations in the preterm fetus may be responsible for several recent provocative observations in exposed neonates. Cystic cerebral lesions have been reported in neonates exposed to indomethacin.[189] Observations of altered cerebral blood flow in exposed fetuses, with resultant tricuspid insufficiency, may explain these lesions.[190] A greater than normal incidence of necrotizing enterocolitis has also been described in indomethacin-exposed neonates, and suggests an altered splanchnic blood flow as the source of the condition.[191] An association between IVH and indomethacin tocolysis has also been suggested.[191] These complications appear to be related to indomethacin therapy lasting for more than 48 hours or continued administration of the drug within 24 hours of delivery, or both.

A greater than normal incidence of patent ductus arteriosus in indomethacin-exposed infants has also been observed.[191,192] Minor alterations in neonatal hemostasis due to indomethacin-induced platelet dysfunction have been described,[193] but usually resolve as the drug is excreted. A theoretical concern for displacement of bilirubin from albumin-binding sites has been voiced.[194]

Recently, a new class of prostaglandin synthetase inhibitors with minimal transplacental transfer have been introduced as tocolytic agents.[195] Preliminary studies suggest that these agents cause minimal alterations in amniotic fluid dynamics and flow velocities through the ductus arteriosus. The capacity of the first such new drug, sulindac, to effectively treat preterm labor without producing undesirable side effects remains to be seen.

In summary, prostaglandin synthetase inhibitors represent a powerful class of tocolytic agents with demonstrable efficacy. However, emerging concerns for fetal-neonatal safety have since limited their clinical use. Sulindac, after further evaluation, may prove to be a useful agent. In the meantime, selected and judicious use of indomethacin as a rescue tocolytic agent seems justified. Limiting its clinical use to a short course of therapy before 32 weeks' gestation, and attempting to discontinue treatment before delivery, may provide an acceptable margin of safety.

CALCIUM-CHANNEL BLOCKING AGENTS

Physiologic Effects

The actions of nifedipine are nonselective and can thus cause relaxation of both visceral and vascular smooth muscle. It is not unreasonable to expect a diminution in systemic blood pressure and reflex tachycardia when nifedipine is used. Additionally, headache and cutaneous flushing should be expected. Figure 17-1 depicts blood pressure changes following sublingual and oral dosing with nifedipine. While some of the changes are statistically significant, as indicated in the figure, they represent minimal changes in the cardiovascular system.[196] The effect of nifedipine on serum levels of sodium, potassium, chloride, any bicarbonate, and the ion

---

Maternal Risks of Potential Calcium-Channel Blocker-Specific Complications

Hypotension

Tachycardia

Altered cardiac conduction

Cutaneous vasodilation

Fluid retention

Hypocalcemia

Hypoglycemia

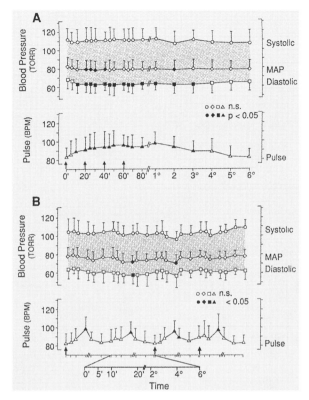

Fig. 17-1. Effects of nifedipine on systolic and diastolic blood pressure, mean arterial pressure (MAP), and pulse rate. **(A)** Sublingual nifedipine. Vertical arrows, timing of administration of 10 mg of nifedipine. **(B)** Oral nifedipine. Vertical arrows, timing of administration of 20 mg of nifedipine. Values expressed as mean ± standard deviation (SD). Solid symbols, a *P* value of less than 0.05 as compared with baseline values; n.s., not significant. (From Ferguson et al,[196] with permission.)

gap have also been evaluated.[196] No significant changes occurred in these parameters; however, when serial glucose and hematocrit determinations were obtained, the glucose was noted to increase to a mean value of 111 mg% (probably reflecting glucose and intravenous crystalloid infusate), and the hematocrit fell from 34 to 31.5 vol%. This most likely represents a hemodilutional change.

In the report of Ferguson and colleagues,[197] side effects were significantly more common in patients receiving ritodrine (18 of 38) than in those receiving nifedipine (5 of 38). The ritodrine treatment group demonstrated chest pain and nausea and vomiting

as the most common side effects; in three cases it was necessary to discontinue the infusion. In the nifedipine group, however, headache and flushing were the most common complaints. Chest pain and pressure associated with pyrosis were encountered in one patient in the nifedipine group, but none of the patients required discontinuation of nifedipine tocolysis. Glock and Morales[198] reported that 41 percent of their study patients experienced transient hypotension lasting less than 15 minutes after an initial sublingual dose of nifedipine, despite having received a prior fluid bolus of 500 ml of crystalloid.[198] It is therefore important to carefully monitor hemodynamic parameters in any patients receiving nifedipine. In their study, Glock and Morales[198] noted that side effects associated with magnesium sulfate often required its discontinuation, while discontinuation of nifedipine was not necessary in the nifedipine study group.

Fetal-Neonatal Side Effects

The potential effects of any tocolytic agent on the fetus must be carefully considered before using it. Unfortunately, there is no substantial body of data on fetal exposure to nifedipine tocolysis. Transplacental passage of nifedipine does occur and, not surprisingly, the highest levels are found in the neonate when the interval from maternal ingestion to delivery was relatively short.[199] When 5 hours or more had elapsed from the most recent maternal nifedipine dose, neonatal nifedipine levels were 6 ng/ml or less in all instances.

Studies of Ulmsten[200] and Read and Welby[201] were reassuring in the findings on fetal and neonatal follow-up after nifedipine exposure. In the report by Ferguson and colleagues,[197] none of the variables

---

Fetal-Neonatal Risks of Potential Calicum-Channel Blocker-Specific Complications

Tachycardia

Altered uteroplacental blood flow

Limited experience to date

of perinatal outcome, including stillbirths, neonatal deaths, incidence of respiratory distress syndrome (RDS), ventilator treatment at 2 and 4 weeks, IVH, Apgar scores below 7 at 1 or 5 minutes, or birth weight showed any difference from their usual values. Similarly, Meyer et al[202] found no difference in the mean Apgar scores of neonates exposed to nifedipine and those exposed to ritodrine, and no change in the mean systolic to diastolic pressure values in Doppler recordings of umbilical artery pressure. Mari et al[203] performed Doppler studies in the middle cerebral artery, renal artery, ductus arteriosis, and umbilical artery in 11 fetuses whose mothers were treated for preterm labor with nifedipine. No differences in any of the measured values were found when post-nifedipine Doppler studies were compared with pre-nifedipine studies. These authors also noted that maternal umbilical artery Doppler waveforms did not change, and that nifedipinee does not adversely effect uteroplacental or fetal blood flow as evaluated by Doppler ultrasound in the doses used for treatment of preterm labor, as previously suggested. Further reassuring information pertaining to fetal and neonatal tolerance of nifedipine has recently been provided by Murray and colleagues.[204] In their historic prospective study, nifedipine was associated with the fewest maternal side effects when compared with other tocolytic agents, and in no case did nifedipine need to be discontinued because of a maternal side effect. Fetal surveillance testing and neonatal outcome failed to reveal deleterious in utero effects of nifedipine.[204]

Ferguson et al[205] have also evaluated neonatal bilirubin production and response after tocolysis with nifedipine for preterm labor. They studied total bilirubin production in vivo, as indexed by carboxyhemoglobin levels, of infants whose mothers had received ritodrine or the calcium-channel blocker nifedipine for tocolysis. No differences were detected in the carboxyhemoglobin levels of the two groups of infants. Furthermore, Ferguson and colleagues found no difference in the number of infants in the two groups who transiently exhibited low glucose levels (≤ 40 mg/dl), transient decreases in mean arterial pressure, or increases in heart rate in the neonatal period.

Potential Non-pharmacologic Complications of Tocolytic Therapy

Maternal sepsis

Chorioamnionitis

Deep venous thrombosis

Pulmonary embolism

Aspiration pneumonitis

Prolonged Ileus

Dermatosis

Postural neuropathies

Malnourishment

Psychosocial adjustments

NONPHARMACOLOGIC COMPLICATIONS OF TOCOLYSIS

Nonpharmacologic complications occur in women subjected to prolonged or repeated courses of tocolysis. During these treatment periods, subtle physiologic complications can go unrecognized and unheeded while health care providers focus on the mechanics of therapy. Psychological hardships are also imposed on these women and their families during these potentially trying times. Prescribing physicians must be aware of the impact of recommendations for tocolysis on the general health and lifestyle of these patients. The overall effects of extended bed rest, prolonged hospitalization, uncertainty of fetal outcome, and drug-induced side effects must sometimes seem overwhelming to these patients and their physicians. It is the duty of practitioners to be attentive to the human needs of patients who are willing to endure these hardships for the sake of the unborn.

CONCLUSIONS

The consequences of tocolysis for mother and child are diverse and wide-ranging. It is clear that some clinical benefit can be derived from these treatment strategies, but the safety of the varying classes of tocolytic agents remains a concern. Selective and judicious use of these powerful medications can reduce the overall risk to exposed mothers and children. Vigilant application of tocolysis is also a prudent strategy for reducing risk in the pregnancies in which it is used. The potential benefit of pharmacologic management of preterm labor can be realized if the practioner has knowledge of the clinical protocols and potential complications outlined in this chapters and Chapter 16.

None of the currently available tocolytic agents is ideal, and the development of a safe, well-tolerated, and effective medication for tocolysis needs to be pursued. Until such a medication is available, it will be necessary for the clinician to apply the available therapeutic agents in a safe and effective manner to minimize the unfavorable impact of these nonselective drugs. The adage of primum non nocere is best heeded when prescribing tocolytics in the treatment of preterm labor.

REFERENCES

1. Benedetti TJ: Maternal complications of parenteral beta-sympathomimetic therapy for premature labor. Am J Obstet Gynecol 145:1, 1983
2. Besinger RE: A systematic review of adverse events documented in the use of currently available treatment of preterm labor. Res Clin Forum 16(3):80, 1994
3. Schwarz R, Retzke U: Cardiovascular effects of terbutaline in pregnant women. Acta Obstet Gynecol Scand 62:419, 1983
4. Wagner JM, Morton MJ, Johnson KA et al: Terbutaline and maternal cardiac function. JAMA 246:2697, 1981
5. Bieniarz J, Ivankovich A, Scommegna A: Cardiac output during ritodrine treatment in premature labor. Am J Obstet Gynecol 118:910, 1974
6. Finley J, Katz M, Rojas-Perez M et al: Cardiovascular consequence of beta-agonist tocolysis: An echocardiographic study. Obstet Gynecol 64:787, 1984
7. Price PH: Review of betamimetic drugs for tocolysis. Special report to FDA public meeting on re-evaluation of ritodrine labelling. October 28, 1992
8. Blickstein I, Zalel Y, Katz Z et al: Ritodrine-induced pulmonary edema unmasking underlying peripartum cardiomyopathy. Am J Obstet Gynecol 159:332, 1988
9. Ron-El R, Caspi E, Herman A et al: Unexpected cardiac pathology in pregnant women treated with beta-adrenergic agents (ritodrine). Obstet Gynecol 61: 10S, 1983
10. Edoute Y, Blumenfeld Z, Bronstein M et al: Peripartum congestive cardiomyopathy and endocardial fibroelastosis associated with ritodrine treatment. J Reprod Med 32:793, 1987
11. Mercer LJ, Aisenbrey G: Atrial myxoma as a complication of tocolytic therapy: a case report. J Reprod Med 30:561, 1985
12. Reichman J, Goldman JA: Pulmonary edema after ritodrine infusion for premature labor in a patient with mitral value disease. Acta Obstet Gynecol Scand 60:87, 1981
13. Hadi HA, Abdulla AM, Fadel HE et al: Cardiovascular effects of ritodrine tocolysis: a new noninvasive method to measure pulmonary capillary pressure during pregnancy. Obstet Gynecol 70:608, 1987
14. Bremme K, Eneroth P, Carsjo BM et al: Blood pressure regulation in third-trimester pregnant women receiving tocolytic terbutaline infusion. Int J Obstet Gynecol Reprod Biol 23:53, 1986
15. Hanssens M, Keirse MJ, Symonds EM: Activation of the renin-angiotensin system during ritodrine treatment in preterm labor. Am J Obstet Gynecol 162: 1048, 1990
16. Spellacy WN, Cruz AC, Buhi WC et al: The acute effects of ritodrine infusion on maternal metabolism: measurement of levels of glucose, insulin, glucagon, triglycerides, cholesterol, placental lactogen and chorionic gonadotropin. Am J Obstet Gynecol 131:637, 1978
17. Kirkpatrick C, Quenon M, Desir D: Blood anions and electrolytes during ritodrine infusion in preterm labor. Am J Obstet Gynecol 138:523, 1980
18. Caldwell G, Scougall I, Boddy K et al: Fasting hyperinsulinemia hypoglycemia after ritodrine therapy for preterm labor. Obstet Gynecol 70:478, 1987
19. Jovanovic R: Serial serum potassium and glucose levels during treatment of premature labor with oral terbutaline. Int J Gynaecol Obstet 23:399, 1985
20. Main EK, Main DM, Gabbe SG: Chronic oral terbutaline tocolytic therapy is associated with maternal glucose intolerance. Am J Obstet Gynecol 157:644, 1987
21. Foley MR, Landon MB, Gabbe SG et al: Effect of prolonged oral terbutaline therapy on glucose tolerance in pregnancy. Am J Obstet Gynecol 168:100, 1993
22. Main DM, Main EK, Strong SE et al: The effect of oral ritodrine therapy on glucose tolerance in pregnancy. Am J Obstet Gynecol 152:1031, 1985
23. Miodovnik M, Peros N, Holroyde JC et al: Treatment

of premature labor in insulin dependent diabetic women. Obstet Gynecol 65:621, 1985

24. Lenz S, Kuhl C, Wang P et al: The effect of ritodrine on carbohydrate and lipid metabolism in normal and diabetic pregnant women. Acta Endocrinol 92:669, 1979

25. Halpren EW, Soifer NE, Haenel LC: Ketoacidosis secondary to oral ritodrine use in a gestational diabetic patient: report of a case. J Am Osteopath Assoc 88: 241, 1988

26. Mordes D, Kreutner K, Metzger W et al: Dangers of intravenous ritodrine in diabetic patients. JAMA 248: 973, 1982

27. Hill WC, Katz M, Kitzmiller JL et al: Tocolysis for the insulin-dependent diabetic woman. Am J Obstet Gynecol 148:1148, 1984

28. Berstein IM, Catalano PM: Ketoacidosis in pregnancy associated with the parenteral administration of terbutaline and betamethasone. A case report. J Reprod Med 35:818, 1990

29. Cano A, Martinez P, Parilla JJ et al: Effects of intravenous ritodrine on lactate and pyruvate levels: role of glycemia and anaerobiosis. Obstet Gynecol 66:207, 1985

30. Desir D, VanCoovorden A, Kirkpatrick C et al: Side effects of drugs: ritodrine-induced acidosis in pregnancy. BMJ 2:1194, 1978

31. Young DC, Toofanian A, Leveno KJ: Potassium and glucose concentrations without treatment during ritodrine tocolysis. Am J Obstet Gynecol 145:105, 1982

32. Cotton DB, Strassner HT, Lipson LG et al: The effects of terbutaline on acid base, serum electrolytes, and glucose homeostasis during the management of preterm labor. Am J Obstet Gynecol 141:617, 1981

33. DiRenzo GC, Anceschi MM: Renin activity, aldosterone levels and urinary sodium and potassium excretion under tocolytic therapy with salbutamol. Eur J Obstet Gynec Reprod Biol 13:43, 1981

34. Bremme K, Eneroth R, Hagenfeld L et al: Changes in maternal serum aldosterone, potassium and prolactin levels during beta-receptor agonist treatment in third trimester pregnancies. Horm Metab Res 14: 198, 1982

35. Cano A, Tovar I, Parrilla JJ et al: Metabolic disturbances during intravenous use of ritodrine: increased insulin levels and hypokalemia. Obstet Gynecol 65: 356, 1985

36. Kawarabayashi T, Tsukamoto T, Kishikawa T et al: Changes in serum calcium, magnesium, cyclic AMP and monoamine oxidase levels during pregnancy and under prolonged ritodrine treatment for preterm labor. Gynecol Obstet Invest 28:132, 1989

37. Behling K, Bleichert A, Scarperi M: A method for the measurement of tremor and a comparison of the effects of tocolytic betamimetics. Eur J Appl Physiol Occup Physiol 39:203, 1978

38. Katz M, Robertson PA, Creasy RK: Cardiovascular complications associated with terbutaline treatment for preterm labor. Am J Obstet Gynecol 139:605, 1981

39. Benedetti TJ: Life threatening complications of betamimetic therapy for preterm labor inhibition. Clin Perinatol 13:843, 1986

40. Carpenter RJ Jr, Decuir P: Cardiovascular collapse associated with oral terbutaline tocolytic therapy. Am J Obstet Gynecol 148:821, 1984

41. Schneider EP, Jonas E, Tejani N: Detection of cardiac events by continuous electrocardiogram monitoring during ritodrine infusion. Obstet Gynecol 71:361, 1988

42. Fink BJ, Wever T: Direct current conversion of maternal supraventricular tachycardia developed during the treatment of a pregnant heroin addict with ritodrine. Acta Obstet Gynecol Scand 60:521, 1981

43. Faidley CK, Dix PM, Morgan MA et al: Electrocardiographic abnormalities during ritodrine administration. South Med J 83:503, 1990

44. Shin YK, Kim YD: Ventricular tachyarrythymias during cesarean section after ritodrine therapy: interactions with anesthetics. South Med J 81:528, 1988

45. Simpson JI, Giffin JP: A glycopyrrolate-ritodrine drug-drug interaction. Can J Anaesth 35:187, 1988

46. Sherer DM, Nawrocki MN, Thompson HO et al: Type I second-degree AV block during ritodrine therapy for preterm labor. Am J Perinatol 8:150, 1991

47. Dean H, Berliner S, Garfinkel D et al: Sinus bradycardia following ritodrine withdrawal. JAMA 247:1810, 1982

48. Hudgens DR, Conradi SE: Sudden death associated with terbutaline sulfate infusion. Am J Obstet Gynecol 169:210, 1993

49. Tye KH, Desser KB, Benchimull A: Angina pectoris associated with use of terbutaline for premature labor. JAMA 244:692, 1980

50. Yink YK, Tejani MS: Angina pectoris as a complication of ritodrine hydrochloride therapy in premature labor. Obstet Gynecol 60:385, 1982

51. Michalak D, Klein V, Marquette GP: Myocardial ischemia: a complication of ritodrine tocolysis. Am J Obstet Gynecol 146:861, 1983

52. Ben-Shlomo I, Zohar S, Marmor A et al: Myocardial ischemia during intravenous ritodrine treatment: is it so rare? Lancet 2:917, 1986

53. Meinen K: Radioimmunoassay procedure of serum

myoglobin in case of a long-term tocolysis with B-sympathomimetics. Gynecol Obstet Invest 12:37, 1981

54. Hadi HA, Albazzaz SJ: Cardiac isoenzymes and electrocardiographic changes during ritodrine tocolysis. Am J Obstet Gynecol 161:318, 1989

55. Hendricks SK, Keroes J, Katz M: Electrocardiographic changes associated with ritodrine-induced maternal tachycardia and hypokalemia. Am J Obstet Gynecol 154:921, 1986

56. Cohen GR, O'Brien WF, Knuppel RA: ST segment depression in paired electrocardiograms and serum electrolytes in pregnant women receiving intravenous ritodrine. J Reprod Med 33:768, 1988

57. Mulders LG, Boers GH, Prickartz-Wijdevald MM et al: A study of maternal ECG characteristics before and during intravenous tocolysis with beta-sympathomimetics. Effect of IV tocolysis on maternal ECG characteristics. Acta Obstet Gynecol Scand 66:417, 1987

58. Leveno KJ, Cunningham FG: Beta-adrenergic agonists for preterm labor. N Engl J Med 327:349, 1992

59. Benedetti TJ, Caritis SN: Treatment of preterm labor with beta-adrenergic agonist ritodrine. N Engl J Med 327:1758, 1992

60. Hankins GD: Complications of beta-sympathomimetic tocolytic agents. p. 223. In Clark SL, Cotton DB, Hankins GDV, Phelan JP (eds): Critical Care Obstetrics. 2nd Ed. Blackwell Scientific, Boston, 1991

61. Robertson PA, Herron M, Katz M et al: Maternal morbidity associated with isoxsuprine and terbutaline in the treatment of preterm labor. Eur J Obstet Gynecol Reprod Biol 11:371, 1981

62. Hatjis CG, Swain M: Systemic tocolysis for premature labor is associated with an increased incidence of pulmonary edema in the presence of maternal infection. Am J Obstet Gynecol 159:723, 1988

63. Taslimi MM, Sibai BM, Amon E et al: A national survey on preterm labor. Am J Obstet Gynecol 160:1352, 1989

64. Besinger RE and Niebyl JR: The safety and efficacy of tocolytic agents for the treatment of preterm labor. Obstet Gynecol Surv 45:415, 1990

65. Canadian Preterm Labor Investigation Group: Treatment of preterm labor with the beta-adrenergic agonist ritodrine. N Engl J Med 327:308, 1992

66. Schrier RW, Lieberman R, Ufferman RC: Mechanism of antidiuretic effect of beta adrenergic stimulation. J Clin Invest 51:97, 1972

67. Lammintausta R, Erkkola R: Effect of long-term salbutamol treatment on renin-aldosterone system in twin pregnancy. Acta Obstet Gynecol Scand 58:447, 1979

68. Grospietsch G, Fenske M, Girndt J et al: The renin-angiotensin-aldosterone system, antidiuretic hormone levels and water balance under tocolytic therapy with fenoterol and verapamil. Int J Gynaecol Obstet 17:590, 1980

69. Spatling L, Staisch KJ, Huch R et al: Effects of ritodrine and betamethasone on metabolism, respiration and circulation. Am J Perinatol 3:41, 1986

70. Philipsen T, Eriksen PS, Lynggard F: Pulmonary edema following ritodrine-saline infusion in premature labor. Obstet Gynecol 58:304, 1981

71. Gupta RC, Foster S, Romano PM et al: Acute pulmonary edema associated with the use of oral ritodrine for premature labor. Chest 95:479, 1989

72. Rosene KA, Featherstone JH, Benedetti TJ: Cerebral ischemia associated with parenteral terbutaline use in pregnant migraine patients. Am J Obstet Gynecol 143:405, 1982

73. Nighoghossian N, Neuschwander P, Sonnet ML et al: Neurological manifestations in the vertebral-basilar system suggesting pregnancy toxemia [french]. Rev Fr Gynecol Obstet 86:119, 1991

74. Catanzarite VA, McHargue AM, Sandberg EC et al: Respiratory arrest during therapy for premature labor in a patient with myasthenia gravis. Obstet Gynecol 64:819, 1984

75. Sholl JS, Hughey MJ, Hirschman RA: Myotonic muscular dystrophy associated with ritodrine tocolysis. Am J Obstet Gynecol 151:83, 1985

76. Essed GG, Sels JP, Menheere PP: Changes in thyroid status in pregnant women treated with ritodrine. Eur J Obstet Gynecol Reprod Biol 26:113, 1987

77. Lotgering FK, Lind J, Huikeshoven FJM et al: Elevated serum transaminase levels during ritodrine administration. Am J Obstet Gynecol 155:390, 1986

78. Rachagan SP, Raman S, Sivanesaratnam V et al: Intestinal obstruction following previous myomectomy and the use of beta-sympathomimetics in pregnancy. Eur J Obstet Gynecol Reprod Biol 22:99, 1986

79. Ikushima Y, Kobayashi H, Imaishi K et al: Ritodrine-induced agranulocytosis. Arch Gynecol Obstet 248:53, 1990

80. Alcena V: Severe hemolytic anemia, leukemoid reaction, hypokalemia and transient hepatitis associated with the administration of ritodrine hydrochloride. Am J Obstet Gynecol 144:852, 1982

81. Bosnyak S, Baron JM, Schreiber J: Acute cutaneous vasculitis associated with prolonged intravenous ritodrine hydrochloride. Am J Obstet Gynecol 165:427, 1991

82. Shenker L: Effect of isoxsuprine on fetal heart rate and fetal electrocardiogram. Obstet Gynecol 26:104, 1965

83. Stawder RW, Barden TP, Thompson JF et al: Fetal cardiac effects of maternal isoxsuprine infusion. Am J Obstet Gynecol 89:792, 1964

84. Brosset P, Ronayette D, Pierce MC et al: Cardiac complications of ritodrine in mother and baby. Lancet 1:1461, 1982

85. Hermansen MC, Johnson GL: Neonatal supraventricular tachycardia following prolonged maternal ritodrine administration. Am J Obstet Gynecol 149:798, 1984

86. Sharif DS, Huhta JC, Moise KJ et al: Changes in fetal hemodynamics with terbutaline treatment and premature labor. J Clin Ultrasound 18:85, 1990

87. Rasanen J: The effects of ritodrine infusion on myocardial function and fetal hemodynamics. Acta Obstet Gynecol Scand 69:487, 1990

88. Weidinger H, Wiest W, Schleich A et al: The effects of betamimetic drugs used for tocolysis on the fetal myocardium. J Perinat Med 4:280, 1976

89. Bohm N, Alder CP: Focal necrosis, fatty degeneration and subendocardial nuclear polyploidization of myocardium in newborns after beta-sympathomimetic suppression of premature labor. Eur J Pediatr 136:149, 1981

90. Ingmarsson I, Arulkumaran S, Kottegoda SR et al: Complications of betamimetic therapy in preterm labor. Aust NZ J Obstet Gynaecol 25:182, 1985

91. Karlsson K: Beta-receptor agonists in pregnancy. Long-term effects in preterm children. Acta Obstet Gynecol Scand Suppl 108:71, 1982

92. Fletcher SE, Fyfe DA, Case CL et al: Myocardial necrosis in the newborn after long-term maternal subcutaneous terbutaline infusion for suppression of preterm labor. Am J Obstet Gynecol 165:1401, 1991

93. Katz VL, Seeds JW: Fetal and neonatal cardiovascular complications from beta-sympathomimetic therapy for tocolysis. Am J Obstet Gynecol 161:1, 1989

94. Kast A, Hermer M: Beta-adrenoreceptor tocolysis and effects on the heart of fetus and neonate. A review. J Perinat Med 21:97, 1993

95. Nuchpuckdee P, Brodsky N, Porat R et al: Ventricular septal thickness and cardiac function in neonates after in utero ritodrine exposure. J Pediatr 109:687, 1986

96. Assche FA, Aerts L: The effect of beta-sympathomimetics on the fetal endocrine pancreas. Eur J Obstet Gynecol Reprod Biol 15:395, 1982

97. Breitweser JA, Meyer RA, Sperling MA et al: Cardiac septal hypertrophy in hyperinsulinemia infants. J Pediatr 96:535, 1980

98. Brettes JP, Renaud R, Gandar R: A double-blind investigation into the effects of ritodrine on uterine blood flow during the third trimester of pregnancy. Am J Obstet Gynecol 124:164, 1976

99. Jouppila P, Kirkinen P, Koivula A et al: Ritodrine infusion during late pregnancy: effects on fetal and placental blood flow, prostacyclin, and thromboxane. Am J Obstet Gynecol 151:1028, 1985

100. Brar HS, Medearis AL, Devore GR et al: Maternal and fetal blood flow velocity waveform in patients with preterm labor: effects of tocolytics. Am J Obstet Gynecol 72:209, 1988

101. Ylikorkala O, Jouppila P, Kirkinen P et al: Maternal prostacyclin, thromboxane, and placental blood flow. Am J Obstet Gynecol 145:730, 1983

102. Dagbjartsson A, Herbertsson G, Stefansson TS: Beta-adrenoceptor agonists and hypoxia in sheep fetuses. Acta Physiol Scand 137:291, 1989

103. Patriarco MS, Viechnicki BM, Hutchinson TA et al: A study on intrauterine fetal resuscitation with terbutaline. Am J Obstet Gynecol 157:384, 1989

104. Burke MS, Porreco RP, Day D et al: Intrauterine resuscitation with tocolysis. An alternative month clinical trial. J Perinatol 9:296, 1989

105. Humphrey M, Chang A, Gilbert M et al: The effect of intravenous ritodrine on the acid-base status of the fetus during the second stage of labor. Br J Obstet Gynaecol 82:234, 1975

106. Cabero L, Giralt E, Navarro E et al: A betamimetic drug and human fetal lung maturation. Eur J Obstet Gynecol Reprod Biol 9:261, 1979

107. Enhorning G, Chamberlain D, Contreras C et al: Isoxsuprine-induced release of pulmonary surfactant in the rabbit fetus. Am J Obstet Gynecol 129:197, 1977

108. Lipshitz J, Broyles K, Hessler JR et al: Effects of hexoprenaline on the lecithin/sphingomyelin ratio and pressure-volume relationships in fetal rabbits. Am J Obstet Gynecol 139:726, 1981

109. Tzafettas JM, Zurnatzi V, Papaloucas AC: L/S ratio, biochemical and clinical changes after ritodrine intravenous infusion. Eur J Obstet Gynecol Reprod Biol 14:357, 1983

110. Brazy JE, Pupkin MJ: Effects of maternal isoxsuprine administration on preterm infants. J Pediatr 94:444, 1979

111. Huisjes HJ, Touwen BCL: Neonatal outcome after treatment with ritodrine: a controlled study. Am J Obstet Gynecol 147:250, 1983

112. Essed GGM: Neonatal effects of beta-adrenergic

drugs. Eur J Obstet Gynecol Reprod Biol 15:397, 1982

113. Kazzi NJ, Gross TL, Kazzi GM et al: Neonatal complications following in utero exposure to intravenous ritodrine. Acta Obstet Gynecol Scand 66:65, 1987

114. Musci MN, Abbasi S, Otis C et al: Prolonged ritodrine exposure and immediate neonatal outcome. J Perinatol 8:27, 1988

115. Gemelli M, DeLuca F, Manganaro R et al: Transient electrocardiographic changes suggesting myocardial ischemia in newborn infants following tocolysis with beta-sympathomimetics. Eur J Pediatr 149:730, 1990

116. Thorkelsson T, Loughead JL: Long-term subcutaneous terbutaline tocolysis: report of possible neonatal toxicity. J Perinatol 11:235, 1991

117. Epstein MF, Nicholls R, Stubblefield RG: Neonatal hypoglycemia after beta-sympathomimetic tocolytic therapy. J Pediatr 94:449, 1979

118. Procianoy RS, Pinheiro CEA: Neonatal hyperinsulinism after short-term maternal beta-sympathomimetic therapy. J Pediatr 101:612, 1982

119. Westgren M, Carlsson C, Lindholm T et al: Continuous maternal glucose measurements and fetal glucose and insulin levels after ritodrine administration at term. Acta Obstet Gynecol Scand Suppl 108:63, 1982

120. Desgranges TF, Moutquin J, Peloquin A: Effects of maternal oral salbutamol therapy on neonatal endocrine status at birth. Obstet Gynecol 69:582, 1987

121. Hopper AO, Cohen RS, Ostrander CR et al: Maternal beta-adrenergic tocolysis and neonatal bilirubin production. Am J Dis Child 137:58, 1983

122. Gemelli M, Manganaro R, Mami C et al: Effects of tocolytic therapy with ritodrine on the occurrence of neonatal hyperbilirubinemia [italian]. Minerva Pediatr 37:207, 1985

123. Ochikubo CG, Sunshine SE, Vreman HJ et al: The effect of ritodrine hydrochloride on bilirubin production in neonatal rats. Pediatr Pharmacol 5:247, 1986

124. Andersen G, Friis-Hansen B: Hypercholesterolemia in neonates: occurrence after antepartum treatment with betamethasone-phenobarbital-ritodrine for the prevention of respiratory distress syndrome. Pediatrics 62:8, 1978

125. Groome LJ, Goldenberg RL, Cliver SP: Neonatal periventricular-intraventricular hemorrhage after maternal beta-sympathomimetic tocolysis. Am J Obstet Gynecol 167:873, 1992

126. Pranikoff J, Helmchen R, Evertson L: Tocolytic therapy and intraventricular hemorrhage in the neonate. Am J Obstet Gynecol 164:511, 1991

127. Laros RK, Kitterman JA, Heilbron DC et al: Outcome of very low birthweight infants exposed to beta-sym-

pathomimetics in utero. Am J Obstet Gynecol 164: 1657, 1991

128. Hansen NB, Oh W, LaRochelle F et al: Effects of maternal ritodrine administration on neonatal renal function. J Pediatr 103:774, 1983

129. Herrera AJ, Macaraeg AL: Maternal ritodrine hydrochloride therapy associated with transient leukemoid reaction in the infant. South Med J 79:78, 1986

130. Polowczyk D, Tejani M, Lauersen N et al: Evaluation of seven-to-nine-year-old children exposed to ritodrine in utero. Obstet Gynecol 64:485, 1984

131. Hadders-Algra M, Touwen BCL, Huisjes JH: Long-term follow up of children prenatally exposed to ritodrine. Br J Obstet Gynaecol 93:156, 1986

132. Thiagarajah S, Harbert GM Jr, Bourgeois FJ: Magnesium sulfate and ritodrine hydrochloride: systemic and uterine hemodynamic effects. Am J Obstet Gynecol 153:666, 1985

133. Petrie RH: Tocolysis using magnesium sulfate. Semin Perinatol 5:266, 1981

134. Beall MH, Edgar BW, Paul RH et al: A comparison of ritodrine, terbutaline, and magnesium sulfate for the suppression of preterm labor. Am J Obstet Gynecol 153:854, 1985

135. Wilkins IA, Lynch L, Mehalek KE et al: Efficacy and side effects of magnesium sulfate and ritodrine as tocolytic agents. Am J Obstet Gynecol 159:685, 1988

136. Armson BA, Samuels P, Miller F et al: Evaluation of maternal fluid dynamics during tocolysis therapy with ritodrine hydrochloride and magnesium sulfate. Am J Obstet Gynecol 167:758, 1992

137. Elliott JP, O'Keefe DF, Greenberg P et al: Pulmonary edema associated with magnesium sulfate and betamethasone administration. Am J Obstet Gynecol 134: 717, 1979

138. Semchyshyn S, Zuspan FP, O'Shaughnessy R: Pulmonary edema associated with the use of hydrocortisone and a tocolytic agent for the management of preterm labor. J Reprod Med 28:47, 1983

139. Schere DM, Cialone PR, Abramowicz JS et al: Transient symptomatic subendocardial ischemia during intravenous magnesium sulfate tocolysis. Am J Obstet Gynecol 166:33, 1992

140. Snyder SW, Cardwell MS: Neuromuscular blockade with magnesium sulfate and nifedipine. Obstet Gynecol 161:35, 1989

141. Digre KB, Varner MW, Schiffman JS: Neuroophthalmologic effects of intravenous magnesium sulfate. Am J Obstet Gynecol 163:1848, 1990

142. Cruikshank DP, Pitkins RM, Donnelly E et al: Urinary

magnesium, calcium and phosphate excretion during magnesium sulfate infusion. Obstet Gynecol 58: 430, 1981

143. Smith LG, Burns PA, Schanler RJ: Calcium homeostasis in pregnant women receiving long-term magnesium sulfate therapy. Am J Obstet Gynecol 167:45, 1992

144. Cholst IN, Steinberg SF, Tropper PJ et al: The influence of hypermagnesemia on serum calcium and parathyroid hormone levels in human subjects. N Engl J Med 310:1221, 1984

145. Spital A, Greenwell R: Severe hyperkalemia during magnesium sulfate therapy in two pregnant drug abusers. South Med J 84:919, 1991

146. Parsons MT, Owens CA, Spellacy WN: Thermic effects of tocolytic agents: decreased temperature with magnesium sulfate. Obstet Gynecol 69:88, 1987

147. Hill WC, Gill PJ, Katz M: Maternal paralytic ileus as a complication of magnesium sulfate tocolysis. Am J Perinatol 2:47, 1987

148. Thorp JM, Katz VL, Campbell D et al: Hypersensitivity to magnesium sulfate. Am J Obstet Gynecol 161: 889, 1989

149. Canez MS, Reed KL, Shenker L: Effect of maternal magnesium sulfate treatment on fetal heart rate variability. Am J Perinatol 4:167, 1987

150. Stallworth JC, Yeh SY, Petrie AH: Effect of magnesium sulfate on fetal heart rate variability and uterine activity. Am J Obstet Gynecol 140:172, 1981

151. Peaceman AM, Meyer BA, Thorp JA et al: The effect of magnesium sulfate tocolysis on the fetal biophysical profile. Am J Obstet Gynecol 161:771, 1989

152. Hankin GDV, Hammond TL, Yeomans ER: Amniotic cavity accumulation of magnesium with prolonged magnesium sulfate tocolysis. J Reprod Med 36:446, 1991

153. Hallak M, Berry BM, Madincea F et al: Fetal serum and amniotic fluid magnesium concentrations with maternal treatment. Obstet Gynecol 81:185, 1983

154. Savory J, Monif GRG: Serum calcium levels in cord sera of the progeny of mothers treated with magnesium sulfate for toxemia of pregnancy. Am J Obstet Gynecol 110:556, 1971

155. McGuinnes GA, Weinstein MM, Cruikshank DP et al: Effects of magnesium sulfate treatment on perinatal calcium metabolism. II. Neonatal responses. Obstet Gynecol 56:595, 1980

156. Rasch DK, Huber PA, Richardson CJ et al: Neurobehavioral effects of neonatal hypermagnesium. J Pediatr 100:272, 1982

157. Koenigsberger MR, Rose JS, Berdon WE et al: Neonatal hypermagnesemia and the meconium-plug syndrome. N Engl J Med 286:823, 1972

158. Lamm CI, Norton KI, Murphy RJ et al: Congenital rickets associated with magnesium sulfate infusions for tocolysis. J Pediatr 113:1078, 1988

159. Holcomb WL, Sheckelford GD, Petrie RH: Magnesium tocolysis and neonatal bone abnormalities: a controlled study. Obstet Gynecol 78:611, 1991

160. Zuckerman H, Shalev E, Gilad G et al: Further study of the inhibition of premature labor by indomethacin. Part II. Double-blind study. J Perinat Med 12: 25, 1984

161. Steiger RM, Boyd EL, Powers DR et al: Acute maternal renal insufficiency in premature labor treated with indomethacin. Am J Perinatol 10:381, 1993

162. Walker MP, Cantrell CJ: Maternal renal impairment after indomethacin tocolysis. J Perinatol 13:461, 1993

163. Collins E, Turner G: Maternal effects of regular salicylate ingestion in pregnancy. Lancet 2:335, 1955

164. Stuart MJ, Gross SJ, Elrad HJ et al: Effects of acetylsalicylic acid ingestion on maternal and neonatal hemostasis. N Engl J Med 307:909, 1982

165. Freidman ZVE, Whitman V, Maisels MI et al: Indomethacin disposition and indomethacin-induced platelet dysfunction in premature infants. J Clin Pharmacol 18:272, 1978

166. Gerson A, Abbasi S, Johnson A et al: Safety and efficacy of long-term tocolysis with indomethacin. Am J Obstet Gynecol 7:71, 1990

167. Reiss U, Atad J, Rubinstein I et al: The effect of indomethacin in labor at term. Int J Gynaecol Obstet 14: 369, 1976

168. Durandy A, Brami C and Griscelli C: The effects of indomethacin administration during pregnancy on women's and newborns' T-suppressor lymphocyte activity and on HLA class II expression by newborns' leukocytes. Am J Reprod Immunol Microbiol 8:94, 1985

169. Naden RP, Iliya CA, Arant BS et al: Hemodynamic effects of indomethacin in chronically instrumented pregnant sheep. Am J Obstet Gynecol 151:484, 1985

170. Mari G, Kirshon B, Wasserstrum N et al: Uterine blood flow velocity waveforms in pregnant women during indomethacin therapy. Obstet Gynecol 76:33, 1990

171. Cantor B, Tyler T, Nelson RM et al: Oligohydramnios and transient neonatal anuria. A possible association with the maternal use of prostaglandin synthetase inhibitors. J Reprod Med 24:220, 1980

172. Itskovitz J, Abramovich H, Brandes JM: Oligohy-

dramnios, meconium and perinatal death concurrent with indomethacin treatment in human pregnancy. J Reprod Med 24:137, 1980

173. Veersema D, de Jong OA, van Wijck JAM: Indomethacin and the fetal renal nonfunction syndrome. Eur J Obstet Gynecol Reprod Biol 16:113, 1983

174. Uslu T, Ozcan FS, Aydin C: Oligohydramnios-induced by maternal indomethacin therapy. Int J Clin Pharmacol 30:230, 1992

175. Morales WJ, Smith SG, Angel JL et al: Efficacy and safety of indomethacin versus ritodrine in the management of preterm labor: a randomized study. Obstet Gynecol 74:567, 1989

176. Bivins HA, Newman RB, Fyfe DA et al: Randomized trial of oral indomethacin and terbutaline sulfate for the long-term suppression of preterm labor. Am J Obstet Gynecol 169:1065, 1993

177. Kirshon B, Moise KJ, Wasserstrum N et al: Influence of short-term indomethacin therapy fetal urine output. Obstet Gynecol 72:51, 1988

178. Kirshon B, Moise KL, Mari G et al: Long-term indomethacin therapy decreases fetal urine output and results in oligohydramnios. Am J Obstet Gynecol 8:86, 1991

179. Mari G, Moise KJ, Deter RL et al: Doppler assessment of the renal blood flow velocity waveform during indomethacin therapy for preterm labor and polyhydramnios. Obstet Gynecol 75:199, 1990

180. Goldenberg RL, Davis RO, Baker RC: Indomethacin-induced oligohydramnios. Am J Obstet Gynecol 160:1196, 1989

181. Moise KJ, Huhta JC, Sharif DS et al: Indomethacin in the treatment of preterm labor. Effects on the fetal ductus arteriosus. N Engl J Med 319:327, 1988

182. Moise KJ: Effect of advancing gestational age on the frequency of fetal ductal constriction in association with maternal indomethacin use. Am J Obstet Gynecol 168:1350, 1993

183. Goodie BM, Dossetor JFB: Effect on the fetus of indomethacin given to suppress labor. Lancet 2:1187, 1979

184. Hallack M, Reiter AA, Ayres NA et al: Indomethacin for preterm labor: fetal toxicity in a dizygotic twin gestation. Obstet Gynecol 78:911, 1991

185. Saenger JS, Mayer DC, D'Angelo LJ et al: Ductus-dependent fetal cardiac defects contraindicate indomethacin tocolysis. J Perinatol 12:41, 1992

186. Levin DL, Fixler DE, Morriss FC et al: Morphologic analysis of the pulmonary vascular bed in infants exposed in utero to prostaglandin synthetase inhibitors. J Pediatr 92:478, 1978

187. Gerson A, Abbasi S, Johnson A et al: Safety and efficacy of long-term tocolysis with indomethacin. Am J Obstet Gynecol 7:71, 1990

188. Rudolph AM: The effects of nonsteroidal anti-inflammatory compounds on fetal circulation and pulmonary function. Obstet Gynecol 58:635, 1981

189. Baerts W, Fretter WP, Hop WC et al: Cerebral lesions in preterm infants after tocolytic indomethacin. Dev Med Child Neurol 32:910, 1990

190. Mari G, Moise KJ, Deter RL et al: Doppler assessment of the pulsitility index of the middle cerebral artery during constriction of the fetal ductus after indomethacin therapy. Am J Obstet Gynecol 161:1528, 1989

191. Norton ME, Merill J, Cooper BA et al: Neonatal complications after administration of indomethacin for preterm labor. N Engl J Med 329:1602, 1993

192. Atad J, Lissak A, Rofe A et al: Patent ductus arteriosus after prolonged treatment with indomethacin during pregnancy. Int J Obstet Gynecol 25:73, 1987

193. Freidman ZVE, Whitman V, Maisels MI et al: Indomethacin disposition and indomethacin-induced platelet dysfunction in premature infants. J Clin Pharmacol 18:272, 1978

194. Rasmussen LF, Wennberger RP: Displacement of bilirubin from albumin binding sites by indomethacin. Clin Res 25:2, 1977

195. Carlan SJ, O'Brien WF, O'Leary TD et al: Randomized comparative trial of indomethacin and sulindac for the treatment of refractile preterm labor. Obstet Gynecol 79:223, 1992

196. Ferguson JE II, Dyson DC, Holbrook RH Jr et al: Cardiovascular and metabolic effects associated with nifedipine and ritodrine tocolysis. Am J Obstet Gynecol 161:788, 1989

197. Ferguson JE II, Dyson DC, Schutz T et al: A comparison of tocolysis with nifedipine or ritodrine: analysis of efficacy and maternal, fetal, and neonatal outcome. Am J Obstet Gynecol 163:105, 1990

198. Glock JL, Morales WJ: Efficacy and safety of nifedipine versus magnesium sulfate in the management of preterm labor: a randomized study. Am J Obstet Gynecol 169:960, 1993

199. Ferguson JE II, Schutz T, Pershe R et al: Nifedipine pharmacokinetics during preterm labor tocolysis. Am J Obstet Gynecol 161:1485, 1989

200. Ulmsten U: Treatment of normotensive and hypertensive patients with preterm labor using oral nifedipine, a calcium antagonist. Arch Gynecol 236:69, 1984

201. Read MD, Welby DE: The use of a calcium antagonist (nifedipine) to suppress preterm labor. Br J Obstet Gynaecol 98:933, 1986

202. Meyer WR, Randall HW, Graves WL: Nifedipine versus ritodrine for suppressing preterm labor. J Reprod Med 35:649, 1990

203. Mari G, Kirshon B, Moise KJ et al: Doppler assessment of the fetal and uteroplacental circulation during nifedipine therapy for preterm labor. Am J Obstet Gynecol 161:1514, 1989

204. Murray C, Haverkamp AD, Orleans M et al: Nifedipine for treatment of preterm labor: a historic prospective study. Am J Obstet Gynecol 167:52, 1992

205. Ferguson JE II, Schutz TE, Stephenson DK: Neonatal bilirubin production after preterm labor tocolysis with nifedipine. Dev Pharmacol Ther 12:113, 1989

Chapter 18

Asthma

Thomas C. C. Peng

Asthma, estimated to affect 1 to 4 percent and possibly up to 10 percent of gravid women, is one of the most common disorders in pregnancy.[1] It is defined by the American Thoracic Society's Joint Committee on Pulmonary Nomenclature as "disease characterized by an increased responsiveness of the airways to various stimuli, manifested by slowing of forced expiration, which changes in severity either spontaneously or as a result of therapy." In general, asthma is a reversible obstructive pulmonary disorder, but still accounts for 4,000 deaths a year. Status asthmaticus is severe asthma not responsive to intensive treatment after 30 to 60 minutes, and occurs in 0.15 to 0.2 percent of pregnant women. The National Asthma Education Program, a working group convened by the U.S. National Institutes of Health, National Heart, Lung, and Blood Institute (NHLBI) has noted a trend of increasing prevalence, morbidity, and mortality from asthma in pregnancy, and has concluded that addressing the undertreatment of asthma may reverse this trend.[2] Therefore, it is important to understand the appropriate evaluation of asthma and to institute effective treatment for it. With appropriate management, pregnancies in asthmatic patients can have normal or near normal outcomes.[3]

Intrapartum management of asthma is the focus of this chapter, but its appropriate antepartum management makes intrapartum management all the easier. This chapter discusses the pathophysiology, evaluation, pharmacotherapy, and medical management of chronic asthma and acute exacerbations of it during the antepartum and intrapartum periods.

PATHOPHYSIOLOGY

Asthma is a disease marked by reversible bronchospasm, the pathophysiology of which is related to hyperreactive airways and inflammation. It bears repeating that inflammation is a critical element in the pathology of the disease. Edema, cellular infiltration of the bronchial mucosa and submucosa, and an eosinophilic exudate with inflammatory cells and desquamated bronchial epithelial cells in the bronchial lumen are consistent findings in postmortem studies of patients who have died from asthma.[4]

Goals of Management of Asthma During Pregnancy

1. Prevention of exacerbations and status asthmaticus
2. Maintenance of normal or near normal maternal pulmonary function and oxygenation
3. Promotion of normal pregnancy outcomes, fetal growth, and delivery of a healthy infant

---

Factors that can provoke an acute exacerbation of chronic asthma include respiratory infections, environmental irritants (e.g., cigarette smoking), cold air, exercise, and allergens such as pet dander, pollen, and house mites. Extrinsic asthma, seen more commonly in children, usually a results from exposure to allergens, leading to IgE-mediated degranulation of mast cells with release of inflammatory mediators. A focus on removing or ameliorating identified allergens may reduce exacerbations of asthma in these patients. Intrinsic asthma, seen more commonly in adults, is associated with atopy, and allergens are generally not identifiable as precipitating factors.

Initially, bronchial smooth muscle contraction results in bronchospasm and reduces air flow. Subsequently, inflammatory mediators such as histamine, slow reacting substance-A, leukotrienes, eosinophilic chemotactic factor, and platelet activating factor are released, with the end result of vasodilation, leaking capillaries, extravasation of extracellular fluid, bronchial edema, increased mucus production, mucus plugging, bronchial smooth muscle hypertrophy, and bronchial muscle contraction, further reducing bronchial compliance and increasing obstruction to airflow.

EFFECTS OF PREGNANCY ON ASTHMA

Summarized studies of 1,087 asthmatic pregnant women noted that 36 percent had improvement of pulmonary function, 41 percent demonstrated no alteration, and 23 percent experienced a worsening of asthma.[5,6] At least, 43 percent of pregnant women experienced one exacerbation of asthma. Most exacerbations tend to occur in the second half of pregnancy and appear to behave similarly from one pregnancy to another in the same patient.[5,6] Exacerbations appear less often and are less severe in the last 4 weeks of pregnancy.[6] Exacerbations during labor and delivery are uncommon, being estimated to occur in 10 percent of asthmatic pregnant patients. These episodes tend to be mild, with most exacerbations reversed with inhaled bronchodilating agents.[6] Although it is difficult to predict which individual pregnancy will suffer an exacerbation, the risk increases with the severity of asthma.

EFFECT OF ASTHMA ON PREGNANCY

Two large epidemiologic studies have documented the adverse effect of asthma on pregnancy. In 1972, a published study of 381 pregnancies in asthmatic women, compared with a control group of 112,530 pregnancies in nonasthmatic women, noted a statistically significant increase in preterm birth, low birth weight, neonatal mortality, decreased mean birth weight, and labor complications in the asthmatic patients.[7] Data from the Collaborative Perinatal Project found a statistically significant higher perinatal mortality rate in 277 asthmatic pregnant women compared with 30,861 normal pregnant women.[8] In one case controlled study in which pregnant patients were matched for age and parity, pre-eclampsia was increased among asthmatic patients, especially for those with severe asthma.[9] Use of steroids in the treatment of asthma has been linked to an increased prevalence of gestational diabetes and insulin-dependent diabetes mellitus.[10]

Fetal growth has been strongly linked to the course of asthma, occurrence of acute antepartum exacerbations and degree of obstructive airflow. Pregnancies complicated by antepartum status asthmaticus are at much greater risk of yielding infants who are small for their gestational age and growth retarded fetuses, as compared to pregnancies without such an episode.[11] These same risks have been noted in steroid-dependent asthma.[12] A Kaiser-Permnante prospective study of asthma and pregnancy noted a direct relationship between the maternal forced expiratory volume in the first second of expiration (FEV_1) and the risk of low fetal birth weight.[13] From these studies, one can conclude that maintaining normal or near normal pulmonary function and preventing status asthmaticus and exacerbations of asthma should have beneficial effects on fetal growth and pregnancy outcome.

Fetal mortality occurs in cases of asthma during pregnancy and is probably the result of severe bronchospasm and hypoxia. Maternal respiratory alkalosis may accentuate fetal hypoxemia, possibly as a result of reduced uterine blood flow, decreased venous return, and an alkaline-induced leftward shift of the fetal oxyhemoglobin dissociation curve.[2] Maternal mortality has also been reported in association with asthma.

Table 18-1. Objective Signs of Severe Acute Asthmatic Exacerbation

Clinical symptoms and signs of breathlessness, use of accessory muscles, difficulty with speech
FEV_1 <1 L (or <25% of predicted)
PEFR <100 L/min

	pH	PO_2	PCO_2
Arterial blood gas patterns			
Normal	7.4–7.45	95–106	28–35
Mild exacerbation	↑	Normal	↓
Severe exacerbation	Normal	↓	Normal
Respiratory failure	↓	↓	↑

OBJECTIVE EVALUATION

The classic symptoms of asthma are wheezing, cough, chest tightness, and dyspnea. However, these subjective symptoms and many of the clinical signs, discussed later, do not correlate well with the severity of bronchospasm. Therefore, objective evaluation is a necessary and important element in the management of asthma (Table 18-1). This includes pulmonary function testing, measurement of peak expiratory flow, and arterial blood gas analysis.

Pulmonary function tests are useful in the assessment of asthma. In pregnancy, there is normally an increase in the tidal volume with an associated increase in minute ventilation, and decrease in forced vital capacity, residual volume, and functional residual capacity. Forced expiratory volumes and flows are not different from those of nonpregnant women.

Pulmonary function tests are useful for establishing a diagnosis in less typical presentations of asthma, such as isolated nocturnal cough; they are also useful in establishing baseline pulmonary function and assessing the severity of an acute exacerbation. Such tests are noninvasive and should be used liberally for these purposes. Assessment of asthma with pulmonary function tests demonstrates an obstructive pattern, with a reduced rate of expiratory air flow predominantly affecting small airways. Progressive involvement eventually involves the larger airways with a concomitant decrease in FEV_1. The forced vital capacity is decreased, although this is proportionally less than the decrease in FEV_1. As a result, the FEV_1/FVC ratio is below 0.75, as is typical in obstructive pulmonary disease. A general hallmark of the severity of an exacerbation is an FEV_1 of less than 1 L. This degree of reduced expiratory flow is correlated with hypoxemia.[14] The correlation is not absolute, as hypoxemia, with an arterial partial pressure of oxygen (PaO_2) of less than 60 mm Hg, has been noted in asthmatic adults with an FEV_1 exceeding 1 L.[14]

Peak expiratory flow rate (PEFR), as measured by simple hand-held devices, represents a clinically useful correlate of FEV_1, although it is not as sensitive for the detection of airway disease. The PEFR is not a diagnostic tool but is useful in the clinical assessment of disease severity in patients with confirmed asthma. A normal PEFR is 380 to 550 L/min, but each patient should establish her own baseline for comparison. Pregnancy does not affect the PEFR. In general, a 10 to 20 percent variation in PEFR from baseline would represent a significant change. A PEFR below 100 L/min would suggest severe obstruction and possible impending respiratory distress.

In pregnancy, the normally increased minute ventilation is associated with a higher PaO_2 (100 to 106 mm Hg), a lower arterial partial pressure of carbon dioxide ($PaCO_2$) (28 to 35 mm Hg), and a slightly more alkaline pH (7.40 to 7.45) than are seen in nonpregnant women. Near term, the PaO_2 falls slightly to 90 to 100 mm Hg as the result of an increased critical closing volume. During the early phase of bronchospasm, a mild ventilation/perfusion (V̇/Q̇) mismatch occurs. Oxygenation is maintained with a mild decrease in PCO_2 and mild respiratory alkalosis. As bronchospasm worsens, V̇/Q̇ mismatch intensifies, alveolar hypoventilation worsens, and CO_2 retention occurs. The PCO_2 begins to increase and "normalize." In pregnancy, the normal values (lower PCO_2, higher pH, and higher PO_2) yield a different threshold for interpretation. A $PaCO_2$ of 35 to 40 mm Hg, while less ominous in a nonpregnant asthmatic patient, may in pregnancy signify impending respiratory failure. Some authors suggest that a PCO_2 above 35 mm Hg and a pH below 7.35 should be considered evidence of respiratory failure in pregnancy. Clearly, patients with this blood gas pattern need to be observed closely in an acute care setting, such as a labor-and-delivery unit, that can provide optimal monitoring of both mother and fetus. Ultimately, without intervention, progressive bronchospasm may lead to hypoxemia, acidosis, respiratory failure, and potentially maternal and fetal death.

Pulse oximetry is useful in monitoring oxygenation once the severity of asthma has been determined. It should not be used to replace evaluation by arterial blood gas analysis, since it yields no information about pH or PCO_2, both of which are useful parameters for defining respiratory failure.

PHARMACOTHERAPY

Pharmacotherapy is one arm in the effective management of asthma, which also includes patient education and objective monitoring of disease activity. Appropriate pharmacotherapy in pregnancy will depend on its clinical effectiveness, adverse side effects, and teratogenic potential. The patient should be taught that while most of the pharmacologic agents used for treating asthma have been used safely in pregnancy, none has been proved to be absolutely safe. Of the drugs used in the treatment of asthma, experience with β-adrenergic agonists, methylxanthines, and glucocorticoids has been greater in pregnancy than that with such agents as atropine, ipratropium, and cromolyn. Atropine and ipratropium (an atropine derivative) are useful bronchodilators with comparatively few side effects, but experience with their use in pregnancy is minimal. This discussion focuses on the first three classes of drugs mentioned above (Table 18-2). Most of the data related

Table 18-2. Pharmacotherapy for Acute Exacerbations of Asthma

Drug	Route of Administration and Dose
Parenteral β-agonists	Epinephrine 0.2–0.5 ml of 1:1,000 dilution, SC Repeat q15–20min, limit to three doses OR Terbutaline 0.25 mg SC Repeat once in 15–20 minutes
Inhaled β-agonists by nebulizer	Albuterol 0.5 ml of 0.5% solution in 2–3 ml of normal saline OR Metaproterenol 0.3 ml of 5% solution in 2–3 ml of normal saline Administered ≤q20–30min for three doses and then q1h until desired response
Corticosteroids	Methylprednisolone 1 mg/kg bolus IV 6–8h OR Hydrocortisone 2 mg/kg bolus IV q4h OR Hydrocortisone 2 mg/kg bolus IV, followed by 0.5 mg/kg/hr continuous infusion
Methylxanthines	Loading dose Theophylline 5 mg/kg or aminophylline 6 mg/kg, IV (patients not chronically medicated with methylxanthine preparation) Maintenance dose Theophylline 0.4 mg/kg/hr or aminophylline 0.5 mg/kg/hr, adjusted to serum levels of 8–12 μg/mL

(Adapted from National Asthma Education Program[2])

to the efficacy of these drugs have been established in nonpregnant asthmatic patients.

β₂-Selective Agonists

β₂-Selective agonists are considered the drugs of first choice in the management of asthma. β₂-Receptors occur on bronchial smooth muscle, mast cells, and secretory cells in the respiratory tract.[15] When these receptors are stimulated by β-adrenergic agonists, adenylate cyclase is activated and cyclic adenosine monophosphate (cAMP) accumulates, leading to bronchodilation, decreased mucus production, and stabilization of mast cells. Drugs with selective β₂ effects include terbutaline, metaproterenol, albuterol, and isoetharine, all of which can be supplied in metered-dose inhalers (MDI), a common form of administering these medications.

Use of the β₂ agents appears to be safe in pregnancy. In one study pregnancy outcomes in terms of perinatal mortality, congenital anomalies, preterm birth, growth retardation, complications of labor and delivery, neonatal complications, and postpartum bleeding were similar in pregnancies involving asthmatic patients using β₂ inhalers and in those involving patients not using inhalers and nonasthmatic controls.[16] Well-controlled asthma generally requires minimal use of inhaled β₂-selective agonists. An increase in their use may be a sign of deteriorating control. β₂ agents such as terbutaline may also be administered orally or parenterally.

Nonselective sympathomimetic drugs such as epinephrine stimulate β₁- β₂-, and α-receptors in both the respiratory tract and cardiovascular system. α-Receptor stimulation reduces vascular congestion and mucosal edema. No long-term fetal effects have been noted with the use of these agents, although there is concern about a theoretical effect of α-receptor-mediated vasoconstriction and its effect on uteroplacental perfusion. Epinephrine continues to be favored by some authors in the emergent treatment of acute exacerbations of asthma. Because of its β₁-stimulating effect, the presence of coronary artery disease, heart failure, or arrythmia should dictate caution in its use. Epinephrine and β₂-selective agonists should not be used simultaneously.

Methylxanthines

A second class of drugs used in treating asthma are the methylxanthines, long a mainstay in management of the disease. Amniophylline and its salt derivative, theophylline (80 percent aminophylline by weight) are methylxanthines that have a bronchodilating effect. Methylxanthines inhibit phosphodiesterase, which degrades cAMP. This was believed to be the mechanism for these drugs' bronchodilating effect in which they were believed to act synergistically with β₂-agonist therapy. However, current studies demonstrate that the level of phosphodiesterase inhibition achieved with the methylxanthines is insufficient to produce bronchodilation.[17] Furthermore, other phosphodiesterase inhibitors do not produce bronchodilation.[15] The mechanism of action of the methylxanthines is unknown. Contrary to previous concepts, they do not act synergistically with β₂-agonists in asthma and do not appear to increase the latter drugs' efficacy, but do appear to increase toxicity.[18]

The toxicity of methylxanthines derives from their effects on other organ systems, including the heart (they are positive inotropes) and central nervous system. Adverse effects include tachycardia, tremor, palpitations, seizures, arrythmia, restlessness, insomnia, and nausea. The therapeutic index for theophylline is quite narrow, and side effects of the drug are common even with careful monitoring of its serum levels. The recommended therapeutic serum level in nonpregnant asthmatic patients is 10 to 20 μg/ml. Serum levels of theophylline are affected by a variety of situations, including cardiac and liver dysfunction, certain drugs such as cimitidine and erythromycin, fever, and hypoxemia. Absorption of theophylline from sustained-release dosage forms may be altered by food and the type of food ingested. In pregnancy, theophylline clearance is affected toward term gestation. Theophylline levels must be monitored in the pregnant patient, since clearance of the drug appears to decrease by as much as 53 percent in the third trimester.[19]

Theophylline has been safely used in pregnancy, although with caution for the adverse effects noted above. No adverse outcomes of pregnancy were noted in the 193 patients exposed to theophylline in the Collaborative Perinatal Project.[2,20] There appears to be no increased risk of fetal developmental problems. Theophylline easily crosses the placenta. Neonatal levels are comparable to maternal levels, although the drug appears to be well tolerated by the fetus.[21] Reported neonatal side effects include jitteriness, tachycardia, and opisthotonus, and can occur in the presence of therapeutic maternal levels of theophylline. Some authors recommend reducing the therapeutic serum level in pregnancy to less than 12 to 14 μg/ml.[2] Because of the side effects, narrow therapeutic index, and the availability of other effective bronchodilators, methylxanthines such as theophylline are no longer considered first-line therapy for asthma.

Glucocorticoids

Glucocorticoids are highly effective anti-inflammatory agents, although widespread use is limited by the side effects. Glucocorticoids reduce edema in bronchial smooth muscle; constrict bronchial microvascular capillaries; reduce fluid extravasation; suppress the recruitment of macrophages, monocytes, and other inflammatory cells; decrease the activity of inflammatory cells; suppress the release of mediators of inflammation; increase the responsiveness of bronchial smooth muscle to β-agonist drugs; and inhibit arachidonic acid metabolism and the synthesis of proinflammatory agents of the lipoxygenase and cyclo-oxygenase pathways.[22]

Steroids with which there has been clinical experience in pregnant asthmatic patients include hydrocortisone, prednisone, methylprednisolone, and beclomethasone. These drugs do not appear to increase the risk of fetal or maternal complications of pregnancy, although the literature on their teratogenic potential is conflicting.[23] Prednisone and prednisolone both cross the placenta. Prednisone crosses readily but is slowly converted by the fetus into the active metabolite prednisolone. Prednisolone, by contrast, crosses the placenta slowly, and fetal levels approximate 10 percent of maternal levels.[7] Maternal side effects of prednisone include weight gain, hypertension, diabetes mellitus, osteoporosis, and suppression of the hypothalamic–pituitary–adrenal axis. Use of this drug in pregnancy should arise from clear indications. Similarly, experience with inhaled steroids such as beclomethasone suggests that they do not increase the risk of adverse pregnancy outcomes but reduce the risk of adverse maternal side effects.[24,11]

Clinical trials demonstrate the efficacy of steroids in improving pulmonary function in asthma. A randomized, double-blind, placebo-controlled clinical trial involving 20 patients with asthma demonstrated a significant improvement in FEV_1 in patients treated with hydrocortisone (2 mg/kg bolus, followed by 0.5 mg/kg/hr for 24 hours).[25] Administration of a single dose of glucocorticoids orally or intravenously begins to improve pulmonary function at 2 hours with a peak effect at 8 hours and a gradual diminution of effect thereafter.[22] Although improvement in function is usually evident after 6 hours, full restoration to normal function generally takes 1 week or longer. Methylprednisolone can be given intravenously, has a five times more potent anti-inflammatory action than hydrocortisone, and penetrates the bronchial mucosa better than prednisone.[22] Prednisone is generally used orally for the chronic management of steroid-dependent asthma.

Inhaled steroids (e.g., beclomethasone) are effective in the chronic management of asthma or in the mildest of exacerbations. They are not effective in the management of acute exacerbations. Inhaled steroids are the preferred choice for chronic steroid therapy. They are minimally absorbed systemically, reduce systemic steroid effects, and can reduce dependence on and the dosage of oral steroids. The most common side effects of inhaled steroids are oral candidiasis, hoarseness, and sore throat. The risk of oral candidiasis can be reduced by an oral rinse after each application of inhaled steroids or the addition of a spacer between the mouth and the MDI. Patients chronically exposed to steroids (which is less likely if their only treatment has been with inhaled steroids) are potentially adrenally suppressed and should receive supplemental steroids in any "stressful" situation, such as labor and delivery, for at least 24 hours.

THE MANAGEMENT OF CHRONIC ASTHMA

Effective management of chronic asthma in the pregnant patient consists of (1) serial monitoring of the severity of disease; (2) serial monitoring of the effect of asthma on the pregnancy; (3) adoption of measures to avoid triggers and stimulants causing bronchospasm; (4) appropriate use of pharmacotherapy, minimizing doses to control symptoms but providing sufficient doses to avoid hypoxia and achieve normalization of pulmonary function; and

(5) patient education. Patient education about the avoidance of triggers and stimulants of bronchospasm creates a partnership in the management of asthma that should lead to early recognition of loss of control of the disease, its early treatment, and a reduction in symptoms, acute exacerbations, and status asthmaticus[2] (Table 18-3).

The initial visit of a pregnant woman with chronic asthma should be used to define the extent of disease and the severity of prior manifestations, including hospitalizations and intubations. The patient's current level of symptoms and physical function (e.g., dyspnea, nocturnal cough) should be assessed, and her medications should be reviewed for safety of use in pregnancy, with the serum levels measured where appropriate. A pulmonary function test and PEFR measurement are strongly recommended to provide baseline function values. A chest radiograph and arterial blood gas analysis are not routinely needed, but should be obtained in cases in which the circumstances dictate (e.g., suspicion of cor pulmonale). The gestational age should be established and confirmed, if necessary, with ultrasonographic fetal biometry.

Serial evaluations of patients' symptoms and objective pulmonary function testing are useful throughout pregnancy, particularly for patients with moderate or severe disease. For instance, patients who develop coughing with inspiration, have persistent nighttime awakenings, or increased wheezing may need additional therapy. Hand-held PEFR devices can be used by the patient to monitor her own baseline pulmonary function.[26] Serial assessment of fetal growth is recommended and can be accom-

Table 18-3. Chronic Asthma

	Mild Asthma	Moderate Asthma	Severe Asthma
Clinical characteristics	Intermittent, brief (<1 hr) wheeze/cough/dypnea, up to 2× weekly Asymptomatic between exacerbations Brief (<½ hr) wheeze/cough/dyspnea with exertion Infrequent (<2×/mo) nocturnal cough/wheeze	Symptoms >1–2×/wk Exacerbations affect sleep or activity level Exacerbations may last several days Occasional emergency care	Continuous symptoms Limited activity Frequent exacerbations Frequent nocturnal symptoms Occasional hospitalization and/or emergency visits
Assessment of pulmonary function (FEV$_1$ or PEFR)	Asymptomatic: ≥80% baseline Symptomatic: varies by ≥20%	60–80% of baseline Varies 20–30% when symptomatic	<60% baseline Highly variable, 20–30% changes while on routine medications and varies >50% during exacerbations
Therapy	Asymptomatic: pretreat PRN with 1–2 puffs of β$_2$-agonist for exposure to exertion, allergen, etc. Symptomatic: β$_2$-agonist (2 puffs, q3–4h) PRN for duration of exacerbation	Inhaled β$_2$-agonist PRN to tid/qid AND Inhaled steroids (2–4 puffs bid) OR Cromolyn (2 puffs qid) Additional therapy includes theophylline, oral β$_2$-agonist	Inhaled steroids (4–6 puffs bid or 2–5 puffs qid) AND Inhaled β$_2$-agonist PRN to qid AND consider Oral steroids daily or alternate-day use with/without, oral sustained-release theophylline and oral β$_2$-agonist
Outcome	Prevent symptoms Reduce PEFR variability Normal activity tolerance	Symptom control Reduce PEFR variability Normal activity tolerance Infrequent exacerbations Reduce nocturnal awakenings Reduce use of PRN inhaled β$_2$-agonist	Improve pulmonary function and reduce PEFR variability Almost normal activity tolerance and reduce nocturnal awakening Reduce frequency of exacerbation, PRN inhaled β$_2$-agonist, oral steroid pulse, and emergency visits

(Adapted from National Asthma Education Program.[2])

plished by physical examination and the use of ultra-sonographic fetal biometry. Surveillance of the fetus after it has achieved a gestational age consistent with viability should especially be considered in patients with exacerbations of asthma, those who require chronic prophylactic therapy, those who have a reduced baseline pulmonary function, and those with moderate to severe disease. Patients can be instructed to count fetal movements and more rigorous fetal heart rate testing may be instituted in those with severe disease, reduced pulmonary function, or fetal indications for this. When combined, these efforts reveal the effectiveness of therapy, maximize the opportunity for early detection of relapse, and permit monitoring of the effect of the disease on pregnancy.

Chronic asthma can be stratified into the categories of mild, moderate, and severe. Mild disease produces infrequent and sporadic symptoms, while severe disease produces more frequent symptoms and requires prophylactic treatment with chronic inhalation therapy, methylxanthines, or steroids. Moderate disease has characteristics intermediate between those of mild and severe disease. Stratification may help in determining the intensity of monitoring during pregnancy.

Mild chronic asthma can be treated as needed with inhaled β_2-adrenergic drugs such as metaproterenol and terbutaline. Moderate chronic asthma, with exacerbations that occur more frequently, requires a scheduled administration of inhaled β_2-adrenergic agents, usually two puffs every 4 to 6 hours. The addition of aerosolized steroids (beclomethasone, 2 puffs) or theophylline may be needed for refractory symptoms. More severe disease requires the addition of oral steroids. In general, a short pulse of high-dose prednisone (i.e., 40 to 60 mg/day with a rapid taper) may be beneficial before instituting maintenance therapy in severe disease.[15] One possible sequence of accelerated pharmacotherapy for the patient with chronic asthma is (1) inhalation of β_2-adrenergic drugs as needed, (2) inhalation of β_2 drugs on a fixed schedule, (3) beclomethasone inhalation, (4) theophylline taken orally, and (5) oral steroids such as prednisone. Long-term steroid use should be tapered to minimal doses and an alternate day schedule whenever possible.

MANAGEMENT OF ACUTE ASTHMATIC EXACERBATIONS

Acute exacerbations of asthma generally present with dyspnea, chest tightness, cough, or wheezing (Fig. 18-1). Although most presentations are obvious, 60 to 70 percent of gravid women experience "normal" dyspnea during pregnancy, and the diagnosis of asthma can sometimes be difficult to confirm. Illnesses that may present with symptoms similar to those of asthma include pulmonary edema, amniotic fluid embolism, pneumonia, chronic obstructive pulmonary disease, upper airway obstruction, cardiac asthma, mitral stenosis, and pulmonary embolism. In general, concurrent clinical findings should allow a rapid differentiation of these various etiologies.

Critical in the initial assessment of the patient is determining the severity of asthma. Although the most reliable method of assessment is spirometric measurement of the FEV_1 or PFER (or both), a history and physical examination are useful adjuncts. The onset, duration, and severity of existing symptoms; the presence of fever; a productive cough; recent steroid use, emergency department visits, or hospitalizations; a history of intubations, all medications currently used; and a recent history of increased use of inhaled or oral bronchodilators should be elicited in taking the history to determine the potential for failure of outpatient therapy and the need for hospitalization. A long history of symptoms and recurrent emergency department visits prior to obstetric admission increase the risk of mucus impaction and hospitalization.

On the physical examination, attention should be directed to the presence of tachypnea, tachycardia, pulsus paradoxus with a 12 mm Hg or greater decrease in systolic blood pressure during inspiration (the mechanism for which is unknown but is believed to be related to increasing negative inspiratory pleural pressures), changes in mentation, and pulmonary auscultatory findings. Disrupted speech secondary to labored breathing is indicative of a severe exacerbation of asthma and generally associated with an FEV_1 of less than 0.45 L.[27] Wheezing is unfortunately not a reliable sign of the severity of asthma. When present throughout the respiratory cycle it is generally significant of greater obstructive

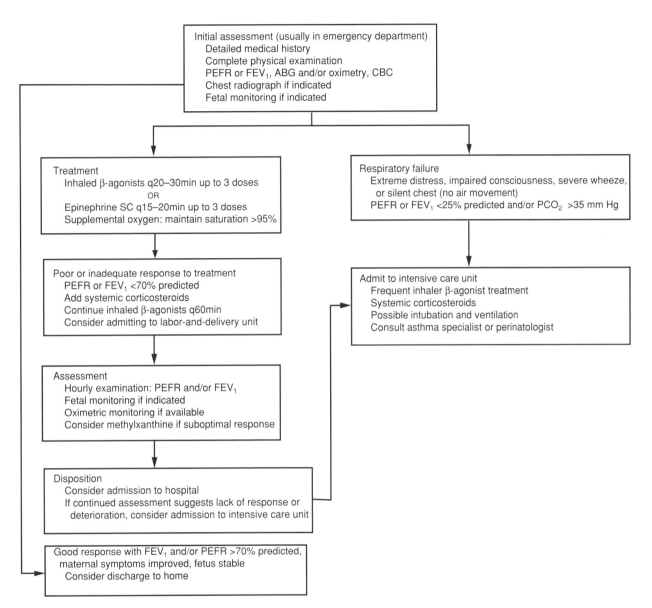

Fig. 18-1. Acute exacerbation of asthma during pregnancy. PEFR, peak expiratory flow rate; FEV$_1$ forced expiratory volume within the first second of expiration; ABG, arterial blood gases; CBC, complete blood count.

disease than is isolated expiratory wheezing. However, wheezing may increase as bronchospasm decreases secondary to increased airflow, and conversely may decrease as obstruction increases secondary to reduced air movement. Two signs of a potentially fatal attack of asthma are central cyanosis and an altered mental status. However, none of these historical factors, symptoms, or signs is wholly reliable or accurate in gauging the severity of an exacerbation.[14]

Objective assessment of pulmonary function and its response to treatment remains the most reliable predictor of the severity of an exacerbation of asthma. Baseline spirometry with assessment of the

FEV_1 or PEFR (or both) should be performed and followed to note the efficacy of treatment. Spirometry can be performed every hour during the acute phase of an asthmatic attack and, when the patient has been stabilized, one to two times a day during the hospitalization. Because FEV_1 and PEFR are effort and volume dependent, it is recommended that the initial baseline values of these parameters be established from the maximum value of three attempts. An FEV_1 of less than 1 L (which generally represents <25 percent of the predicted value for women) and/or a PEFR of less than 100 L/min (generally <20 percent of predicted) are both indicative of severe obstruction. An arterial blood gas analysis is useful and recommended for all but the mildest of exacerbations to determine oxygenation and the risk of respiratory failure on the basis of PCO_2 and pH (Table 18-1). A mild exacerbation is generally associated with hypocapnea, mild alkalosis, and normal or near normal oxygenation. As the severity of bronchospasm increases and FEV_1 decreases, the PCO_2 rises and pH falls, approaching normal nonpregnancy values. It is important to recall that in pregnancy, a normal PCO_2 is 35 mm Hg and a normal pH is 7.4 to 7.45. In a severe exacerbation of asthma the blood gas analysis reveals a pattern of acidosis, hypercarbia, and hypoxemia. A chest radiograph is not routinely indicated, but in the presence of suggestive symptoms or signs is helpful in excluding the possibility of pneumonia or other diagnoses. Routine chest radiographs appear to be of low yield, rarely providing insight into the management of asthma.[15] A complete blood count is helpful in patients with a suspected infection. A serum theophylline assay is helpful in patients previously medicated with theophylline, both to determine the potential etiology of an exacerbation and adequate therapeutic dosing of the drug. The fetal heart rate should be monitored during the evaluation and treatment phases of asthma in pregnancies in which the gestational age is consistent with fetal viability.

Some physicians use a scoring index of seven items derived from the constellation of symptoms, physical findings, and objective testing in asthma to determine the severity of an exacerbation, likelihood of failure of outpatient therapy, and need for hospitalization. Indicators of severe asthma include a pulse exceeding 120 beats/min, a respiratory rate above 30/min, pulsus paradoxus with a pressure above 18 mm Hg, a PEFR below 120 L/min, moderate to severe dyspnea, moderate to severe wheezing, and moderate to severe use of accessory respiratory muscles. An index score of 4 or more indicates a 95 percent probability of relapse and the need for hospitalization.[28] This scoring index is useful but not highly reliable.[15] In general, characteristics that identify the risk of life-threatening deterioration include an improvement of less than 10 percent in FEV_1 or PEFR in the emergency department, an FEV_1 below 25 percent of that predicted or a PEFR below 100 L/min, a prior history of life-threatening exacerbations, and a PCO_2 of 35 mm Hg or more.[2]

Because of the potentially adverse consequences of maternal hypoxia on fetal welfare, a liberal policy of hospitalization of pregnant women with an asthmatic exacerbation is warranted. The initial assessment of an acute exacerbation may occur in the office, but generally occurs in the emergency department or labor-and-delivery unit. If significant improvement has not occurred within a short period, or if a prolonged period of treatment is anticipated before stabilization, assessment should continue in an acute care setting such as the labor-and-delivery unit, where both fetal and maternal welfare can be adequately monitored.

Initial treatment of an acute exacerbation of asthma consists of hydration, oxygenation, and medication. Fluid hydration should not be overly aggressive, although most patients will benefit from an initial liter of physiologic saline. Supplemental oxygen with a low flow rate of 2 to 3 L/min is generally sufficient for oxygenation, and can be titrated according to blood gas measurements and monitored with pulse oximetry or arterial blood gas analysis. Supplemental oxygen should maintain a 95 percent oxyhemoglobin saturation and a PaO_2 above 60 to 70 mm Hg.

The primary therapy is repeated use of a β_2-agonist (inhaled or parenteral) and systemic corticosteroids. β-Agonists are the drugs of first choice in the management of an acute exacerbation, although debate exists over which β-agonist (i.e., epinephrine or β_2-agonists) or route of administration (i.e., parenteral or inhaled) is best (Table 18-2). Subcutaneous epinephrine remains preferred by some investigators, primarily because of its rapidity of action.[29] Epinephrine given subcutaneously in a dose of 0.2 to 0.5 ml of a 1:1,000 dilution provides evident bronchodilation within 5 minutes of its administration. The larger dose is for the heavier patient. The dose may be repeated every 15 to 20 minutes, and it is recommended that treatment be limited to three doses. Terbutaline is an alternative choice. It can be used subcutaneously (0.25 mg, repeated once in 15 to 20 minutes if needed, with a maximum dose of 0.5 mg in 4 hours) or intravenously (6 μg/kg), and also produces effective bronchodilation with significant improvement of the PEFR.[15,30] Terbutaline has a longer duration of action than epinephrine. The parenteral route of administration is preferred, especially with severe bronchospasm, which may prevent the adequate delivery of inhaled agents.

Repetitive inhaled β₂-agonist therapy is also effective and produces incremental bronchodilation. The onset of action of such therapy occurs within 5 minutes of administration. Initial treatment with three doses every 20 to 30 minutes can be given safely in the absence of cardiovascular disease, and can be continued hourly thereafter until the desired response is achieved. Milder exacerbations of asthma may be adequately treated with an inhaled (e.g., via a nebulizer or MDI) β₂-agonist.

Clinical trials show that inhaled β₂-agonists can produce an improvement in pulmonary function, as measured by FEV_1, of similar magnitude to traditional treatment with parenteral epinephrine.[31] In one study of nonpregnant asthmatic patients, intravenous terbutaline produced an improvement in PEFR equal to that with inhaled nebulized terbutaline, but a greater increase in PaO_2.[30]

An improvement of FEV_1 to more than 1.6 to 2.1 L or improvement of the PEFR to more than 300 L/min, would indicate a response to therapy.[28] If β-agonist therapy fails to achieve the desired response within the first hour of its use, adding parenteral steroids will generally ameliorate most refractory attacks. However, the effect of steroids generally does not become manifest for 6 to 8 hours, and β-agonist therapy should therefore be continued. Steroids are an effective second line of therapy because of their anti-inflammatory effect and effectiveness in preventing status asthmaticus and hospitalization in nonpregnant asthmatic patients.[32] Methylprednisolone administered at 125 mg every 6 hours demon-

strates greater efficacy and produces a significantly more rapid response than at lower doses.[34] Prompt use of methylprednisolone, within 30 minutes of the onset of an exacerbation of asthma, may also reduce the rate of hospital admissions.[32] Topical or inhaled glucocorticoids are not indicated, since they are less effective and may not reach the desired site in sufficient quantities to provide the effect needed. Once the exacerbation is controlled, steroids are generally continued parenterally for 48 hours before conversion to the oral route. A general initial daily dose of oral prednisone is 40 to 60 mg. In patients not being treated chronically with steroids, weaning from parenteral therapy can occur rapidly over a 7- to 10-day period. Patients receiving chronic steroid therapy can be weaned to maintenance therapy.

The addition of methylxanthines such as aminophylline to β-agonist therapy is an alternative to steroid therapy, but has not been shown to augment the bronchodilation achieved with β-agonists, and in fact has been shown to increase toxicity.[31,18,33] The initial intravenous loading dose (over 20 to 30 minutes) in patients without prior exposure is 5 to 6 mg/kg of actual body weight rather than ideal body weight, as is recommended in nonpregnant asthmatic patients.[35] The maintenance dose is 0.5 to 0.7 mg/kg/hr IV. Serum levels should be assessed 10 to 12 hours after the initiation of therapy and maintained within the lower range of therapeutic concentrations (i.e., 10 to 15 μg/mL). After successful treatment, aminophylline can be converted to oral theophylline or sustained release preparations.

Mechanical ventilation is indicated with respiratory failure, and has been successfully used with good pregnancy outcomes.[36] Respiratory failure occurs when the patient is unable to maintain a PaO_2 above 60 mm Hg despite maximal therapy, unable to maintain a PCO_2 below 40 mm Hg, or demonstrates respiratory exhaustion.[37] Patients who require mechanical ventilation are at high risk of morbidity, including barotrauma, pneumomediastinum, alveolar hypoventilation, and mortality, at rates reportedly as high as 40 percent.[36] General guidelines for reducing these risks include the use of a large-bore endotracheal tube, volume-cycled ventilator, increasing humidity of inspired air to improve the mobilization of mucus secretions, adequate time for expiration to prevent air trapping, and sedation with possible paralysis to facilitate ventilation.[2] The addition of continuous positive airway pressure (CPAP) can decrease the work of breathing and maximize ventilation. Broncheoalveolar lavage may help in removing mucus plugs, which are often a contributing cause of mortality.[36,38] Extracorporeal membrane oxygenation may be considered as salvage therapy if mechanical ventilation fails.

MANAGEMENT OF THE ASTHMATIC PATIENT IN LABOR AND DELIVERY

In labor, ventilation increases dramatically from 12 L/min late in the third trimester to almost 20 L/min in the first stage of labor, and then progressively to 23 L/min at delivery.[39] Oxygen consumption increases more than twofold, from 281 mL/min to 703 mL/min. The metabolic rate increases from 0.7 to 1.3 kcal/m^2/min. It is obvious that achieving normal or near normal pulmonary function is important for maternal and fetal oxygenation and the conduct of normal labor and delivery. In all asthmatic patients, continuous fetal heart rate monitoring may be helpful for determining the impact of the disease on the fetus during labor and delivery.

In patients with mild asthma who have not had intercurrent deterioration, an initial evaluation of baseline respiratory function with a history, physical examination, and measurement of PEFR or FEV$_1$ (well-controlled disease is indicated by a PEFR/FEV$_1$ ratio $\geq$ 80 percent of baseline) is generally all that is required[2] (Fig. 18-2). Pulse oximetry is a useful adjunct if available. During labor, the fetus serves as an in vivo oximeter. If maternal hypoxemia should ensue, the fetal heart rate pattern will generally be consistent with fetal jeopardy (or frank fetal distress). When the fetal heart rate pattern is no longer reassuring, asthmatic maternal pulmonary dysfunction must be included in the differential of etiologies for such an abnormal heart rate pattern. Supplemental oxygen is not routinely indicated during labor, and its use should generally, be based on obstetric indications.

Evaluation of baseline respiratory function in patients with moderate or severe asthma includes a PEFR or FEV$_1$ measurement. If the physical examination or objective testing demonstrate elements of active obstructive disease, full assessment, with arterial blood gas analysis, pharmacotherapy, and monitoring of drug levels is advisable. Prior maintenance medications are continued. Pulse oximetry and intensive continuous fetal monitoring are recommended. "Stress" doses of steroids (hydrocortisone, 100 mg q8h IV) are given to patients exposed to chronic systemic steroids in the prior 9 months or exposed acutely in the prior 4 weeks, and are continued for 24 hours after delivery.

For asthmatic patients undergoing induction of labor, oxytocin is the preferred agent, although intravaginal or intracervical prostaglandin E$_2$ (PGE$_2$) gel has not been reported to provoke bronchospasm.[2] For patients with postpartum hemorrhage, PGE$_2$ or another uterotonic agent is recommended instead of PGF$_{2d}$, which has been associated with oxyhemoglobin desaturation.[40]

Epidural or spinal anesthesia is the preferred analgesia for asthmatic patients during labor and delivery. Preference is given to narcotics such as fentanyl, with the avoidance of morphine and meperidine, which may stimulate histamine release. For cesarean delivery, epidural or spinal anesthesia is preferred over general anesthesia, since intubation can induce intense bronchospasm. If general anesthesia is required, premedication with atropine may decrease mucus production, and the use of halothane is preferred (for bronchodilation). Forewarning the anesthesiologist about asthmatic patients is necessary to coordinate and deliver optimal care.

SUMMARY

Asthma can pose a serious threat to a normal outcome of pregnancy. The normal physiology of pregnancy alters the parameters of management and treatment such that one cannot universally apply management techniques for nonpregnant patients to those who are pregnant. For these reasons, the obstetrician needs to understand the physiology of pregnancy and the pathophysiology of asthma. Aggressive, objective evaluation and treatment are indicated to optimally manage chronic and acute asthmatic exacerbations. Consideration should be given to the early and aggressive use of steroids for acute exacerbations. Objectives in treatment include maintaining normal or near normal pulmonary function,

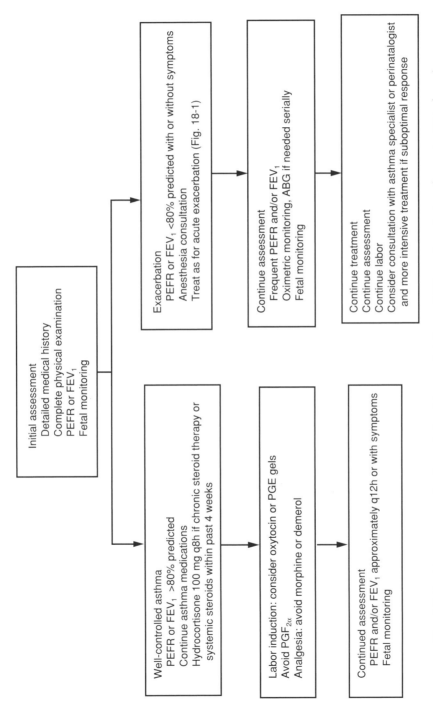

Fig. 18-2. Management of asthma during labor and delivery. PEFR, peak expiratory flow rate; FEV₁ forced expiratory volume within the first second of expiration; ABG, arterial blood gases; PGE, prostaglandin E; PGF₂ₐ, prostaglandin F₂ₐ. (Adapted from National Asthma Educational Program.[2])

Initial assessment
Detailed medical history
Complete physical examination
PEFR or FEV₁
Fetal monitoring

Well-controlled asthma
PEFR or FEV₁ >80% predicted
Continue asthma medications
Hydrocortisone 100 mg q8h if chronic steroid therapy or systemic steroids within past 4 weeks

Labor induction: consider oxytocin or PGE gels
Avoid PGF₂ₐ
Analgesia: avoid morphine or demerol

Continued assessment
PEFR and/or FEV₁ approximately q12h or with symptoms
Fetal monitoring

Exacerbation
PEFR or FEV₁ <80% predicted with or without symptoms
Anesthesia consultation
Treat as for acute exacerbation (Fig. 18-1)

Continue assessment
Frequent PEFR and/or FEV₁
Oximetric monitoring, ABG if needed serially
Fetal monitoring

Continue treatment
Continue assessment
Continue labor
Consider consultation with asthma specialist or perinatalogist and more intensive treatment if suboptimal response

symptomatic relief of bronchospasm, normal fetal growth, and a normal pregnancy outcome.

REFERENCES

1. Clark SL, National Asthma Education Program: Asthma in pregnancy. Obstet Gynecol 82:1036, 1993
2. National Asthma Education Program: Management of asthma during pregnancy. NIH Publication No. 93-3279. National Institutes of Health. U.S. Government Printing Office, Washington, DC, 1993
3. Greenberger PA: Asthma during pregnancy. J Asthma 27:341, 1990
4. Dunnill MS: The pathology of asthma with special reference to changes in bronchial mucosa. J Clin Pathol 13:27, 1960
5. Gluck JC, Gluck PA: The effects of pregnancy on asthma: a prospective study. Ann Allergy 37:164, 1976
6. Schatz M, Harden K, Forsythe A et al: The course of asthma during pregnancy, postpartum, and with successive pregnancies: a prospective analysis. J Allergy Clin Immunol 81:509, 1988
7. Bahna SL, Bjerkdal T: The course and outcome of pregnancy in women with bronchial asthma. Acta Allergol 27:397, 1972
8. Gordon M, Niswander KR, Berendes H, Kantor AG: Fetal morbidity following potentially anoxigenic obstetric conditions. Am J Obstet Gynecol 106:421, 1970
9. Stenius-Aarniala B, Piirila P, Teramo K: Asthma and pregnancy: a prospective study of 198 pregnancies. Thorax 43:12, 1988
10. Perlow JH, Montgomery D, Morgan MA et al: Severity of asthma and perinatal outcome. Am J Obstet Gynecol 167:963, 1992
11. Fitzsimmons R, Greenberger PA, Patterson R: Outcome of pregnancy in women requiring corticosteroids for severe asthma. J Allergy Clin Immunol 78:349, 1986
12. Greenberger PA, Patterson R: The outcome of pregnancy complicated by severe asthma. Allergy Proc 9:539, 1988
13. Schatz M, Zeiger RS, Hoffman CP: Intrauterine growth is related to gestational pulmonary function in pregnancy asthmatic women. Chest 98:389, 1990
14. Corre RA, Rothstein RJ: Assessing severity of adult asthma and need for hospitalization. Ann Emerg Med 14:45, 1985
15. Huff RW: Asthma in pregnancy. Med Clin 73:653, 1989
16. Schatz M, Zeiger RS, Harden K et al: The safety of inhaled β-agonist bronchodilators during pregnancy. J Allergy Clin Immunol 82:686, 1988
17. Rossing TH: Methylxanthines in 1989. Ann Intern Med 110:502, 1989
18. Siegel D, Sheppard D, Gelb A, Weinberg PF: Aminophylline increases the toxicity but not the efficacy of an inhaled beta-adrenergic agonist in the treatment of acute exacerbations of asthma. Am Rev Respir Dis 132:283, 1985
19. Carter BL, Driscoll CE, Smith GD: Theophylline clearance during pregnancy. Obstet Gynecol 68:555, 1986
20. Neff RK, Leviton A: Maternal theophylline consumption and the risk of stillbirth. Chest 97:1266, 1990
21. Labovitz E, Spector S: Placental theophylline transfer in pregnant asthmatics. JAMA 247:786, 1982
22. Morris HG: Mechanisms of action and therapeutic role of corticosteroids in asthma. J Allergy Clin Immunol 75:1, 1985
23. Schatz M, Patterson R, Zeitz S et al: Corticosteroid therapy for the pregnant asthmatic patient. JAMA 233:804, 1975
24. Greenberger PA, Patterson R: Beclomethasone diproprionate for severe asthma in pregnancy. Ann Intern Med 98:478, 1983
25. Fanta CH, Rossing TH, McFadden ER: Glucocorticoid in acute asthma. Am J Med 74:846, 1983
26. Newhouse MT, Dolovich MB: Control of asthma by aerosols. N Engl J Med 315:870, 1986
27. Rees HA, Millar JS, Donald KW: A study of the clinical course and arterial blood gas tensions of patients in status asthmaticus. Q J Med 37:542, 1967
28. Fischl MA, Pitchenik A, Gardner LB: An index predictive of relapse and need for hospitalization in patient with acute bronchial asthma. N Engl J Med 305:783, 1981
29. Greenberger PA, Patterson R: Management of asthma during pregnancy. N Engl J Med 312:897, 1985
30. Renterghem DV, Lamont H, Elinck W et al: Intravenous versus nebulized terbutaline in patients with severe acute asthma: a double-blind randomized study. Ann Allergy 59:313, 1987
31. Fanta CH, Rossing TH, McFadden ER: Emergency room treatment of asthma. Am J Med 72:416, 1982
32. Littenberg B, Gluck EH: A controlled trial of methylprednisolone in the emergency treatment of acute asthma. N Engl J Med 314:150, 1986
33. Fanta CH, Rossing TH, McFadden ER: Treatment of acute asthma. Is combination therapy with sympathomimetics and methylxanthines indicated? Am J Med 80:5, 1986
34. Haskell RJ, Wong BM, Hansen JE: A double-blind, randomized clinical trial of methylprednisolone in status asthmaticus. Arch Intern Med 143:1324, 1983

35. Summer WR: Status asthmaticus. Thorax 87:87s, 1985

36. Scoggin CH, Sahn SA, Petty TL: Status asthmaticus. JAMA 238:1158, 1977

37. Hankins GDV: Acute pulmonary injury and respiratory failure during pregnancy. p. 290, In Clark SL, Phelan JP, Cotton DB (eds): Critical Care Obstetrics. Medical Economics Books, Oradell, NJ, 1991

38. Schreier L, Cutler RM, Saigal V: Respiratory failure in asthma during the third trimester: report of two cases. Am J Obstet Gynecol 160:80, 1989

39. Turner ES, Greenberger PA, Patterson R: Management of the pregnant asthmatic patient. Ann Intern Med 6:905, 1980

40. Hankins GDV, Cunningham FG: Asthma complicating pregnancy. p. 1. In Cunningham FG, MacDonald PC, Gant NF (eds): Williams Obstetrics. Vol. 15. (suppl). Appleton & Lange, E. Norwalk, CT, 1992

Chapter 19

Diabetic Ketoacidosis

Michael F. Greene

Diabetic ketoacidosis (DKA) is a potentially life-threatening emergency for both mother and fetus. In Joslin's[1] original series of 10 pregnancies among seven diabetic women, published 7 years before the discovery of insulin, there were four maternal mortalities, one due to DKA. With modern management, maternal mortality is so rare that the rate of mortality from DKA is impossible to estimate accurately. Associated morbidity, such as adult respiratory distress syndrome (ARDS)[2] and coma due to cerebral edema, do continue to occur.[3] The risk of fetal mortality is also difficult to estimate. A rate of 50 percent, derived from several reported series stretching back over more than two decades, is often quoted.

The increasing rarity of DKA also makes it difficult to estimate its incidence. In a review of series reported in the English language literature between 1965 and 1985, Cousins[4] estimated the incidence of DKA in pregnancy to be 9.3 percent, which is about 10 times the rate in nonpregnant diabetic persons. This rate has been falling steadily, and it is doubtful that the current rate is nearly that high. The decreasing frequency of episodes of DKA inevitably results in decreasing familiarity with the pathophysiology and management of the disorder. Delay in its recognition, or hesitation or timidity in its management, can have lethal consequences.

PATHOPHYSIOLOGY

The development of DKA requires both a relative or absolute deficiency of insulin and a relative or absolute increase in the major counter-regulatory hormone glucagon. These changes can be initiated by failure to take insulin, a major physiologic stress such as an infection, or treatment of premature labor with β-adrenergic agonists with or without concurrent glucocorticoid therapy.[5,6] Both insulin deficiency indirectly and β-stimulation directly increase glucagon secretion. The combined results of hypoinsulinemia and hyperglucagonemia are increased hepatic glucose production and decreased peripheral glucose use, both of which produce hyperglycemia.[7] Furthermore, β-stimulation, either through exogenous β-mimetic agents or endogenous epinephrine release due to stress, inhibits insulin-induced glucose transport into peripheral tissues. Most hepatic glucose production is from gluconeogenesis, using amino acids derived from protein catabolism. The resulting hyperglycemia causes an osmotic diuresis and dehydration characteristic of DKA.

Both hypoinsulinemia and β-stimulation activate lipolysis in adipose tissue, releasing free fatty acids into the circulation. These travel to the liver, where they would simply be re-esterified into triglycerides under normal hormonal circumstances. Hyperglucagonemia, however, which prevails during starvation or uncontrolled diabetes, activates the β-oxidative enzymes in the liver, which metabolize free fatty acids to ketone bodies. Although at high concentrations of acetoacetate and β-hydroxybutyrate, there is some suppression of peripheral ketone-body utilization, it is mainly the overproduction of ketone bodies that is responsible for the hyperketonemia. These ketone bodies are fixed acids that drive down the pH and bicarbonate ion concentration, while accounting almost exclusively for the increased anion gap.

The causes of the water and electrolyte disturbances are complex and result in total body depletion of water, sodium, potassium, chloride, magnesium, phosphate, and bicarbonate. Hyperglycemia causes an osmotic diuresis with loss of large amounts of water. The increased osmotic pressure and loss of volume from the intravascular space draws water from the intracellular space, reducing the serum sodium concentration. Catabolism of muscle protein releases intracellular potassium, while hypoinsulinemia inhibits the sodium–potassium exchange pump in muscle cell membranes, limiting potassium uptake. Stimulated by hypovolemia, the kidneys retain sodium while wasting potassium into the urine. Vomiting associated with DKA results in further loss of water and electrolytes.

PRESENTATION AND DIAGNOSIS

The classic clinical presentation of DKA includes anorexia, nausea, vomiting, polyuria, tachycardia, and abdominal pain or muscle cramps. If sufficiently severe at presentation, the picture could include Kussmaul hyperventilation and signs of volume depletion, such as hypotension and oliguria. There may also be an alteration in mental status from lethargy to coma. Body temperature is normal to reduced. The "fruity" odor of ketones may be noticeable on the patient's breath.

If DKA is suspected on the basis of clinical signs and symptoms, the urine should first be tested for glucose and ketones. If neither is present, the diagnosis is very unlikely. If they are present, the patient's blood should be studied. In a nonpregnant person, a blood glucose of less than 250 mg/dl would make the diagnosis of DKA very unlikely. Pregnant women are well-known, however, to be able to develop DKA at relatively low blood glucose values (200 to 250 mg/dl). Although total body sodium and po-

tassium are profoundly depleted, the serum sodium concentration is usually low-normal and the serum potassium normal to slightly elevated. The serum bicarbonate is, by definition, less than 15 mEq/L. Although the ketone bodies acetoacetate and β-hydroxybutyrate are not usually measured clinically, their presence in excess can be inferred from a large anion gap. Serum osmolarity is usually greater than 300 mOsm/L. The hematocrit is usually elevated as a result of hemoconcentration, and there is a leukocytosis that can be very dramatic. The arterial pH will be less than 7.3, by definition, and the partial pressure of carbon dioxide (PCO_2) will be low.

In a patient known to have type I diabetes, the diagnosis of DKA is usually obvious. Occasionally, a diabetic patient experiencing protracted nausea and vomiting due to morning sickness in early pregnancy or gastroenteritis later in pregnancy can present a confusing picture, with ketonuria that can be mistaken for simple starvation ketosis. In this setting, hyperglycemia should alert the clinician to the possibility of DKA. Patients who clearly have type II non-insulin-dependent diabetes or gestational diabetes may develop DKA during pregnancy.[8] DKA cannot be ruled out just because the patient is not known to have type I diabetes. Rarely, patients not previously known to have diabetes of any sort may present with DKA in pregnancy.

The differential diagnosis includes alcoholic ketoacidosis, which occurs in chronic alcoholism, usually following a binge. It is frequently associated with pancreatitis and the blood glucose is usually less than 150 mg/dl. Occasionally, these patients are hypoglycemic.

PRECIPITATING FACTORS

An attempt should be made to find a cause in every case of DKA. Frequently, the cause is inadequate insulin therapy in the face of an otherwise minor illness. Patients may reduce or omit their insulin doses in the presence of gastroenteritis because they are concerned about the possibility of an insulin reaction due to anorexia, nausea, and vomiting. This is a matter of patient education about the appropriate therapy for "sick days." A careful history and physical examination with appropriate laboratory studies should be done to search for a significant bacterial infection (e.g., pyelonephritis or pneumonia). As mentioned above, leukocytosis is present simply as a result of DKA, but a fever would indicate infection.

Patients using continuous subcutaneous insulin infusion pumps receive only regular insulin. If the pump malfunctions and stops infusing, the patient becomes hypoinsulinemic very quickly because she has no reservoir of longer-acting insulin. She may develop DKA very rapidly. Similarly, a patient receiving insulin only by continuous intravenous infusion during an attempted induction of labor has no intermediate acting reserve. If the induction is unsuccessful and the patient is allowed to sleep overnight before a second day of induction, she should receive some intermediate-acting insulin to carry her through the night. We have seen a patient develop DKA overnight when this was inadvertently omitted.

Tocolytic therapy with β-sympathomimetic agents, with or without concomitant glucocorticoid therapy, can also precipitate DKA. Every attempt should be made to avoid these agents in women with diabetes. Alternatives such as magnesium sulfate or calcium-channel blockers should be considered.

EFFECT ON THE FETUS

Electronic monitoring of the fetal heart rate (FHR) during maternal DKA is frequently associated with the development of nonreassuring FHR patterns.[9,10] Although the pressure to perform a cesarean delivery to extricate a fetus from a situation wherein there is a nonreassuring or even "ominous" FHR pattern may be difficult to resist, this could be a dangerous procedure for an unstable parturient. Furthermore, these patterns do resolve with treatment of the maternal metabolic disorder, without obvious sequelae to the neonate (Fig. 19-1). Reports in the literature are anecdotal because there is not a sufficient volume of such cases to permit a meaningful treatment trial. Most authors recommend vigorous treatment of the maternal metabolic disorder with the fetus in utero, reserving cesarean delivery for mothers in stable condition whose fetuses continue to seem compromised.

TREATMENT
Volume Replacement

Volume replacement and insulin therapy are the two most urgent concerns in treating DKA. The average water volume deficit in established DKA is 3.5 to 7

L, or 5 to 10 percent of body weight, and the average sodium deficit is 350 to 600 mEq. Most patients will be deficient in water in excess of their sodium deficit, and will therefore require some free water in addition to normal saline. Two intravenous lines should be started promptly: one large-bore line for rapid fluid infusion and a second for insulin therapy. Initial treatment should be with normal saline at a rate of 15 to 20 ml/kg/hr, 500 ml/m^2/hr, or approximately 1 L/h for the first 2 hours of the resuscitation. This will rapidly replete the intravascular volume, improving general tissue perfusion and insulin delivery. It will also improve renal perfusion, permitting excretion of glucose in the urine and slowing potassium wasting in the urine. Although provision of some free water will ultimately be necessary, this initial resuscitation should be with isotonic saline because it will restore the circulating volume more quickly and lead to a less rapid decline in osmolarity. It is hypothesized that too rapid a decrease in intravascular osmolarity may lead to intracellular swelling and cerebral edema. A Foley catheter should be placed early in the resuscitation to accurately monitor urine output. Fluid therapy should be reduced in the third and subsequent hours to 7.5 ml/kg/hr, according to the clinical situation and urine output. As the blood glucose level comes down to 300 to 250 mg/dl, the intravenous fluid solution should be changed to 5 percent glucose in water. This will prevent hypoglycemia and provide substrate to suppress lipolysis and ketogenesis. This also serves to supply free water, which is needed to help prevent or correct the hyperchloremic acidosis that would otherwise develop. Intravenous fluids should be continued until all nausea and vomiting have resolved, bowel sounds are present, and the patient is able to tolerate adequate quantities of fluids by mouth.

Insulin Therapy

Insulin replacement therapy should begin as early in the resuscitation process as possible because DKA will not resolve without it. Although it may be given either intramuscularly or subcutaneously, insulin is best administered intravenously in this circumstance.[11] Poor tissue perfusion will result in delayed and erratic absorption from intramuscular and subcutaneous sites, initially delaying response and later leading to more hypoglycemia. Intravenous therapy

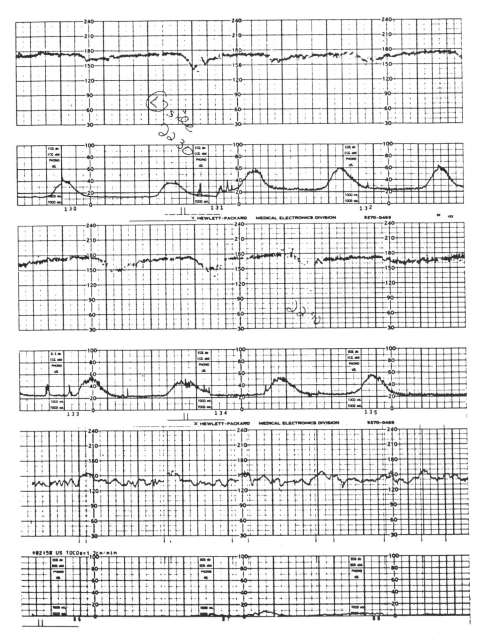

Fig. 19-1. Fetal heart rate and uterine activity monitoring of a patient with acute pyelonephritis precipitating diabetic ketoacidosis **(Upper two panels)** before and **(Lower panel)** after correction of ketoacidosis and treatment of pyelonephritis. (From Rigg and Petrie,[17] with permission.)

should begin with a 10-U bolus of insulin followed immediately with a continuous infusion of 5 to 10 U/h. All therapy during this initial resuscitation should be with regular insulin. Because insulin tends to bind to plastic intravenous tubing, several milliliters of insulin solution should be run through the tubing and discarded, to coat its walls with insulin so that the patient receives the full dose of insulin immediately without loss to the tubing.

All patients in DKA are insulin resistant, but the doses of insulin described above are usually adequate to overcome the resistance and reverse the DKA.[12] If, however, the patient does not show improvement in both the hyperglycemia and anion gap within 2 hours after therapy is begun, very severe insulin resistance is present. In this case, a 20-U intravenous bolus should be given and the infusion rate doubled to 20-U/n. This should be adequate to saturate all insulin receptors and lead to a physiologic response. There is no risk in giving an excessively large intravenous bolus of insulin because it has no effect beyond saturating all receptors, and has a short half-life. For this reason, and because the severely resistant patient cannot be anticipated, some have suggested that all patients be initially treated with a much larger intravenous bolus of 25 to 50 U.

Hyperglycemia and acidosis will resolve much more quickly than the ketonemia and ketonuria of DKA. After the blood glucose level has been normalized, intravenous insulin therapy should be continued with intravenous glucose until the acidosis is resolved. Some authors suggest that intravenous insulin therapy be continued until the ketonuria has resolved. Resolution of the ketonuria, however, may take 24 to 48 hours, which is long after the patient is otherwise apparently recovered and stable. The transition back to routine subcutaneous regular and intermediate-acting insulin should overlap the administration of intravenous insulin.

Potassium Replacement

Although the serum potassium level at presentation in DKA is often high, the mean total body potassium deficit is 200 to 400 mEq. Insulin therapy in the presence of hyperglycemia will drive potassium from the intravascular to the intracellular space. Intravenous potassium replacement should begin 2 to 4 hours

into the resuscitation period as the serum potassium level falls toward the normal range and urine production is demonstrated.[13] Occasionally, patients will present with a low or normal serum potassium, in which case replacement should begin promptly, but with caution, until urine production is demonstrated. For a serum potassium in the physiologic range, replacement should begin at a rate of 30 to 40 mEq/h. In the rare circumstance in which a patient presents with a very low serum potassium, insulin administration should be delayed briefly until 40 mEq of potassium can be infused. Failure to do this could result in a rapid decrease in serum potassium levels on initiation of insulin, with the precipitation of a severe cardiac dysrhythmia.

Inclusion of an electrocardiogram (ECG) as part of the initial evaluation of a patient in DKA will help in rapidly estimating the serum potassium level. Lead II is particularly helpful, with high, peaked T waves and a broadened QRS complex indicating hyperkalemia. Hypokalemia is evidenced by low T waves and the appearance of U waves. Repetition of the ECG during the resuscitation is a convenient way to quickly and roughly reassess the serum potassium level.

Bicarbonate and Phosphate Therapy

It is intuitively appealing to want to treat acidosis with bicarbonate, but such therapy has not been shown to be helpful and is not routinely used. Theoretical potential advantages to bicarbonate administration include a more rapid correction of the extracellular acidosis, minimization of the hyperchloremic acidosis, reduction of cardiac irritability, and an increased responsiveness of the vascular system to pressors. Despite the lack of documented efficacy for bicarbonate administration, all authors recommend its use in the case of "severe" acidosis.[14] The definition of "severe" varies, but is generally defined as a pH below 7.0. If bicarbonate is given, it should be as an intravenous infusion of 1 to 2 mEq/kg over 2 hours, and should be discontinued when the pH reaches 7.20.

Phosphate is depleted in DKA, and serum phosphate levels are usually low due to decreased intake, enhanced catabolism, and urinary loss. Hypophosphatemia can deplete the serum levels of 2,3-diphosphoglycerate and result in a shift of the hemoglobin–oxygen disassociation curve toward more avid oxygen binding and poorer oxygen delivery to tissues. Severe hypophosphatemia (<2 mEq/L) can cause rhabdomyolysis. For these reasons, phosphate replacement would seem desirable.[15] Furthermore, replacing some of the potassium as phosphate rather than chloride can help to minimize the hyperchloremia. By contrast, administration of too much phosphate intravenously can cause hypocalcemia, it is rapidly replaced from dietary sources as soon as the patient starts eating, and its acute intravenous replacement has not been shown to improve outcome in any measurable way. The necessity for the acute intravenous replacement of phosphate is therefore controversial. If potassium phosphate is used, it should not exceed 90 mEq in 24 hours, to avoid hypocalcemia, and the patient's serum calcium levels should be monitored.

SUMMARY

Successful management of DKA does not require an intensive care unit, but it does require a setting in which the patient can be monitored very frequently with a 1:1 nurse/patient ratio. A labor-and-delivery suite is perfectly suitable. Initial evaluation of the patient should include a routine history and detailed inquiry into the possible cause for DKA. The usual investigation of vital signs, physical examination, and documentation of fetal viability or well-being should also include the patient's mental status.[16] The initial laboratory evaluation should include a complete blood count, blood type and irregular antibody screen; serum electrolyte, glucose, blood urea nitrogen (BUN), creatinine, calcium, phosphate, and urine ketone assays; and cultures of blood, urine, and other sites as appropriate. A Foley catheter is very useful for documenting urine output. Two intravenous lines should be started: one a large-caliber line for volume and electrolyte replacement and the second for an insulin infusion. A 12-lead ECG should be obtained if the serum potassium falls significantly outside of the physiologic range. An initial arterial blood pH should be obtained.

As soon as the diagnosis of DKA is made and the necessity for an intensive resuscitation is recognized, a flow sheet should be established at the patient's bedside, on which should be recorded all vital signs,

laboratory data, urine output, fluid, insulin, and other medical therapies, and mental status if appropriate. Capillary blood glucose determinations should be done hourly at the bedside to help guide the resuscitation. It is not particularly helpful to follow ketonuria or ketonemia. Attention should rather be directed at correcting the hyperglycemia and anion gap, and progress in the resuscitation should be assessed on the basis of these measures.

The patient should be kept without oral intake (NPO) until all nausea and vomiting have resolved and bowel sounds are heard. The first dose of subcutaneous regular and intermediate-acting insulin should be given before discontinuing the intravenous insulin infusion. The search for the cause of the DKA episode should be completed, and appropriate therapy or education instituted to prevent recurrence. Although DKA is a metabolic emergency, it is both treatable and largely preventable, and should not result in maternal mortality.

REFERENCES

1. Joslin EP: Pregnancy and diabetes mellitus. Boston Med Surg J 173:841, 1915
2. Breidbart S, Singer L, St. Louis Y, Saenger P: Adult respiratory distress syndrome in an adolescent with diabetic ketoacidosis. J Pediatr 111:736, 1987
3. Winegrad AI, Kern EFO, Simmons DA: Cerebral edema in diabetic ketoacidosis. N Engl J Med 312:1184, 1985
4. Cousins L: Pregnancy complications among diabetic women: review, 1965–1985. Obstet Gynecol Surv 42:140, 1987
5. Thomas DJB, Gill B, Brown P, Stubbs WA: Salbutamol-induced diabetic ketoacidosis. BMJ 2:438, 1977
6. Borberg C, Gillmer MDG, Beard RW, Oakley NW: Metabolic effects of beta-sympathomimetic drugs and dexamethasone in normal and diabetic pregnancy. Br J Obstet Gynaecol 85:184, 1978
7. Flier JS, Moore MJ: The metabolic derangements and treatment of diabetic ketoacidosis. N Engl J Med 309:159, 1983
8. Maislos M, Harman-Bohem I, Weitzman S: Diabetic ketoacidosis: a rare complication of gestational diabetes. Diabetes Care 15:968, 1992
9. Rhodes RW, Ogburn Jr. PL: Treatment of severe diabetic ketoacidosis in the early third trimester in a patient with fetal distress. J Reprod Med 29:621, 1984

10. LoBue C, Goodlin RC: Treatment of fetal distress during diabetic keto-acidosis. J Reprod Med 20:101, 1978

11. Fisher JN, Shahshahani MN, Kitabchi AE: Diabetic ketoacidosis: low-dose insulin therapy by various routes. N Engl J Med 297:238, 1977

12. Luzi L, Barrett EJ, Groop LC et al: Metabolic effects of low-dose insulin therapy on glucose metabolism in diabetic ketoacidosis. Diabetes 37:1470, 1988

13. Santiago JV: Medical Management of Insulin-Dependent (Type I) Diabetes. p 76. 2nd Ed. American Diabetes Association, Alexandria, VA, 1994

14. Morris LR, Murphy MB, Kitabchi AE: Bicarbonate therapy in severe diabetic ketoacidosis. Ann Intern Med 105:836, 1986

15. Keller U, Berger W: Prevention of hypophosphatemia by phosphate infusion during treatment of diabetic ketoacidosis and hyperosmolar coma. Diabetes 29:87, 1980

16. Rosenbloom AL: Intracerebral crises during treatment of diabetic ketoacidosis. Diabetes Care 13:22, 1990

17. Rigg LA, Petrie RH: Fetal biochemical and biophysical assessment. p. 375. In Reece EA, Coustan DR (eds): Diabetes Mellitus in Pregnancy: Principles and Practice. Churchill Livingstone, New York, 1988

Chapter 20

Sickle Cell Disease

Samuel Charache, Mabel Koshy, and Eva Pressman

PATHOPHYSIOLOGY

The term *sickle cell disease* refers to all sickling disorders that produce significant disease under ordinary circumstances. These disorders include sickle cell anemia, hemoglobin SC disease, sickle/β-thalassemia, and such rare conditions as hemoglobin S/O_{Arab} and S/D_{Punjab} disease. For those seeking a general reference on sickle cell disease, Serjeant's text[1] and that edited by Embury et al[2] are recommended. Sickle cell trait does not produce significant disease under ordinary circumstances, and is not included in the rubric. Patients with sickle cell anemia (SS) have two abnormal genes that produce sickle cell β-globin chains; patients with hemoglobin SC disease ("SC") or sickle/β-thalassemia have genes for β^S and either β^C or β^{THAL} globin. Persons with sickle cell trait (AS) have one normal gene (β^A) and one abnormal one (β^S).

Sickle cell disease is caused by the sickling of red blood cells, which is caused by the polymerization of deoxyhemoglobin S. Whether or not a red cell sickles depends on the concentration of deoxyhemoglobin S within it, and the nature of other hemoglobins present. SS red cells contain only hemoglobin S, and require less deoxygenation for sickling than do SC cells. Hemoglobin O_{Arab} fits into polymers more readily than does hemoglobin C, and SO_{Arab} cells sickle more readily than do SC cells. As a consequence, hemoglobin SO_{Arab} disease is as severe as sickle cell anemia, but SC disease is a milder disorder.

Sickle cell disease has two main clinical manifestations: hemolytic anemia and vaso-occlusive episodes. The pathogenesis of the hemolysis is unclear; membrane damage probably plays a central role, but other malign forces (immunologic destruction, physical trauma) may also be involved. By and large, the anemia causes little disability in youth or the childbearing years. Many physiologic adjustments (facilitated unloading of oxygen from red cells, increased cardiac output, enhanced diffusion of oxygen from capillaries to cells) permit such patients to carry on with hemoglobin levels of 50 to 60 percent of normal. Similar maternal (and fetal) adjustments probably permit normal oxygen transport to the fetus in utero.

Vaso-occlusive episodes are primarily caused by impaction of inflexible sickled cells in the microvasculature, abetted by the tendency of sickled cells to adhere to endothelium and to each other. Macroscopic tissue damage (pulmonary infarction, aseptic necrosis of the femoral head) requires either embolization of necrotic bone marrow or tangled sickle cells, simultaneous occlusion of many microvascular channels "feeding" a tissue site, or accumulation of many microscopic injuries.

It is unknown why vaso-occlusive episodes (*sickle cell crisis*) occur when they do. They may have no apparent antecedent or may follow deoxygenation, postoperative atelectesis, or vasospasm (swimming in cold water[3]). Infection, inflammation, and pregnancy may also precipitate crises, but are harder to comprehend as factors precipitating vaso-occlusion; they may involve increased stickiness of red cell membranes or blood vessel walls.[4–6] Still other events that can preceed crises, such as emotional stress, are more difficult to understand in pathophysiologic terms. None of these factors consistently evokes vaso-occlusive attacks, and most painful episodes have no recognizable precipitant.[7]

HISTORY

Clinical History

When sickle cell anemia was first described and for some time thereafter,[8] few patients lived beyond their early twenties, and adults with the disease were unknown in some parts of Africa.[9] Patients died of infection, malnutrition, and severe anemia caused by red cell hypoplasia following infection or folate deficiency. Anesthesia and surgery were associated with high mortality and severe morbidity. Fertility was low, and pregnancy and delivery were associated with risks for both mother and fetus.[10]

Later Experience and Data from the Cooperative Study of Sickle Cell Disease

With the improvement of general public health, infection control, knowledge of nutritional anemia, and availability of transfusion therapy, reports began to appear of unusual longevity of SS patients.[11,12] Neonatal screening, prophylactic penicillin therapy, and the use of antipneumococcal vaccine had striking effects on the survival of children.[13] Improved techniques for anesthesia and postoperative care, better understanding of the intrapartum physiology of the mother and fetus, and the emergence of high-risk obstetric clinics were followed by considerable improvement in the outcome of pregnancy. It remains unclear whether the improvement was due to public health measures and improved care of all patients, or to specific maneuvers such as transfusion and antibiotic therapy.

The true impact of these measures was not fully recognized until data began to appear from the Co-operative Study of Sickle Cell Disease (CSSCD).[14] The mean survival of patients with diagnosed disease today is 40 years, and septuagenarian patients warrant only brief notice[15] in medical journals. Perhaps the most striking finding to date is documentation of the disparity between the stereotype of an SS patient who frequents the emergency department and the great majority of patients, who have only a few crises a year and may be unknown to medical centers.[16] It has become clear that improvement from previous descriptions of the disease is multifactorial: epidemics of typhoid and cholera no longer occur, antiviral vaccines are widely used, access to medical care is better, and more physicians know how to treat sickling disorders. Contemporary management of all aspects of sickle cell disease is concisely described in a publication of the U.S. Public Health Service.[17]

Pregnancy and Childbirth Today

Concurrent improvements in many areas of medicine have been reflected in obstetric practice. Women with sickle cell disease become pregnant, more are delivered of their infants, and most babies of these women survive. A desired pregnancy in a woman with sickle cell disease is no longer a prima facie indication for abortion in the United States; differences in availability of medical care in developing nations are responsible for this qualification. A recent publication of the American College of Obstetricians and Gynecologists[18] presents one set of current opinions on therapy in a judicious manner. Controversies remain and some are listed in the box below.

Pregnancy in Sickle Cell Disease: Controversies

1. Methods of contraception for patients with SS disease
2. Screening and counseling of patients who enroll in obstetric clinics
3. Counseling of women with SS trait detected during the screening process
4. Prophylactic transfusion

Our views on those topics, and others that follow, are predicated on easy and continued communication between obstetrician and internist: no rule works all the time, every patient has (or could have) unique problems, and we are obliged to coordinate our treatment plans if we want the best outcomes.

CONTRACEPTION

There is no general reason to interdict desired pregnancy in patients with sickle cell disease, but accidental or unwanted conceptions pose avoidable risks for both the mother and the child-to-be.[19] Family planning and contraception should be strongly advised by all pediatricians, general practitioners and internists, as well as gynecologists, and all physicians must be prepared to help the patient choose the best personal contraceptive technique.[19] It must be remembered that vaso-occlusive episodes in sickle cell disease are not primarily due to blood coagulation but to the impaction of sickled cells in small vessels. The woman with sickle cell disease does not have a "thrombotic" disorder, and her risk of thrombosis is no greater than that of other women who take oral contraceptives. Liver disease is often considered a contraindication to the use of oral contraceptives, but the jaundice of sickle cell disease is primarily due to hemolysis, and mildly abnormal levels of serum transaminases and alkaline phosphatase reflect processes that are not affected by estrogenic hormones. There is no contraindication to the use of implanted contraceptives (i.e., Norplant).

Tubal ligation in the postpartum period may be recommended for multiparous women and those with previous complicated pregnancies. Tubal ligation should not be recommended as an alternative method of birth control for young patients without children. Indications for such discussion are more compelling for women with sickle cell disease than for women in the general population, but are similar to those for women with hypertension, lupus erythematosus, and diabetes mellitus.

PRENATAL SCREENING AND COUNSELING

Most women with sickle cell anemia know that they have "a blood disease" because of anemia and recurrent pain, but women with SC disease and sickle/thalassemia may not. Neither anemic nor symptomatic beforehand, they sometimes develop severe complications of the disease during or immediately after pregnancy, and it is best to follow them in a high-risk obstetric clinic. In order to detect such patients, some clinics screen all newly entered patients who are at risk for a hemoglobinopathy. If the only reason for screening is concern for the mother, it is sufficient to first use a solubility test (such as Sickle-Quik), which detects sickle cell hemoglobin only, and to then do electrophoresis only on those patients with positive tests, to separate SS, SC, S/Thal, AS, and so on. Women with sickle cell disease are then counseled about risks to themselves and their infant. But if one is also concerned about the fetus, hemoglobin electrophoresis and a multichannel blood count should be done first; the former will pick up hemoglobin C trait in addition to sickling disorders, and the latter will reveal a low mean corpuscular volume (MCV), which could be due to thalassemia trait or iron deficiency. Detection of any hemoglobinopathy would then lead to screening of the father and counseling of the couple about the child's prognosis (and the mother's, if she has sickle cell disease) (Fig. 20-1).

Maternal Risks

Women with sickle cell disease have an increased frequency of all usual complications of pregnancy (see below). They may have more frequent crises than they did before pregnancy, including life-threatening "pneumonia" (more properly called *chest syndrome*, since it is more often due to infarction than to infection in adults), stroke, heart failure, and pyelonephritis. They may require transfusion, and they may have a difficult postpartum course if they require ceasarean section. None of these possibilities interdicts pregnancy, but the mother should be made aware of the risks, if for no other reason than to motivate her to attend a high-risk clinic.

Fetal Risks

If the mother has sickle cell disease, the fetus is at increased risk of spontaneous abortion and intrauterine growth retardation (IUGR). Although there is some evidence for a belief that transfusions can ameliorate the mother's condition, there is no evidence that they can improve the fetus's lot.

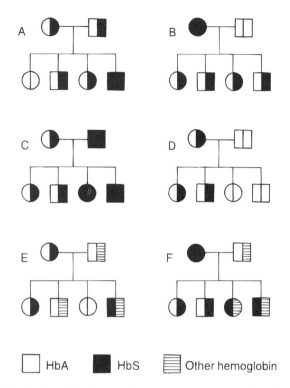

□ HbA   ■ HbS   ☰ Other hemoglobin

Fig. 20-1. Inheritance of common sickling disorders. **(A)** Sickle cell trait x sickle cell trait: in each pregnancy, the risk of having a child with sickle cell anemia is 1:4. **(B)** Sickle cell anemia x normal: all children will have SC trait. **(C)** Sickle cell trait x sickle cell anemia: in each pregnancy, the risk of having a child with SC anemia is 1 in 2. **(D)** Sickle cell trait x normal: no children will have sickle cell anemia. **(E)** Sickle cell trait x another trait (HbC trait, thalassemia trait): in each pregnancy, the risk of having a compound heterozygous child (e.g., S/C disease) is 1 in 4. **(F)** Sickle cell anemia x another trait: no children will have sickle cell anemia, but in each pregnancy the risk of having a compound heterozygous child is 1 in 2.

If both the mother and father are carriers of hemoglobinopathies (e.g., sickle trait and thalassemia trait), the child has a one in four risk of getting both abnormal genes (S/thalassemia, in this case). If the mother has two abnormal genes and the father has a trait, the situation is more complex, yielding an equal likelihood of SC × AS = AS, SS, AC or SC. If the parents want to know the fetus's genotype, prenatal diagnosis using chorionic villi sampling[20,21] can be safely done as early as the 10th week of pregnancy. It is implicit that the couple be made aware

of the medical significance of the various possibilities before the sample is obtained, preferably by a trained counselor. The counselor need not have an advanced degree, but must have demonstrated knowledge of the medical facts in the transmission of hemoglobinopathies and demonstrated ability to communicate with the parents.

ANTEPARTUM MANAGEMENT
By Whom

During pregnancy, a woman with sickle cell disease should be followed in a high-risk obstetric clinic. The patient must know the name of her primary physician if a team is responsible for her outpatient care. A detailed initial consultation with a hematologist experienced in treating patients with hemoglobinopathies should be arranged. Some hematologists prefer monthly follow-up visits, in addition to those in the high-risk obstetric clinic; because the patient's course most often runs smoothly, others prefer less formal interactions between the obstetrician and the hematologist. In either case, instructions to patients should come from only one source. If the patients is already being followed by a hematologist, the hematologist must be made aware that a pregnancy is underway, and should be asked for an opinion before significant decisions are made.

Vitamins and Iron

Women with hemolytic anemia need more folic acid than do normal women, but often consume enough in their diet to meet their needs. Pregnant women with hemolytic anemias, including sickle cell disease, have higher requirements[22] and should be given the 1 mg/day in the form of prescribed prenatal iron-and-vitamin tablets. There is a risk of "covering up" the anemia of pernicious anemia by giving folic acid. Pernicious anemia does occur in young black women,[23] and the physician could be responsible for permitting subacute combined degeneration of the spinal cord to occur. The risk of this however, appears quite small, and the benefits of folate administration are significant.

In patients who have not received many transfusions, iron requirements are no different from those of normal pregnant women. Those who have been extensively transfused probably have increased iron stores, since the only routes for the loss of transfused iron are menstruation and pregnancy. A serum ferritin assay may provide some information, for a low value would be a clear indication for treatment; a very high value (> 500 ng/L) probably should lead to omission of antenatal iron therapy. Remember that iron therapy will not improve the anemia of sickle cell anemia, and although the hydremia of pregnancy usually reduces the patient's hemoglobin concentration somewhat, it does not necessarily impair oxygen transport.

"Obstetric" Complications of Pregnancy

Although improvements in the prenatal care of patients with sickle cell disease have decreased perinatal mortality from more than 50 percent before 1970 to less than 20 percent today, certain complications of pregnancy persist.[24,25] Increased risk of abortion, stillbirth, preterm labor, pregnancy-associated hypertension, and IUGR continue to be reported. Most of these complications can be managed by techniques described in other parts of this book.

Management of Painful Crises

Painful crises may begin slowly as a general aching and gradually become more severe, or they may develop rapidly. Pain may be localized to one or two bones or joints, or patients may "hurt all over." The pain may be mild or may require parenteral narcotics for relief. Sickle cell crisis can be diagnosed only after all more treatable disorders have been excluded. The more common conditions that enter into the differential diagnosis include urinary tract infection, biliary tract disease, appendicitis, other causes of a "surgical abdomen," bacterial or viral pneumonia, pyogenic arthritis, gout, and osteomyelitis. Fever and increased leukocytosis, a common finding in the foregoing conditions, is often seen in uncomplicated sickle cell pain, but temperatures over $39°C$ and white blood cell counts over 25,000/mm^3 are unusual in vaso-occlusive crises. Blood and urine cultures are almost always indicated, and since infections can "trigger" crises, two conditions may coexist.

After treating any complicating condition that may be present, one treats the crisis itself. Moderate doses of parenteral analgesics[26,27] can be given safely; many internists prefer morphine to meperidine because of the epileptogenic effects of the latter's metabolite, normeperidine. Patient-controlled analgesia[28] can work very well, but care must be taken to control the "lockout" that prevents overdosing by the patient. At least some "unexplained" deaths during hospitalization for vaso-occlusive crises[29] may be due to respiratory depression caused by narcotics given by conventional means or by pumps. Adequate pain relief is the goal, but the patient's condition must be assessed frequently to avoid oversedation.

Parenteral fluids should be administered if there is any question about the adequacy of oral intake, but some patients are willing and able to drink adequate volumes of fluid (if they are made available at the bedside). Many severely affected patients have had all of their peripheral veins thrombosed during prior treatments with intravenous fluids; it is well worth the effort to try oral hydration rather than inserting a central venous cannula. Oxygen therapy must be given if it is needed, but is a waste of money and effort if used routinely in all patients with sickle cell crises. Patients who wear their nasal "prongs" on the top of their heads or under their pillows are telling us something: measurement of arterial partial pressure of oxygen (PaO_2) or pulse oximetry should guide oxygen therapy. Raising the PO_2 to abnormally high levels and dissolving a little more oxygen in the plasma of a patient with normal oxygen saturation does no good, and may not be entirely harmless.[30]

Chest Syndrome

A pulmonary infiltrate associated with fever, often alluded to as chest syndrome,[31] warrents separate discussion. The term *chest syndrome* is used because this condition has no known etiologic diagnosis; in adults with sickle cell disease, we often do not know the cause of lung infiltrates. The term *chest syndrome* also tells us that whatever its cause, the condition can progress to a life-threatening severity in which it mimics adult respiratory distress syndrome.[32] SS cells at pH 7.4 begin to sickle at a PO_2 of about 60 mm Hg. If the PaO_2 is lower than this there will be even less oxygen in more peripheral vessels, and the stage is set for generalized sickling. If sickling occurs on the venous side, the inflexible sickled cells will be trapped in the next microvascular network they meet, the lung, which makes oxygenation still worse, with grim consequences.

If the PaO_2 is above 70 mm Hg, and preferably above 80 mm Hg, or pulse oximetry yields saturations of greater than 85 percent, one can rely on nasal oxygen and repetitive measurements of either of these parameters. If measurements are lower, a higher inspired oxygen fraction (FiO_2) and a face mask should be used; if this does not work, preparation should be made for immediate exchange transfusion (see below) and probable transfer of the patient to an intensive care unit. Pediatricians sometimes see immediate improvement in oxygenation following exchange transfusion[33]; internists usually do not (perhaps because the pathogenesis is different), but we often see no further progression after an adequate exchange transfusion in what initially looked like a very bad situation. Whether an immediate exchange transfusion is performed, some hematologists think that occurrence of chest syndrome is probably an indication for chronic transfusion until delivery.

For the patient with a small infiltrate who does not appear seriously ill, has no pathogens in the sputum, and has adequate oxygenation, it is not necessary to give antibiotics immediately if close observation can be assured. Most of the time one does treat, with a drug effective against both *Streptococcus pneumoniae* and *Hemophilus influenza*, realizing that it may be unnecessary but afraid not to use it. Cefuroxime is a reasonable drug to use. The dosage is 750 mg IV every 8 hours if renal function is normal.

Stroke

Stroke due to occlusion of large intracranial vessels is a problem in children; both vaso-occlusion and subarachnoid hemorrhage occur in young adults.[34] The pathogenesis of either type of event is unclear.[35] There is fairly convincing evidence that chronic transfusion therapy can prevent recurrent stroke in children,[36] although stroke has been reported as a complication of transfusion[37] (perhaps because excessive increases in hematocrit cause increased blood viscosity). In an adult, including a pregnant woman, every effort must be made to detect a treatable vascular lesion. There are few data to guide one in deciding whether and how long to transfuse an adult for stroke, and opinions of hematologists are mixed.

Chronic Transfusion Therapy

Blood transfusion has very definite risks[25]: major and minor transfusion reactions, transmission of blood-borne disease, and alloimmunization[38] cannot be completely eliminated, although the risk of the last can be reduced if one uses blood from black donors.[39,40] A low hemoglobin concentration in a patient with sickle cell disease usually is not an indication for transfusion; inability to carry out daily activities, marked fatigue, dyspnea, tachycardia, and headaches usually are indications for transfusion.[33]

Many hematologists caring for adult patients think that maintaining more than 50 percent of normal cells in the circulation (pediatricians would say > 70 percent) sometimes prevents vaso-occlusive episodes in patients with sickle cell disease.[33] Few physicians understand either how or why this exerts a beneficial effect, and most think that letting an SS patient's hemoglobin level get above 14 g/dl can be dangerous because of possible hyperviscosity syndrome unless virtually all sickle cells have been replaced.

Given these beliefs, the lack of understanding of the mechanisms, and knowledge of the hazards of transfusion, the real questions are whether transfusion should be undertaken in an effort to *prevent* problems for the mother or the child. Opinions differ among obstetricians,[41–45] there are numerous anecdotes pro and con,[45–48] and only one controlled study[24] that does not provide all the needed answers. Without proof of the efficacy of transfusion through an extensive controlled trial, our practice has been that summarized in the box below.

Decision-Making Protocol for Chronic Transfusion Therapy

If the patient's crises are no more severe or frequent during pregnancy than they were antepartum, do not transfuse

If the patient has no more symptoms that could be due to anemia than do other women at her stage of gestation, do not transfuse

(Continues)

If crises become more severe or more frequent, or the patient develops even a mild episode of chest syndrome, perform exchange transfusion and maintain more than 50 percent normal red cells until delivery

If the patient is in labor and is unexpectedly found to require cesarean section, proceed after notifying the anesthesiologist that an epidural or spinal anesthetic is preferred. Be sure that the operating room is kept warm, that the recovery room staff and nurses on the postpartum unit know that pulmonary precautionary measures (coughing, turning, deep breathing, incentive spirometry) must be followed meticulously. Giving 1 or 2 U of red cells will accomplish little or nothing vis-a-vis sickling, and unnecessarily exposes the patient to the risks of transfusion

If cesarean section is anticipated and the patient has no pre-existing lung disease, proceed as above. If pulmonary function is already compromised, plan exchange transfusion prior to delivery

If the decision is made to undertake chronic transfusion therapy, the patient will probably need about 2 U of red cells every 4 weeks. The first follow-up transfusion should be scheduled about 1 month after the exchange, the percentage of HbS in the patient's blood should be measured before starting the transfusion and blood known not to be from sickle trait donors should be used (see above). When the percentage of HbS result comes back in a few days, the next transfusion should be scheduled based on that number (if it was <40 percent, every 4.5 weeks may be sufficient; if it was >50 percent a transfusion may be necessary every 3 to 3.5 weeks).

Technique for Exchange Transfusion

The goal of exchange transfusion in sickling disorders is to achieve more than 50 percent normal red cells (Fig. 20-2). There is no sense in measuring the percentage of hemoglobin (HbS) before transfusion; it will be about 100 percent in an untransfused SS

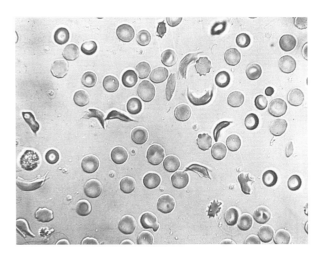

Fig. 20-2. Proportion of sickle cells after transfusion is most accurately estimated by measuring the percentage of HbS in a hemolysate by electrophoresis or chromatography. At night or on a weekend, sickle cells can be counted in a sickle cell preparation (a small drop of blood mixed with sodium metabisulfite solution and sealed with petroleum jelly or stopcock grease under a cover slip). After incubation for at least 2 hours, sickled forms are easily distinguished from normal (transfused) cells, and their proportion can be estimated by counting at least 400 cells.

patient, 70 percent in a patient with S/thalassemia, and 50 percent in a patient with SC disease. If the patient's hemoglobin level were 5.5 g/dl, transfusion to a level of 11 g/dl would accomplish the goal, assuming precautions were taken to avoid fluid overload. If the patient's initial hemoglobin level were 10 g/dl, transfusion to a hemoglobin level exceeding 20 g/dl (>50% normal cells) would be dangerous, and exchange transfusion would be necessary.

If a cell separator is available for exchange transfusion, and venous access is adequate, this provides the neatest and fastest way to perform the process, although it is about twice as expensive as a manual exchange. "Recipes" for the exchange have been published.[49] Some of us prefer to use blood that has been screened to eliminate sickle trait (AS) units; measurement of the proportion of HbS (the proportion of the patient's remaining red cells) is the easiest way to guage the efficacy of the exchange. The odds of a unit being positive for sickle trait are very low (<1 percent), and the precaution may be unnecessary.

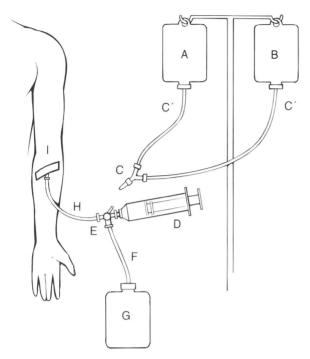

Fig. 20-3. Apparatus used for manual exchange transfusion: A, 0.9 percent sodium chloride solution; B, normal red cells; C, Y-connector and C', tubing clamps; D, 50-ml syringe; E, three-way stopcock; F, plasma transfer set with spike and needle adapter (e.g., Baxter 4C2240). G, Blood bag containing anticoagulant, or empty blood bag. H, Extension tube. I, 16-gauge plastic venous cannula. When blood is being removed, the syringe is connected to the stopcock; when red cells or sodium chloride solution are being infused, the Y-connector is connected to the stopcock.

If the exchange must be done manually (Fig. 20-3), the technique involved depends on the patient's hemoglobin concentration, the urgency of the situation, and the patient's blood volume (about 70 ml/kg). Three examples involving patients weighing 55 kg illustrate the problems.

1. *Transfusion prior to elective cesarean section; hemoglobin level 8 g/dl:* Sickle cells have a much shorter survival than normal cells. Two units of packed cells should be transfused per week for 3 to 4 weeks, measuring the percentage of HbA before each transfusion. Transfusion will depress the patient's production of new sickle cells, the old cells will be destroyed, and the percentage of HbA will

gradually reach the desired level without the need for removing any of the patient's own blood. Because the process requires more blood and takes longer, it is somewhat more expensive than a manual exchange transfusion.

2. *Transfusion for acute chest syndrome: hemoglobin level 8 g/dl:* Five units of red cells should be cross-matched; the blood bank should be asked to remove some of the preservative solution in the units to a hematocrit of about 60 percent. A large (16-gauge) intravascular cannula and a 50-ml syringe should be used to remove 500 ml of blood from the patient. Next, 400 ml of 0.9 percent sodium chloride solution should be infused. The first unit of red cells should be hung, ready to infuse. Then, 500 ml of blood should be removed from the patient and 5 U of packed cells should be infused. The total volume of blood removed is 1,000 ml; the total volume of saline infused is usually about 600 ml; and the total volume of red cells infused is about 1,600 ml. The final hemoglobin level should be about 13 g/dl.

3. *Transfusion to prevent increasingly severe crisis: hemoglobin level 13 g/dl (SC disease):* On day −1, 500 ml of blood should be removed on an outpatient basis; the patient should force fluids at home. On day 0, the patient should be admitted; 7 U of red cells should be cross-matched; 500 ml of blood should be removed; and fluids should be forced. On day 1, 500 ml of blood should be removed and 400 ml of 0.9 percent sodium chloride solution should be infused. Then, an additional 500 ml of blood should be removed and 1 U of red cells without any preservative removed should be infused. An additional 500 ml of blood should then be removed and 5 U of red cells (with preservative removed as above) should be infused. The total blood volume withdrawn on day 1 is 1,500; the total saline solution infused is about 800 ml; and the total volume of red cells infused is about 2,000 ml. On day 2, the hemoglobin level and the percentage of HbS should be checked. If necessary, more blood should be removed or the final unit of blood (unit 7) should be infused (or both).

Intrauterine Growth Retardation

Recent studies have demonstrated an incidence of IUGR of 14 to 42 percent in patients with sickle cell disease.[42,50,51] The etiology of fetal growth retardation is not completely understood, but it is believed to be secondary to vaso-occlusive events in the placental circulation. Severe anemia or chronic hypoxemia may be associated with low birth weight, but there are scant data to implicate these factors in the growth retardation of SS disease. Recurrent intravascular sickling may lead to microinfarctions of the placenta and impaired transfer of nutrients to the fetus. This in turn results in impaired fetal growth.

The diagnosis of IUGR is based on a birth weight below the 10th percentile for gestational age. Prenatally this is assessed by an estimated fetal weight based on the ultrasonographic biometric parameters of biparietal diameter, head circumference, abdominal circumference, and femur length.[52] Ultrasonography alone, however, has low sensitivity and specificity, especially in the late second and early third trimesters. Recently, Doppler velocimetry and systolic/diastolic ratios of umbilical artery blood flow have been used to evaluate placental function in fetuses suspected of having IUGR. Application of this technology to patients with sickle cell disease appears to improve the accuracy of diagnosis of IUGR.[51,53]

There is no specific therapeutic or preventive treatment for IUGR disease. Prophylactic transfusions, although they may decrease maternal symptomatology, have not been shown conclusively to decrease the incidence of IUGR.[24,42,54] Standard therapy consisting of bed rest and a high calorie/high protein diet, is usually employed. Fetal assessment should be initiated with nonstress tests, biophysical profiles, fetal movement counts, and serial sonograms for measurement of fetal growth.[18] Delivery is mandated if results of fetal testing become ominous or there is no evidence of any fetal growth over a 2- to 3-week period. Exchange transfusion has been employed in some cases of IUGR, but there is no convincing evidence that it is effective in accelerating fetal growth or relieving fetal distress.

INTRAPARTUM MANAGEMENT

Most women with sickle cell disease will present no unusual problems at the time of delivery, and can be managed uneventfully. Adequate oxygenation must be maintained, and epidural or spinal anesthesia are preferred over inhalation techniques. The patient who has been receiving chronic transfusion therapy usually needs no additional blood if she has been followed closely in clinic. If she has not, there usually is not adequate time to get more than a hematocrit result back from the laboratory before delivery; the hematologist who has been working with the obstetrician in following the patient should be asked for advice. Painful crises during labor, if they can be distinguished from labor pains, should be treated as other crises. Management of the unanticipated cesarean section is discussed above.

NEONATAL DIAGNOSIS

Most states now require screening of all newborns for sickle cell disease. Techniques, pitfalls, and problems with such plans are discussed in a recent Clinical Practice Guideline published by the Agency for Health Care Policy and Research of the U.S. Public Health Service.[55] All infants should be screened, but is essential that offspring of women with sickle cell disease be tested, since they must have one abnormal gene and could have two.

Essential Features of a Screening Program

Screening of all newborns

Acceptable laboratory techniques employed by laboratories that participate in proficiency testing programs

Repeat testing of all infants with suspected disease, often involving evaluation by a pediatric hematologist

Medical follow-up of the infant by a physician who will be responsible for starting penicillin prophylaxis and later administration of pneumococcal vaccine

Education of the parents about the nature and prognosis of the child's illness, their responsibilities for the child's care, and counseling about future pregnancies

POSTPARTUM COUNSELING

At the postpartum visit, it should be made clear to the patient that her internist or generalist is now responsible for her care, and that physician should be informed of the shift in responsibility. The need for contraception should be reviewed. The patient should be reminded that no form of contraception prevents sexually transmitted disease. If competent to do so, the obstetrician should review genetic risks for future pregnancies.

FUTURE THERAPIES WITH ANTI-SICKLING AGENTS

Experimental therapy of sickle cell disease with hydroxyurea[56] is beginning to move into practice. Study protocols may demand the use of contraception by men and women taking this drug,[57] but in actual practice a slightly more liberal view is appropriate.[58] Large doses of hydroxyurea are teratogenic in animals,[59,60] the drug is a mutagen,[61] and we strongly advise against pregnancy during its use. Nevertheless, pregnancies do occur in patients using hydroxyurea. No existing data suggest that the doses used to treat sickle cell disease can cause problems for children of the partners of men taking the drug; we do advise our male patients that there may be a risk if pregnancy occurs. Female patients are at greater risk, and although normal children have been born to women taking hydroxyurea through pregnancy,[62,63] we advise abortion for such patients.

SUMMARY

Pregnancy in women with sickle cell disease should be managed by obstetricians in high-risk clinics, with the advice of hematologists. Pregnancy should not be interdicted in women with sickle cell disease, since most gestations among such patients are uneventful; unwanted pregnancies should be avoided by thorough contraceptive counseling. Prenatal diagnosis is available, should the patient's partner be a carrier of a hemoglobinopathy. Prescription prenatal iron-and-vitamin pills contain adequate amounts of both folic acid and iron, and no more of these nutrients need be given. Routine prophylactic transfusion is not indicated for pregnant women with sickle cell

disease, but should be considered for such acute events as chest syndrome and stroke, or if the frequency or severity of vaso-occlusive crises increases beyond what is observed antepartum.

REFERENCES

1. Serjeant GR: Sickle Cell Disease. Oxford University Press, New York, 1992
2. Einbury SH, Hebbel RH, Mohandas N, Steinberg MH (eds): Sickle Cell Disease: Scientific Principles and Clinical Practice. Raven Press, New York, 1994
3. Resar LMS, Oski FA: Cold water exposure and vaso-occlusive crises in sickle cell anemia. J Pediatr 118: 407, 1991
4. Smith BD, La Celle PL: Erythrocyte-endothelial cell adherence in sickle cell disorders. Blood 68:1050, 1986
5. Hebbel RP, Boogaerts MAB, Eaton JW, Steinberg MH: Erythrocyte adherence to endothelium in sickle-cell anemia: a possible determinant of disease severity. N Engl J Med 302:992, 1980
6. Platt OS: Easing the suffering caused by sickle cell disease. N Engl J Med 330:783, 1994
7. Francis RB, Johnson CS: Vascular occlusion in sickle cell disease: current concepts and unanswered questions. Blood 77:1405, 1991
8. Kobak AJ, Stein PJ, Daro AF: Sickle cell anemia in pregnancy. a review of the literature and report of six cases. Am J Obstet Gynecol 41:811, 1941
9. Labie D, Richin C, Pagnier J et al: Hemoglobins S and C in Upper Volta. Hum Genet 65:300, 1984
10. Fort AT, Morrison JC: Motherhood with sickle cell and sickle-C disease is not worth the risk. South Med J 65:531, 1972
11. Sydenstricker VP, Kemp JA, Metts JC: Prolonged survival in sickle cell disease. Am Practit 13:584, 1962
12. Charache S, Richardson SN: Prolonged survival of a patient with sickle cell anemia. Arch Intern Med 113: 844, 1964
13. Vichinsky E, Hurst D, Earles A, et al: Newborn screening for sickle cell disease: effect on mortality. Pediatrics 81:749, 1988
14. Platt OS, Brambilla DJ, Rosse WF et al: Mortality in sickle cell disease: life expectancy and risk factors for early death. N Engl J Med 330:1639, 1994
15. Steinberg MH: Sickle cell anemia in a septuagenarian. Br J Haematol 710:297, 1989
16. Platt OS, Thorington BD, Brambilla DJ et al: Pain in sickle cell disease: rates and risk factors. N Engl J Med 325:11, 1991

17. Charache S, Lubin B, Reid CD: Management and therapy of sickle cell disease. National Institutes of Health Publication No. 89-2117, U.S. Government Printing Office, Washington, DC, 1989
18. Hemoglobinopathies in pregnancy. Technical Bulletin No. 185. American College of Obstetricians and Gynecologists, Washington, DC, 1993
19. Howard RJ, Lillis C, Tuck SM: Contraceptives, counselling, and pregnancy in women with sickle cell disease. BMJ 306:1735, 1993
20. Charache S, Lubin B, Reid CD: Leg ulcers. p. 30. In: Management and Therapy of Sickle Cell Disease. National Institutes of Health Publication No. 84-2117. U.S. Government Printing Office, Washington, DC, 1984
21. Old JM, Fitches A, Heath C et al: First-trimester fetal diagnosis for haemoglobinopathies: report on 200 cases. Lancet 2:763, 1986
22. Willoughby MLN: An investigation of folic acid requirements in pregnancy. Br J Haematol 13:503, 1967
23. Carmel R, Johnson CS: Racial patterns in pernicious anemia. Early age at onset and increased frequency of intrinsic-factor antibody in black women. N Engl J Med 298:647, 1978
24. Koshy M, Burd L, Wallace D et al: Prophylactic red-cell transfusions in pregnant patients with sickle cell disease: a randomized cooperative study. N Engl J Med 319:1447, 1988
25. Koshy M, Chisum D, Burd L et al: Management of sickle cell anemia and pregnancy. J Clin Apheresis 6:230, 1991
26. Foley KM: The practical use of narcotic analgesics. Med Clin North Am 66:1091, 1982
27. Acute Pain Management Guideline Panel: Acute Pain Management: Operative or Medical Procedures and Trauma. Clinical Practice Guideline. Center for Research Dissemination and Liason, Agency for Health Care Policy and Research, U.S. Public Health Service, Rockville, MD, 1992
28. White PF: Use of patient-controlled analgesia for management of acute pain. JAMA 259:243, 1988
29. Parfrey NA, Moore GW, Hutchins GM: Is pain crisis a cause of death in sickle cell disease? Am J Clin Pathol 84:209, 1985
30. Embury SH, Garcia JF, Mohandas N et al: Effects of oxygen inhalation on endogenous erythropoietin kinetics, erythropoiesis, and properties of blood cells in sickle cell anemia. N Engl J Med 311:291, 1984
31. Charache S, Scott JC, Charache P: Acute chest syndrome in adults with sickle cell anemia. Arch Intern Med 139:67, 1979
32. Charache S, Phillips S: Sickle cell anemia. p. 42. In

Glew RH, Peters SP (eds): Clinical Studies in Medical Biochemistry. Oxford University Press, New York, 1987
33. Wayne AS, Kevy SV, Nathan DG: Transfusion management of sickle cell disease. Blood 81:1109, 1993
34. Anson JA, Koshy M, Ferguson L, Crowell RM: Subarachnoid hemorrhage in sickle-cell disease. J Neurosurg 75:552, 1991
35. Adams RJ, Nichols FT, McKie VC et al: Cerebral infarction in sickle cell anemia: mechanism based on CT and MRI. Neurology 38:1012, 1988
36. Ohene-Frempong K: Stroke in sickle cell disease: demographic, clinical, and therapeutic considerations. Semin Hematol 28:213, 1991
37. Buchanan GR, Bowman WP, Smith SJ: Recurrent cerebral ischemia during hypertransfusion therapy in sickle cell anemia. J Pediatr 103:921, 1983
38. Rosse WF, Gallagher D, Kinney TR et al: Transfusion and alloimmunization in sickle cell disease. Blood 76:1431, 1990
39. Vichinsky EP, Earles A, Johnson RA et al: Alloimmunization in sickle cell anemia: the results of transfusion with racially unmatched blood. N Engl J Med 322:1617, 1990
40. Sosler SD, Jilly BJ, Saporito C, Koshy M: A simple, practical method for reducing alloimmunization in patients with sickle cell disease. Am J Hematol 43:103, 1993
41. Perry KG, Jr., Morrison JC: Hematologic disorders in pregnancy. Obstet Gynecol Clin North Am 19:783, 1992
42. Cunningham FG, Pritchard JA, Mason R: Pregnancy and sickle cell hemoglobinopathies: results with and without prophylactic transfusions. Obstet Gynecol 62:419, 1983
43. Morrison JC, Schneider JM, Whybrew WD et al: Prophylactic transfusions in pregnant patients with sickle hemoglobinopathies: benefit versus risk. Obstet Gynecol 56:274, 1980
44. Tuck SM, James CE, Brewster EM et al: Prophylactic blood transfusion in maternal sickle cell syndromes. Br J Obstet Gynecol 94:121, 1987
45. Keeling MM, Lavery JP, Clemons AU et al: Red cell exchange in the pregnancy complicated by a major hemoglobinopathy. Am J Obstet Gynecol 138:185, 1980
46. Ricks P Jr: Further experience with exchange transfusion in sickle cell anemia and pregnancy. Am J Obstet Gynecol 100:1087, 1968
47. Nagey DA, Garcia J, Welt SI: Isovolumetric partial exchange transfusion in the management of sickle cell

disease in pregnancy. Am J Obstet Gynecol 141:403, 1981

48. Rhimi Z, Marpeau L, Achite N et al: Drepanocytose majeure et grossesse. Transfusions prophylactiques systematiques. J Gynecol Obstet Biol Reprod 21:701, 1992

49. Piomelli S, Seaman C, Ackerman K et al: Planning an exchange transfusion in patients with sickle cell syndromes. Am J Pediatr Hematol/Oncol 12:268, 1990

50. Tuck SM, White JM: Pregnancy in sickle cell disease in the UK. Br J Obstet Gynecol 90:112, 1983

51. Anyaegbunam A, Langer O, Brustman L et al: Third-trimester prediction of small-for-gestational-age infants in pregnant women with sickle cell disease. Development of the ultradop index. J Reprod Med 36: 577, 1991

52. Morrison JC, Blake PG, McCoy C et al: Fetal health assessment in pregnancies complicated by sickle hemoglobinopathies. Obstet Gynecol 61:22, 1983

53. Anyaegbunam A, Morel M-IG, Merkatz IR: Antepartum fetal surveillance tests during sickle cell crisis. Am J Obstet Gynecol 165:1081, 1991

54. Miller JM Jr, Horger EO III, Key TC, Walker EM Jr: Management of sickle hemoglobinopathies in pregnant patients. Am J Obstet Gynecol 141:237, 1981

55. Sickle Cell Disease Guideline Panel: Sickle Cell Disease: Screening, Diagnosis, Management, and Counseling in Newborns and Infants. Clinical Practice Guideline No. 6. Publication No. 93-0562. Agency for Health Care Policy and Research, U.S. Public Health Service, Rockville, MD, 1993

56. Charache S, Dover GJ, Moore RD et al: Hydroxyurea: effects on hemoglobin F production in patients with sickle cell anemia. Blood 78:212, 1992

57. Charache S, Terrin ML, Moore RD et al: Design of the multicenter study of hydroxyurea. Controlled Clin Trials (in press)

58. Tertian G, Tchernia G, Papiernik E, Elefant E: Hydroxyurea and pregnancy. Am J Obstet Gynecol 266: 1868, 1992

59. Scott WJ, Ritter EJ, Wilson JG: DNA synthesis inhibition and cell death associated with hydroxyurea teratogenesis in rat embryos. Dev Biol 26:306, 1971

60. DeSesso JM, Goeringer GC: The nature of the embryo-protective interaction of propyl gallate with hydroxyurea. Reprod Toxicol 4:145, 1990

61. Timson J: Hydroxyurea. Mutat Res 32:115, 1975

62. Delmier A, Rio B, Bauduer F et al: Pregnancy during myelosuppressive treatment for chronic myelogenous leukemia. Br J Haematol 82:783, 1992

63. Jackson N, Shukri A, Ali K: Hydroxyurea treatment for chronic myeloid leukaemia during pregnancy. Br J Haematol 85:203, 1993

Chapter 21

Role of Maternal Transport in Modern Obstetrics

John P. Elliott

The goal of obstetric care is to guide the pregnant woman safely through her gestation, manage her labor and delivery, and obtain the best outcome possible for both the woman and her infant. This care is provided in many different ways in different cultures, varying from local care (in the woman's home) to more centralized systems involving travel to a common location (a hospital or birthing center) to deliver. The practicality of bringing patients to a centralized delivery center awaited advances in modes of human travel, as distance and speed of travel determined where services could be provided. Innovations in patient transport were driven mostly by military needs to treat wounded soldiers, but were eventually adapted to civilian medical care. Momentous technologic advances occurred with the invention of the automobile, airplane, and helicopter, each of which improved the important factor of speed in getting to a medical care facility.

Military evacuations of wounded soldiers became accepted practice during the Korean War, which demanded the use of helicopters because of a lack of landing fields for fixed-wing aircraft. Front-line regionalized centers were established as helicopters brought casualties to mobile army surgical hospitals (MASH). These units stabilized patients and provided initial lifesaving medical and surgical care. Survivors were then flown to back-line hospitals, which provided more sophisticated and specialized care. Survival improved dramatically with this triage and transport concept in a regionalized system of medical care, and during the Vietnam conflict, greater than 95 percent survival was achieved for wounded personnel who reached the MASH hospitals alive.

The benefit of stabilization and fast transport by helicopter was demonstrated in the civilian trauma setting by Baxt and Moody.[1] They compared the outcome of 150 patients involved in blunt trauma who were transported by land vehicles with that of 150 other patients transported by helicopter. There was a 52 percent reduction in mortality in the helicopter transport group, according to predicted mortality rates based on trauma scores. In perinatal care, these concepts were first applied to the management of sick neonates. An excellent review of the history of neonatal transport is provided by Butterfield.[2]

In 1899, Dr. Joseph Bolivar DeLee[3] transported premature infants in "incubators" from the vicinity of Chicago into the Chicago Lying-In Hospital for care. The equipment and personnel involved in the transport of sick babies improved as the pace of neonatal care in general improved in the 1960s and 1970s. Heat and oxygen were important concepts applied during the initial transports, which were done in ground ambulances. Roget et al[4] first described the transport of sick neonates by helicopter in France in 1964, demonstrating the safety and decreased time of transport with helicopters.

The availability of well-equipped transport vehicles facilitated the development of regionalization for newborn care. Problems with early transport incubators encouraged the transport of pregnant women to specialized neonatal facilities, with delivery occurring in those facilities and the mother serving as the "ideal incubator." The twin demands of speed and distance were now applied to a more unpredictable situation—the risk of labor and possible delivery occurring during the trip. Full-service maternal transport also benefited from the advances of air travel.

Thus, it was the availability of fast, safe transport vehicles that allowed the development of perinatal centers to provide care to mothers and neonates at increased risk of morbidity or mortality. Regionalization of perinatal care in the United States was motivated first by the desire to provide appropriate care to high-risk mothers and infants in order to reduce morbidity and mortality, and second by the impracticality and cost of attempting to provide these services in all hospitals for all possible maternal-neonatal complications. In 1975, Ryan[5] published the recommendations of the Committee on Perinatal health (made up of representatives of the American Academy of Family Practice [AAFP], American Acad-

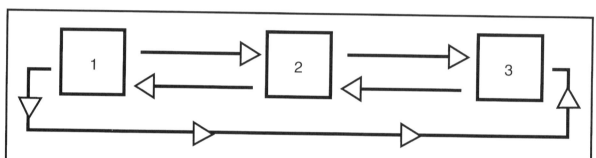

LEVEL 1 to LEVEL 2:

Complicated cases not requiring intensive care

LEVEL 1 to LEVEL 3:

Complicated cases requiring intensive care

LEVEL 1—RESPONSIBILITIES

1. Uncomplicated maternity and neonatal care for areas not served by other units
2. Emergency management of unexpected complications

Special Services

1. Early indentification of high-risk patients
2. Preventive and social services

LEVEL 2 to LEVEL 3:

Complicated cases requiring intensive care (e.g., labor <34 weeks'

gestation, severe isoimmune disease, severe medical complications, anticipated need for neonatal surgery)

LEVEL 2—RESPONSIBILITIES

1. Complete maternity and neonatal care for uncomplicated and most high-risk patients

Special Services

1. 15-minute start-up time for cesarean section
2. 24-hour in-house anesthesia for obstetrics
3. Short-term assisted ventilation of newborn
4. 24-hour clinical laboratory services
5. 24-hour radiology services
6. 24-hour blood bank services
7. Fetal monitoring
8. Special care nursery

LEVEL 3 or LEVEL 2 to HOSPITAL OF ORIGIN:

For growth and development of infants no longer requiring intensive care

LEVEL 3—RESPONSIBILITIES

1. Complete maternity and neonatal care plus intensive care of intrapartum and neonatal high-risk patients

Special Services

1. 24-hour consultation service for region
2. Coordination of transport system
3. Development and coordination of educational program for region
4. Data analysis for region

Fig. 21-1. Schematic showing transport among the three levels of care with explanations of the requirements and responsibilities of each level.

emy of Perinatologists [AAP], American College of Obstetricians and Gynecologists [ACOG], and the American Medical Association [AMA]), which formalized regionalization and encouraged designation of level I, II, and III perinatal facilities. The levels of care provided and responsibilities of the hospitals in the regional system are outlined in Figure 21-1. Regionalization of care allows society to save resources by not duplicating the purchase of expensive equipment in many small hospitals, but more importantly it effectively allows appropriate development of the skills necessary to deal with these special circumstances by physicians, nurses, respiratory technicians, ultrasound technicians, and other relevant personnel. The volume of patients in a regionalized system also allows maintenance of these skills. The broad framework for regionalization is the concept that perinatal care requiring complex technology should be available to every patient within a designated region, but will not be available within each hospital. The level of care provided within individual hospitals is determined by the availability of technology, skilled nursing and medical personnel, and other related support services. When transport becomes necessary, the issue is not quality of care but rather the level of available technology and support.

REGIONALIZATION IN OBSTETRICS

Any major change in health-care delivery requires documentation of its efficacy. Many studies have compared neonates whose mothers were transported antepartum to a tertiary perinatal care center to those transported after birth.[6-12] Conclusions supported by these studies include increased survival, decreased short- and long-term morbidity, and decreased cost of hospitalization for infants transported in utero and delivered at a tertiary care center. Questions have been raised about the validity of these studies because of possible selection bias. Delaney-Black et al[13] found that maternal transports were more frequently associated with a maternal risk factor (pregnancy-induced hypertension [PIH], antepartum bleeding, prolonged rupture of membranes, or chorioamnionitis) than were neonatal transports. One or more acute complications of pregnancy occurred twice as often among the ante-

natally referred mothers. Miller and colleagues[14] evaluated maternal and neonatal transport in the entire population in their area, evaluating the perinatal denominator for the first time.

The perinatal denominator was completely identified by including patients who died before transport, were transported to other facilities, or remained at the hospital of delivery for care. The study supported maternal transport before delivery for premature infants. Despite having greater risk factors, the antepartum transported patients experienced a significantly lower mortality by delivering at a tertiary care facility. Population-based studies in the Netherlands also validated better outcomes for maternally transported patients at risk than for neonatally transported patients.[15-18] The compiled evidence supports in utero transfer of patients at risk of a poor neonatal outcome.

INDICATIONS FOR MATERNAL TRANSPORT

Maternal transport to a tertiary facility should be considered when (1) the circumstances immediately available to the patient are not sufficient to deal with the patient's actual or predicted obstetric, medical, or surgical complications; or (2) there is reasonable expectation of the birth of one or more infants who may require more intensive neonatal care than that available at the patient's current location; or (3) the patient's obstetric, medical, or surgical circumstances require continuous attendance by trained personnel not available at the patient's current location. The reasons for maternal transport may differ in various regions of the United States. In Georgia, Kanto et al[19] reported primarily fetal indications for transport, although 28 percent of the cases in their study were referred for maternal indications. This contrasts with data from Colorado,[13] which documented significantly more maternal complications in cases of maternal transport than in neonatal transport. The investigators concluded that "It appears that pregnancy complications affecting the mother rather than fetal risk determined maternal delivery site in both of our study populations." Knox and Schnitker[20] found that over 90 percent of the maternal transports in their referral population were done for risk of prematurity, with 78 percent of patients actually in preterm labor (PTL), but they stress that early consultation and referral of appropriate patients removes these (other maternal indications) from the need for acute transport. Low[21] compiled data for air transport of maternal patients in the United States. Of 463 patients transported within a 6-month study period, the reasons for transport were prematurity in 330 (71 percent) cases, hemorrhage in 79 (17 percent), PIH in 41 (9 percent), and eclampsia in eight 8 (2 percent). Our experience in an urban referral area in Long Beach, California[22] gave the following breakdown of gestational ages at transport: 31 percent were less than 30 weeks, 47 percent were between 30 and 34 weeks, and 22 percent were of more than 34 weeks' gestation. The last group of transports were presumably for maternal reasons.

It is clear that the philosophy of the region must be to provide the appropriate level of care for each patient. Establishing the diagnosis of preterm labor early, when transport can be safely arranged, is very important. Knox[20] reported excellent success in Minneapolis with the transport of patients over long distances (>40 miles) and in cases of advanced cervical dilatation (>4 cm). Elliott et al[23] reviewed the cases of 1,080 patients transported for preterm labor in an 18-month period in northern Arizona. Fifty-four (5 percent) were 7 cm or more dilated at the time of the call for transport. A decision was made not to transport 5 patients, and the other 49 were successfully transported to one of three tertiary hospitals in Phoenix. There were no deliveries en route. Low[21] documented one delivery in 463 transports. It is clear that with adequately trained transport crews exercising some caution, transport to a tertiary care center can be performed for any diagnosis, with active labor, with advanced cervical dilatation, and over considerable distances. Successful in utero transport depends on consultation between the referring and tertiary care physicians. The standard of care calls for transport in all but extremely unstable circumstances.

MODE OF TRANSPORT

Coordinators of maternal transport must consider several factors when selecting an appropriate vehicle for transport. The first of these are whether to use a private car, ground ambulance, helicopter, or fixed-wing airplane. There are differences in speed and in the personnel that accompany the transport. For long distances, fixed-wing aircraft would be useful; for shorter distances the choice of vehicle is outlined in Table 21-1. In Long Beach[22] we found that shorter-distance flights are slightly more expensive by helicopter than by ground ambulance. At a distance of about 10 miles the costs are equal, and at distances beyond 10 miles the helicopter is cheaper than ground ambulance. The experience of the personnel accomplishing the transport is also important. Obstetric flight nurses will have more experience and better judgment than cross-trained adult-trauma flight nurses, and will be more comfortable transporting patients in advanced preterm labor.[23] Regardless of background, a transport nurse doing maternal transports should have the skills listed in the box. The decision to transport a patient in utero or to deliver at the referring hospital and stabilize

---

Necessary Skills for Transport Team Nurses

The registered nurse on the transport team must be proficient in the following minimum skills as they relate to the care of high-risk mothers and infants:

In-depth physical assessment of the gravid woman and her fetus

Newborn assessment and resuscitation

Advanced airway management, including intubation of newborns and adults

Peripheral intravenous catheter insertion and therapy

Foley catheter placement

Vaginal examination including sterile speculum examination

Administration of tocolytic medications

Fetal heart rate monitoring and interpretation of the heart rate tracing

Emergency delivery

Exceptional interpersonal skills

Table 21-1. Appropriate Transport for Obstetric Complications

Reason for Transport	Car	Ambulance	Helicopter
Low risk of complication en route			
Diabetes mellitus, controlled	Yes	Yes	No
Fetal demise (uncomplicated)	Yes	No	No
Mild to moderate pre-eclampsia	Yes	Yes	Sometimes
Placenta previa without bleeding	Yes	Yes	Sometimes
Preterm premature rupture of membranes (no labor)	Yes	Yes	Sometimes
Rh isoimmunization	Yes	No	No
Moderate to high-risk of complication en route			
Abnormal fetal lie	No	Yes	Yes
Diabetes mellitus out of control or ketoacidosis	No	Yes	Yes
Eclampsia or severe pre-eclampsia	No	Yes	Yes
Placental abruption	No	Yes	Yes
Placental previa bleeding actively	No	Yes	Yes
Preterm premature rupture of membranes in labor	No	Yes	Yes
Premature labor[a]	No	Yes	Yes
Referring physician desire to transport for any reason	Yes	Yes	Yes
Severe maternal medical complications (cardiovascular, renal, etc.)	No	Yes	Yes

[a] Patient in premature labor with cervix dilated ≥6 cm should be transported only by helicopter with an accompanying physician.

and transport the infant is made by the referring and receiving physicians. Factors that are considered are the potential benefits of transport and the risks involved compared with the benefits and risks of not transporting; the skill of the transport team; inherent risks in the problem necessitating transport; distance to the receiving hospital; and finally, the support available if transport is not undertaken (e.g., the availability of a respirator for a premature infant, the ability to perform a cesarean section.)

Safe transport of the pregnant woman requires some experience and thought by the transport personnel. Katz and Hansen[24] stress three important principles in maternal transport: (1) the use of left lateral tilt rather than the supine position to avoid aortocaval compression by the uterus (especially in trauma transports); (2) adequate volume replacement to ensure adequate uterine perfusion; and (3) use of supplemental oxygen. The fetal status should be monitored during transport. Fetal heart rate can be ascertained with a Doppler ultrasound instrument, or more information about fetal status can be gained by using a fetal heart rate monitor.[25] Poulton and Kisicki[26] documented that only 2 percent of transport programs in the United States use fetal heart rate monitoring during transport, and that only 29 percent evaluated the fetal status with a Doppler instrument. Monitoring the fetal status is important because simple interventions may improve oxygen delivery to the fetus (e.g., increased oxygen delivery by mask, increased fluids, position change). An additional benefit of knowing the status of the fetus is that it allows the transport team to alert the receiving hospital to have an appropriate team available to respond in situations involving possible fetal distress.

In our transport program, the tocolytic drug of choice is intravenous magnesium sulfate. This is an extremely efficacious agent, especially for short-term goals such as transport.[27] We start magnesium sulfate even if labor is not established to ensure safe transport over long distances. Knox[20] also recommends magnesium sulfate because of its low toxicity and capacity for use in hypertensive or bleeding patients in whom β-mimetic drugs are contraindicated. We recommend a 6-g loading dose (over 15 to 20 minutes), followed by maintenance therapy at 3 g/h, with adjustments upward or downward depending on the therapeutic response. Subcutaneous doses of terbutaline (0.25 mg) can supplement the magnesium sulfate. β-Sympathomimetic drugs have also been used successfully for transport over long distances in Australia.[28] The drug used was salbutamol.

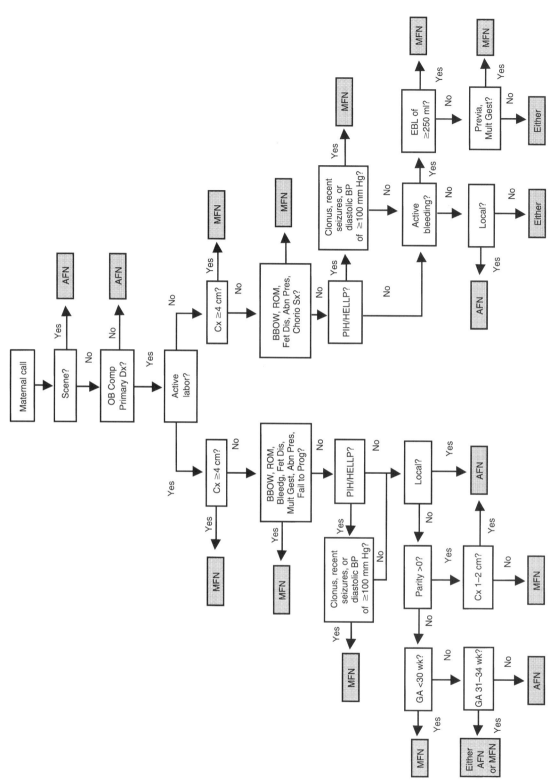

Fig. 21-2. Algorithm for maternal transport triage. AFN, adult flight nurse; MFN, maternal flight nurse; Scene, scene; BBOW, bulging bag of water; ROM, rupture of membranes; Chorio, chorioamnionitis; Abn pres, abnormal presentation.

Twenty-six percent of patients had a change in their cervical examination findings during transport, and 62 percent had no change. Twelve percent did not have cervical examinations done for obstetric reasons. There was one delivery during transport, of a patient dilated 2 cm at the start of transport.

The transport team composition varies in different programs. At Samaritan Airevac we use a combination of maternal flight nurses, adult flight nurses, neonatal flight nurses, respiratory therapists, and physicians assistants. Before the flight, the team is chosen by the perinatologist who is acting as medical director, and by the appropriate flight nurse (maternal or adult cross-trained). Figure 21-2 shows a triage tree that has been developed as a guideline for the appropriate level of nursing skill necessary on each flight. A second team member is chosen on the basis of the risk of delivery in flight or possible maternal respiratory complications. Some programs require that physicians accompany transports, but our experience and that of Reedy et al[29] document safe transport of maternal patients with a nurse transport team that relies on data gathering, assessment, nursing judgment, and stabilization of the patient. Safety during transport is critical because the environment for delivery in the transport vehicle is usually inferior to that in the referring hospital.

ROLE OF THE REFERRING HOSPITAL

Many obstetric complications are of sudden onset or are not recognized in early stages by patients or health-care providers. In most level I and level II hospitals, the labor-and-delivery area is the center for the initial evaluation and treatment of obstetric complications. It is important that initial diagnosis and stabilization of the patient occur quickly. Premature labor and premature ruptured membranes constitute the bulk of diagnoses prompting maternal transport. Early diagnosis and treatment with bed rest, hydration, and tocolytic drugs may have a beneficial effect on the ability to transport the patient. It must not be assumed that transport is only for delivery. Aggressive tocolysis may allow delay of delivery for 48 hours, even with advanced cervical dilatation. This would allow steroids to be administered, which could improve the outcome in cases involving premature delivery.

Regionalization can be influenced by level I hospitals using risk scoring and then considering delivery at a level II or III hospital, depending on risk and distance. Sokol and associates[30] evaluated a risk-scoring system to determine whether it could be used in a clinical setting to identify patients at increased risk of poor neonatal outcome. In this study, 50 percent of the patient population was at low risk of poor neonatal outcome, based on antepartum risk screening. Forty percent of this group developed risk factors in labor, and these were associated with 16 percent of perinatal deaths. The 50 percent of patients who were classified as having a high antepartum risk for poor neonatal outcome were also split about 50-50 on the score for intrapartum risk. High risk in both categories was associated with a perinatal mortality rate of 93.4 per 1,000 births, which was statistically significantly different from that in the other risk groups. This risk-scoring system should be applied in a regionalized perinatal system to at least identify low-risk patients, who would receive appropriate care in level I facilities, although even these facilities must be staffed and equipped to deal with obstetric emergencies (placental abruption, ruptured uterus, prolapsed cord). Berg and colleagues[31] have confirmed that even for infants weighing more than 2,500 g, the highest neonatal mortality rate was observed at level I hospitals. This study also examined risk scores and outcomes.

Why are these patients at increased risk of poor neonatal outcome at level I hospitals? The United States Office of Technology Assessment evaluated the cost and effectiveness of neonatal intensive care units (NICUs).[32] It identified three main reasons for the lack of use of this technology: (1) most importantly, a lack of awareness on the part of physicians of the improvement in outcome with delivery at a facility of the appropriate level; (2) the desire of physicians or hospitals to be viewed as capable of providing a complete range of services; and (3) financial inability of women to pay for the high cost of neonatal intensive care. Level I hospitals often do not have the volume of patients necessary to permit the provision of an on-site emergency response capability.

Richardson et al[33] investigated how obstetricians make referral decisions, concluding that medical considerations were the predominant ones affecting transport (class and degree of control of diabetics, quality of the nursery, and the presence of PIH). There is a small but real influence of financial and social factors, which may play a role in borderline cases. A maternal transport index (MTI)[34] was developed to assist in decision-making about maternal transport. The MTI was a comparison of outcomes of individual medical conditions based on the site of treatment. This scoring system needs to be evaluated in a clinical situation to prove its usefulness.

What is necessary at the referring hospital to assist in smooth transfer to the receiving facility? Once a patient has been identified who would benefit from care at a level III facility, communication with that facility and the receiving physician is necessary to prepare for smooth transfer. The patient and her family need both physical and psychological transfer to a new facility and new care providers. The labor and delivery staff and physician of the referring hospital need to explain the need for transfer and a general idea of what to expect. It is not advisable to give any treatment plan because it may change at the tertiary care hospital, and expectations may create a difficult psychological and emotional adjustment for the patient.

In consultation with the perinatologist at the level III center, therapy may be initiated at the referring hospital and continued during transport. Indications for consultation or transport in the Tennessee Perinatal Care System for level I facilitates and level II hospitals are given in the boxes below.[35] The family needs to be given information about where the mother is being sent, how to get there, and whether someone may accompany the patient during transport. Positive information about the quality of the receiving hospital and its nurses and physicians will help give the patient confidence in the transfer system.

THE TERTIARY CARE HOSPITAL: A REGIONAL ROLE

The level III hospital has the equipment and staff to care for normal pregnancies, but can also manage the most complicated and life-threatening complications with confidence. Obstetricians and pediatricians are receiving better training and using new technologies in their practice. Specialists have evolved in both areas who care for mothers and neonates at increased risk of a poor outcome. Perinatologists and neonatologists are available at level III hospitals to manage such pregnancies and the neonates delivered from them. Nursing has also developed subspecialties, with neonatal intensive care nursing and perinatal nurse specialists contributing to the tertiary care team. The labor-and-delivery nurse at the tertiary care center is familiar with the increased acuity of transport patients and is capable of handling the increased volume of patients created by transfer. In many regional systems the labor-and-delivery nurses are also the transport nurses, applying their skills and experience outside the hospital in the transport environment.

Four general categories of patients are transported to tertiary care centers: (1) those at risk of delivering a premature infant, (2) anomalous fetuses, (3) patients with serious maternal illness or injury, and (4) patients with diagnostic dilemmas or who represent unusual cases.

The most immediate impact of maternal transport on a tertiary care hospital is the volume and acuity of patients it creates. In a mature regionalized referral system in northern Arizona, a state with a population of about 4 million, approximately 1,000 maternal transports per year are brought to the three tertiary care hospitals in Phoenix. There are also about 500 neonatal transports. Approximately 60 percent of these maternal transports come to Good Samaritan Regional Medical Center/Phoenix Children's Hospital, resulting in approximately 50 transports per month, or 1.5/day, arriving in the hospital's labor-and-delivery unit.

Seventy to eighty percent of transports involve expected premature delivery. In the absence of contraindications (e.g., documented fetal pulmonary maturity, chorioamnionitis, fetal distress, advanced cervical dilatation [≥8 cm dilated] or life-threatening maternal or fetal disease, aggressive tocolysis is continued at the tertiary hospital. This is true even for patients with apparent failed tocolysis at the referring facility. Several factors allow the perinatologist to continue tocolysis. The first is that the NICU is available in the event of failure of therapy. Second, obstetricians frequently give a subtherapeutic dose of a tocolytic drug or do not give the drug for an adequate amount of time. Third, a tocolytic drug

Indications for Maternal Consultation or Transfer: Level I Facilities

Antepartum
  Maternal History
    Diagnosed abnormalities of genital tract
    Medical indication for termination of previous pregnancy
Neonate more than 4,000 g at term or any large-for-gestational-age neonate
    Neonate who required more than routine observation or care
    Neonate with known or suspected genetic or familial disorder
    Preterm labor (<37 weeks) or low-birth-weight neonate (<2,500 g)
    Previous cesarean section
    Previous stillbirth, neonatal loss, or two or more abortions
    Severe emotional problems associated with previous pregnancy or delivery
    Suspected incompetent cervix
  Medical/surgical complications
    Cardiac disease
    Chemical abuse
    Diabetes mellitus
    Hematologic disorder
    Hypertension
    Infection
    Malignancy
    Musculoskeletal abnormality
    Neurologic disorder
    Nutritional abnormality
    Other endocrine disorders
    Psychiatric disorder
    Pulmonary disease
    Renal disease
    Surgical emergency
    Trauma
  Obstetric complications
    Age under 16 or over 35 years
    Elective induction of labor or elective cesarean section
    Exposure to teratogens
    Fetal demise
    Glucose intolerance
    Height under 150 cm (60 in)
    Hyperemesis

    Inappropriate fetal growth for gestational age
    Isoimmunization
    Multiple gestation
    Persistent anemia
    Post-term gestation (>42 weeks)
    Pre-eclampsia or eclampsia
    Prepregnant weight under 45 kg (approximately 100 lb) or over 90 kg (approximately 200 lb)
    Preterm cervical dilatation without uterine contraction
    Preterm rupture of membranes with or without uterine contraction
    Rupture of membranes at term for more than 12 hours without labor or evidence of amnionitis or sepsis at any time
    Sexually transmitted disease
    Suspected ectopic pregnancy
    Suspected fetopelvic disproportion
    Suspected missed abortion
    Suspected polyhydramnios or oligohydramnios
    Urinary tract infection
    Vaginal bleeding
Intrapartum
  Abnormal bleeding
  Abnormal presentation
  Desultory labor
  Meconium in amniotic fluid
  Multiple gestation
  Pre-eclampsia or eclampsia
  Preterm (<37 weeks) cervical dilatation with uterine contractions
  Rupture of membranes at term for more than 12 hours or evidence of amnionitis or sepsis at any time
  Suspected fetal distress
  Suspected fetopelvic disproportion
  Uterine atony
Postpartum
  Abnormal bleeding
  Pre-eclampsia or eclampsia
  Sepsis
  Thromboembolic disease

(From Troiano,[35] with permission)

Indications for Maternal Consultation or Transfer: Level II Facilities

Antepartum
  Medical-surgical complications
    Cardiac disease
    Chemical abuse
    Hematologic disorder
    Insulin-dependent diabetes mellitus
    Malignancy
    Musculoskeletal abnormality
    Neurologic disorder
    Other endocrine disorders
    Pulmonary disease
    Renal disease
    Surgical emergency
    Trauma
  Obstetric complications
    Inappropriate fetal growth for gestational age
    Isoimmunization
    Medical or obstetric indication for preterm (<34 weeks) delivery
    Multiple gestation (preterm or >2)
    Preterm cervical dilatation without uterine contraction
    Preterm rupture of membranes with or without uterine contraction
    Severe pre-eclampsia or eclampsia
    Suspected fetal anomalies

Intrapartum
  Preterm (<34 weeks) cervical dilatation with uterine contraction
  Severe pre-eclampsia or eclampsia with or without hematologic complications
  Severe or unresponsive sepsis

Postpartum
  Severe pre-eclampsia or eclampsia with or without hematologic complications
  Severe or unresponsive sepsis
  Thromboembolic disease

(From Troiano,[35] with permission)

---

may have been discontinued for a side effect, which can either be tolerated with support for the patient or overcome by changing drugs. Fourth, the perinatologist may be more comfortable using tocolytic drugs in combination, a situation in which complications and side effects are increased.[36] Our tocolytic drug of choice in virtually all circumstances is magnesium sulfate. The recommended loading dose for suppression of preterm labor is a 6-g bolus given over a period of 20 minutes and followed by a constant infusion of 3 g/hr IV. If contractions continue, the magnesium sulfate infusion is increased to obtain a serum magnesium level of 5.5 to 7.5 mg/dl. This may require infusion at a rate of 4 or 5 g/hr for some period. The labor-and-delivery nurses should be very comfortable with this aggressive use of tocolysis and should be able to work with the patient to help her tolerate its side effects (flushing, nausea, headache, muscle weakness, visual disturbances). They should also be comfortable in assessing the patient being treated with magnesium sulfate (reflexes, respirations, urine output). The goal of tocolysis must be determined by the clinical situation. In some circumstances it may be to gain 48 hours before delivery to allow antenatal corticosteroids to be given to the mother to reduce respiratory distress syndrome (RDS) or intraventricular hemorrhage (IVH) in the neonate. Elliott[27] provides data on the delay of delivery by cervical dilatation through the aggressive use of magnesium sulfate in singleton and twin pregnancies with intact and ruptured membranes.

If tocolysis fails or is contraindicated, the management of labor and delivery in a preterm gestation differs from that in a term pregnancy. The goal is to atraumatically deliver an infant that is not acidotic and is not hypothermic, with the neonatal resuscitation team present at the delivery. How does preterm labor differ from labor in a term pregnancy? In general, labor is shorter in preterm gestations. Preterm fetuses do not tolerate the contractions of labor as well as those in term pregnancies, probably because of inadequate fat and glycogen stores. Cord compression is more likely to cause hypoxia and acidosis in premature infants than in term fetuses, and acidosis can develop very quickly. Electronic fetal heart rate monitoring should be used and the physician should understand the signs of fetal intolerance of labor. If possible, the physician should avoid rupturing membranes in a premature gestation. Narcotic analgesia should be used sparingly, but epidural anesthesia is believed to be well tolerated. Delivery is also different with more cesarean sections done in premature deliveries. A significantly greater number of breech and other malpresenting fetuses, multiple gestations, and instances of significant maternal disease and fetal intolerance of labor contribute to the 30 to 50 percent cesarean section rate. Vacuum extraction and forceps deliveries should be avoided because of possible trauma to the premature fetal head. Crenshaw et al[37] recommend cesarean section in circumstances of (1) fetal distress unresponsive to conservative treatment, (2) breech presentation and gestational age of less than 32 weeks, or (3) delivery for maternal or fetal indications and a closed, firm cervix.

The second group of patients who will arrive in the labor-and-delivery unit of a tertiary hospital are those with acute maternal medical complications. Elliott and colleagues[38] documented that in a 20-month study period, Samaritan Airevac transported 1,541 maternal patients, of whom 360 (23.4 percent) had critical care diagnoses. Fifty-two percent had hypertensive crises, 36 percent had hemorrhage, 6 percent had trauma, and 3 percent had respiratory compromise. These patients should be cared for in the labor-and-delivery unit rather than in a traditional medical-surgical intensive care unit (ICU). At Good Samaritan Regional Medical Center, the labor-and-delivery unit has been transformed into an obstetric ICU. Two large rooms are used as ICU rooms, although all nine labor rooms have monitors for invasive central monitoring lines. The concept of a maternal-fetal ICU (MF-ICU), established on a labor-and-delivery unit and staffed by a team of healthcare providers, including a perinatologist, medical intensivist, anesthesiologist, obstetrics resident, obstetric ICU nurse, and respiratory therapist is being advanced, with preliminary results demonstrating outcomes equal to those with traditional medical ICU care.[39] In comparing outcome in the MF-ICU with previous outcome in the medical ICU, patients were kept alive for a longer period of time before death, although there was no difference in mortality (21.7 per 100,000 births versus 22.1 per 100,000 births). The hope in establishing MF-ICUs is that with more experience, mortality will fall. The labor-

and-delivery nurse must receive special training in ICU techniques, including the setting up of invasive lines and monitoring and interpreting the parameters provided by a Swan-Ganz catheter.[40] Obstetric nurses have a better understanding of the physiology of the pregnant patient than do ICU nurses, and therefore should be part of the team, especially before delivery, when the fetus assumes an importance equal to that of the mother. Some situations may put the fetus at a disproportionately greater risk than the mother. These would include abdominal trauma to the mother, severe pre-eclampsia, fetal-maternal hemorrhage, eclampsia, diabetic ketoacidosis, and maternal respiratory compromise from any cause.

Transports for fetal anomalies are managed in the labor-and-delivery unit on the basis of the potential viability of the neonate. Often, pediatric subspecialists (neurosurgery, pediatric surgery, cardiology, endocrinology, neurology) are involved during the immediate neonatal period. The timing of delivery may be important, and the route of delivery should be determined in consultation with the perinatologists, neonatologists, and pediatric subspecialists involved in a particular case.

Finally, difficult diagnostic dilemmas and unusual cases may be transported. These include cases of maternal fever of unknown origin, maternal malignant diseases (leukemia, lymphoma), high-order multiple gestations (triplets, quadruplets), pregnancies with an acardiac twin, cases of twin-twin transfusion syndrome or hydrops fetalis, and others. The management of these cases should be individualized.

The concept of regionalization, which allows the delivery of specialized care to all patients who need it, demands three more components for completion. Communication from the perinatologist to the referring physician will keep the latter knowledgeable[41] about a referred case so that inquiries from local family members can be answered. Outreach education by the perinatal team is necessary to elevate the standard of care practiced in level I and level II hospitals. This will assist these facilities in providing better care in the 40 percent of cases with potentially bad outcomes that cannot be predicted in time to transport the mother. The final component of this regionalized system is neonatal back transport of appropriate infants.[42–44]

CHALLENGES FOR THE FUTURE

With the growth of regionalization of care over the past 25 years, there is now a movement toward de-regionalization. Level II hospitals are hiring neonatologists and neonatal nurse practitioners, and in some cases telling physicians and the community that they can keep premature deliveries to a minimum of 28 weeks gestation. There is a notable lack of outcome-based data with which to address this issue, but it is terribly important from an economic and also from an outcome standpoint. Hickok et al[45] presented Washington State data from 1980 to 1990 on birth weight-specific mortality for 43,832 live-born infants weighing less than 2,500 g. After 1988 these investigators detected a shift in the location of birth of infants weighing 1,500 to 1,999 g toward nontertiary care hospitals. For infants weighing less than 2,000 g, delivery at a nontertiary care hospital was associated with significantly higher mortality from preventable conditions.

Can level II hospitals employ neonatologists and achieve the same outcome as tertiary care hospitals? Additional outcome data are needed to adequately address this question, but a New Zealand study[46] has interesting implications. In a 6-year study period from 1984 to 1989, 40 infants born at the National Women's Hospital in Auckland had to be transported from that level III hospital to other level III facilities in the region because of inadequate space. Forty stable inborn infants requiring transport were matched with 80 controls that were also inborn and remained at the National Women's Hospital. The investigators concluded that the transported infants were adversely affected by the transport. They had worse respiratory function, grew less well during the neonatal period, had more IVH, and had worse neurologic outcomes. The investigators were unable to determine whether the adverse outcome of transported infants was due to the transport itself or to possible differences in neonatal care practices in the different level III centers. Field et al[47] presented data indicating that the size of the neonatal nursery is important in determining outcome.

Factors that will affect the ability of an obstetrician/gynecologist to care for a patient in the labor-and-delivery unit of a level II hospital must be considered separately from differences in level III neonatal nurseries. Many level II facilities lack the availability of a 24-hour obstetric anesthesiologist in their labor-and-delivery units. Critical care patients are less frequent in these centers and managing invasive lines is more problematic. The level II center may not be a level I trauma center. Laboratory support may not be adequate. Fetal lung maturity studies, coagulation studies, serum magnesium assays, and scalp pH determinations must be done in a timely manner. Blood banking must cover any and all blood types at any time, including need for large volumes of factor therapy. The availability of ultrasound examination is necessary on the labor-and-delivery unit rather than in the radiology department. It is helpful for the obstetrician to be able to use the machine directly, rather than having to wait for a technician to be called from home and a radiologist called to interpret the sonogram. It is important to be able to perform a cesarean section as quickly as possible, and the entire team needed for this must be available within the hospital. The obstetrician should be present during labor. These patients cannot be managed by a nurse, with the physician arriving in time to catch the baby. The tertiary care center usually has available investigational protocols that might be appropriate for a particular patient and which would not be available at a level II facility. Finally, I believe that the perinatologist makes a difference—call it greater experience with cases requiring urgent care (collected wisdom)—that is of intangible benefit for diagnostic and therapeutic interventions. As a result of extra years of training, the perinatologist has certain skills that the average obstetrician does not have. These include skills in the interpretation of ultrasonograms, the performance of invasive procedures (choronic villi sampling, cordocentesis, fetal surgery), abdominal cerclage, therapeutic amniocentesis, and expertise in tocolysis. There is an element of judgment involved in managing high-order multiple gestations, delayed-interval delivery of multiple gestations, interpretation of fetal monitor strips,[48] and other procedures. The most important quality that a perinatologist may add to the outcome of these pregnancies is constant availability. Preterm patients are notoriously unpredictable, experiencing chronic abruptions, placenta previa, labor in cases of preterm premature rupture of membranes, and development of fetal intolerance of labor. The average obstetrician/gynecologist cannot be constantly available. It is consistency that provides for good outcomes and maintenance of skills. Neither obstetricians nor labor-and-delivery nurses can maintain their skills without a steady volume of patients. Physician and nursing judgments about labor and delivery are critical to outcome, and in high-risk situations, the patient deserves the best care available.

If outcome data support the delivery of premature infants (<2,000 g) at level II hospitals, then regionalization should be modified accordingly. Until that concept is validated, however, transport to a regional tertiary care hospital should be the standard for women at risk of complications of pregnancy.

REFERENCES

1. Baxt WG, Moody P: The impact of a rotorcraft aeromedical emergency care service on trauma mortality. JAMA 249:3047, 1983
2. Butterfield LJ: Historical perspectives of neonatal transport. Pediatr Clin North Am 40:221, 1993
3. Cone TE: History of the Care and Feeding of the Premature Infant. Little Brown, Boston, 1985
4. Roget J, Beaudoing A, Gilbert Y: Le transport héliporté des prématurés. Maternité 13:418, 1964
5. Ryan GM: Toward improving the outcome of pregnancy. Obstet Gynecol 46:375, 1975
6. Modanlou GD, Dorchester WL, Thorosian A et al: Antenatal versus neonatal transport to a regional perinatal center. A comparison between matched pairs. Obstet Gynecol 53:725, 1979
7. Merenstein GB, Pettett G, Woodall J et al: An analysis of air transport results in the sick newborn. II. Antenatal and neonatal referrals. Am J Obstet Gynecol 128:520, 1977
8. Mirata T: Increased handicaps in transported very low birth-weight infants, abstracted. Clin Res 27:125A, 1979
9. Gortmaker S, Sobol A, Clark C et al: The survival of very low-birth weight infants by level of hospital of birth: a population study of perinatal systems in four states. Am J Obstet Gynecol 153:517, 1985
10. Harris BA, Wirtschafter DD, Huddleston JF, Perlis W: In utero versus neonatal transportation of high-risk perinates: a comparison. Obstet Gynecol 57:496, 1981
11. Harris TR, Isaman J, Giles HR: Improved neonatal survival through maternal transport. Obstet Gynecol 52:294, 1978

12. Anderson CL, Aladjem S, Ayuste O et al: An analysis of maternal transport within a suburban metropolitan region. Am J Obstet Gynecol 140:499, 1981
13. Delaney-Black V, Lubchenco LO, Butterfield J et al: Outcome of very-low-birth-weight infants: are populations of neonates inherently different after antenatal versus neonatal referral? Am J Obstet Gynecol 160:545, 1989
14. Miller TC, Densberger M, Krogman J: Maternal transport and the perinatal denominator. Am J Obstet Gynecol 147:19, 1983
15. Verloove-Vanhorick SP, Verwey RA, Ebeling MC et al: Mortality in very preterm and very low birth weight infants according to place of birth and level of care: results of a neonatal collaborative survey of preterm and very low birth weight infants in the Netherlands. Pediatrics 81:404, 1988
16. Kollée LA, Verloove-Vanhorick SP, Verwey RA et al: Maternal and neonatal transport: results of a national collaborative survey of preterm and very low birth weight infants in the Netherlands. Obstet Gynecol 72:729, 1988
17. Kollée LA, Brand R, Schreuder AM et al: Five-year outcome of preterm and very low birth weight infants: a comparison between maternal and neonatal transport. Obstet Gynecol 80:635, 1992
18. Kollée LA, Eskes TK, Peer PG, Koppes JF: Intra- or extrauterine transport? Comparison of neonatal outcomes using a logistic model. Eur J Obstet Gynecol Reprod Biol 20:393, 1985
19. Kanto WP, Bryant J, Thigpen J et al: Impact of a maternal transport program on a newborn service. South Med J 76:834, 1983
20. Knox GE, Schnitker KA: In-utero transport. Clin Obstet Gynecol 27:11, 1984
21. Low RB, Martin D, Brown C: Emergency air transport of pregnant patients: the national experience. J Emerg Med 6:41, 1988
22. Elliott JP, O'Keeffe DF, Freeman RK: Helicopter transportation of patients with obstetric emergencies in an urban area. Am J Obstet Gynecol 143:157, 1982
23. Elliott JP, Sipp TL, Balazs KT: Maternal transport of patients with advanced cervical dilatation—to fly or not to fly? Obstet Gynecol 79:390, 1992
24. Katz VL, Hansen AR: Complications in the emergency transport of pregnant women. South Med J 83:7, 1990
25. Elliott JP, Trujillo R: Fetal monitoring during emergency obstetric transport. Am J Obstet Gynecol 157:245, 1987
26. Poulton TJ, Kisicki PA: Physiologic monitoring during civilian air medical transport. Aviat Space Environ Med 58:367, 1987

27. Elliott JP: Magnesium sulfate as a tocolytic agent. Am J Obstet Gynecol 147:277, 1983
28. Tsokos N, Newnham JP, Langford SA: Intravenous tocolytic therapy for long distance aeromedical transport of women in preterm labour in Western Australia. Asia-Oceania J Obstet Gynaecol 14:21, 1988
29. Reedy NJ, Kupfer B, Bozzelli JE, Depp R: Maternal-fetal transport: a nurse team. Obstetr Gynecol Neonatal Nurs 13:91, 1982
30. Sokol RJ, Rosen MG, Stojkov J, Chik L: Clinical application of high-risk scoring on an obstetric service. Am J Obstet Gynecol 128:652, 1977
31. Berg CJ, Druschel CM, McCarthy BJ et al: Neonatal mortality in normal birth weight babies: does the level of hospital care make a difference? Am J Obstet Gynecol 161:86, 1989
32. Neonatal intensive care for low birthweight infants: Costs and effectiveness. Health Technology Case Study 38. U.S. Office of Technology Assessment, Washington, DC, 1987
33. Richardson DK, Gabbe SG, Wind Y: Decision analysis of high-risk patient referral. Obstet Gynecol 63:496, 1984
34. Strobino DM, Frank R, Oberdorf MA et al: Development of an index of maternal transport. Med Decis Making 13:64, 1993
35. Troiano NH: Applying principles to practice in maternal-fetal transport. Perinat Neonatal Nurs 2:20, 1989
36. Ferguson JE, Holbrook H, Stevenson DK et al: Adjunctive magnesium sulfate infusion does not alter metabolic changes associated with ritodrine tocolysis. Am J Obstet Gynecol 156:103, 1987
37. Crenshaw C, Payne P, Blackmon L et al: Prematurity and the obstetrician. Am J Obstet Gynecol 147:125, 1983
38. Elliott JP, Foley MR, Young L, Balazs KT et al: Transport of obstetrical care patients to tertiary centers. J Reprod Med (in press)
39. Kirshon B, Hinkely CM, Cotton DB, Miller J: Maternal mortality in a maternal-fetal medicine intensive care unit. J Reprod Med 35:25, 1990
40. Berkowitz RL, Rafferty TD: Invasive hemodynamic monitoring in critically ill pregnant patients: role of Swan-Ganz catheterization. Am J Obstet Gynecol 137:127, 1980
41. Boehm FH, Haire MF: One-way maternal transport: an evolving concept. Am J Obstet Gynecol 134:484, 1979
42. Pittard WB: Economics of neonatal back transport in South Carolina. J South Carolina Med Assoc 82:397, 1986
43. Bose CL, LaPine TR, Jung AL: Neonatal back-transport. Med Care 23:14, 1985
44. Gates M, Shelton S: Back-transfer in neonatal care. Perinat Neonatal Nurs 2:39, 1989
45. Hickok D: Deregionalization of care: Impact on birthweight-specific mortality. Am J Obstet Gynecol (in press)
46. Harding JE, Morton SM: Adverse effects of neonatal transport between level III centres. J Paediatr Child Health 29:146, 1993
47. Field D, Hodges S, Mason E, Burton P: Survival and place of treatment after premature delivery. Arch Dis Child 66:408, 1991
48. Helfand M, Morton K, Veland K: Factors involved in the interpretation of fetal monitor tracings. Am J Obstet Gynecol 151:737, 1985

Chapter 22

Electronic Fetal Monitoring

Lawrence D. Devoe and Bruce A. Work

More than a quarter of a century has passed since electronic fetal monitoring (EFM) was first applied to the task of continuous intrapartum observation.[1] The scientific basis for the clinical use of EFM was based almost entirely on descriptive studies begun during the preceding decade.[2,3] These and subsequent studies sought to define the components and "patterns" of the fetal heart rate (FHR) baseline in subjects receiving continuous intrapartum monitoring, and to correlate these physiologic findings with their subsequent perinatal outcomes. There were no prospective, randomized controlled studies of the diagnostic value or clinical efficacy of these data. In the years following this, when intrapartum EFM was used in obstetric management, there was concomitant decline in perinatal death rates.[4] In retrospect, it is most probable that the emergence of neonatal intensive care units (NICUs) contributed significantly to these improved infant survival rates. Declines in antenatal stillbirth rates reflected improved access to prenatal care, better therapies for common medical or obstetric complications in pregnancy, and the increasing numbers of specialists trained in the treatment of high-risk pregnancies.

The use of EFM was associated with an increased cesarean section rate.[5,6] Neutra and colleagues,[7] among others, suggested that this increase in the cesarean section rate might have been due less to the use of EFM itself than to the population in whom it was applied (i.e., patients at higher risk of intrapartum complications). Growing concerns with therapeutic and economic implications of EFM led to a widely publicized critical evaluation of the technique in 1978 by Banta and Thacker.[8] Their report was aimed at evaluating the efficacy and safety of EFM for some or all labors. They observed that although few randomized controlled trials of EFM had been reported, its relatively low sensitivity, coupled with the low prevalence of adverse intrapartum events or neonatal outcomes, should at least lead clinicians to question the value of universal EFM. In view of the increased medical and social costs associated with EFM, they concluded

> whether or not the results of published studies are comparable to those found in the majority of obstetric services is a question that warrants study prior to the spread of a new technology such as EFM. . . . The most recent argument for the use of EFM instead of auscultation is the shortage of trained nurse-midwives and the tedious nature of auscultation. It is a sad commentary on the quality of obstetric services in this country if we are unable to provide human support for all women in labor. However, . . . replacement of nurse monitoring by EFM is an acceptable practice from the standpoint of the technology.

A contemporary U.S. National Institutes of Health (NIH) Task Force Consensus Statement[9] was prepared in 1979 on the use of intrapartum methods of detecting fetal distress. The Task Force recommended the use of EFM principally for pregnancies with established risk factors, but concluded that "the uncertain status of knowledge about EFMs benefits and risks should prompt, rather than limit, discussion of the technique by patients and providers of medical care." By inference, the Task Force also recommended intermittent FHR auscultation as an acceptable intrapartum alternative for low-risk patients.[9] Parenthetically, these recommendations contributed to the basic guidelines in the most recent American College of Obstetricians and Gynecologists (ACOG) Technical Bulletin[10] on intrapartum FHR monitoring, as noted below.

In short order, Hobbins and colleagues[11] offered a rebuttal that responded to the issues raised by Banta and Thacker. The success or failure of their criticism rests on the concession that "Although ideally the data would be best obtained by RCT [randomized controlled trial], there will definitely be problems [due to anticipated difficulty in establishing such trials] . . . More study is required to establish the cost and benefit of EFM. In the meantime, let us use the modality wisely."

In the next few years, other trials of EFM were reported. In 1987, Thacker[12] published a meta-analysis of seven prospective, randomized controlled trials that compared EFM with intermittent FHR auscultation. He could not attribute any "statistically significant" benefit to the use of EFM while cesarean section rates were significantly higher in most groups undergoing EFM. In 1989, the Oxford Database of Perinatal Trials included additional studies in their meta-analyses,[13] thereby implying that the controversy surrounding the value of EFM would probably continue into the present decade. Further, the ACOG position papers and technical bulletins have not entirely resolved the "monitoring problem" for those continuing to provide obstetric care to low- and high-risk pregnancies. Thus, for example, its most recent assessment states that: "Previously, it had been presumed that continuous electronic fetal monitoring would be more sensitive and accurate than intermittent auscultation in detecting heart rate patterns that indicate significant compromise. This presumption has not been supported by recent randomized prospective studies, however."[10]

The current controversy about the use of EFM is centered on the issues of:

1. FHR interpretation and associated problems with clinical correlations
2. Observer reliability and reproducibility
3. Whether patient selection for application should be routine (universal) or selective (based on specific indications)
4. Contextual application of EFM data

Before tackling these issues, we would like to establish some ground rules for this chapter. First, it would be far too easy to expose the alleged shortcomings of EFM. In presenting the few satisfactory studies that have sought to evaluate EFM objectively, we try to make evenhanded appraisals of their validity and biases. In working toward a proper clinical positioning of EFM, we also examine studies that, although lacking the obvious power of randomized clinical trials, make what we believe are meritorious positive or negative points about its use.

Our intrinsic preconception is that the most effective use of EFM or, for that matter, any diagnostic tool demands a fundamental understanding of the machines on which it is based and the data they attempt to report. It is beyond the intent of this chapter to present a detailed review of EFM hardware or an interpretation of its output. However, any discussion of the problems and pitfalls of EFM must point out that these basic issues should be understood and incorporated into the training of end users. At the conclusion we hope to achieve a fair perspective of intrapartum EFM as it evolves toward the next century. As clinical investigators who have been involved in the development, promulgation, and use of this modality since its inception, we dedicate this assignment to those who are learning the art and science of intrapartum care and to whom we will sign over our patients in the labor-and-delivery suite.

FHR BASELINE INTERPRETATION AND CLINICAL CORRELATION

Before the development of systems capable of providing continuous electronic recording of FHR and maternal uterine activity, an intrinsic clinical value was assigned to the observed FHR and its relationship to uterine activity during labor.[1] Although rigorous studies of how these observations influenced or altered perinatal outcome are lacking, it remains the perception of obstetricians that there is practical merit in registering the baseline FHR and its alterations before, during, or after uterine contractions. Relatively few studies have been done to assess the accuracy of "manual" as opposed to electronic cardiotocography. This important issue is covered in a subsequent section.

Two main routes of investigation are available for ascertaining the intrinsic value of FHR observation. The first involves examining the correlation of all baseline elements of the FHR with accepted standard measures of perinatal outcome. The second involves either working forward from index cases of FHR monitoring in which the worst possible outcomes might be anticipated (i.e., those with the highest degrees of apparent FHR abnormality) or working backward from index cases with the worst neonatal outcomes to their intrapartum FHR records. The following section presents data from representative studies that correlate FHR elements with Apgar scores, umbilical cord arterial pH, or perinatal outcomes.

The FHR baseline has been defined, since the inception of its continuous electronic recording, by several elements that together form the visual patterns from which normal or abnormal conditions of the fetal-placental unit are inferred. Taken individually, these elements are

1. *Baseline rate:* the dominant group of heart periods over time, conventionally in epochs of 10 minutes or longer
2. *Baseline variability:* fluctuation of the rate over short intervals ("beat-to-beat") or longer intervals (cyclic oscillations in amplitude and frequency)
3. *Accelerations:* periodic, transient increases in rate, usually lasting 15 to 30 seconds, and associated with fetal movements or uterine contractions
4. *Decelerations:* periodic, transient decreases in the baseline rate, that accompany contractions at various points (early, late, or variable)

Taken collectively, these FHR baseline elements have been grouped into descriptive patterns that range from "reassuring" or "normal" through "suspicious" or "equivocal," "ominous," "sinister" or "preterminal," to "agonal" or "terminal." The difficulties in translating these semantic levels of FHR interpretation are substantial and have contributed to major problems in comparative analyses of earlier studies performed at a variety of institutions.

In the early 1970s, Cibils[14–18] began a series of meticulous analyses that correlated the FHR baseline rate and its accelerations, and decelerations, and other alterations with the clinical outcomes of 1,304 singleton fetuses monitored for at least 1 hour before delivery. Among the virtues of these studies were that the population typified in its gestational age range and distribution (7 percent <37 weeks, 10 percent >42 weeks, 83 percent >37 and <42 weeks), parity (56 percent primigravid, 44 percent multigravid), and medical problems the populations encountered by many clinicians who were using EFM. Abnormalities of fetal heart rate (mostly tachycardias) occurred in 15 percent of cases and abnormalities in baseline variability in 20 percent. Most patients (54 percent) exhibited some type of FHR deceleration, of which variable decelerations were the most common (24 percent). Some of the more salient clinical correlations are summarized in Table 22-1.

Table 22-1. Clinical Correlations of FHR Decelerations and Perinatal Outcome

FHR Feature	Rate[a]	Intrapartum Fetal Distress	5-Minute Apgar <7	Perinatal Death
Early decelerations	19†	5	2	0.4
Variable decelerations	24	23[b]	4[b]	2.2[b]
Late decelerations	11	50[b]	12[b]	7.0[b]

[a] All data are expressed as percentages.
[b] Data are significantly different from control subjects without decelerations.
(Data from Cibils[14–18].)

Table 22-2.   Correlation Between FHR Patterns in the First and Final 30 Minutes of EFM with 5-Minute Apgar Score

Pattern	First 30 Minutes		Last 30 Minutes	
	No.	5-Minute Apgar <7 (%)	No.	5-Minute Apgar <7 (%)
Normocardia	1,882	3.6	1,525	3.5
Tachycardia (marked)	8	25.0	16	19.0
Bradycardia (marked)	0	0	98	6.1
Variability				
Normal	1,516	2.6	1,323	2.1
<5 beats/min	437	10.3[a]	551	9.1[a]
<6 osc/min	65	26.2[a]	93	23.7[a]
<5 beats/min and <6 osc/min)	39	28.2[a]	50	24.0[a]
Accelerations				
Normal >5/30 min	1,455	2.6	1,196	2.3
<5/30 min	537	8.4[a]	792	6.7[a]
Decelerations				
None	1,634	3.6	594	1.9
Early	93	4.3	325	4.0
Variable	239	5.9[a]	988	4.8[a]
Late	31	29.0	89	19.5[a]
Prolonged	86	4.7	48	4.2

[a] $P < 0.05$ when compared with normal group within each category.
(From Krebs et al,[19] with permission.)

Krebs et al[19] performed a detailed analysis of the initial and final 30 minutes of continuous direct FHR monitoring in 2,000 cases, and correlated their observations with 1- and 5-minute Apgar scores. At least one-half of these patients were categorized as "in some risk category" (Table 22-2). This study showed that initial FHR recordings were relatively poor predictors of Apgar scores unless there were multiple FHR abnormalities; that the frequency of FHR abnormalities increased near delivery; that the most "ominous" abnormalities were very rare; and that most infants exhibiting FHR abnormalities attained normal 5-minute Apgar scores. Although most contemporary analysts would demand other objective perinatal outcomes this study typifies the problems inherent in using early or late intrapartum FHR data to predict neonatal condition.

In the early 1970s there was a prevailing opinion (which remains popular) that a meaningful relationship existed between fetal acid–base balance and specific FHR variables or patterns. Kubli et al[20] had shown that fetal scalp blood pH decreased progressively with the evolution of FHR decelerations (Table 22-3). Similarly, Tejani et al[21] observed that an increasing total area under the tracings of variable or late decelerations bore a significant relationship to the likelihood of a fetal scalp pH below 7.25. Fleischer et al[22] reported a significant temporal relationship between the appearance of late or variable FHR decelerations or decreased variability and the development of acidosis, defined as an umbilical artery blood pH below 7.25. In this small series, acidosis

Table 22-3.   Correlation of FHR Patterns and Fetal Scalp Blood pH

FHR Pattern	pH Value (Mean ± SD)
No decelerations, mild variable decelerations, early decelerations	7.30 ± .04
Moderate variable decelerations	7.26 ± .04
Mild late decelerations, moderate late decelerations	7.21 ± .06
Severe variable decelerations, severe late decelerations	7.13 ± .07

(From Kubli et al,[20] with permission.)

occurred within 115 minutes after the start of late decelerations, within 145 minutes after the start of variable decelerations, and within 185 minutes after the start of decreased variability in 50 percent of each group with such abnormalities. As their study group had entered labor with apparently normal FHR tracings, they concluded that a critical period of 90 to 120 minutes precedes acidosis in most appropriately grown fetuses who develop these types of FHR abnormalities. Low et al[23] compared 8-hour-long FHR tracings in 200 pairs of high-risk fetuses matched for maternal medical and obstetric complications and gestational age. According to umbilical cord blood gas analyses, one member of each pair developed metabolic acidosis in labor while the other had normal acid–base status at delivery. Frequencies of bradycardias, tachycardias, decreased variability, and absent FHR accelerations were similar in both groups. The incidences of total, variable, and late decelerations were significantly higher in the group developing metabolic acidosis, but only for the last hour before delivery. However, the probability of developing metabolic acidosis was only 25 percent in the presence of marked total decelerations and 48 percent in the presence of late decelerations in this preselected population.

Other efforts have been made to relate specific patterns of FHR baseline elements to long-term measures of infant and child development. Painter et al[24] reported one of the few studies in the American literature that undertook a long-term follow-up of children whose intrapartum FHR tracings contained moderately severe variable, severe variable, or late decelerations. They tracked 50 children born of full-term pregnancies whose developmental and neurologic status was evaluated at ages of 1 year and 6 to 9 years. At birth, 68 percent of infants with moderately severe to severe FHR abnormalities had abnormal neurologic examinations, as opposed to 17 percent of infants with normal patterns. At 1 year, 18 percent of infants with moderately severe to severe FHR abnormalities and none of those with normal tracings had abnormal neurologic examinations. At ages 6 to 9 years only two (14%) infants in the group with the most severe FHR abnormalities (N = 14) had persistent neurologic abnormalities: one had neurosensory hearing loss and the other a probable dysmorphic syndrome. It should be noted

that, in this study, severely abnormal FHR patterns were present for up to 16 hours with apparently normal subsequent outcomes.

Since a purported goal of intrapartum FHR interpretation is to alert clinicians to evolving intrauterine conditions that predispose the fetus to hypoxia or, even worse, asphyxia, the relative lack of predictive power of FHR findings conveyed by studies such as those cited above should prompt serious concern. It could be alleged that these discrepancies might reflect the impact of intervention, thereby interrupting the natural history of fetal–placental compromise. Consequently, there has been interest in working backward from index cases in which there has been obvious neurologic damage or developmental delay (or both) to the FHR tracings that preceded delivery.

Many of these retrospective reports are confounded by the inclusion of significantly preterm infants whose neurologic outcomes might be strongly influenced by early neonatal problems.[25] Another obvious problem with this literature is the lack of standard terminologies or criteria for FHR interpretation. If the focus is restricted to studies that included term infants and in which a case-controlled blind review of FHR tracings was performed, only the studies of Minchom et al[26] and Keegan et al[27] totalling 96 cases of morbidity, would qualify. Their positive predictive values of FHR monitoring for predicting neonatal seizures ranged from 0.02 to 0.3 percent.

Rosen and Dickinson[28] reported on a selected group of 55 neurologically impaired infants whose intrapartum FHR records had been collected and reviewed over two decades. Three analysis periods of FHR recording were identified: (1) onset (first 10 minutes); (2) interval (of variable length); and (3) end (last 10 minutes). Their findings are summarized in Table 22-4. Their careful review shows no obvious FHR pattern that typifies the infant who will develop subsequent serious neurologic impairment. While about 50 percent of the cases in their review had some abnormality at the onset of monitoring, raising the possibility of pre-existing lesions, 16 percent had no abnormal FHR events throughout the record.

Not all infants exposed to hypoxia or asphyxia during labor will have serious sequelae, as already

Table 22-4. Temporal Distribution of FHR Abnormalities in 55 Cases of Severe Neonatal Neurologic Morbidity

Pattern	Onset		Interval		End	
	Present	Absent	Present	Absent	Present	Absent
Variable decelerations	11	44	11	44	24	31
Late decelerations	13	42	14	41	22	33
Late and variable decelerations	6	49	7	48	14	41
Bradycardia	3	52	2	53	9	46
Tachycardia	3	52	3	52	2	53
Decreased variability	19	36	21	34	20	35

(From Rosen and Dickinson,[28] with permission.)

suggested. Nonetheless, if these conditions could be anticipated at the earliest possible time, measures might be undertaken to obviate or minimize potential adverse outcomes. Most of our prospective knowledge on the appearance of these patterns is probably (and fortunately) not derived from human experiments but from controlled studies of ovine and nonhuman primate models. A so-called critical oxygenation/circulatory threshold has been postulated, based on graded experiments with uterine blood flow reduction.[29,30] Below this threshold, cerebral and cardiac oxygenation are maintained secondary to compensatory shunting; above it, there is myocardial failure. Cohn and colleagues[31] demonstrated that bradycardia is an initial cardiovascular response to acute hypoxia or asphyxia; more prolonged asphyxia (i.e., 10 to 15 minutes' duration) may be accompanied by tachycardia and loss of variability or late decelerations (or both). Late FHR decelerations that accompany reduced FHR variability have been shown in chronic sheep models to reflect hypoxic myocardial depression, and are not significantly modified by the administration of atropine.[32] In humans, Paul et al[33] showed that the maintenance of long-term variability helped to discriminate fetuses with otherwise abnormal FHR patterns but without intrapartum acidemia or depressed Apgar scores. Systematic, controlled human studies examining responses of late decelerations to therapeutic maneuvers are lacking.

The ultimate index of FHR abnormality might be expected from analytic reviews of terminal or agonal FHR patterns in infants with autopsy-proven hypoxic or asphyxial injury. Understandably, such reports are small and heterogeneous. Cibils[16] reviewed agonal tracings of infants who were stillborn or died within 8 hours of delivery. No consistent pattern preceding death or delivery was identified, much as in the case of Rosen and Dickinson's survey of neurologically injured infants. However, Cibils noted different evolutions of agonal patterns, depending on whether the fetuses were preterm (<37 weeks), term, or post-term (>42 weeks). Parer has attempted an overview of terminal patterns based on collected observations of the FHR tracings of fetuses with confirmed in utero asphyxia[34]:

1. The baseline rate tends to be above 150 beats/min (also see Cibils[16])
2. Short-term variability is ultimately lost in all cases
3. Long-term variability is decreased in most cases
4. Sinusoidal patterns occur in one-third of cases
5. Preterminal patterns may start with undulating, smooth decelerative baselines or without periodic change
6. Preterm fetuses appear to be different and often show profound periodic changes (also see Cibils[16])

In summary, this section has dealt with some of the problems, that have always accompanied EFM. These problems go to the very foundation of this modality and expose its obvious scientific weaknesses. The discrepancies between observed FHR patterns and anticipated fetal outcomes, or between observed neonatal outcomes and preceding FHR patterns, should not vitiate several important points. First, there is a large body of collected experience which, if understood and heeded, can lead clinicians to make a preliminary assessment of intrapartum fetal status, based on FHR patterns, that aids, subsequent decision-making. Next, it is possible to assign a status of good intrapartum health that would be very unlikely to warrant sudden and dramatic intervention. Furthermore, most abnormal FHR patterns that evolve during the monitoring process appear to permit sufficient time for contextual assessment of the patient and formulation of a rational treatment plan. Isolated FHR abnormalities are common and should neither distract the obstetrician or nurse nor provoke a panic response that may endanger the mother or fetus. Finally, appropriate follow-up of worrisome or suspicious FHR tracings should involve consulting observers who have considerable clinical experience and who are likely to have previously encountered similar cases.

RELIABILITY AND REPRODUCIBILITY

Whether the standard of care for some or most parturients should entail intermittent FHR auscultation or EFM, a problem common to both situations is the variability, fallibility, and unreliability of the human observer who makes an auditory or visual assessment of the FHR. Miller et al[35] polled a panel of relatively experienced observers who "auscultated" FHR tapes, recorded their findings, and then compared these with the actual EFM record. (Table 22-5) Their results suggest that systematic errors occur when human observers are rated against mechanical note-takers. These auscultation errors ranged from 18 percent for decreased variability in late decelerations to 37 percent for late decelerations with good variability. Matching of the auscultated FHR to the printed FHR pattern produced even poorer correlations. While the authors concluded that "failure to recognize classic patterns of fetal distress . . . is unacceptable in modern obstetrics," would such discrepancies be truly important for clinical management?

The reliability and reproducibility of baseline FHR interpretation has become a recurring concern of other investigators.[36–41] Although many studies have focused on antepartum records and have sought to determine areas of agreement and disagreement among observers, several points have clearly emerged:

1. There is a reasonably high level of intraobserver agreement with regard to the baseline rate, accelerations, and most decelerations in the FHR tracing
2. There is a lower level of interobserver agreement for these same variables in the FHR tracing
3. Even lower levels of intra- and interobserver agreement occur for variability in amplitude or oscillatory frequency
4. Stochastic methods of assessing baseline variability correlate poorly with its standard visual assessment
5. The reliability of FHR assessment among observers declined as the levels or categories for discrimination increased

Table 22-5. Auscultatory Assessment versus Electronic Recording of FHR

Pattern	Auditory Identification of Auditory Signal		Visual Identification of Auditory Signal	
	Physicians (N = 16)	Nurses (N = 16)	Physicians (N = 16)	Nurses (N = 16)
None	16[a]	15	9	12
Accelerations	10	13	12	13
Saltatory	6	2	11	8
Early decelerations	10	8	11	10
Variable decelerations	12	12	8	9
Late decelerations (good variability)	10	10	9	9
Late decelerations (poor variability)	14	12	10	11

[a] Number of correct responses.
(Data from Miller et al[35].)

The importance of the observer factor in the application of EFM to subsequent management and decision-making cannot be overemphasized. Prospective studies of sufficient size to test the impact of observer reproducibility and reliability on subsequent clinical management are virtually nonexistent. Since the best use of the information in the FHR tracing depends on its accurate and consistent interpretation, this is a problem that should already have been resolved.

Alternative approaches to standard visual assessment of the intrapartum FHR record are being considered. Dawes et al[42] performed a preliminary study of 136 patients evaluated during labor with a computerized system for FHR detection and baseline analysis. While their results did not support the use of algorithmic determination of baseline variation as a good predictor for neonatal acidemia, it should be noted that this was a small study with only 15 cases of severe acidemia (by their criteria). Subsequently, Pello and associates[43] reported on 400 cases of term labor in which computerized FHR analysis was performed with the same system. They were unable to identify fetuses at risk of birth acidemia, even with objective identification and quantitation of all common baseline variables. Although disappointing in themselves, efforts such as this should encourage others to investigate objective, reproducible, com-

puter-assisted systems to reduce the likelihood that the raw FHR signal is either misread or incorrectly analyzed by observers of varying expertise and experience.

PATIENT SELECTION AND IMPACT ON MATERNAL-INFANT OUTCOMES

Our initial criterion was that the use of EFM should be based on the best scientific or clinical evidence for its effectiveness. Although there are many ways of acquiring such data, most investigators would agree that randomized clinical trials provide the greatest power. Unfortunately, relatively few trials have been conducted in selected or unselected low- or high-risk labors in which EFM alone has been compared wit intermittent ascultation. Because a number of these trials have used ancillary management tools (e.g., fetal scalp blood pH determinations), their outcomes might have been affected by the additional data thus provided. Endpoints chosen for comparing EFM with intermittent auscultation also have varied among the studies. Most offer intervention rates (cesarean section or vaginal operative deliveries) for presumed fetal distress, some measure of infant outcome (Apgar score, survival, neurologic complications), and associated maternal characteristics.

Table 22-6 summarizes trials in which EFM alone

Table 22-6. Randomized, Controlled Studies of EFM Versus Intermittent Auscultation for Maternal and Infant Outcomes in High-risk Populations

Study	Sample Size	Operative Delivery[a]			Deaths[a]		1-Minute Apgar[a]		NICU[a]	Neonatal Seizures
		All	All CS	FDCS	IP	All	<4	<7		
All high risk										
Haverkamp[48]	242/241[b]	41/39	16/7	7/1	0/0	0/0	6/5	18/14	14/11	0.9/0.9
Haverkamp[49]	233/232	45/29	18/6	7/.4	0/0	0/0	4/4	12/12	10/12	0.8/0.8
Neldam[51]	482/487	23/17	6/4	1.6/1.4	0/0.2	0/0.2	1/1	6/6	10/10	0/0
All low risk										
Kelso[50]	253/251	38/35	9/4	1.6/1.2	0/0	0/0.4	2/3	9/9	17/17	0/0.4
EFM/pH option										
High risk										
Renou[45]	175/175	63/52	22/14	9/5	0/0.6	0.6/0.6	2/3	16/14	6/17	0/2
Low risk										
Wood[52]	445/482	31/23	4/2	NA	0/0	0.2/0	1/1	8/8	13/10	0/0
MacDonald[44]	6,530/6,554	10/8	2/2	0.4/0.1	0.05/0.03	0.2/0.2	4/4	0.9/0.9	8/8	0.2/0.4

Abbreviations: CS, cesarean section; FDCS, cesarean section for fetal distress; IP, intrapartum; NICU, admission to neonatal intensive care unit; NA, not available.
[a] Expressed as percentages.
[b] In all columns, figures are study group/control group.

was compared with intermittent auscultation, and includes sample sizes, outcomes for operative delivery, mortality, 1-minute Apgar score, NICU admission, and neonatal seizures. These studies include patient populations that ranged from entirely high-risk to all risk categories. Several also incorporated fetal scalp blood pH determination as an optional tool. Higher rates of all operative deliveries, all cesarean sections, and cesarean sections for fetal distress were seen consistently in the EFM groups. These differences were smallest in the largest trial, performed by MacDonald et al[44] at the National Maternity Center in Dublin. Mortality rates were strikingly similar in all the trials, and intrapartum fetal death was rare in any of them. Neonatal outcomes were quite similar for corrected mortality, Apgar score, NICU admission, and seizure activity, with the exception of the trials conducted by Renou et al[45] and MacDonald,[44] in which higher rates of the latter two outcomes occurred in the intermittent auscultation group. Again, it should be noted that adverse neonatal outcomes were uncommon in the EFM and intermittent auscultation groups, whether the parturients were judged to be at initially high risk or low risk.

Among the specially selected studies, that of Leveno and colleagues[46] involved a sample size considerably greater than in any of the previously cited trials (Table 22-7). In this study the investigators offered universal EFM and selected high-risk EFM in alternate months without a control intermittent auscultation group.. Nonetheless, their outcomes, when comparing practices of EFM, were very similar in all respects to those in the studies cited previously.

Luthy et al[47] reported on a group of preterm fetuses whose increased rate of adverse outcomes might have been be anticipated from the complications of premature birth alone (Table 22-7). This study failed to show that the use of EFM reduced the occurrence of any adverse outcomes.

By contrast, Table 22-8 summarizes several non-randomized, controlled observational reports that represent in aggregate nearly 90,000 patients. A meta-analysis of these trials cannot be properly conducted because of the differences in inclusion criteria and intervention strategies. However, it is interesting to note that the relative risk of intrapartum fetal death in the EFM groups was 0.2 of that in the non-EFM groups. Similarly, the relative risk of neonatal death in the EFM groups was 0.38 of that in the non-EFM groups. These differences and their consistent direction appear to have clinical relevance, and were noted in virtually all of the reports analyzed.

Is it possible to account for the differences between the prospective randomized controlled trials and nonrandomized studies? Do these differences reflect investigational biases rather than true clinical efficacy? In response to the first question, the nonrandomized studies were generally conducted during an earlier period when there were inherent differences in antepartum and intrapartum practice with regard to EFM. That an EFM learning curve based on clinical experience began to appear is supported by the descriptive report of Boehm et al.[59] They compared cesarean section rates for fetal distress in the years before and after liberal adoption of EFM in their institution. They were unable to doc-

Table 22-7. Studies of EFM for Maternal and Infant Outcomes in Specially Selected Populations

Study	Sample Size	Operative Delivery[a]			Deaths[a]		1-Minute Apgar[a]		NICU[a]	Neonatal Seizures[a]
		All	All CS	FDCS	IP	All	<4	<7		
Leveno[b,46]	17586/17409[d]	NA	11/10	2.6/2.1	NA	1.5/1.7	NA	NA	2.6/2.5	0.3/0.3
Luthy[c,47]	122/124	28/23	15.6/15	8.2/5.7	1/1	12/14	7.4/3.2	NA		5.7/5.7

[a] Expressed as percentages.
[b] Alternate months universal group versus selective group respectively.
[c] EFM versus intermittent auscultation for 26 to 32 weeks and 700 to 1751 g.
[d] In all columns, figures are study group/control group.
Abbreviations: CS, cesarean section; FDCS, cesarean section for fetal distress; IP, intrapartum; NICU, admission to neonatal intensive care unit; NA, not available.

Table 22-8. Nonrandomized Controlled Observational Studies of EFM

Study	Sample No.	Intrapartum Stillbirths		Neonatal Deaths	
		No.	Rate	No.	Rate
Paul[4]	6,686/21,100	4/29	0.6/1.4	36/139	5.4/6.7
Tutera[5]	608/6,179	1/37	2/6	0/49	0/8.0
Shenker[53]	1,950/11,599	1/14	0.5/1.2	6/128	3.1/11.0
Koh[54]	286/794	1/5	3.5/6.3	1/3	3.5/3.8
Edington[55]	2,102/5,597	1/26	0.5/4.6	9/63	4.3/11.3
Lee[56]	3,529/4,323	1/16	0.3/3.7	21/56	6.0/13.0
Amato[57]	4,226/2,981	1/9	0.2/3.0	4/24	0.9/5.7
Johnstone[58]	7,312/9,099	3/11	0.4/1.2	NA	NA
Total	26,699/61,670	13/147	0.5/2.4	77/462	3.3/8.5

ument any change in cesarean section rate attributable to overdiagnosis of fetal distress, in that its percentage of contribution to all cesarean sections was no different during these two periods. Further, during the late 1970s and early 1980s, antenatal screening and diagnostic tests for fetal compromise proliferated. The consequences of extensive antepartum FHR testing were an apparent reduction in antepartum stillbirth and overall perinatal mortality rates in high-risk populations.[60] More frequent antepartum screening also raised the likelihood that obstetricians would exclude the most compromised fetuses from exposure to intrapartum monitoring, while increasing the likelihood that a more selective group would be offered intrapartum EFM as a result of the prior identification of risk factors. Although this attractive hypothesis could explain some of the differences in the groups studied, it would be extremely difficult to validate for all reports.

A plausible explanation for the apparent lack of differences in outcomes in the randomized controlled trials is the nature of care administered to the intermittent auscultation groups. Very close observation, unitary staff/patient ratios, and other, possibly hidden biases in care might have contributed to similarities in obstetric outcomes. These biases are virtually impossible to detect without reviewing details of all patient records, or to avoid completely when trials are not blinded and when investigators intentionally seek to prove the equivalence of two treatments. General improvements in the treatment

of obstetric and medical disorders and in care of the sick neonate have also occurred since the inception of the earliest trials. These advances not only reduce the likelihood of poor outcomes in high-risk pregnancies, but also might require enrollments of patients larger than those actually studied.

We could conclude, from the best available randomized controlled trials that any improvement in perinatal outcome attributable to EFM alone or supplemented with the scalp pH option is of a much lower order of magnitude than suggested by the optimistic data reported in the nonrandomized studies. Were this true, then none of the published randomized controlled trials would be adequate in size to reject the null hypothesis (α-error). Conversely, it is unlikely that randomized controlled trial of adequate size (i.e., enrolment greater than 50,000) will be undertaken any time in the near or remote future. This puts the obstetric community in the unenviable position of having a technology that holds pride of place by virtue of its longevity, but for which the scientific data necessary to establish its benefits for all parturients, regardless of risk category, are lacking.

FUTURE DIRECTIONS AND SUMMARY

A 1979 U.S. National Institute of Child Health and Development (NICHD) consensus report[9] listed a series of recommendations for the future evaluation of EFM. Some of those most pertinent to the discussion in this chapter are summarized below:

1. Research on effects of intrapartum hypoxia on fetal and neonatal evolution, with emphasis on the prognostic values of intrapartum assessment methods
2. Identification of risk factors for fetal distress best managed with EFM, with prospective early recognition of patients who would receive the most benefit from this technique
3. Additional randomized controlled trials of EFM in various high-risk categories, with the inclusion of scalp blood pH sampling
4. Development of accurate, noninvasive or invasive intrapartum tools for assessing fetal well-being

A final caveat in the NICHD consensus report's recommendations was that "no technologic innovation to assess fetal health and distress should be introduced into clinical practice without carefully designed and executed clinical evaluations which include randomized controlled trials of the potential risks, benefits and limitations."

Fifteen years have passed since the publication of this report, with few of its recommended goals having been thoroughly realized or satisfactorily resolved. Research into the effects of fetal hypoxia during labor is difficult to perform prospectively or ethically on humans. The retrospective reports summarized previously represent small, usually uncontrolled series that only hint at the limitations of current EFM techniques in prompting diagnoses and interventions. Although most clinicians agree that high-risk populations can be identified through good antenatal screening and continuing assessment, the actual benefits from applying EFM to any of the specific subgroups of these populations remains unknown. Labor admission testing has been attempted, using both stimulated and unstimulated FHR tracings and amniotic fluid assessments.[61–63] These analyses, while promising, have not been validated prospectively by studies of sufficient size.

The few randomized controlled trials of EFM in high-risk patients that have appeared since the NIH report are summarized in the preceding section. It is clear that they have not succeeded in demonstrating the unquestioned superiority of EFM for any high-risk patient category. Most recently, Vintzileos and associates[64] reported a randomized controlled trial conducted in Greece that enrolled patients in all risk categories but that did not provide backup pH monitoring. The main differences in group outcomes were higher rates of oxytocin use and operative intervention with EFM, but a significantly lower rate of perinatal hypoxia-related deaths than with intermittent auscultation. The study was interrupted before total enrollment was completed, and consecutive recruitment was not employed, thereby introducing potential entry and treatment biases. Although the need for large and well-conducted RCTs continues, it is not clear that this need will be met any time soon.

Developments in new technologies for noninvasive fetal assessment have been limited. In addition to labor admission testing, there has been interest in applying other antepartum modalities to intrapartum assessment, including vibroacoustic stimulation (VAS),[62] biophysical profile testing,[65] and fetal umbilical artery Doppler velocimetry.[63] Smith et al[66] have shown that VAS may have benefit in reducing the need for fetal scalp blood sampling; however, prospective larger trials of this technique are lacking. Neither biophysical profile testing nor umbilical artery Doppler velocimetry have been shown to provide benefit for the intrapartum assessment of fetal condition.

Augmentation of invasive EFM capabilities has been attempted by continuous pH,[68] transcutaneous oxygen partial pressure (PO_2)[69] and more recently, fetal pulse oximetry recording.[70] While the first two modalities have not proved useful, there is reason to hope that technologic improvements in scalp oximetry transducers will enable future studies of its risk versus benefit to be conducted in the United States. The recent adaptation of the direct FHR signal to electrocardiographc (ECG) processing that discriminates trends in the S-T segment also seems to be a potentially valuable approach to better use of EFM data. Westgate et al[71] in a prospective, randomized trial, showed that the additional information conveyed by the S-T waveform was associated with lower rates of intervention for fetal distress, fewer cases of metabolic acidosis, and low 5-minute Apgar scores.

This chapter began with the premise that a controversy exists regarding the use of EFM in current intrapartum practice that could be approached from several perspectives. We made no pretense that sufficient data were available to resolve this controversy to universal satisfaction. Careful review of the medical-scientific basis for using and interpreting EFM shows that many potential avenues for revolving the controversy have been explored but not thoroughly exploited.

It is apparent that EFM has not fulfilled the high expectations promised in early reported series. However, a large clinical experience correlating baseline FHR with frequently and rarely encountered intrapartum problems has been acquired. A physiologic understanding of normal and abnormal FHR alterations has been achieved that establishes their relevance to fetal condition. The accuracy and limitations of various FHR parameters in establishing intrauterine fetal well-being and compromise have been determined. The shortcomings and unreliability of human observers have been measured and reported. Finally, the settings in which EFM should be considered for screening fetal condition have been described, if not convincingly established.

The current evidence for the clinical role of EFM continues to support the conservative suggestions of the 1979 NIH task force:

1. EFM is not a global window into fetal condition but rather a limited aid to screening for fetal health and disease throughout the intrapartum period. It requires backup and augmentation through other modalities (e.g., scalp blood pH testing) for its optimal utilization. Even so, there is no other tool now available that has been shown to be more applicable, accessible, or accurate.

2. EFM requires skilled and knowledgeable interpretation by end users. The broad range of patterns associated with good and poor outcomes, as well as their biologic bases, should be well known or at least accessible through expert consultation. Interpretive errors will inevitably reduce the potential value of these data and may lead to unnecessary interventions. Good, continuing clinical education of physicians and nurses can minimize, if not entirely prevent, the occurrence of such mistakes.

3. EFM may be associated with higher rates of intervention through either operative vaginal or abdominal delivery for conditions other than fetal distress. The explanations for these outcomes vary, but suggest that the designation of "high risk" in monitored patients may create a pressure to intervene that is not perceived in intermittent auscultation groups. All the randomized controlled trials of EFM, except the trial conducted by MacDonald and colleagues[44] report this effect but cannot explain it completely.

4. EFM should be considered in the overall context of pregnancy. Intrapartum problems are more prevalent in high-risk than in low-risk groups. Within groups of high-risk patients, however, intrapartum risks may increase or decrease as functions of numerous factors (e.g., gestational age, fetal weight centile, medications required). There are no good data to suggest how best to scale or weight the contributions of modifying factors to adjust risk following findings of abnormal intrapartum FHR patterns. It has been observed that in apparently low-risk pregnancies, the appearance of FHR abnormalities (e.g., late or variable decelerations) may antecede acidosis by a considerable period (>1 hour).[22] Similar data are not well established for high-risk patients.

5. EFM is a mechanical modality. Although it may not be conclusively superior to intermittent auscultation, it enables a single observer to maintain vigilance over more than one patient at a time from a single station. This is an important consideration for economies of staffing and the realities of hiring and maintaining cadres of diligent, well-educated, and experienced clinicians. It also implies that the level of assistance it can offer will remain limited by the attention, knowledge, and interpretive acumen of the observer, who is the actual monitor, rather than the electronic monitor, which is only an uninformed, unintelligent device.

We are convinced by the evidence presented, and in some areas by lack of such evidence, that EFM must and will change rather significantly during the current decade. It will undergo inevitable changes in hardware, improved central monitoring, and computerized archival and retrieval capabilities.

Functionally, such changes may be helpful but will probably make little impact on labor outcomes. What will make an impact is the emergence of "intelligent" perinatal information systems capable of providing expert insights to users who are novices, or assisting experienced users who are busy or fatigued. In such systems, EFM may be a component part that would be augmented by complete patient records and larger information archives. We are reasonably certain that some developments in physiologic probes will continue and may practically supplement, if not replace, conventional EFM. Finally, and most critically, the effort to educate clinical users of EFM in its proper application and understanding is vital and should benefit from multimedia didactics, accessible central data banks of archived examples, and interactions with intelligent systems.

REFERENCES

1. Goodlin RC: History of fetal monitoring. Am J Obstet Gynecol 133:323, 1979
2. Swartwout JR, Campbell WE, Williams LG: Observations on the fetal heart rate. Am J Obstet Gynecol 82: 301, 1961
3. Caldeyro-Barcia R: Estudio de la anoxia fetal intrauterina mediante el ECG fetal y el registro continuo de la frecuencia cardiaca fetal. 3rd Cong Lat-Am Obstet Ginecol (Mexico) 2:388, 1958
4. Yeh S-Y, Diaz F, Paul RH: Ten-year experience of intrapartum fetal monitoring in Los Angeles County/ University of Southern California Medical Center. Am J Obstet Gynecol 143:496, 1982
5. Tutera G, Newman RL: Fetal monitoring: its effect on the perinatal mortality and cesarean section rates and its complications. Am J Obstet Gynecol 122:750, 1975
6. Hughey MJ, LaPata RE, McElin TW et al: The effect of fetal monitoring on the incidence of cesarean section. Obstet Gynecol 49:513, 1977
7. Neutra RR, Greenland S, Friedman EA: Effect of fetal monitoring on cesarean section rates. Obstet Gynecol 55:175, 1980
8. Banta HD, Thacker SB: Assessing the costs and benefits of electronic fetal monitoring. Obstet Gynecol Surv 34:627, 1979
9. Task Force on Predictors of Fetal Distress, NICHD Consensus Development Conference on Antenatal Diagnosis. p. 1. In Antenatal Diagnosis. U.S. National Institutes of Health Publication No. 79-1973, Bethesda, MD,
10. Intrapartum fetal heart rate monitoring. Technical Bulletin No. 132. American College of Obstetricians and Gynecologists, Washington DC, 1989
11. Hobbins JC, Freeman R, Queenan JT: The fetal monitoring debate. Obstet Gynecol 54:103, 1979
12. Thacker S: The efficacy of intrapartum electronic fetal monitoring. Am J Obstet Gynecol 156 , 1987
13. Grant A: Monitoring the fetus during labor. p. 846. In Chalmers I, Enkin M, Keirse MJNC (eds): Effective Care in Pregnancy and Childbirth. Oxford University Press, Oxford, 1989
14. Cibils L: Clinical significance of fetal heart rate patterns during labor. I. Baseline patterns. Am J Obstet Gynecol 125:290, 1976
15. Ciblis L: Clinical significance of fetal heart rate patterns during labor. II. Late decelerations. Am J Obstet Gynecol 123:473, 1975
16. Cibils L: Clinical significance of fetal heart rate patterns during labor. IV. Agonal patterns. Am J Obstet Gynecol 129:833, 1977
17. Cibils L: Clinical significance of fetal heart rate patterns during labor. V. Variable decelerations. Am J Obstet Gynecol 132:791, 1978
18. Cibils L: Clinical significance of fetal heart rate patterns during labor. I. Early decelerations. Am J Obstet Gynecol 136:392, 1980
19. Krebs HB, Petres RE, Dunn LJ et al: Intrapartum fetal heart rate monitoring. I. Classification and prognosis of fetal heart rate patterns. Am J Obstet Gynecol 113: 762, 1979
20. Kubli FW, Hon EH, Khazin AF, Takemura H: Observations on heart rate and pH in the human fetus during labor. Am J Obstet Gynecol 104:1190, 1969
21. Tejani N, Mann LI, Bhakthavathsalan A, Weiss RR: Correlation of fetal heart rate-uterine contraction patterns with fetal scalp blood pH. Obstet Gynecol 46: 392, 1975
22. Fleischer A, Schulman H, Jagani N et al: The development of fetal acidosis in the presence of an abnormal tracing. I. The average for gestational age fetus. Am J Obstet Gynecol 144:55, 1982
23. Low JA, Cox MJ, Karchmar EJ et al: The prediction of intrapartum fetal metabolic acidosis by fetal heart rate monitoring. Am J Obstet Gynecol 139:299, 1981
24. Painter MJ, Scott M, Hirsch RP et al: Fetal heart rate patterns during labor: neurologic and cognitive development at six to nine years of age. Am J Obstet Gynecol 159:854, 1988
25. Ellison PH, Foster M, Sheridan-Pereira M, MacDonald D: Electronic fetal heart rate monitoring, auscultation and neonatal outcome. Am J Obstet Gynecol 164: 1281, 1991

26. Minchom P, Niswander K, Chalmers I et al: Antecedents and outcomes of very early neonatal seizures in infants born at or after term. Br J Obstet Gynaecol 94: 431, 1987

27. Keegan KA, Waffarn F, Quilligan EJ: Obstetric characteristics and fetal heart rate patterns of infants who convulse during the newborn period. Am J Obstet Gynecol 153:732, 1985

28. Rosen MG, Dickinson JC: The paradox of electronic fetal monitoring: more data may not enable us to predict or prevent infant neurologic morbidity. Am J Obstet Gynecol 168:745, 1993

29. Jones MD, Sheldon RE, Peeters LL et al: Fetal cerebral oxygen consumption at different levels of oxygenation. J Appl Physiol 43:1080, 1977

30. Parer JT: The effect of acute maternal hypoxia on fetal oxygenation and umbilical circulation in sheep. Eur J Obstet Gynecol Reprod Biol 10:125, 1980

31. Cohn HE, Sacks EJ, Heymann MA, Rudolph AM: Cardiovascular responses to hypoxemia and acidemia in fetal lambs. Am J Obstet Gynecol 120:817, 1974

32. Harris JL, Krueger TR, Parer JT: Mechanisms of late decelerations of the fetal heart rate during hypoxia. Am J Obstet Gynecol 144:491, 1982

33. Paul RH, Suidan AK, Yeh S-Y et al: Clinical fetal monitoring. VII. The evaluation and significance of intrapartum baseline FHR variability. Am J Obstet Gynecol 123:206, 1975

34. Parer JT: Handbook of Fetal Heart Rate Monitoring. WB Saunders, Philadelphia, 1983

35. Miller FC, Pearse KE, Paul RH: Fetal heart rate pattern recognition by the method of auscultation. Obstet Gynecol 64:332, 1984

36. Nielsen PV, Stigsby B, Nickelson C, Nim J: Intra- and inter-observer variability in the assessment of intrapartum cadiotocograms. Acta Obstet Gynecol Scand 66: 421, 1987

37. Lotgering FK, Wallenberg HCS, Schouten JA: Interobserver and intraobserver variation in the assessment of antepartum cardiotocograms. Am J Obstet Gynecol 144:701, 1982

38. Borgatta L, Shrout PE, Divon MY: Reliability and reproducibility of nonstress test readings. Am J Obstet Gynecol 159:554, 1988

39. Trimbos JB, Keirse MJNC: Observed variability in assessment of antepartum cardiotocograms. Br J Obstet Gynaecol 85:900, 1978

40. Escarcena L, McKinney RD, Depp R: Fetal baseline heart rate variability estimation. Am J Obstet Gynecol 1335:615, 1979

41. Hage ML: Interpretation of nonstress tests. Am J Obstet Gynecol 153:490, 1985

42. Dawes GS, Rosevear SK, Pello LC et al: Computerized analysis of episodic changes in fetal heart rate variation in early labor. Am J Obstet Gynecol 165:618, 1991

43. Pello LC, Rosevear SK, Dawes GS et al: Computerized fetal heart rate analysis in labor. Obstet Gynecol 78: 602, 1991

44. MacDonald D, Grant A, Sheridan-Pereira M, et al: The Dublin randomized controlled trial of intrapartum fetal heart rate monitoring. Am J Obstet Gynecol 152: 524, 1985

45. Renou P, Chang A, Anderson I, Wood C: Controlled trial of fetal intensive care. Am J Obstet Gynecol 126: 470, 1976

46. Leveno KJ, Cunningham FG, Nelson S et al: A prospective comparison of selective and universal electronic fetal monitoring in 34,995 pregnancies. N Engl J Med 315:615, 1986

47. Luthy DA, Shy KK, van Belle G et al: A randomized trial of electronic fetal monitoring in preterm labor. Obstet Gynecol 69:687, 1987

48. Haverkamp AD, Thompson HE, McGee JG, Cetrulo C: The evaluation of continuous fetal heart rate monitoring in high-risk pregnancy. Am J Obstet Gynecol 125:310, 1976

49. Haverkamp AD, Orleans M, Langendoerfer S et al: A controlled trial of different effects of intrapartum fetal monitoring. Am J Obstet Gynecol 134:399, 1979

50. Kelso IM, Parsons RJ, Lawrence GF et al: An assessment of continuous fetal heart rate monitoring in labor: a randomized trial. Am J Obstet Gynecol 131: 526, 1978

51. Neldam S, Osler M, Hansen PK et al: Intrapartum fetal heart rate monitoring in a combined low- and high-risk population: a controlled clinical trial. Eur J Obstet Gynecol Reprod Biol 23:1, 1986

52. Wood C, Renou P, Farrell E et al: A controlled trial of fetal heart rate monitoring in a low-risk obstetric population. Am J Obstet Gynecol 141:527, 1981

53. Shenker L, Post RC, Seiler JS: Routine electronic monitoring of fetal heart rate and uterine activity during labor. Obstet Gynecol 46:185, 1975

54. Koh KS, Greves D, Yung S et al: Experience with fetal monitoring in a university teaching hospital. Can Med Assoc J 112:455, 1975

55. Edington PT, Sibanda J, Beard RW: Influence on clinical practice of routine intrapartum fetal monitoring. BMJ 3:341, 1975

56. Lee WK, Baggish MS: The effect of unselected intrapartum fetal monitoring. Obstet Gynecol 47:516, 1976

57. Amato JC: Fetal monitoring in a community hospital: a statistical analysis. Obstet Gynecol 50:269, 1977

58. Johnstone FD, Campbell DM, Hughes GJ: Antenatal care: has continuous intrapartum monitoring made any impact on fetal outcome? Lancet 1:1298, 1978

59. Boehm FH, Davidson KK, Barrett JM: The effect of electronic fetal monitoring on the incidence of cesarean section. Am J Obstet Gynecol 140:295, 1981

60. Devoe LD: The nonstress test. Obstet Gynecol Clin North Am 17:111, 1990

61. Ingemarsson I, Arulkumaran S, Ingemarsson E et al: Admission test: a screening test for fetal distress in labor. Obstet Gynecol 68:800, 1986

62. Sarno AP, Ahn MO, Phelan JP, Paul RH: Fetal acoustic stimulation in the early intrapartum period as a predictor of subsequent fetal condition. Am J Obstet Gynecol 162:762, 1990

63. Sarno AP, Ahn MO, Harbinder SB et al: Intrapartum Doppler velocimetry, amniotic fluid volume and fetal heart rate as predictors of subsequent fetal distress. Am J Obstet Gynecol 161:1508, 1989

64. Vintzileos AM, Antsaklis A, Varvarigos I et al: A randomized trial of intrapartum electronic fetal heart rate monitoring versus intermittent auscultation. Obstet Gynecol 81:899, 1993

65. Sassoon DA, Castro LC, Davis JL et al: The biophysical profile in labor. Obstet Gynecol 76:360, 1990

66. Smith CV, Nguyen HN, Phelan JP, Paul RH: Intrapartum assessment of fetal well-being: a comparison of fetal acoustic stimulation with acid-base determinations. Am J Obstet Gynecol 155:726, 1986

68. Young BK, Katz M, Klein SA: The relationship of heart rate patterns and tissue pH in the human fetus. Am J Obstet Gynecol 134:685, 1979

69. Aarnoudse JG, Huisjes HJ, Gordan H et al: Fetal subcutaneous scalp pO_2 and abnormal heart rate during labor. Am J Obstet Gynecol 153:565, 1985

70. Johnson N, Johnson VA, Fisher J et al: Fetal monitoring with pulse oximetry. Br J Obstet Gynecol 948:36, 1991

71. Westgate J, Harris M, Curnow JSH, Greene KR: Plymouth randomized trial of cardiotocogram only versus ST waveform plus cardiotocogram for intrapartum monitoring in 2400 cases. Am J Obstet Gynecol 169:1151, 1993

Chapter 23

Amniotic Fluid Dynamics and Modulation

Thomas H. Strong, Jr.

Until relatively recently, amniotic fluid was largely ignored as a contributor to fetal well-being. Contemporary obstetricians now routinely study it to determine fetal karyotype or pulmonary maturity status, and to aid in the diagnosis of chorioamnionitis. Amniotic fluid has many vital functions during gestation. It serves to protect the umbilical cord from compression and to cushion the fetus from external trauma. It plays a role in the development of the fetal body habitus and pulmonary system, has bacteriostatic properties, affords some degree of fetal skin lubrication, and may play a role in fetal nutrition and temperature maintenance. As the amniotic cavity is only a potential space, sufficient quantities of amniotic fluid also permit regular fetal activity by preventing the uterus from collapsing against the fetus.

The volume of fluid that occupies the amniotic space represents a complex interplay between mother and fetus. It is the manifestation of a dynamic interaction between processes that tend to increase the amniotic fluid volume and those that tend to decrease it. Because a variety of obstetric complications are associated with amniotic fluid volumes that fall outside the normal range, amniotic fluid volume is also an indirect, subacute marker of fetal status. Therefore, the fetus that enters labor with an abnormal amniotic fluid volume may be at increased risk of a suboptimal outcome. An understanding of the processes that affect amniotic fluid volume is important for obstetricians who seek to optimize labor outcomes of their patients through modulation of this parameter.

AMNIOTIC FLUID INDEX

Amniotic fluid volume progressively increases until the end of the second trimester. Thereafter, it remains relatively stable until term.[1-5] During this interval, roughly 3.5 L/hr/day of fluid pass between maternal and fetal compartments, with complete turnover of amniotic fluid occurring perhaps every 3 hours.[6,7] Beyond 37 weeks' gestation, amniotic fluid volume gradually diminishes.[3-5]

Although it is generally agreed that an abnormal amniotic fluid volume is associated with higher rates of adverse perinatal outcome, there has been less than a consensus about the definition of such a volume. Although many techniques for quantifying amniotic fluid have been developed since the introduction of ultrasonography, no single technique had achieved widespread acceptance until relatively recently. The amniotic fluid index (AFI), or "four quadrant" amniotic fluid assessment, is a semiquantitative method that has gradually gained favor in the obstetric and radiologic communities.[8] The AFI assessment is a method for estimating amniotic fluid volume that offers the advantages of objectivity, reproducibility, and a level of simplicity that make it easy to learn and teach.[9,10] In addition, the AFI permits serial assessments of amniotic fluid volume throughout pregnancy or labor. Since its introduction, the AFI has become the standard technique for objectively communicating clinical data pertaining to amniotic fluid volume.

Determination of the AFI in a given patient entails

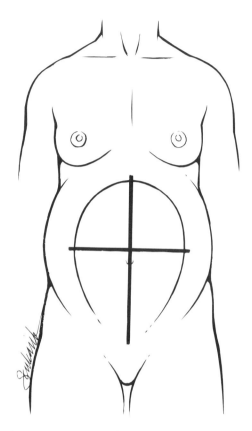

Fig. 23-1. Four-quadrant diagram of the uterus.

summing the deepest vertical fluid pocket (in centimeters) from each of four uterine quadrants (Fig. 23-1). The quadrants are described by the maternal linea nigra and an imaginary perpendicular line located at miduterine height.

Amniotic Fluid Index Technique Summary

Proper technique
  Mother
    Placed supine with shoulders and hips aligned
    Bladder empty
  Uterus: divided into 4 imaginary quadrants (Fig. 23-1)

(Continues)

Vertical axis: maternal linea nigra
Horizontal axis: imaginary line at miduterine height (generally in the vicinity of the maternal umbilicus in the term pregnancy)
  Ultrasound transducer
    Held in longitudinal or transverse maternal plane, whichever provides the clearest view of amniotic fluid pockets
    Held perpendicular to floor at all times (Figure 23–2)

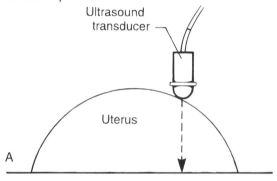

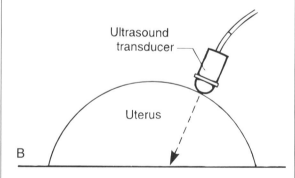

Fig. 23-2. (A) Proper and **(B)** improper ultrasound transducer orientation.

  Measurements
    Deepest vertical, cord-free amniotic fluid pocket in each quadrant
    A given pocket is measured only once, even if visible from a different quadrant

Inappropriate technique
  Use on multiple gestations
  Inclusion of fetal bladder volume in the AFI sum

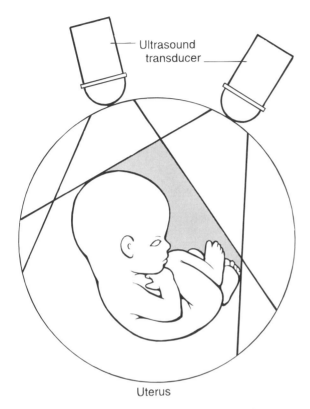

Fig. 23-3. Overlapping sonographic views of the same amniotic fluid pocket.

Whereas the original guidelines for AFI determination stipulated that the ultrasound transducer be held in a longitudinal plane at all times, there are some instances in which amniotic fluid pockets may be more readily visualized when the transducer is held in a different orientation.[8] Moreover, Strong and Lovelace[11] found that AFI values obtained with the ultrasound transducer held in a transverse orientation are no different than those obtained with the standard, longitudinal technique.

Overlapping sonographic views between adjacent quadrants can occasionally result in redundant fluid pocket measurements and falsely elevated AFI values (Fig. 23-3). Although concerted efforts to keep the ultrasound transducer perpendicular to the floor during AFI assessment (Fig. 23-2) can reduce redundant fluid pocket measurements, the risk of this error still exists, especially if a curvilinear or sector scanning transducer is used. By using alternating transducer orientations on alternating uterine quad-

rants, as shown in Figure 23-4, fluid pocket redundancy may be reduced and accuracy increased.

Normal and abnormal amniotic fluid volumes have been defined with the AFI technique. The published work of several authors indicates that the mean AFI at term ranges from 12 to 16 cm, whereas an AFI of 8 cm represents the fifth percentile of AFI values.[10,12–14] Moore and Cayle[10] have developed normal AFI ranges for each week of gestation beyond 15 weeks. While somewhat more specific than the above parameters, their age-associated ranges are generally in step with previous reports. Typically, however, clinical outcomes are not adversely affected until the AFI falls to 5 cm or less.[14,15]

AMNIOTIC FLUID FLUXES

The fetal urinary system is the major contributing source of amniotic fluid. Relatively large amounts of fluid are also secreted into the amniotic cavity from the fetal lung. In the setting of intact membranes, fetal swallowing is the primary avenue of amniotic fluid egress from the amniotic space. However, passage of amniotic fluid across the surface of the placenta into the fetal circulation (intramembranous pathway) and across the amniochorion into the maternal circulation (transmembranous pathway) may augment outflow of fluid from the amniotic cavity somewhat. The amniotic fluid volume that ulti-

---

Amniotic Fluid Pathways in Late Pregnancy[a]

Into amniotic space
   Fetal urination
   Fetal pulmonary secretions
   Other fetal secretions
      Lacrimal
      Salivary
      Sweat

Out of amniotic space
   Fetal swallowing
   Intramembranous
   Transmembranous

[a]In order of relative contribution.

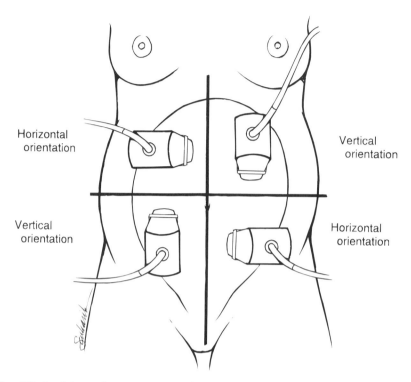

Horizontal
orientation

Vertical
orientation

Vertical
orientation

Horizontal
orientation

Fig. 23-4. Schema for minimizing redundant amniotic fluid pocket measurements.

mately accumulates in a given pregnancy represents the difference in net inward versus net outward fluid fluxes. Although many pathophysiologic processes may be at play, polyhydramnios and oligohydramnios can frequently be traced to a disruption of the alimentary or urinary tracts, respectively. A variety of medications may also alter amniotic fluid balance. Furosemide, for example, may temporarily increase amniotic fluid volume, while nonsteroidal anti-inflammatory drugs and angiotensin-converting enzyme inhibitors may decrease it.

AMNIOTIC FLUID PRODUCTION

Fetal Micturition

Amniotic fluid production in the latter half of pregnancy depends largely on fetal urination, a process that begins at approximately 8 to 11 weeks of gestation.[16,17] Following fetal epithelial keratinization at roughly 20 to 25 weeks, transdermal passage of fluid into the amniotic space ceases, leaving the fetal uri-

nary system as the primary source of amniotic fluid.[18] At term, fetal urinary output exceeds 1 L/day.[19] Any pathophysiologic process that affects fetal urine production may adversely affect amniotic fluid volume.

In the normal human adult, urinary output is an indirect but clinically useful method for assessing intravascular fluid status. In the setting of intravascular fluid depletion, hypoperfusion of the kidneys will ultimately result in decreased urine production. A similar situation exists with the fetus, although its intravascular fluid status depends on uteroplacental perfusion. Since the vast majority of amniotic fluid is fetal urine, the status of the uteroplacental unit may be reflected by the amniotic fluid volume. Postdatism and fetal growth retardation, two conditions commonly associated with uteroplacental insufficiency, are often complicated by reduced amniotic fluid volume. Oligohydramnios has been associated with increased frequencies of nonreactive nonstress tests, variable fetal heart rate (FHR) decelerations, meconium staining, cesarean delivery for fetal distress, and low Apgar scores.[14,15] Therefore, it would appear that amniotic fluid volume provides important information about uteroplacental status, and may have utility in identifying the patient at risk of a suboptimal outcome of labor.

Pulmonary Secretion

From early in gestation, fluid flows into the amniotic cavity from the fetal lungs.[20] While some of this fluid is swallowed, a considerable amount ultimately makes its way into the amniotic space.[20] Several animal studies suggest that the average pulmonary fluid outflow is roughly 10 percent of body weight per day.[21–24] Nevertheless, disruption of this system alone is not usually associated with oligohydramnios.

Other Sources

The volume of fluid produced by fetal lacrimal, salivary, and sweat glands is unknown but probably inconsequential.

AMNIOTIC FLUID EGRESS

Fetal Swallowing

Fetal deglutition is the major route by which amniotic fluid is removed from the amniotic cavity.[25] Swallowing begins at approximately 8 weeks of gestation.[26] Up to 500 ml/day leaves the amniotic space via this route, a volume that is significantly less than that produced by the fetal urinary system.[27,28] Although this discrepancy may be a function of errors in experimental measurement, it is nevertheless likely that daily fetal urine volumes exceed daily fetal deglutition volumes.[25]

Fluid Movement Across Membranes

The amniotic surface of the fetal membranes is composed entirely of cells with microvilli that protrude into the amniotic cavity.[16] Tortuous intercellular channels formed from complex interdigitations that occur at the cell wall borders may also be noted.[16] Abnormalities in the ultrastructure of the amnion have been identified in pregnancies complicated by abnormal amniotic fluid volumes, suggesting that the amnion plays a role in amniotic fluid volume regulation.[29–31] Moreover, the amnion appears to be affected by various pregnancy-associated hormones. Decidual prolactin has been shown to promote transfer of fluid out of the amniotic space: injection of this substance into the amniotic space in fetal monkeys will decrease amniotic fluid volume.[32] Conversely, some cases of polyhydramnios have been associated with reduced concentrations of prolactin in the amniotic fluid.[33] Decidual prolactin appears to be stimulated by hyperosmotic amniotic fluid and progesterone.[34,35]

A variety of reports suggest that fluid may pass into the vessels on the fetal surface of the placenta (intramembranous fluid movement). While the exact volume of fluid that exits the amniotic space in this fashion is unclear, intramembranous absorption averages approximately 200 ml/day in sheep fetuses.[36–38] A small volume of fluid may also traverse the amniochorion and enter maternal blood vessels in the decidua. Ovine studies have suggested that transmembranous fluid movement accounts for only 10 ml/day.[39,40]

A normal, static amniotic fluid volume represents a dynamic process that has its influx and efflux components in equilibrium. Certain pathophysiologic processes may adversely increase or decrease amniotic fluid volume. It has been proposed that when one component of flux is compromised, the remaining pathways actually adjust their fluid flow rates so as to maintain amniotic fluid volume stability.[25] Indeed, polyhydramnios occurs in less than half of cases of alimentary tract obstruction.[41]

Effect of Maternal Hydration on Amniotic Fluid Volume

A variety of studies suggests that both the volume and composition of amniotic fluid are highly regulated during gestation via many disparate mechanisms. In the karyotypically and anatomically normal fetus with intact membranes, the most important factor for maintaining normal fetal fluid homeostasis is transplacental flow of fluid between mother and fetus. Maternal dehydration may produce an increase in fetal plasma osmolality that results in fetal vasopressin secretion and an increase in fetal urine concentration.[42,43] Fetal vasopressin may also be secreted in response to hypoxia, umbilical cord compression, and fetal blood loss.[44,45] Indeed, the nonstressed fetus tends to produce hypo-osmolar urine.[46] Sherer et al[47] reported a case of severe maternal dehydration that was associated with oligohydramnios despite intact membranes. With successful rehydration of the mother, sonographic re-evaluation demonstrated that the amniotic fluid volume had normalized.

It would appear that the uterus, even during pregnancy, is a relatively low priority organ with regard to maternal blood flow, and that in times of significant physical stress (i.e., maternal disease, heavy physical exertion, dehydration) uterine blood flow is diverted to more vital organs.[48–54] Conversely, reduction of significant maternal physical stressors may result in redistribution of blood flow to the uterus and improvement in amniotic fluid volume.

AMNIOTIC FLUID VOLUME DURING LABOR

The intrapartum period is fraught with risk for the parturient and her fetus. In the setting of an abnormal amniotic fluid volume, perinatal risks are increased. For instance, amniorrhexis in the patient with polyhydramnios is associated with increased risk of fetal malpresentation, umbilical cord prolapse, and placental abruption. Relative to intrapartum problems posed by oligohydramnios, however, polyhydramnios is generally of less concern to the parturient and her obstetrician.

Protection against umbilical cord compression is probably the most important function of a normal amniotic fluid volume during pregnancy, and particularly during labor. Umbilical cord compression is a common intrapartum occurrence and a cause for concern, especially when the compression is severe, prolonged, and repetitive. It has long been a goal to identify the gravid woman destined to develop ominous FHR tracings during labor. Although knowledge of the mother's antenatal course is always useful in this endeavor, Westgren and colleagues[55] demonstrated that 10 percent of "low-risk" pregnancies ultimately develop ominous FHR patterns that require scalp blood pH assessment or operative intervention. Moreover, Hobel et al[56] found that 20 percent of their low-risk gravid women develop intrapartum complications despite a carefully formulated selection program. Thus, there would appear to be a subpopulation at risk of fetal morbidity that cannot be readily identified antenatally.

The concept of a fetal "admission test" performed early in the course of labor has recently been described.[57] While a variety of parameters have been advanced as markers for the fetus at risk of intrapartum morbidity, it appears that amniotic fluid volume is one of the variables most reliably related to outcome among normal fetuses.[14,15] As mentioned earlier, oligohydramnios in the antenatal period has been associated with many perinatal problems, including abnormal antepartum FHR patterns. Thus, it should follow that an evaluation of amniotic fluid volume in early labor may predict fetal morbidity. Indeed, when AFI assessment was applied to the early intrapartum period as a fetal admission test, Sarno et al[15] found that an AFI value of 5 cm or less was associated with a significant risk of abnormal FHR patterns later in labor, cesarean delivery for fetal distress, and low Apgar scoring.[15]

Most patients who develop oligohydramnios do so secondary to ruptured membranes.[15] It would therefore appear that a low-risk antenatal course provides no assurance that the intrapartum period will also be of low risk. An evaluation in early labor to identify the fetus with a suboptimal amniotic fluid volume would be preferable to antenatal risk assessment, since it would permit an immediate, updated assessment of fetal risk.

MODULATING THE AMNIOTIC FLUID VOLUME

A variety of physiologic, pathologic, and iatrogenic processes can alter the amniotic fluid volume. By modifying these processes, the obstetrician may optimize the amniotic fluid volume immediately before or during labor.

Noninvasive Techniques

Modifying the Hemodynamics of the Mother and Fetus

During pregnancy, maternal plasma volume increases, reaching an amount that is 30 to 50 percent above that in the nongravid state by the 24th week of pregnancy. Red blood cell volume also increases, but more slowly. The net result is that the maternal hematocrit gradually falls as gestation advances. This process is probably the result of normal pregnancy-associated changes in maternal physiology. Several common pregnancy complications appear to be associated with a reduced or absent maternal volume expansion, including fetal growth retardation and oligohydramnios.[58–62] Indeed, a number of studies have described a direct relationship between birth weight and the magnitude of increase in maternal plasma volume, suggesting that adequate maternal plasma expansion is essential for normal fetal growth.[63,64] Therefore, in the healthy, adequately nourished gravid woman, a moderately low hematocrit is a manifestation of increased plasma volume. By contrast, a relatively high hematocrit may suggest inadequately increased plasma volume and may indicate increased risk of a suboptimal pregnancy outcome.[64] In the setting of pregnancy complications such as fetal growth retardation or oligohydramnios, taking measures to increase maternal plasma volume may be beneficial. Several techniques for achieving this increase have been described, including bed rest, maternal hydration, and subtotal immersion.

Bedrest

A considerable volume of intravascular fluid can pass into the extracellular space of the lower extremities in the physically active gravid woman as a result of increased hydrostatic pressure within blood vessels of the legs. When the gravid woman is placed in the left lateral recumbent position in the third trimester of pregnancy, Starling forces are modified and extracellular fluid gradually re-enters and expands the intravascular space. As a result, a modest decrease in maternal hematocrit may be seen. Additionally, systemic vascular resistance decreases and blood flow to maternal viscera (including the uterus and kidneys) increases. Clinically, a concomitant decrease in maternal blood pressure and increase in maternal urine production can be appreciated when the pregnant woman is placed on her left side.

Maternal Rehydration

The final common pathway of many pregnancy complications is fetal growth retardation, oligohydramnios, and occasionally, fetal demise. Frequently, sonographic assessment of the fetus and placenta will demonstrate accelerated placental maturation and increased resistance to blood flow through the uteroplacental unit. Many women who demonstrate these pregnancy complications have intravascular fluid depletion.[64] Not infrequently, increased peripheral vascular resistance may also be noted. Direct expansion of maternal intravascular volume has been shown to decrease maternal systemic vascular resistance and increase cardiac output.[65–69] Indeed, Karsdorp and associates found that absent end-diastolic umbilical artery flow reappeared after acute maternal volume expansion, while Kilpatrick et al found

that maternal ingestion of large volumes of fluid produced a significant increase in amniotic fluid volume.[70,71] Therefore, it would appear that maternal hydration may improve maternal and fetal fluid status to the point at which an increase in amniotic fluid volume occurs. When combined with left lateral recumbency, significant improvements in uteroplacental blood flow may be noted. Unfortunately, the effect of bed rest or maternal hydration appears to be transient, and in some cases ineffective for the patient with severe disease.[72]

Subtotal Immersion Therapy

All therapeutic modalities used in the management of oligohydramnios seek to optimize uteroplacental blood flow. Bed rest, the mainstay of treatment, is associated with a transfer of 500 ml of blood to the intrathoracic circulation, an increase in cardiac and renal function, and a corresponding natriuresis and diuresis.[72] However, some of these responses attenuate over time.[72] As the underlying maternal disease process progresses and uteroplacental insufficiency worsens, bed rest alone frequently becomes inadequate for plasma volume expansion. Administration of large volumes of fluid, as mentioned above, may further augment intravascular volume, but can be impractical for the patient, especially if the fluid is administered orally.

Katz and associates[73] have shown that immersion of pregnant women in shoulder-deep water can reduce dependent edema. The technique hydrostatically forces extravascular fluid into maternal blood vessels, producing an intravascular infusion that begins within 7 seconds of shoulder immersion.[74] More importantly, subtotal immersion produces a significant decrease in mean arterial pressure, suggesting that systemic vascular resistance is reduced.[73] Khosla and DuBois[75] suggest that the hemodynamic responses produced by immersion are equivalent to those created by the infusion of 2 L of isotonic saline. The acute volume expansion that results from immersion appears to alter maternal cardiovascular dynamics in the same fashion as intravenous hydration, and may also favorably affect uteroplacental blood flow. In contrast to bed rest, subtotal immersion is associated with a transfer of approximately 750 ml of blood to the intrathoracic circulation and a renal response that does not attenuate.[72,74] Moreover, Epstein[74] suggests that immersion therapy may have

Physiologic Effects of Immersion[a]

Extravascular fluid forced into maternal vessels

Plasma volume increases

750 ml of blood shifts from legs to chest

Heart size increases 30 percent

Central venous pressure increases 30 percent

Systemic vascular resistance decreases 30 percent

Mean arterial pressure decreases

Sodium excretion increases

Diuresis

[a]Synonyms: head-out immersion, hydrotherapy, subtotal immersion.

an affect on cardiovascular dynamics that is 50 to 100 percent greater than that of bed rest. Strong[76] reported that oligohydramnios was reversed in patients undergoing immersion therapy, suggesting that this modality may be an effective technique for augmenting amniotic fluid volume in a noninvasive fashion.

Immersion in sufficiently deep water causes an increase in net inward Starling forces. In effect, the hydrostatic force of deep water overwhelms net outward Starling forces and pushes extravascular fluid back into maternal vessels.[73] Because hydrostatic pressure increases by 22.4 mm Hg for each 12 inches of depth, the effect of immersion therapy will be proportional to the water depth. Indeed, most reports of immersion suggest that a significant clinical effect is not noted until the patient's shoulders are immersed, a water depth that is generally of 3 to 4 feet. Patients undergoing subtotal immersion therapy at our institution undergo two to three 30-minute sessions daily at a water temperature of 34 to 37°C. Owing to the large, rapid fluid shifts that accompany subtotal immersion, the technique is probably best avoided in patients with heart failure or mitral or aortic stenosis. Additionally, the technique is not used in patients with ruptured membranes or open skin lesions. Immersion therapy generally will not reverse

oligohydramnios when the underlying pathophysiology is unrelated to uteroplacental insufficiency.[76]

Invasive Techniques

Intrapartum Amnioinfusion

Amnioinfusion has recently received considerable attention in the obstetric literature. A growing body of data suggests that infusion of fluid into the amniotic space may have utility for a variety of indications during labor, and that this simple, inexpensive modality may deserve consideration for properly selected patients. Although several permutations of the technique have been described, including meconium dilution, the common therapeutic goal is expansion of the amniotic fluid volume.

Traditionally, variable FHR decelerations have been managed by uterine displacement, intravenous fluid boluses, oxygen, and discontinuation of oxytocin. Since the first report of this technique in 1983, amnioinfusion has been shown to be generally more successful for preventing or eliminating intrapartum variable FHR decelerations than standard resuscita-

Table 23-1. Clinical Trials of Amnioinfusion

Study	Year	Result
Miyazaki[77]	1983	Effective in 74% (no control group)
Miyazaki[78]	1985	Fewer FHR decelerations ($P = 0.001$)
Nageotte[79]	1985	Fewer FHR decelerations ($P < 0.001$)
Owen[80]	1990	Nonsignificant decrease in FHR decelerations; less endometritis ($P = 0.01$)
Strong[81]	1990	Less meconium ($P = 0.04$), fewer severe FHR decelerations. ($P = 0.04$), less bradycardia ($P = 0.05$), fewer operative deliveries for fetal distress ($P = 0.002$)
MacGregor[82]	1991	Nonsignificant decrease in FHR decelerations
Nageotte[83]	1991	Fewer FHR decelerations ($P = 0.01$)
Schrimmer[84]	1991	Less operative delivery for fetal distress ($P = 0.0001$); less amnionitis/endometritis ($P = 0.002$)
Chauhan[85]	1992	Nonsignificant decrease in FHR decelerations

tive techniques (Table 23-1). Because it can take at least 10 minutes to achieve sufficient expansion of amniotic fluid volume, some obstetricians advocate amnioinfusion for women at risk before the onset of severe FHR decelerations. In several published reports, obstetric outcomes were significantly better among women with oligohydramnios who underwent prophylactic amnioinfusion.[79,80,81,83,86] However, a report by Cook[87] suggests that prophylactic and therapeutic amnioinfusions may be equally effective. Notwithstanding, it appears that expanding the amniotic fluid volume better protects the umbilical cord against compression during labor. Several studies also suggest that amnioinfusion may reduce the risk of infection in the peripartum period.[80,88]

Candidates

The presence of repetitive variable decelerations in the FHR is currently the most common indication for amnioinfusion during labor.[89] Nevertheless, am-

nioinfusion is not justified in all instances in which decelerative FHR patterns are present. Because late decelerations in the FHR result from a pathophysiologic mechanism that differs from that responsible for variable FHR decelerations, amnioinfusion is contraindicated in their presence. Theoretically, by increasing intrauterine pressure, amnioinfusion may further compromise uteroplacental blood flow. When fetal acidosis cannot be ruled out, delaying delivery to perform amnioinfusion is unwarranted. Amnioinfusion used in the wrong setting may delay appropriate treatment by falsely reassuring the obstetrician.

Technique

The most important tool for administering amnioinfusion is the hollow intrauterine pressure catheter (IUPC) (Figs. 23-5 and 23-6). Before inserting the IUPC, it is connected to a bag of amnioinfusate solu-

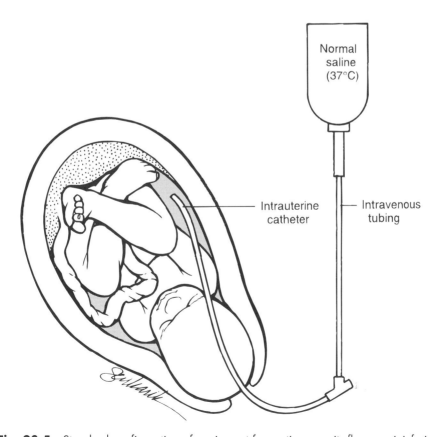

Fig. 23-5. Standard configuration of equipment for routine, gravity-flow amnioinfusion.

Contraindications to Intrapartum Amnioinfusion

Absolute contraindications
  Active maternal genital herpes infection
  Diminished FHR variability or reactivity
  Fetal scalp pH below 7.20
  Late decelerations in the FHR
  Placenta previa or placental abruption

Relative contraindications
  Fetal anomalies
  Impending delivery
  Multiple gestations
  Prior cesarean delivery

---

tion by intravenous extension tubing. To avoid the potential risk of air embolism, the system should be flushed before its insertion into the uterus. A fetal scalp electrode is also recommended.

When the amnioinfusion bottle is suspended 3 to 4 feet above the uterus, the rate of infusion will approach 20 ml/min.[90] Instead of using gravity flow for amnioinfusion, fluid may also be continuously administered with an infusion pump. A fluid warmer may also be added. However, these accessories complicate the technique considerably. Gravity flow amnioinfusion offers the advantage of simplicity and economy. In addition, fluid infused in this manner is delivered in discreet volumes and then stopped, thereby decreasing the risk of uterine overdistension. Several studies have noted that the AFI will increase an average of 4 cm for every 250 ml of fluid infused into the uterus by gravity flow.[91,92]

To avoid the possibility of vagally-induced fetal bradycardia, some obstetricians advise that the amnioinfusate solution be warmed to 37°C before administration. It is also prudent to monitor uterine activity during the amnioinfusion sequence, but there is no clear advantage of internal pressure monitoring over external tocodynamometry.

Intrapartum Amnioinfusion Technique

Cervical examination
  Rule out cord prolapse, meconium, impending delivery
  Artificial rupture of membranes, if necessary
  Place fetal scalp electrode

Intrauterine pressure catheter (IUPC) insertion
  Hollow variety IUPC
  Aseptic technique
  Insertion after IUPC has been flushed with saline

Normal saline
  Warmed to 37°C
  Connect saline bag to IUPC via intravenous extension tubing

Infusion
  Infusion pump option
    10 to 20 ml/min bolus (800 ml maximum)
    3 ml/min maintenance
    Discontinue for uterine hypertonus or bleeding
    Monitor uterine activity
  Gravity flow option
    Saline bag 4 feet above catheter tip
    10 to 20 ml/min bolus; administer in discrete 250 to 500 ml doses, as needed
    Discontinue for uterine hypertonus or bleeding
    Monitor uterine activity
  Re-boluses
    For AFI below 8 cm
    For reappearance or worsening of variable FHR decelerations following large vaginal fluid losses

---

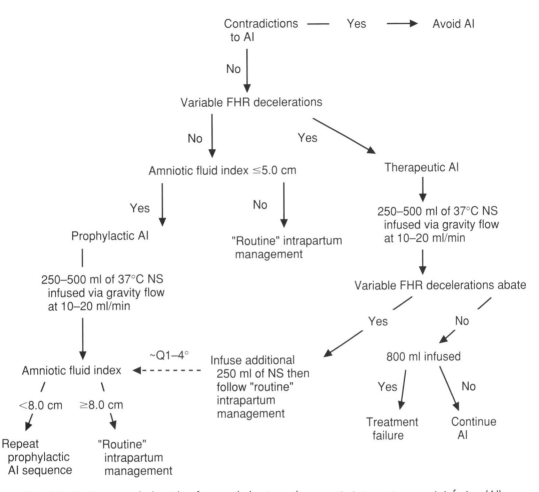

Fig. 23-6. Suggested algorithm for prophylactic or therapeutic intrapartum amnioinfusion (AI).

Meconium Dilution

The meconium aspiration syndrome is a potentially lethal neonatal condition that may occur when thick, tenacious meconium is present in the amniotic space. Intrauterine lavage has been described in the obstetric literature as a technique for diluting and lavaging meconium during labor (Table 23-2). To accomplish this, Wenstrom and Parsons[94] amnioinfused 1 L of saline every 6 hours during labor in patients with meconium-stained amniotic fluid, while Sadovsky et al[93] used a continuous infusion technique. In a number of reports, the occurrence of meconium below the neonatal vocal cords was significantly less common among women receiving prophylactic intrapartum amnioinfusion. However, oth-

ers have noted less promising outcomes. In vitro studies suggest that meconium may enhance bacterial growth in amniotic fluid in a dose-dependent fashion.[102] Therefore, meconium lavage might theoretically reduce the potential for chorioamnionitis as well. No reports have yet been published on this topic.

Prelabor Amnioinfusion

While it appears that intrapartum amnioinfusion may reduce the frequency and severity of umbilical cord compression during labor among fetuses with oligohydramnios, the cervix must be sufficiently dilated to permit insertion of a hollow IUPC, and the fetal membranes must be ruptured. Mandelbrot and

Table 23-2. Clinical Trials of Meconium Dilution

Study	Year	Result
Sadovsky[93]	1989	Less meconium below neonatal vocal cords ($P < 0.05$); less need for positive pressure ventilation ($P < 0.05$)
Wenstrom[94]	1989	Less meconium below neonatal vocal cords ($P < 0.05$)
Nageotte[95]	1990	No significant difference between study and control groups
Hensleigh[96]	1991	37% with meconium below neonatal vocal cords
Macri[86]	1992	Less meconium below neonatal vocal cords (RR = 0.12); less aspiration syndrome (RR = 0.09)
Parsons[97]	1992	Authors conclude amnioinfusion not useful
Cialone[98]	1994	Less meconium below neonatal vocal cords ($P < 0.001$); less aspiration syndrome ($P < 0.05$)
Spong[99]	1994	No significant difference between study and control groups
Eriksen[100]	1994	Less meconium below neonatal vocal cords ($P = 0.02$)
Usta[101]	1994	No significant difference between study and control groups

Abbreviation: RR, relative risk.

colleagues[103] suggested that transabdominal amnioinfusion before labor induction in gravid women with oligohydramnios may be a promising alternative.

Eglinton[104] noted that the malpresenting fetus with an AFI of 5 cm or lower has a poor prognosis for successful external cephalic version. Perhaps transabdominal amnioinfusion could also improve the prospect for successful fetal rotation in this situation by increasing amniotic fluid volume. However, no published reports exist of this potentially useful technique.

Amnioinfusate Solution Types

Most reported applications of amnioinfusion have used normal saline or Ringer's lactate solutions. Imanaka and Ogita[105] reported their successful experience with infusing amino acid solutions into the amniotic cavities of human fetuses with preterm, premature membrane rupture. No untoward effects were reported. Blakemore and associates[106] successfully infused a mixture of Ringer's lactate and a 10 percent dextrose solution for seven fetuses with severe oligohydramnios in the antepartum period, with good results.

Risks and Side Effects

Amnioinfusion appears to be associated with few risks. Uterine hyperactivity, or tetany, has been described in a single report.[92] The obstetric literature does not support anecdotal reports that labor progresses more rapidly following amnioinfusion.[99,107] One case of uterine overdistension has been described in a woman who underwent amnioinfusion (via continuous infusion pump) with no untoward effects.[108] Although isolated reports of these complications exist, amnioinfusion has not been associated with increased rates of amniotic fluid embolism, placental abruption, uterine rupture, umbilical cord prolapse, amnionitis, or maternal cardiopulmonary compromise.[78,81,99,109–111] Other reported complications do not appear to be directly related to amnioinfusion itself, but are associated with membrane rupture or insertion of the intrauterine pressure device.

Amnioinfusion is relatively contraindicated in the setting of multiple fetuses or a uterine scar. However, several reports of small numbers of cases have not suggested that amnioinfusion with twin gestations or during an attempted vaginal birth after cesarean section was associated with a suboptimal outcome.[111–114] One case of uterine scar disruption in association with amnioinfusion has been reported, but it is not clear whether the disruption preceded or followed the amnioinfusion procedure.[78] The most common clinical finding at the time of uterine rupture is a decelerative FHR pattern.[115] Because repetitive FHR decelerations are also the most common indication for amnioinfusion, one must entertain the possibility of antecedent disruption of a uterine scar when considering amnioinfusion for candidates for vaginal birth after cesarean section (VBAC). Strong and associates[113] have suggested that in the absence of vaginal leakage, failure of amnioinfusion to increase the amniotic fluid volume in a laboring woman with a prior cesarean delivery may suggest uterine rupture.

SUMMARY

A variety of intricate, incompletely understood systems influence amniotic fluid volume. The actual volume of amniotic fluid that surrounds a given fetus represents a complex interplay between mother and fetus, and a balance between the opposing processes of fluid influx and egress. Although amniotic fluid plays many important roles, its most important function during the intrapartum period is protection of the umbilical cord from compression. Women who enter labor with reduced amniotic fluid volume are at increased risk of a suboptimal outcome. However, amniotic fluid volume may be estimated sonographically, and fetuses with oligohydramnios may be identified. Amniotic fluid volume may be optimized before or during labor by modifying maternal hemodynamics or with amnioinfusion. The former technique is most practical before labor, while the latter is generally better suited to the intrapartum period.

REFERENCES

1. Mandelbaum B, Evans TN: Life in the amniotic fluid. Am J Obstet Gynecol 104:365, 1969
2. Gadd RL: The volume of the liquor amnii in normal and abnormal pregnancies. J Obstet Gynaecol Br Commonw 73:11, 1966
3. Beischer NA, Brown JB, Townsend L: Studies in prolonged pregnancy. III. amniocentesis in prolonged pregnancy. Am J Obstet Gynecol 193:496, 1969
4. Queenan JT: Amniocentesis. p. 201. In Queenan JT (ed): Management of High Risk Pregnancy. Medical Economics Books, Oradell, NJ, 1985
5. Queenan JT, Thompson W, Whitfield CR et al: Amniotic fluid volumes in normal pregnancies. Am J Obstet Gynecol 114:34, 1972
6. Hutchinson DL, Gray MJ, Plenti AA: The role of the fetus in the water exchange of the amniotic fluid of normal and hydramniotic patients. J Clin Invest 38:971, 1959
7. Vosburgh GH, Flexner LB, Cowie DB et al: The rate of renewal in woman of the water and sodium of the amniotic fluid as determined by tracer techniques. Am J Obstet Gynecol 46:1156, 1948
8. Phelan JP, Smith CV, Broussard P et al: Amniotic fluid volume assessment using the four quadrant technique in the pregnancy between 36 and 42 weeks. J Reprod Med 32:540, 1987
9. Rutherford SE, Phelan JP, Smith CV et al: The four quadrant assessment of amniotic fluid volume: interobserver and intraobserver variation. J Reprod Med 32:597, 1987
10. Moore TR, Cayle JE: The amniotic fluid index in normal human pregnancy. Am J Obstet Gynecol 162:1168, 1990
11. Strong TH, Lovelace GS: The impact of transducer orientation upon the amniotic fluid index abst. Society of Perinatal Obstetricians, Fourteenth Annual Meeting, 1994, Abstract 144. Am J Obstet Gynecol 170:317, 1994
12. Jeng C-J, Jou T-J, Wang KG et al: Amniotic fluid index measurement with the four-quadrant technique during pregnancy. J Reprod Med 35:674, 1990
13. Phelan JP, Ahn MO, Smith CV et al: Amniotic fluid index measurements during pregnancy. J Reprod Med 32:601, 1987
14. Rutherford SE, Phelan JP, Smith CV, Jacobs N: The four-quadrant assessment of amniotic fluid volume: ad adjunct to antepartum fetal heart rate testing. Obstet Gynecol 70:353, 1987
15. Sarno AP, Ahn NO, Phelan JP: Intrapartum amniotic fluid volume at term. Association of ruptured membranes, oligohydramnios and increased fetal risk. J Reprod Med 35:719, 1990
16. Wintour EM, Shandley L: Effects of fetal fluid balance on amniotic fluid volume. Sem Perinatol 17:158, 1993
17. Abramovich DR, Page KP: Pathways of water transfer between liquor amnii and the Feto-placental unit at term. Eur J Obstet Gynaecol 3:155, 1973
18. Phelan JP: Amniotic fluid assessment and significance of contaminants. p. 777. In Reece EA, Hobbins JC, Mahoney MJ, Petrie RH (eds): Medicine of the Fetus and Mother. JB Lippincott, Philadelphia, 1992
19. Rabinowitz R, Peters MT, Vyas S et al: Measurement of fetal urine production in normal pregnancy by real-time ultrasonography. Am J Obstet Gynecol 161:1264, 1989
20. Harding R: Fetal lung liquid. p. 42. In Brace RA, Ross MG, Robillard JE (eds): Fetal and Neonatal Body Fluids: The Scientific Basis for Clinical Practice. Perinatology Press, Ithaca, NY, 1989
21. Adamson TM, Brodecky V, Lambert TF et al: The production and composition of lung liquids in the in utero foetal lamb. p. 208. In: Foetal and Neonatal Physiology. Cambridge University Press, Cambridge, 1975
22. Mescher EJ, Platzker A, Ballard PL et al: Ontogeny of tracheal fluid, pulmonary surfactant, and plasma

corticoids in the fetal lamb. J Appl Physiol 39:1017, 1975

23. Oliver RE, Strang LB: Ion fluxes across the pulmonary epithelium and the secretion of lung liquid in the foetal lamb. J Physiol 241:327, 1974

24. Lawson EE, Brown ER, Torday JS et al: The effect of epinephrine on tracheal fluid flow and surfactant efflux in fetal sheep. Am Rev Respir Dis 118:1023, 1978

25. Gilbert WM, Brace RA: Amniotic fluid volume and normal flows to and from the amniotic cavity, Sem Perinatol 17:150, 1993

26. Romero R, Pilu G, Jeanty P et al (eds): The gastrointestinal tract and intradominal organs. In: Prenatal Diagnosis of Congenital Anomalies. p. 234. Appleton & Lange, E. Norwalk, CT, 1988

27. Abramovich DR, Garden A, Jancial L et al: Fetal swallowing and voiding in relation to hydramnios. Obstet Gynecol 54:15, 1979

28. Pritchard JA: Deglutition by normal and anencephalic fetuses. Obstet Gynecol 25:289, 1965

29. Hebertson RM, Hammond ME, Bryson MJ: Amniotic epithelial ultrastructure in normal, polyhydramnic, and oligohydramnic pregnancies. Obstet Gynecol 68: 74, 1986

30. Pollard SM, Symonds EM, Aye NN: Scanning electron microscopic appearances in the amnion in polyhydramnios and oligohydramnios. Br J Obstet Gynaecol 86:228, 1979

31. Wang T, Reale E, Schneider J: Amnionepithel bei hydramnion. Fortsch Med 97:1009, 1979

32. Josimovich JB, Merisko K, Boccella L: Amniotic prolactin control over amniotic and fetal extracellular water and electrolytes in the rhesus monkey. Endocrinology 100:564, 1977

33. Tyson JE, Hwant P, Guyda H et al: Studies of prolactin secretion in human pregnancy. Am J Obstet Gynecol 113:14, 1972

34. Anderson JR, Borggard B, Ornvold K et al: The effect of hyposmotic and sodium chloride hyperosmotic environments on the secretion and synthesis of prolactin from human decidua in vitro. Acta Endocrinol 100:623, 1982

35. Daly DC, Maslar IA, Riddick DH: Term decidua response to estradiol and progesterone. Am J Obstet Gynecol 145:679, 1983

36. Gilbert WM, Brace RA: The missing link in amniotic fluid volume regulation: intramembranous absorption. Obstet Gynecol 74:748, 1989

37. Gilbert WM, Brace RA: Novel determination of filtration coefficient of ovine placenta and intramembranous pathway. Am J Physiol 259:1281, 1990

38. Jang PR, Brace RA: Amniotic fluid composition changes during urine drainage and tracheoesophageal occlusion in fetal sheep. Am J Obstet Gynecol 167:1732, 1992

39. Anderson DF, Faber JJ, Parks CM: Extraplacental transfer of water in the sheep. J Physiol (Lond) 406: 75, 1988

40. Anderson DF, Borst HJP, Boyd RDH et al: Filtration of water from mother to conceptus via paths independent of fetal placental circulation in sheep. J Physiol (Lond) 431:1, 1990

41. Lloyd JR, Clatworthy HW: Hydramnios as aid to the early diagnosis of congenital obstruction of the alimentary tract: a study of the maternal and fetal factors. Pediatrics June:903, 1958

42. Bell RJ, Congiu M, Hardy KJ et al: Gestation-dependent aspects of the response of the ovine fetus to the osmotic stress induced by maternal water deprivation. Q J Exp Physiol 69:187, 1984

43. Schreyer P, Sherman DJ, Ervin MG et al: Maternal dehydration: impact on ovine amniotic fluid volume and composition. J Dev Physiol 13:283, 1990

44. Ervin MG: Perinatal fluid and electrolyte regulation: role of arginine vasopressin. Semin Perinatol 12:134, 1988

45. Robillard JE, Smith FG, Nakamura KT et al: Fetal renal function regulation of water and electrolyte excretion. p. 66. In Brace RA, Ross MG, Robillard JE (eds): Fetal and Neonatal Body Fluids: The Scientific Basis for Clinical Practice. Perinatology Press, Ithaca, NY, 1989

46. Wintour EM, Bell RJ, Congui M et al: The value of urine osmolality as an index of stress in the ovine fetus. J Dev Physiol 7:347, 1985

47. Sherer DM, Cullen JBH, Thompson HO, Woods JR: Transient oligohydramnios in a severely hypovolemic gravid woman at 35 weeks gestation, with fluid reaccumulating immediately after intravenous maternal hydration. Am J Obstet Gynecol 162:770, 1990

48. Brinkman CRG III, Erkkola R, Nuwayhid B et al: Adrenergic vasoconstrictor receptors in the uterine vascular bed. p. 113. In Moawad AH, Lindheimer MD (eds): Uterine and Placental Blood Flow. Masson Publishing, New York, 1982

49. Oakes GK, Walker AM, Ehrenkranz et al: Uteroplacental blood flow during hyperthermia with and without respiratory alkalosis. J Appl Physiol 41:197, 1976

50. Bell AW, Hales JRS, Fawcett AA et al: Contribution of the uterus to circulatory requirements of exercise and heat stress in pregnant sheep. p. 377. In Hales JRS (ed): Thermal Physiology. Raven Press, New York, 1984

51. Lotgering FK, Gilbert RD, Longo LD: Exercise response in pregnant sheep: oxygen consumption, uterine blood flow, and blood volume. J Appl Physiol 55:834, 1983

52. Hohimer AR, Bissonnette JM, Metcalfe J et al: Effect of exercise on uterine blood flow in the pregnant pygmy goat. Am J Physiol 246:H207, 1984

53. Wasserstrum N, Rudelstorfer R, Khoury A et al: Effects of elevation of maternal oxygen consumption of system and uterine hemodynamics, abstracted. Presented at the Thirty-first Annual Meeting of the Society for Gynecologic Investigation, San Francisco, 1984

54. Greiss FC: Uterine vascular response to hemorrhage during pregnancy. Obstet Gynecol 27:549, 1966

55. Westgren M, Ingemarsson E, Ingemarsson I et al: Intrapartum electronic fetal monitoring in low-risk pregnancies. Obstet Gynecol 56:301, 1980

56. Hobel C, Hyvarienen M, Okana D et al: Prenatal and intrapartum high risk screening. Am J Obstet Gynecol 117:1, 1973

57. Ingemarsson I, Arulkumaran S, Paul RH et al: Admission test: a screening test for fetal distress in labor. Obstet Gynecol 68:800, 1986

58. Hytten FE, Paintin DB: Increase in plasma volume during normal pregnancy. J Obstet Gynaecol Br Commonw 70:402, 1965

59. Retief FP, Brink AJ: A study of pregnancy anemia: blood volume changes correlated with other parameters of hemopoietic efficiency. J Obstet Gynaecol Br Commonw 74:683, 1967

60. Pirani BBK, Campbell DM, MacGillivray I: J Obstet Gynaecol Br Commonw 80:884, 1973

61. Gibson HM: Plasma volume and glomerular filtration rate in pregnancy and their relation to differences in fetal growth. J Obstet Gynaecol Br Commonw 80:1067, 1973

62. Goodlin RC, Anderson JC, Gallagher TF: Relationship between amniotic fluid volume and maternal plasma volume expansion. Am J Obstet Gynecol 146:505, 1983

63. Gallery EDM, Saunders DM, Hunyor SN et al: The relationship between plasma volume expansion and intrauterine fetal growth in normal and hypertensive pregnancy. Aust NZ J Obstet Gynaecol 19:179, 1979

64. Goodlin RC, Quaife MA, Dirksen JW: The significance, diagnosis and treatment of maternal hypovolemia as associated with fetal/maternal illness. Semin Perinatol 5:163, 1981

65. Ultrych M, Hofman J, Heil Z: Cardiac and renal hyperresponsiveness to acute plasma volume expansion in hypertension. Am Heart J 68:293, 1964

66. Lund-Johnson P: Hemodynamics in early essential hypertension—still an area of controversy. J Hypertens 3:209, 1983

67. Schalekamp MADH, Krauss XH, Schalekamp-Kuyken MPA et al: Studies on the mechanism of hypernatriuresis in essential hypertension in relation to measurement of plasma renin concentration, body fluid compartments and renal function. Clin Sci 41:219, 1971

68. Safar ME, London GM, Levenson JA et al: Rapid dextran infusion in essential hypertension. Hypertension 1:615, 1979

69. Birkenhager ED, De Leeuw PW, Schalekamp MADH: Control Mechanisms in Essential Hypertension. Elsevier, Amsterdam, 1982

70. Kilpatrick SJ, Safford K, Pomeroy T et al: Maternal hydration increases amniotic fluid index. Obstet Gynecol 78:1098, 1991

71. Karsdorp VHM, van Vugt JMG, Dekker GA, van Geijn HP: Reappearance of end-diastolic velocities in the umbilical artery following maternal volume expansion: a preliminary study. Obstet Gynecol 80:679, 1992

72. Goodlin RC, Hoffman KLE, Williams NE, Buchan P: Shoulder out immersion in pregnant women. J Perinat Med 12:173, 1984

73. Katz VL, Ryder RM, Cefalo RC et al: A comparison of bed rest and immersion for treating the edema of pregnancy. Obstet Gynecol 75:147, 1990

74. Epstein M: Renal effects of head-out water immersion in man: implications for an understanding of volume homeostasis. Physiol Rev 58:529, 1978

75. Khosla SS, DuBois AB: Osmoregulation and interstitial fluid changes in humans during water immersion. Am J Physiol 241:686, 1981

76. Strong TH: Reversal of oligohydramnios with subtotal immersion: a report of five cases. Am J Obstet Gynecol 169:1595, 1993

77. Miyazaki FS, Nevarez F: Saline amnioinfusion for relief of variable or prolonged decelerations: a preliminary report. Am J Obstet Gynecol 146:670, 1983

78. Miyazaki FS, Nevarez F: Saline amnioinfusion for relief of repetitive variable decelerations: a prospective randomized study. Am J Obstet Gynecol 153:301, 1985

79. Nageotte MP, Freeman RK, Garite TJ, Dorchester W: Prophylactic intrapartum amnioinfusion in patients with preterm premature rupture of membranes. Am J Obstet Gynecol 153:557, 1985

80. Owen J, Henson BV, Hauth JC: A prospective randomized study of saline solution amnioinfusion. Am J Obstet Gynecol 102:1146, 1990

81. Strong TH, Hetzler G, Sarno AP, Paul RH: Prophylactic intrapartum amnioinfusion: a randomized clinical trial. Am J Obstet Gynecol 162:1370, 1990

82. MacGregor SN, Banzhaf WC, Silver RK, Depp R: A prospective, randomized evaluation of intrapartum amnioinfusion: fetal acid-base status and cesarean delivery. J Repro Med 36:69, 1991

83. Nageotte MP, Bertucci L, Towers CV et al: Prophylactic amnioinfusion in pregnancies complicated by oligohydramnios: a prospective study. Obstet Gynecol 77:677, 1991

84. Schrimmer DB, Macri JC, Paul RH: Prophylactic amnioinfusion as a treatment for oligohydramnios in laboring patients: a prospective, randomized trial. Am J Obstet Gynecol 165:972, 1991

85. Chauhan SP, Rutherford SE, Hess LW et al: Prophylactic intrapartum amnioinfusion for patients with oligohydramnios, a prospective randomized study. J Reprod Med 37:817, 1992

86. Macri CJ, Schrimmer DB, Leung A et al: Prophylactic amnioinfusion improves outcome of pregnancy complicated by thick meconium and oligohydramnios. Am J Obstet Gynecol 167:117, 1992

87. Cook V, Spinnato JA: Prophylactic versus therapeutic amnioinfusion, abstracted (no. 236). In the Proceedings of the Society of Perinatal Obstetricians, Thirteenth Annual Meeting, 1993. Am J Obstet Gynecol 168:363, 1993

88. Major CA, de Veciana M, Asrat T et al: The impact of amnioinfusion on maternal and neonatal morbidity in pregnancies complicated by preterm premature rupture of the membranes and amnionitis, abstracted (no. 399). In the Proceedings of the Society of Perinatal Obstetricians, Twelfth Annual Meeting, 1992. Am J Obstet Gynecol 166:385, 1992

89. Strong TH: Amnioinfusion with preterm, premature rupture of membranes. Clin Perinatol 19:399, 1992

90. Miyazaki FS: Relieving variable decelerations. Contemp Obstet Gynecol 29:23, 1987

91. Strong TH, Hetzler G, Paul RH: Amniotic fluid volume change following amnioinfusion of a fixed volume. Am J Obstet Gynecol 45:284, 1990

92. Posner MD, Ballagh SA, Paul RH: The effect of amnioinfusion on uterine pressure and activity: a preliminary report. Am J Obstet Gynecol 163:813, 1990

93. Sadovsky Y, Amon E, Bade ME, Petrie RH: Prophylactic amnioinfusion during labor complicated by meconium: a preliminary report. Am J Obstet Gynecol 161:613, 1989

94. Wenstrom KD, Parsons MT: The prevention of meconium aspiration in labor using amnioinfusion. Obstet Gynecol 73:647, 1989

95. Nageotte MP, Bertucci L, Towers CV et al: Prophylactic amnioinfusion for thick meconium: a prospective study, abstracted (no. 68). In the Proceedings of the Society of Perinatal Obstetricians, Tenth Annual Meeting. 1990

96. Hensleigh P, Loots M, Hilsinger L: Complications associated with amnioinfusion for meconium, abstracted (no. 259). In the Proceedings of the Society of Perinatal Obstetricians, Eleventh Annual Meeting, 1991. Am J Obstet Gynecol 164:317, 1991

97. Parsons MT, Parsons AK, Angel JL: The failure of routine amnioinfusion in patients with thick meconium to eliminate the occurrence of meconium aspiration syndrome, abstracted (no. 472). In the Proceedings of the Society of Perinatal Obstetricians, Twelfth Annual Meeting, 1992. Am J Obstet Gynecol 166:405, 1992

98. Cialone PR, Sherer DM, Ryan RM, Sinkin RA, Abramowicz JS: Amnioinfusion during labor complicated by particulate meconium-stained amniotic fluid decreases neonatal morbidity. Am J Obstet Gynecol 170:842, 1994

99. Spong CY, Ogundipe OA, Ross MG: Prophylactic amnioinfusion for meconium-stained amniotic fluid, abstracted (no. 46). In the Proceedings of the Society of Perinatal Obstetricians, Fourteenth Annual Meeting, 1994. Am J Obstet Gynecol 170:285, 1994

100. Eriksen N, Hostetter M, Parisi V: Prophylactic amnioinfusion in pregnancies complicated by thick meconium, abstracted (no. 246). In the Proceedings of the Society of Perinatal Obstetricians, Fourteenth Annual Meeting, 1994. Am J Obstet Gynecol 170:344, 1994

101. Usta IM, Mercer BM, Aswad NK, Sibai BM: The impact of a policy for meconium-stained amniotic fluid. In the Proceedings of the Society of Perinatal Obstetricians, Fourteenth Annual Meeting, 1994. Am J Obstet Gynecol 170:391, 1994

102. Florman AL, Teubner D: Enhancement of bacterial growth in amniotic fluid by meconium. J Pediatr 74:111, 1969

103. Mandelbrot L, Dommergues M, Dumez Y: Pre-partum transabdominal amnioinfusion for severe oligohydramnios. Acta Obstet Gynecol Scand 71:124, 1992

104. Eglinton GS: The role of external version in modern obstetrics. p. 500. In Phelan JP, Clark SL (eds): Cesarean Delivery. Elsevier Publishers, New York, 1988

105. Inamaka M, Ogita S: New technologies for management of PROM Obstet Gynecol Clin North Am 19(2):365, 1992

106. Blakemore K, Pressman E, McGowan K et al: "Amni-

olyte": a physiologic solution for artificial amniotic fluid, abstracted (no. 194). In the Proceedings of the Society of Perinatal Obstetricians, Thirteenth Annual Meeting, 1993. Am J Obstet Gynecol 168:353, 1993

107. Macri CJ, Schrimmer DB, Greenspoon JS et al: Amnioinfusion does not affect the length of labor. Am J Obstet Gynecol 167:1134, 1992

108. Tabor BL, Maier JA: Polyhydramnios and elevated intrauterine pressure during amnioinfusion. Am J Obstet Gynecol 156:130, 1987

109. Dibble L, Elliott JP: Possible amniotic fluid embolism associated with amnioinfusion. J Matern Fet Med 1: 263, 1992

110. Miyazaki FS: Concern about saline amnioinfusion. Am J Obstet Gynecol 155:227, 1987

111. Wenstrom KD, Andrews WW, Maher JE: Prevalence, protocols and complications associated with amnioinfusion, abstracted (no. 235). In the Proceedings of the Society of Perinatal Obstetricians, Fourteenth Annual Meeting, 1994. Am J Obstet Gynecol 170:341, 1994

112. Strong TH, Howard MJ, Wade BK et al: Intrapartum amnioinfusion in twin gestations: a preliminary report. J Reprod Med 38:397, 1993

113. Strong TH, Vega JS, O'Shaugnessey MJ et al: Amnioinfusion among women attempting vaginal birth after cesarean delivery. Obstet Gynecol 79:673, 1992

114. Cook V, Roy W, Spinnato JA: Amnioinfusion and vaginal birth after cesarean section, abstracted (no. 373). In the Proceedings of the Society of Perinatal Obstetricians, Fourteenth Annual Meeting, 1994. Am J Obstet Gynecol 170:379, 1994

115. Rodriguez MH, Masaki DI, Phelan JP et al: Uterine rupture: are intrauterine pressure catheters useful in the diagnosis? Am J Obstet Gynecol 161:666, 1989

Chapter 24

Scalp Blood pH and Cord Blood Gases

John W. C. Johnson

Much of the energy and financial resources expended by health-care providers in the management of labor and delivery is directed toward preventing hypoxic-acidemic injury to the fetus. Over the years, careful intrapartum fetal management is credited with a decrease in the frequency of fetal acidemia and a concomitant decline in perinatal mortality.[1] To effectively prevent and treat abnormal states of fetal oxygenation, it is important to have a clear understanding of fetal homeostasis and normal acid–base balance.[2–4] A brief review of fetal oxygenation and acid–base physiology introduces this chapter.

BASIC ACID–BASE PHYSIOLOGY

For normal growth and development, the human fetus depends primarily on two substrates: oxygen and glucose. Both are generally available in ample quantity, but acute deficiencies of oxygen are more frequently encountered and pose more serious consequences for the fetus than does an acute deficiency of glucose.

Oxygen is transferred across tissue planes by passive diffusion. Therefore, the oxygen tension within any oxygen supply compartment is the key to transference of oxygen "downstream," or to tissues with lesser oxygen tension. In comparison to the adult, the fetus appears to be significantly disadvantaged.

At sea level, the ambient air has an oxygen partial pressure (PO_2) of 149 mm Hg. After incomplete equilibration and some venous admixture, arterial blood emerges from the maternal heart with a PO_2 of 95 to 100 mm Hg. This high PO_2 ensures adequate oxygen transfer to extravascular adult tissues. But much lower PO_2 driving pressures are available for diffusion to fetal tissues (Fig. 24-1). Uterine arterial blood perfuses the intervillous space (IVS), where venous admixture results in a mean oxygen pressure of approximately 40 mm Hg. From a fetal respiratory standpoint, the IVS is similar to the intra-alveolar space of the adult. An intra-alveolar PO_2 of 40 mm Hg in the adult is equivalent to residence at an altitude of 33,000 feet. This finding prompted Eastman to describe the normal fetal oxygen status as "Mount Everest in Utero."[5] Because of the occurrence of shunting and venous admixture, the oxygenated blood normally perfusing fetal tissues may have PO_2 values ranging from 25 to 35 mm Hg. After equilibrating with fetal tissues, blood returns to the placenta in the umbilical arteries with a PO_2 of about 15 mm Hg.

Fortunately, there are mechanisms that enable the fetus to tolerate momentarily even lower PO_2 values and still continue with normal growth and development. Some of the recognized compensatory mechanisms are (1) increased blood hemoglobin concentrations, which result in a greater capacity to carry

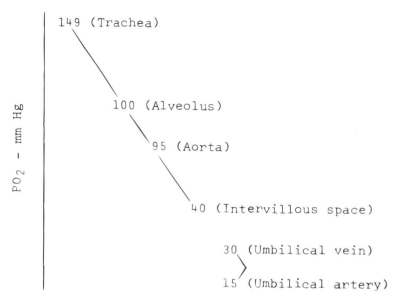

Fig. 24-1. Graphic depiction of change in oxygen partial pressure (PO$_2$) (driving gradient) from maternal inspired air to fetal tissues.

oxygen; (2) increased cardiac output (three times adult cardiac output), which permits an increase in oxygen pickup; (3) a unique red blood cell hemoglobin, hemoglobin F, that facilitates even more oxygen loading in the IVS; and (4) a special vascular circuitry that provides delivery of more oxygenated blood to higher priority tissues (heart and brain).

From the fetal standpoint, the most important determinant of oxygen supply is clearly the delivery of adequate quantities of oxygen to the IVS by the mother. When this fails and the usual compensatory mechanisms are insufficient to provide adequate oxygen, aerobic metabolism (Eq. 1) is followed by anaerobic metabolism (Eq. 2) in fetal tissues.

Aerobic metabolism:
$$C_6H_{12}O_6 \text{ (glucose)} + 6O_2 \leftrightarrows 6CO_2 + 6H_2O$$
$$(1)$$

Anaerobic metabolism (Embden-Meyerhoff pathway):
$$C_6H_{12}O_6 \text{(glucose)} + \text{hypoxemia} \rightarrow \text{lactate}^- + H^+$$
$$(2)$$

The protons (H$^+$) produced by anaerobic metabo-

lism promote acidemia. Severe acidemia may lead to organ malfunction and even death.

Carbon dioxide is a major product of aerobic metabolism. Through the action of erythrocytic carbonic anhydrase, it combines with water to form the weak acid H$_2$CO$_3$:

$$CO_2 + H_2O \rightleftarrows H_2CO_3 \rightleftarrows H^+ + HCO_3^- \quad (3)$$

The principles of acid–base equilibrium describing the interrelationship of carbon dioxide with carbonic acid are best described by the Henderson–Hasselbach equation:

$$pH = pK_1 + \log \frac{[HCO_3^-]}{[S \times PCO_2]} \quad (4)$$

This equation yields the pH of a carbonic acid solution (plasma) with carbon dioxide dissolved in solution, where K_1 is the dissociation constant. The bicarbonate concentration is represented by [HCO$_3^-$] and S is the solubility coefficient for carbon dioxide in plasma. S × PCO$_2$ equals the concentration of dissolved carbon dioxide, which substitutes for the negligible quantity of H$_2$CO$_3$.

Substituting pregnancy values for bicarbonate and carbon dioxide pressure and 6.1 for pK_1 in the Henderson-Hasselbach equation results in

$$pH = 6.1 + \log\frac{21}{(0.3)(35)} \qquad (5)$$
$$pH = 7.4$$

The excess $[H^+]$ ions produced by anerobic metabolism are removed from the system in several ways. The removal of excessive carbon dioxide by diffusion across the placenta to the mother tends to drive the reaction to the left (Eq. 3) away from carbonic acid. Retention of the bicarbonate ion $[HCO_3^-]$ by the fetus also tends to drive the reaction to the left.

Another important method of correcting $[H^+]$ imbalance is the buffer system. Buffers are solutions of weak acids and their salts, which resist the change in pH caused by adding or removing protons. The most important fetal buffers are bicarbonate (plasma) and hemoglobin (erythrocytes), which together constitute 70 percent of the blood's total buffering capacity.

The lactic acid produced by anaerobic metabolism (Eq. 2) can be buffered by the bicarbonate–carbonic acid buffer system as follows:

$$Lactate^- + H^+ + Na^+ + HCO_3^- \leftrightarrows Na\ lactate$$
$$+ H_2CO_3 \qquad (6)$$
$$H_2CO_3 \rightleftarrows h_2O + CO_2$$

$[H^+]$ is removed by conversion to carbonic acid and then to water and carbon dioxide. Carbon dioxide is excreted by diffusion across the placenta to the mother.

The fetus experiencing impaired respiratory gas exchange may demonstrate compensatory cardiovascular reflex mechanisms that appear to ameliorate the effects of hypoxemia and acidemia. These are complex, integrated cardiovascular events that have collectively been designated as the "diving reflex." This series of cardiovascular changes has been shown to occur in diving or breath-holding mammals. Many of these same changes may occur in the human fetus in respiratory stress (i.e., bradycardia) or vasodilation of vital regions (central nervous system, heart, placenta, and adrenals), with a concomitant reduction in the perfusion (vasoconstriction) of less vital areas such as the lung, gastrointestinal tract, kidneys, and limbs. Often, these changes occur in absolutely normal fetuses during normal labor.

Generally speaking, normal labor is characterized by a mild impairment of fetal respiratory gas exchange across the placenta, secondary to uterine contractions. This results in a mildly progressive acidosis in the fetus during labor and at the time of delivery. This is a normal, physiologic response of the fetus to the stresses of labor and delivery. Mean values of pH, PO_2, PCO_2, and base excess for term infants at several different institutions are summarized in Table 24-1.[6–9] It is reassuring to find that

Table 24-1. Vaginal Term Deliveries

	Selected		Unselected	
	Throp et al[6] (n = 1,924)	Yeomans et al[8] (n = 148)	Eskes et al[7] (n = 3,711)	Riley et al[9] (n = 3,522)
UA pH	7.24 (0.07)[a]	7.28 (0.05)	7.23 (0.07)	7.27 (0.07)
UA PO_2	18 (7)	18 (6)	X	18.4 (8)
UA PCO_2	56 (9)	49 (8)	X	50.3 (11)
UA BE	−4 (3)	X	−13 (4)	−2.7 (2.8)
UV pH	7.32 (0.06)	7.35 (0.05)	7.32 (0.07)	7.34 (0.06)
UV PO_2	29 (7)	29 (6)	X	28.5 (8)
UV PCO_2	44 (7)	38 (6)	X	40.7 (8)
UV BE	−3 (2)	X	−6 (3)	−2.4 (2)

Abbreviations: UA, umbilical arterial; UV, umbilical venous; SD, standard deviation; PO_2, partial pressure of oxygen in millimeters of mercury; PCO_2, partial pressure of carbon dioxide in millimeters of mercury; BE, base excess in milliequivalents per liter; X, no data provided.
[a] Mean (± SD).

Table 24-2. Vaginal Preterm Delivery[a,b] (n = 1,015)

UA pH	7.28 (0.09)
UA PO$_2$	19.1
UA PCO$_2$	50.2
UA BE	−2.5
UV pH	7.35 (0.8)
UV PO$_2$	27.9
UV PCO$_2$	41.7
UV BE	−2.1

[a] See Table 24-1 for abbreviations.
[b] Numbers in parentheses are the mean ± SD.
(Adapted from Riley and Johnson,[9] with permission.)

the values from different institutions are so similar. Values for preterm infants have been reported to be similar to those of term infants.[9] (Table 24-2).

FETAL ACIDOSIS

Importance of Detection

In modern obstetric experience, the presence of fetal acidemia is usually a consequence of subnormal fetal respiratory gas exchange. Fetal acidemia is thus a signal that fetal respiratory gas exchange is impaired. The severity of the acidemia is an indication of the extent of the impairment. In the great majority of cases of acidemia, the fetus compensates for and tolerates the stress without demonstrable adverse effects. Occasionally, however, the severity of acidemia is such that organ injury may occur.

Until very recently, a common question asked by obstetricians and neonatologists was "How severe must fetal acidemia be to cause increased mortality and morbidity?" Since then there have been independent studies from three large academic institutions reporting that in term fetuses, there is no increased mortality nor major morbidity until the extent of fetal acidosis reaches an umbilical arterial pH of less than 7.00.[10-12] It is surprising that the healthy term fetus appears to cope so successfully with such severe acidemia. It is extraordinary that three independent studies would identify the same cut off value for meaningful acidosis in the term fetus. One institution has demonstrated that acidosis and injury have a dose–response relationship[11] (Fig 24-2 and 24-3); the more severe the acidemia below a pH of 7.00, the more likely the neonate is to have major organ injury and complications. Among these complications are those involving the central nervous system, cardiovascular system, kidneys, and gastrointestinal system. It is important to cite several caveats with regard to this. First, not all fetuses with umbilical arterial pH values below 7.00 suffer mortality or significant morbidity; at least 50 to 60 percent recovered without major morbidity.[11] Second, the medical care provided at these three academic centers probably was excellent. Other institutions may not be able to provide comparable obstetric, resuscitative, and neonatal expertise and therefore might experience perinatal mortality and major neonatal morbidity at a lesser degree of acidosis. Third, most of the infants observed in these studies

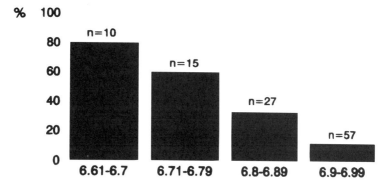

Fig. 24-2. Umbilical arterial pH at delivery and frequency of hypoxic encephalopathy; n = 109. (Data from Goodwin et al.[11])

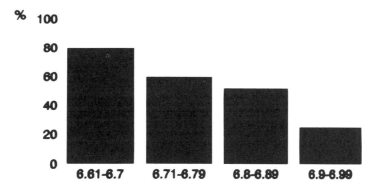

Fig. 24-3. Umbilical arterial pH at delivery and frequency of neonatal cardiac, renal, or pulmonary morbidity; n = 109. (Data from Goodwin et al.[11])

were healthy before the acute intrapartum acidemia. Fetuses chronically stressed before labor (i.e., premature, growth retarded, anomalous) may not tolerate such extreme degrees of acidosis. Finally, whether it is clinically safe and cost effective to withhold delivery until an umbilical arterial pH of 7.00 is reached remains to be confirmed. Lesser degrees of acidosis may be associated with lesser degrees of morbidity, which may result in more costly neonatal care.

Whether fetal acidosis and hypoxemia can cause cerebral palsy is a question of considerable debate.[13] Despite the introduction and implementation of careful fetal monitoring and fetal scalp sampling over the past 20 years in many different countries, the frequency of cerebral palsy has remained essentially unchanged. The frequency of fetal death has decreased strikingly, but there has still been no dramatic improvement in the frequency of cerebral palsy. While there is no obvious explanation for the unchanging frequency of cerebral palsy over the past several decades, it may be that its frequency is increasing among low birth weight infants, many of whom formerly failed to survive the birth process. Perhaps such an increase is negated by a relative decrease in asphyxia-related cerebral palsy occurring in the term infant.

The laboratory and clinical evidence that fetal acidosis and hypoxia may predispose to cerebral palsy is inconclusive. The rhesus studies of Myers[14] demonstrate that partial asphyxia may eventually lead to long-term static lesions that resemble the lesions of cerebral palsy seen in the human infant, but which are not exactly the same. Several institutions have demonstrated that severe acidemia in the term fetus is associated with a higher frequency of neurologic complications, including seizures. Seizures occurring in the newborn infant are generally considered a harbinger of cerebral palsy.[13] Volpe[15] and other pediatric neurologists are convinced that hypoxic ischemic injury sustained by the fetus during the intrapartum period can eventually lead to major neurologic handicaps, including cerebral palsy.

A recent study by Goldenberg and colleagues[16] evaluating the relationship of neonatal complications to neurologic sequelae found that a low cord bicarbonate level, the presence of intraventricular hemorrhage (IVH), and a patent ductus arteriosus were all associated with increased neurologic handicaps, including cerebral palsy. Low and co-workers[17] also demonstrated an increased frequency of central nervous system complications in association with severe fetal metabolic acidosis. Other investigators, however, have failed to demonstrate a similar relationship.[18]

In a careful retrospective case-control study, Richmond et al[19] found that abnormal fetal heart rate (FHR) recordings were identified more frequently in children with subsequent cerebral palsy. After assessing the obstetric management of their patients, the authors concluded that the elimination of suboptimal management of fetal distress might reduce the prevalence of cerebral palsy by 16 percent.

The bulk of evidence indicates that intrapartum hypoxemic acidemia is an infrequent cause of hypoxic encephalopathy. In such cases, the umbilical arterial pH at delivery is expected to be less than 7.00. Both the American College of Obstetricians and Gynecologists (ACOG) and the American Academy of Pediatrics (AAP) have reported that specific criteria must be met before intrapartum hypoxemic acidemia can be considered as the cause of neurologic sequelae.[20,21]

Criteria for the Diagnosis of Severe Fetal Hypoxic Insult

Profound metabolic or mixed acidemia (pH less than 7.00) in an umbilical cord arterial blood sample, if obtained

Persistent Apgar score of 0 to 3 for longer than 5 minutes

Evidence of neonatal neurologic sequelae (e.g., seizures, coma, or hypotonia)

Multiorgan system dysfunction (one or more of the following: cardiovascular, gastrointestinal, hematologic, pulmonary, or renal system)

(Data from refs. 20 and 21.)

It becomes a primary objective of the health-care provider to prevent this degree of severe acidemia from occurring in the fetus. Knowledge of the causes of fetal acidosis and the timely diagnosis of severe fetal acidosis are paramount to the fulfillment of this objective.

Etiology of Fetal Acidemia

Most fetal acidemia detected in modern obstetric care is related to a primary reduction in fetomaternal gas exchange rather than secondary to maternal acidemia. Fetal hypercarbia occurs in conjunction with fetal hypoxemia. The latter leads to an increase in lactic acid and metabolic acidosis.

In simplest terms, fetal respiratory compromise occurs because of one of three abnormalities: (1) inadequate fetal perfusion of the placenta; (2) inadequate maternal perfusion of the placenta; or (3) a reduction in diffusion of respiratory gases across the placenta. Examples of abnormalities causing reduced fetal perfusion of the placenta include umbilical cord occlusion, fetal anemia, and reduced fetal cardiac output (sepsis). Disorders causing abnormalities in the maternal delivery of respiratory gases to the placenta include abnormal maternal blood gas values (maternal hypoxemia or hypercarbia) and reduced placental perfusion (reduced maternal cardiac output, maternal uterine vascular disease, excessive uterine tone). Since the placenta is the organ for respiratory gas exchange between mother and fetus, reduced placental exchange may also compromise the fetus (abruption, multiple infarctions, inflammation, villous edema).

Potential iatrogenic causes of fetal acidemia include excessive oxytocin administration, excessive amnioinfusion, maternal or fetal drug overdose, and drug anaphylaxis. Possible complications related to anesthesia include hypotension secondary to conduction anesthesia and hypoxia or hypercarbia secondary to maternal ventilation problems. Moreover, any combination of these maternal, fetal, and placental problems can coexist, possibly resulting in more severe impairment of fetal respiratory gas exchange than any single factor.

Intrapartum Screening

Whereas normal FHR findings are very reassuring, with a very low false-negative rate, abnormal FHR findings require careful assessment. Often such findings are present in very normal fetuses. The sensitivity of abnormal FHR patterns in revealing fetal acidemia is modest, and the false-positive rate is estimated to be 56 percent[22] (Table 24-3). Important variables contributing to the high false-positive rate include differences in individual fetal responses to stress and differences in the duration and severity of respiratory stress. Of the many changes induced by stress, bradycardia, FHR decelerations, and loss of FHR variability are the main ones that may be detected by electronic or auscultatory monitoring. The variable responsiveness of individual fetuses is not predictable. Therefore, disagreement often exists among maternal-fetal medicine experts about the significance of various electronic fetal monitoring (EFM) findings.[25] This is understandable in view

Table 24-3. Accuracy of Clinical Observations in Diagnosing Fetal Acidosis

Clinical Measure	Sensitivity (%)	Specificity (%)	False-Positive Results (%)	False-Negative Results (%)
Apgar score <7 at 1 minute[a]	46	84	62	12
Apgar <4 at 5 minutes[b]	8	99	73	2
Meconium[b]	31	86	95	2
Abnormal fetal heart rate pattern[a]	62	84	56	9
Severe newborn encephalopathy[b]	24	92	78	7

[a] Fetal acidemia defined as umbilical arterial pH <7.0.[23]
[b] Fetal acidemia defined as umbilical arterial buffer base <34 mmol/L.[24]
(Adapted from Johnson et al,[22] with permission.)

of the often unknown severity and duration of stress and the variable fetal response to it.

Intrapartum Monitoring Observer Variability (Four Obstetricians, 50 Traces)

Intraobserver variability   21%

Interobserver Variability   69%

Accuracy, overall   59%

(Data from Nielsen et al.[25])

The measurement of fetal scalp blood pH appears to be the most accurate method of identifying the fetal implications of abnormal FHR traces.[26–28] Because of the skills and laboratory facilities required to perform fetal scalp blood sampling and pH determination, other methods of fetal assessment have been sought. Clark and Paul[29] reported that FHR acceleration in response to fetal scalp stimulation could be used as a substitute for fetal pH testing. They reported that fetuses with a scalp pH of 7.20 or higher always exhibited FHR accelerations. Even among those fetuses that did not respond to scalp stimulation with accelerations, 61 percent had reassuring scalp pH values. Clark and Paul maintained that fetal scalp blood pH determination remains a valuable clinical tool in select cases, but that its use in clinical practice should be de-emphasized. They concluded that the well-informed clinician could detect fetal distress from the electronic monitor results, and that fetal blood pH studies were needed in only a few cases.

Edersheim[30] reported that fetal vibroacoustic stimulation (VAS) applied to the maternal abdominal surface could be used instead of scalp stimulation to test for fetal reactivity. A positive response was found only in association with a fetal scalp pH over 7.20. Nearly 92 percent of fetuses that failed to register an FHR acceleration were noted to have pH values above 7.20.

Additional studies have now been reported of the effectiveness of VAS in identifying fetuses with a scalp pH of less than 7.20.[31,32] Totaling the results noted among 378 cases subjected to intrapartum VAS in four studies, one finds a sensitivity of 89.2 percent and a specificity of 65.5 percent[30,33–35] (Table 24-4). However, although these studies suggest that VAS might avert the need for fetal scalp blood sampling in 61 percent of cases, they also suggest that 10 percent of acidemic fetuses might be overlooked. The findings are weakened by the fact that only 28 (7.4 percent) of all the fetuses in these four studies were acidemic.

Additional methods studied for the intrapartum assessment of fetal status in conjunction with EFM have included the injection of warm saline via an

Table 24-4. Vibroacoustic Stimulation (VAS) and Fetal pH <7.20 (7.4%)[a]

	pH <7.20	pH ≥7.20	Total
VAS −	25	120	145
VAS +	3	230	233
Total			378

[a] Sensitivity, 89.2%; specificity, 65.5%; positive predictive value, 17.1%; negative predictive value, 98.7%.

intrauterine pressure catheter, and continuous scalp tissue electrode measurement of pH, PO_2, or PCO_2.[36] Doppler studies[37] and tissue temperature studies are also under investigation. At present, none of these techniques has gained acceptance over fetal scalp blood sampling and VAS.

FETAL SCALP BLOOD SAMPLING

Fetal capillary blood pH, as determined by fetal scalp blood sampling, has excellent agreement with arterial pH values[38] (Fig. 24-4). Other measures of fetal respiratory status, such as blood PO_2 or PCO_2, have been studied but do not appear to correlate as well with outcome as does scalp blood pH. Most experts would agree that whenever there is a strong

suspicion of significant fetal respiratory compromise, fetal scalp sampling for pH is helpful. Obvious indications would be repetitive late FHR decelerations or severe variable decelerations that do not respond to corrective measures. Prolonged absence of short-term variability in FHR or a persistent sinusoidal pattern are generally also considered indications for fetal pH assessment. Patterns that are unusual and difficult to interpret should also be considered as indicating the possible need for scalp pH determination.

In the case of persistent late decelerations or severe variable decelerations, the pH should be reassessed every 20 to 40 minutes, depending on the FHR pattern and the expected time of delivery. If the pH is found to be 7.20 or less, delivery is indicated. A fetal pH that is observed to decline below a value of 7.00 will be associated with a significantly increased risk of perinatal death or infant morbidity.[10-12] The scalp pH value indicating the need for intervention has been set at the higher value of 7.20. In view of the recent establishment of a fetal pH of 7.00 as the cutoff for adverse outcome, it has been suggested that the scalp pH cutoff value could be set below 7.20. However, time must be allowed to prepare the patient for operative delivery and to provide suitable anesthesia. The leeway provided by the scalp pH cutoff value of 7.20 seems to have worked well in reducing the number of infants ultimately born with a pH of 7.00. Any change in this 7.20 cutoff should be carefully studied and documented as safe before being implemented.

Artifactual alterations in pH are possible and must be considered. As mentioned previously, primary maternal alkalosis (hyperventilation) or acidosis may cause spurious fetal scalp pH values. On the rare occasion when maternal acid–base derangement is suspected (maternal seizures, dehydration, sepsis, hyperventilation), it can be confirmed by ascertaining that the pH of a free-flowing maternal venous blood sample (obtained without a tourniquet) is within 0.1 pH units of the fetal scalp blood pH.[39] Larger pH differences between mother and fetus are indicative of primary fetal acid–base derangements.

Fetal blood sampling should not be done when the mother has genital herpetic infection or human immunodeficiency virus (HIV) infection, or when the

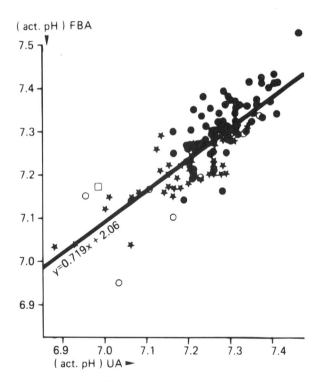

Fig. 24-4. Coefficient of correlation between fetal scalp sample pH in second stage and umbilical arterial pH at delivery was r = 0.82. Closed circles, spontaneous delivery (n = 72); stars, vacuum extraction (n = 37); open circles, vaginal delivery from breech presentation (n = 9); open squares, cesarean section (n = 1). (From Boenisch and Saling,[38] with permission)

fetus has a suspected blood dyscrasia (such as Von Willebrand's disease or hemophilia).

Technique

The technique of fetal scalp sampling for pH was introduced by Saling[40] in 1967. If the cervix is dilated to at least several centimeters, the vertex is well applied to the cervix, and the membranes are ruptured, the patient may be a suitable candidate for fetal scalp blood sampling.[1] The mother is placed in the lithotomy position or in the Sims position. A lighted endoscope is inserted through the cervix and applied snugly to the fetal scalp. The fetal scalp is prepared with an antiseptic solution and silicone gel is then applied to the scalp, since this facilitates parting the hair and makes the fetal skin more accessible. At this point a 2-mm special blade is used to incise the skin, and as blood forms on the skin surface it is collected immediately in a heparinized glass capillary tube. The silicone gel also aggregates the blood into a large droplet, which aids sample collection. Standard clinical laboratory techniques are used to assess the pH of the sample. Repeated samples are obtained at each sampling session so that duplicate determinations are possible. Sampling from the fetal buttocks in the case of breech presentation has also been reported to be satisfactorily performed. In general, a fetal scalp blood pH of 7.20 or less warrants prompt delivery.

It is important to observe the site of scalp sampling carefully during several contractions, to be sure that there is no persistent bleeding. There have been reported cases of significant fetal hemorrhage from scalp sampling. Other complications related to scalp sampling include infection and neonatal bleeding. Worrisome bleeding may also be encountered when vacuum extraction delivery is used in infants who have had scalp sampling.

UMBILICAL BLOOD ACID–BASE STUDIES

The arguments for routine umbilical blood acid–base studies at delivery have been previously enumerated.[6,22,41] It is clear that such studies provide the most accurate method for quantifying an infant's acid–base status at delivery. It is well documented that the Apgar score, the presence of abnormal FHR patterns, and the presence of meconium staining are poor clinical proxies for fetal acidosis, yielding high false-positive rates (Table 24-3). When umbilical blood acid–base studies have been done routinely, they have permitted determination of the extent to which fetal acidemia is associated with adverse long-term outcomes. As noted above, there have been three large studies demonstrating that a pH value below 7.00 is associated with a significant increase in perinatal complications.[10–12] Similar cutoff values need to be determined for infants born prematurely.[42,43]

Umbilical blood acid–base studies can also serve as objective, scientific measures of the efficacy of various antepartum and intrapartum interventions designed to improve fetal outcome. Moreover, umbilical blood acid–base studies provide indications of the mechanisms responsible for acidosis.[44,45] Both experimental and clinical evidence indicates that a comparison of pH values in the umbilical artery and umbilical vein can be used to determine whether fetal acidemia is due primarily to reduced fetoplacental perfusion or reduced maternoplacental perfusion. In general, large gradients are seen with impaired fetoplacental perfusion, as demonstrated in a case of acute cord prolapse (Table 24-5). The large differences in the blood pH values for the two vessels also demonstrate the importance of being sure that an umbilical arterial sample is obtained in assessing the fetus. Should an umbilical venous sample be obtained rather than an umbilical arterial sample, the acid–base status of the fetus could be misjudged. Small differences between umbilical arterial and ve-

Table 24-5. Cord Blood Values in Umbilical Cord Prolapse

	Umbilical Artery	Umbilical Vein
pH	6.85^a	7.31
PCO_2 (mm Hg)	113^a	50
PO_2 (mm Hg)	19	23
HCO_3^- (mEq/L)	18.8^a	24.3
BE (mEq/L)	-12.5^a	-0.7
Oxygen saturation (%)	9^a	33.1
Oxygen content (vol%)	1.5^a	5.4

Abbreviations: PCO_2, partial pressure of carbon dioxide; PO_2, partial pressure of oxygen; HCO_3 bicarbonate; BE, base excess.
^{a} Beyond 2 SD from mean value.

nous blood are more indicative of reduced maternal perfusion of the placenta.

Two of the most common arguments against cord blood gas analyses are that they are costly and that abnormal values could place the obstetrician at risk of litigation. In today's climate of hospital cost setting, most laboratory units charge sums well above the actual expense. True costs for cord blood gas analysis are estimated to be in the $5 to $15 range, but charges range from $20.00 to $150.00 per analysis. There is good reason to expect that cord blood gas studies might fend off litigation in cases of maloccurrence (personal communication, Huddleston J, Emory University; and Yun H, Jersey City Medical Center). Studies indicate that 85 percent of cases of cerebral palsy are associated with normal 5-minute Apgar scores.[46] Although abnormal fetal monitoring traces may be seen in such cases, umbilical blood acid–base studies can best substantiate appropriate intrapartum care. The money saved by the prevention of one major award could pay for cord blood gas analyses in 70,000 to 100,000 deliveries.[22] What about the medicolegal risks of abnormal cord blood values? The occurrence of significant fetal acidemia (pH <7.00) at term delivery is generally quite rare, occurring in approximately 0.2 to 0.3 percent of cases.[11] Even if such a low pH was unexpectedly discovered at delivery, current opinion indicates that severe umbilical blood acidemia is not sufficient in itself to make the diagnosis of significant hypoxic insult; the clinical findings must also be compatible.[21,47] By contrast, failure to obtain an umbilical blood pH value would not preclude the diagnosis of intrapartum hypoxic encephalopathy if the neonatal clinical findings and neonatal intensive care pH findings were abnormal. Other, more likely causes of such findings would be antepartal or neonatal complications that might be difficult to differentiate from intrapartum complications without reassuring cord blood values. It is important to emphasize that at least 85 to 90 percent of all cerebral palsy cases are not thought to be related to intrapartum problems. Currently, the best means available to exclude intrapartum causation is the documentation of a normal umbilical arterial pH value. There is little to lose and much to be gained by scientific documentation of fetal status with umbilical blood acid–base studies at delivery. It is believed that umbilical blood acid-

Table 24-6. Frequency of Cord Blood Analysis Among 143 Academic Centers

Frequency (% Deliveries)	United States (%)	Canada (%)
<25	39.8	40.1
25–50	23.4	13.3
51–75	10.2	13.3
>75	26.6	33.3

(Adapted from Johnson and Riley,[48] with permission.)

base studies will be more helpful than harmful to obstetricians. In a 1992 survey of academic centers, the majority response was one of approval for cord blood studies.[48] All 128 of the responding academic centers used cord blood analysis at some deliveries. Thirty-five percent applied these studies to over half of their deliveries (Table 24-6).

Technique

Immediately on delivery of the infant, a segment of cord approximately 15 to 30 cm long should be doubly clamped. To ensure good vessel filling, one should clamp the cord close to the infant and then strip (milk) the cord from the placenta toward that first clamp. Subsequently, a second clamp is placed 10 to 35 cm distal to the first clamp. The samples are collected in prelabeled and preheparinized syringes, with care taken to exclude air bubbles. The samples are then taken to the laboratory for prompt analysis, and the results are posted in the patient's chart.

The specific details of and recommendations for collection of cord blood gas samples have been described in several previous publications.[9,44] Collecting samples from both umbilical vessels is important. It assures that the umbilical arterial pH has been obtained, which is the most accurate measure of fetal pH. If the umbilical venous sample is the only one obtained, it may not be sufficiently accurate to extrapolate to the fetal acid-base status. Obtaining both an umbilical arterial and venous sample may also help in determining the cause of fetal acidemia (poor fetal or poor maternal perfusion of the placenta).

Obtaining the umbilical arterial sample is not always easy because of small vessels, poorly filled vessels, a short cord, excessive Wharton's jelly, and other technical problems. In a recent study of umbilical arterial sampling by experienced personnel, errors in sampling technique were found in 8 to 10 percent of cases.[9] Cord arterial and venous samples may be augmented by placental vessel sampling if the latter is done shortly after delivery.

UNIVERSITY OF FLORIDA PROTOCOL

In the Labor and Delivery Unit of the University of Florida Medical Center, fetal scalp blood sampling for pH assessment is used on a liberal basis. Approximately 4 to 6 percent of patients have such sampling done during the course of labor management. The sampling is done in cases of nonreassuring FHR characteristics that do not respond to the usual supportive measures. This includes bradycardia, persistent severe variable decelerations, persistent late decelerations, persistent loss of beat-to-beat variability, and FHR monitor tracings of puzzling configuration. If the fetal scalp blood sample has a pH below 7.20, delivery is expedited.

In addition to these policies relating to fetal scalp blood sampling umbilical cord arterial and venous blood samples are routinely obtained for blood gas analyses at the time of every delivery. All fetal scalp blood pH determinations and cord blood acid–base determinations are posted in the mother's chart. The pressures of managed care competition may require alterations in these current policies.

CONTROVERSIES

Necessity of Fetal Scalp Blood Sampling

Most authorities would agree that the prevention of severe fetal acidemia during labor and delivery is one of the most important goals of intrapartum ob-

stetric care. Today, the presence of fetal acidemia during labor is most accurately determined by fetal scalp blood pH determination. Even though the procedure has faults and a few risks, it is the "gold standard" for quantifying intrapartum fetal acidemia.

The major obstetric texts in the United States,[1,3,4] and ACOG Technical Bulletin No. 127 on the assessment of fetal and newborn acid-base status,[47] describe fetal scalp blood pH determinations and indicate that it is a useful procedure in reducing the complications of fetal acidemia. British and Scandinavian reports maintain that scalp blood testing is also an important means of reducing the cesarean section rate. Grant,[49] in a meta-analysis of prospective studies (although not directly comparative studies), found that EFM with fetal scalp blood sampling for pH was associated with a 52 percent reduction in the risk of cesarean section over EFM without scalp blood sampling (Figs. 24-5 and 24-6).

Nielsen et al,[57] in a retrospective review of national data, concluded that the reduction of the annual cesarean section rate to 10.8 percent in Sweden in 1990 could be ascribed in large part to the widespread use of scalp blood sampling for pH during labor. It is generally agreed that scalp blood sampling for pH improves both the sensitivity and specificity of FHR monitoring.[49]

By contrast, Goodwin,[58] Clark[59] and others have concluded from retrospective studies that fetal scalp blood sampling for pH determination is not needed to maintain a low cesarean section rate or a low frequency of perinatal asphyxial complications. These authors have suggested that such sampling has little

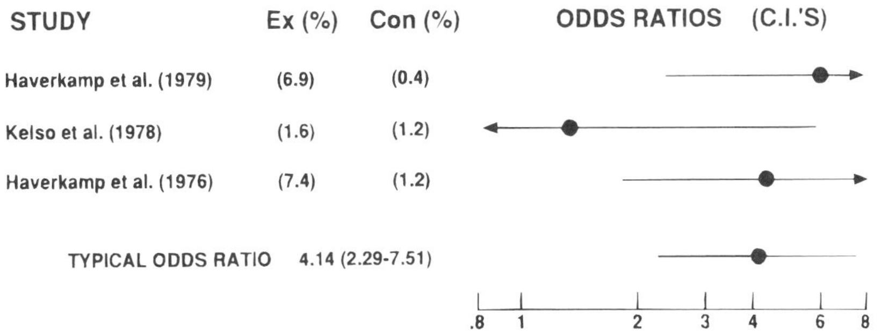

Fig. 24-5. Meta-analyses of electronic fetal monitoring without fetal scalp blood pH study (Ex) versus intermittent auscultation (Con) and cesarean section rates for fetal distress. C.I.'s, confidence intervals. (Data from Haverkamp et al[50,51] and Kelso et al.[50,51] and Kelso et al.[52]) (Adapted from Grant,[49] with permission.)

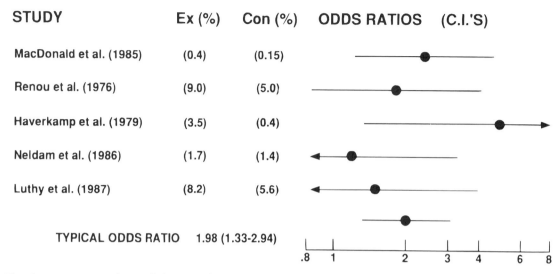

Fig. 24-6. Meta-analyses of electronic fetal monitoring with fetal scalp blood pH study (Ex) versus intermittent auscultation (Con) and cesarean section rates for fetal distress. C.I.'s confidence intervals. (Data from MacDonald et al,[53] Renou, et al,[54] Haverkamp et al,[51] Neldam et al,[55] and Luthy.[56]) (Adapted from Grant,[49] with permission.)

utility in current intrapartum management, provided that clinicians are well informed about the reassuring and nonreassuring aspects of fetal monitor tracing characteristics, including the response to fetal stimulation. They cite a number of clinical reports suggesting that the response to fetal stimulation (either scalp stimulation or VAS) can be used as a proxy for scalp blood sampling for pH determination. Most studies have reported that fetal reactivity signifies a fetal pH of 7.20 or higher. Failure of the fetus to react to stimulation may or may not signify a pH below 7.20. The large, prospective randomized studies that would permit the conclusion that fetal scalp blood sampling for pH determination and fetal stimulation are equivalent or that one is better than the other as a method of fetal assessment have not been done. Fetal scalp sampling for pH determination must be considered the gold standard for intrapartum assessment until additional studies are done to verify the validity of fetal stimulation studies.

In the circumstance in which fetal scalp blood sampling cannot be done, the clinician should use either the VAS or scalp stimulation test as recommended.[29,58] In circumstances of persistent FHR abnormalities in which the fetus fails to respond to stimulation, the clinician should resort to expedient delivery, as also recommended.[29,58]

Necessity of Umbilical Arterial Acid–Base Analysis for Every Delivery

It has been estimated that in the United States, approximately $500 is spent per obstetric patient to prevent the occurrence of severe fetal acidemia.[22] If one accepts the dictum that the prevention of fetal acidemia is a major objective of obstetric management, then assessing the extent of acidemia experienced by each fetus up to the time of delivery is important in documenting how effectively one has met that goal. Cord acid–base studies are an important measure of the quality of such obstetric care. Also, this accurate and objective assessment of fetal acid–base status provides important clinical information to the obstetrician, pediatrician, and anesthesiologist.[22,60] Despite certain known limitations of these studies, they seem to be highly regarded within North American academic centers in terms of their clinical and medicolegal benefits and cost effectiveness[48] (Fig. 24-7). One very recent example of the benefits of routine cord blood pH studies is the determination among term fetuses of the umbilical artery pH cutoff value consistent with fetal hypoxic injury. Three separate centers have ascertained that umbilical artery pH values must be less than 7.00 before hypoxic consequences are aggravated in the

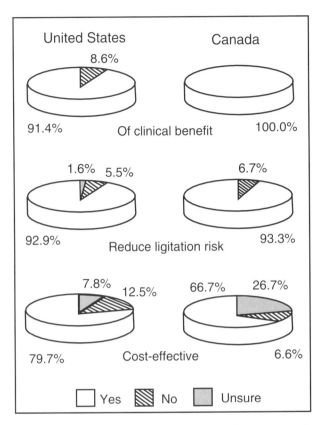

Fig. 24-7. Results of a questionnnaire to chairpersons of academic Obstetric and Gynecology departments of North America concerning attitudes about umbilical cord blood acid—base studies. (From Johnson and Riley,[48] with permission.)

Rather, such values describe the type and extent of respiratory compromise experienced by that fetus in labor and delivery. The corresponding values for all or most deliveries serve as an excellent measure of the overall quality of intrapartum care. Over time, this feedback may be expected to improve the quality of care. Cord acid–base values for a given case may also reduce the risk of litigation in the event of a poor neonatal or infant outcome. The recent ACOG Committee Opinion on the utility of umbilical cord blood acid–base assessment[63] suggested that umbilical cord segments be collected after each delivery, but that they be used for blood pH analysis only if a serious abnormality arises in the delivery process or there is a serious neonatal problem persisting beyond the first 5 minutes after delivery. Although this may be considered a cost-effective approach to the utility of cord blood gas analysis, it fails to provide important follow-up information about the obstetric care of those neonates who do not have cord blood studies. The cost of cord blood acid–base analysis seems to be worth the quality assessment of any obstetric management that is provided. Also, it is important to consider that 85 percent of infants who ultimately develop cerebral palsy are reported to have normal Apgar scores at 5 minutes.[46] From a medicolegal standpoint, failure to document a normal acid–base status at delivery could prove expensive. Additional large studies would assist in determining the overall cost-effectiveness of umbilical cord blood acid–base studies.

term neonate.[10–12] This is probably one of the most important advances in decades in terms of understanding fetal oxygen needs and acid–base physiology. It will have important implications in the diagnosis and management of fetal intrapartum status.

However, not all obstetric units may find it appropriate to provide the resources for such studies in all deliveries. A number of authorities would agree that this is acceptable.[61,62] Perkins and co-workeres,[62] in a retrospective analysis of 3,807 deliveries, of which 3,365 had cord blood acid–base studies, concluded that routine cord blood pH sampling at delivery was not cost effective. Cord blood acid–base studies done at delivery are not expected to improve the outcome of the obstetric care just provided.

REFERENCES

1. Petri RH: Intrapartum fetal evaluation. p. 457. In Gabbe SG, Niebyl JR, Simpson JL (eds): Obstetrics: Normal and Problem Pregnancies. 2nd Ed. Churchill Livingstone, New York, 1991
2. Blechner JN: Maternal-fetal acid-base physiology. Clin Obstet Gynecol 36:3, 1993
3. Boylan PB, Parisi VM: Fetal acid-base balance. p. 349. In Creasy RK, Resnik R (eds): Maternal-Fetal Medicine. 3rd Ed. WB Saunders, Philadelphia, 1994
4. Gilstrap LC, Cunningham GF: Umbilical cord blood acid-base analysis. In: Williams Obstetrics. 19th Ed. (Suppl 4). Appleton & Lange, E. Norwalk, CT. Dec 1993/Jan 1994
5. Eastman NJ: Mount Everest in utero. President's Address. Am J Obstet Gynecol 67:701, 1954

6. Thorp JA, Sampson JE, Parisi VM et al: Routine umbilical cord blood gas determinations? Am J Obstet Gynecol 161:600, 1989

7. Eskes TK, Jongsma HW, Houx PC: Percentiles for gas values in human umbilical cord blood. Euro J Obstet Gynecol Reprod Biol 14:341, 1983

8. Yeomans ER, Hauth JC, Gilstrap LC et al: Umbilical cord pH, pCO_2, and bicarb following uncomplicated term vaginal deliveries. Am J Obstet Gynecol 151:798, 1985

9. Riley WJ, Johnson JWC: Collecting and analyzing cord blood gases. Clin Obstet Gynecol 36:13, 1993

10. Goldaber KG, Gilstrap LC, Leveno KJ et al: Pathologic fetal acidemia. Obstet Gynecol 78:1103, 1991

11. Goodwin TM, Belai I, Hernandez P et al: Asphyxial complications in the term newborn with severe umbilical acidemia. Am J Obstet Gynecol 167:1506, 1992

12. Winkler CL, Haugh JC, Tucker JM et al: Neonatal complications at term as related to the degree of umbilical artery acidemia. Am J Obstet Gynecol 164:637, 1991

13. Nelson KB, Ellenbereg JH: Antecedents of cerebral palsy. N Engl J Med 315:81, 1986

14. Myers RE: Two patterns of perinatal brain damage and their conditions of occurrence. Am J Obstet Gynecol 112:246, 1972

15. Volpe JJ: Neurology of the Newborn. 2nd Ed. WB Saunders, Philadelphia, 1987

16. Goldenberg R, Gaudier F, Nelson K et al: The relationship of maternal and neonatal characteristics to major handicap $\geq$ one year of age. Am J Obstet Gynecol 170:372, 1994

17. Low JA, Panagiotopoulos C, Derrick EJ: Newborn complications after intrapartum asphyxia with metabolic acidosis in the term fetus. Am J Obstet Gynecol 170:1081, 1994

18. Socol ML, Garcia PM, Riter S: Depressed apgar scores, acid-base status, and neurologic outcome. Am J Obstet Gynecol 170:991, 1994

19. Richmond S, Niswander K, Snodgrass A, Wagstaff I: The obtetric management of fetal distress and its association with cerebral palsy. Obstet Gynecol 83:643, 1994

20. Fetal distress and birth asphyxia. Committee Opinion No. 137. American College of Obstetricians and Gynecologists, Washington, DC, 1994

21. Guidelines for Prenatal Care. 3rd Ed. American Academy of Pediatrics, Elk Grove Village, IL; American College of Obstetricians and Gynecologists Washington, DC, 1992

22. Johnson JWC, Richards DS, Wagaman RA: The case for routine umbilical blood acid-base studies at delivery. Am J Obstet Gynecol 162:621, 1990

23. Page FO, Martin JN, Palmer SM et al: Correlation of neonatal acid-base status with Apgar scores and fetal heart rate tracings. Am J Obstet Gynecol 154:1306, 1986

24. Low JA: The role of blood gas and acid-base assessment in the diagnosis of intrapartum fetal asphyxia. Am J Obstet Gynecol 159:1235, 1988

25. Nielsen PV, Stigsby B, Nickelsen C, Nim J: Intra- and inter-observer variability in the assessment of intrapartum cardiotocograms. Acta Obstet Gynecol Scand 66:421, 1987

26. Adamsons K, Beard RW, Cosmi EV et al: The validity of capillary blood in the assessment of the acid-base state of the fetus. p. 175. In Adamsons K (ed): Diagnosis and Treatment of Fetal Disorders. Springer-Verlag, New York, 1968

27. Bowe ET, Beard RT, Finster M et al: Reliability of fetal blood sampling. Am J Obstet Gynecol 107:279, 1970

28. Zalar RW, Quilligan EJ: The influence of scalp sampling on the cesarean section rate for fetal distress. Am J Obstet Gynecol 135:239, 1979

29. Clark SL, Paul RH: Intrapartum fetal surveillance: the role of fetal scalp sampling. Am J Obstet Gynecol 153:717, 1985

30. Edersheim TG, Hutson JM, Druzin ML, Kogut EA: Fetal heart rate response to vibratory acoustic stimulation predicts fetal pH in labor. Am J Obstet Gynecol 157:1557, 1987

31. Richards DS, Cefalo RC, Thorpe JM et al: Determinants of fetal heart rate response to vibroacoustic stimulation in labor. Obstet Gynecol 71:535, 1988

32. Anyaegbunam AM, Ditchik A, Stoessel R, Mikhail MS: Vibroacoustic stimulation of the fetus entering the second stage of labor. Obstet Gynecol 83:963, 1994

33. Ingermarsson I, Arulkumaran S: Reactive fetal heart rate response to vibroacoustic stimulation in fetuses with low scalp blood pH. Br J Obstet Gynecol 96:562, 1989

34. Polzin GB, Blakemore KJ, Petrie RH, Amon E: Fetal vibro-acoustic stimulation: magnitude and duration of fetal heart rate accelerations as a marker of fetal health. Obstet Gynecol 72:621, 1988

35. Umstad M, Bailey C, Permezel M: Intrapartum fetal stimulation testing. Aust NZ J Obstet Gynaecol 32:222, 1992

36. Boos R, Ruttgers H, Muliawan D et al: Continuous measurement of tissue pH in the human fetus. Arch Gynecol 226:183, 1978

37. Fairlie FM, Lang GD, Sheldon CD: Umbilical artery

flow velocity waveforms in labour. Br J Obstet Gynaecol 96:151, 1989

38. Boenisch H, Saling E: The reliability of pH-values in fetal blood samples: a study of the second stage. J Perinat Med 4:45, 1976

39. Bowen LW, Kochenour NK, Rehm NE, Woolley FR: Maternal-fetal pH difference and fetal scalp pH as predictors of neonatal outcome. Obstet Gynecol 67:487, 1986

39. Saling E, Schneider D: Biochemical supervision of the foetus during labour. J Obstet Gynecol Br Commonw 74:799, 1967

41. Richards DS, Johnson JWC: The practical implications of cord blood acid-base studies. Clin Obstet Gynecol 36:91, 1993

42. Behnke M, Eyler FD, Conlon M et al: The relationship between umbilical cord and infant blood gases and developmental outcome in very low birth weight infants. Clin Obstet Gynecol 36:73, 1993

43. Dickinson JE, Eriksen NL, Meyer BA et al: The effect of preterm birth on umbilical cord blood gases. Obstet Gynecol 79:575, 1992

44. Boesel RR, Olson AE, Johnson JWC: Umbilical cord blood studies help assess fetal respiratory status. Contemp Obstet Gynecol 28:63, 1986

45. Gordon A, Johnson JWC: Value of umbilical blood acid-base studies in fetal assessment. J Reprod Med 30:329, 1985

46. Freeman JM, Nelson KG: Intrapartum asphyxia and cerebral palsy. Special articles. Pediatrics 82:240, 1988

47. Assessment of fetal and newborn acid-base status. Technical Bulletin No. 127. American College of Obstetricians and Gynecologists, Washington, DC, 1989

48. Johnson JWC, Riley WJ: Cord blood gas studies: a survey. Clin Obstet Gynecol 36:99, 1993

49. Grant A: Monitoring the fetus during labour. p. 846. In Chalmers I, Enkin M, Keirse MJNC (eds): Effective Care in Pregnancy and Childbirth. Oxford University Press, New York, 1989

50. Haverkamp AD, Thompson HE, McFee JG, Cetrulo C. The evaluation of continuous fetal heart rate monitoring in high-risk pregnancy. Am J Obstet Gynecol 125:310, 1976

51. Haverkamp AD, Orleans M, Langendoerfer S et al: A controlled trial of the differential effects of intrapartum fetal monitoring. Am J Obstet Gynecol 134:399, 1979

52. Kelso IM, Parsons RJ, Lawrence GF et al: An assessment of continuous fetal heart rate monitoring in labor—a randomised trial. Am J Obstet Gynecol 131:526, 1978

53. MacDonald D, Grant A, Sheridan-Pereira M et al: The Dublin randomised trial of intrapartum fetal heart monitoring. Am J Obstet Gynecol 152:524, 1985

54. Renou P, Chang A, Anderson I, Wood C: Controlled trial of fetal intensive care. Am J Obstet Gynecol 126:470, 1976

55. Neldam S, Osler M, Hansen PK et al: Intrapartum fetal heart rate monitoring in a combined low- and high-risk population: a controlled clinical trial. Eur J Obstet Gynecol Reprod Biol 23:1, 1986

56. Luthy DA, Shy KK, van Belle G et al: A randomised trial of electronic fetal monitoring in preterm labor. Obstet Gynecol 69:687, 1987

57. Nielsen TF, Olausson PO, Ingemarsson I: The cesarean section rate in Sweden: the end of the rise. Birth 21:34, 1994

58. Goodwin TM, Milner-Masterson L, Paul RH: Elimination of fetal scalp blood sampling on a large clinical service. Obstet Gynecol 83:971, 1994

59. Clark SL, Gimovsky ML, Miller FC: The scalp stimulation test: a clinical alternative to fetal scalp blood sampling. Am J Obstet Gynecol 148:274, 1984

60. Goldaber KG, Gilstrap LC: Correlations between obstetric clinical events and umbilical cord blood acid-base and blood gas values. Clin Obstet Gynecol 36:47, 1993

61. Goodlin RC, Freedman WL, MDFee JG, Winter SD: The neonate with unexpected acidemia. J Reprod Med 39:97, 1994

62. Perkins RP, Weaver PA, Sweeney WJ: Questioning the practice of routine umbilical cord blood pH sampling at delivery. J Matern Fet Med 2:191, 1993

63. Utility of umbilical cord blood acid-base assessment. Committee opinion No. 138. American College of Obstetricians and Gynecologists, Washington, DC, 1994

Chapter 25

Active Management of Labor

Ellice Lieberman and Fredric D. Frigoletto, Jr.

Active management, a standardized method of labor management, was introduced during the 1960s at the National Maternity Hospital in Dublin, Ireland[1] to shorten the length of labor in nulliparous women. The humanitarian motivation underlying its implementation is clear from the first publication on the subject by O'Driscoll et al[1] in 1969, which began with the following statement:

> Prolonged labor presents a picture of mental anguish and physical morbidity which often leads to surgical intervention and may produce a permanent revulsion to childbirth. . . . The harrowing experience is shared by relatives, and by doctors and nurses to the extent that few complications so tarnish the image of obstetrics.

The name *active management of labor* was chosen for the practice because its proponents asserted that for shorter labors to be achieved, the obstetrician needed to become an active director controlling the course of labor, rather than being a passive observer "waiting in the hope that it may conclude within a reasonable period of time."[2] The active role of the obstetrician was defined to include the careful diagnosis of labor and subsequent constant monitoring of its progress, with prompt intervention according to standard principles in the case of unsatisfactory progress.[1,2] As measured by the duration of labor,

the program at the National Maternity Hospital has been successful; nearly all nulliparous women deliver within 12 hours of admission.[3]

O'Driscoll et al also maintain that standardization of practice is an essential prerequisite to maximizing the quality of care provided to patients.[3] Active management therefore provides specific guidelines for the management of all aspects of normal labor. Criteria exist for the diagnosis of labor, monitoring and management of its progress, and indications for cesarean section. The type of nursing care that patients will receive is also spelled out. All these principles are also incorporated into childbirth classes so that women will understand the process that awaits them once labor begins.

As practiced at the National Maternity Hospital, active management of labor is also very standardized with regard to the responsibilities of specific personnel. Each member of the care-giving team has a precise role to fulfill, and a clear chain of command exists.[3,4] At any given time there is a single nurse-midwife in charge of the labor unit. The midwife in charge is responsible for the management of all aspects of normal labor and delivery; staff midwives act as her personal assistants and she also supervises resident physicians. The midwife in charge consults with senior physicians as needed.

In a 1983 publication, O'Driscoll et al[5] observed that from 1965 to 1980, the cesarean section rate in the United States rose from less than 5 percent to over 15 percent, while during that same period the cesarean delivery rate at the National Maternity Hospital remained stable at under 5 percent. Given this, they suggested the use of active management to safely reduce the number of cesarean deliveries in the United States.[5,6] There has been considerable debate surrounding the safety and potential efficacy of such a protocol as a means of reducing the rate of cesarean delivery in the United States. This chapter reviews the basic tenets of the protocol for the active management of labor as practiced at the National Maternity Hospital, and then reviews the evidence for and against its safety and efficacy as a means of reducing the cesarean section rate.

ACTIVE MANAGEMENT PRINCIPLES

Population

Data on the active management of labor from the National Maternity Hospital are generally limited to the population of women who are nulliparous with a singleton infant in a cephalic presentation, and who have had a spontaneous onset of labor. This method of reporting reflects three clear distinctions about labor at the National Maternity Hospital:

1. The dissimilarity between nulliparous and multiparous labor: nulliparous labor tends to be longer and more subject to failure to progress. In addition, the practices involved in active management assume that the nulligravid uterus is virtually immune to rupture (except as a result of manipulation) regardless of the dose of oxytocin used[3]
2. The difference between induced labor and labor of spontaneous onset: specifically, induced labor tends to be longer and the risk of cesarean section higher[3]
3. The distinction between the management of normal labor and treatment of obstetric abnormalities such as malposition: for the purposes of labor management, multiple pregnancies are included as obstetric abnormalities and are not subject to active management[3]

Protocol Components

Active management of labor can be thought of as having three main components: (1) criteria for the diagnosis of labor, (2) methods of labor manage-

ment, and (3) one-to-one nursing care. In addition to the aspects of active management that occur during labor, childbirth education is considered a vital part of the active management approach. The principles of active management presented below are applied only to nulliparous women in spontaneous labor with singleton infants in a cephalic presentation, who have no obstetric abnormalities.

Diagnosis

At the National Maternity Hospital, the determination of whether a woman is in labor is made by the nurse-midwife in charge, and must be made within 1 hour of admission to the labor unit. Painful uterine contractions alone do not provide sufficient evidence to justify a diagnosis of labor. The diagnosis of labor is made only when such contractions are accompanied by bloody show, rupture of the membranes, or full cervical effacement.[3,6] As a precaution, women presenting at the labor unit who do not meet these criteria are admitted to the antenatal ward until the next day, at which time they are discharged if labor has not begun.[3]

The correct diagnosis of labor is considered to be the single most important determination in the conduct of labor, as an incorrect diagnosis will lead to inappropriate treatment. Accepting the diagnosis of labor in a woman in whom labor has not begun will result in an increased likelihood of her requiring a cesarean section. By contrast, if the diagnosis of labor is rejected for a woman actually in labor, the error will become apparent. Such an error will present no problem to the mother so long as she has been admitted to the hospital for observation.[3]

Management

Rupture of Membranes

The membranes are artificially ruptured 1 hour after the diagnosis of labor is made,[3] to permit assessment of the quantity of fluid and the presence of meconium. A normal volume of clear amniotic fluid indicates that fetal distress is unlikely, assuming that delivery occurs within a reasonable period and that no labor complications (such as placental abruption or cord prolapse) occur.[4] Rupture of the membranes itself may accelerate labor and must be performed before treatment with oxytocin, which is administered only in the presence of clear amniotic fluid.[3]

Progress During the First Stage of Labor

Early progress in labor is carefully monitored. After admission, pelvic examinations are performed at intervals of 1 hour for the first 3 hours. Subsequent examinations are performed at intervals of no longer than 2 hours. Whenever possible, all examinations should be performed by a single individual, to minimize interobserver variation in measurement.[3]

Satisfactory progress in the first stage of labor is assessed solely on the basis of advancement of cervical dilatation, which is recorded on a partogram[6] (Fig. 25-1). Dilatation is expected to proceed at a rate of at least 1 cm/hr once the membranes have been ruptured.[4] In the nulliparous patient, slower progress is most often the result of inefficient uterine action.[3] In the absence of medical contraindications, labor that fails to progress at the foregoing rate is treated with oxytocin according to the regimen described below.

Progress During the Second Stage of Labor

During the second stage of labor, progress is measured by fetal descent and rotation.[6] This stage of labor is divided into two phases. The first phase is the time from full dilatation until the fetal head reaches the pelvic floor; the second phase extends from the head reaching the pelvic floor to delivery of the infant.[3] The first phase of the second stage (descent) is viewed as a natural extension of the first stage of labor. Its onset is liable to go unnoticed unless a vaginal examination happens to be performed. If the fetal head is high in the pelvis, the woman who has no urge to push should not be encouraged to do so.[3] If the fetal head fails to descend, oxytocin treatment may be useful.

Causes of Dystocia

Dystocia, or failure of labor to progress, is diagnosed when the cervix fails to dilate at least 1 cm/hr during the first stage of labor, or when the fetal head fails to descend during the second stage of labor.[3] Assuming that labor was correctly diagnosed, three possible causes for failure to progress are possible (excluding malpresentations and hydrocephalus): inefficient

uterine action, an occiput-posterior position, and cephalopelvic disproportion. In the nulliparous patient, dystocia, especially early in labor, is most often the result of inefficient uterine action. Secondary arrest of labor after previously satisfactory progress may be due to an occiput-posterior position or cephalopelvic disproportion, although inefficient uterine action is still the most common cause. To differentiate between the possible explanations, oxytocin is administered. If satisfactory progress of labor resumes with the administration of oxytocin, the diagnosis of inefficient uterine action is confirmed. Only if satisfactory progress is not restored with oxytocin can the diagnosis of malposition (in the presence of an occiput-posterior position) or cephalopelvic disproportion be made.

Administration of Oxytocin

Both primary and secondary failure of labor to progress are treated with oxytocin unless its use is contraindicated. Oxytocin may not be administered until the membranes have been ruptured and the amniotic fluid is noted to be clear.[3,4] It may only be used when there is a singleton fetus in a vertex position and there is no evidence of fetal distress.[6] In the presence of nonreassuring fetal heart rate (FHR) patterns, fetal blood sampling is performed to ascertain fetal distress.[4]

Oxytocin is administered in a consistent dosage and rate. The initial rate of administration is 6 mU/min, and the rate is increased by 6 mU/min every 15 minutes to a maximum rate of administration of 40 mU/min. The maximum total dose administered is 10 U and the maximum duration of administration is 6 hours.[3]

One-to-one Nursing Care

Each pregnant patient is provided with a personal nurse who remains with her throughout the course of labor. While this nurse monitors progress during labor, her primary role is to provide emotional support. The founders of active management believe that the presence of a figure who is well informed as well as sympathetic is the only means of providing the mother with proper guidance and support. Practically, this level of support is possible only in a setting in which the duration of labor is limited.[3]

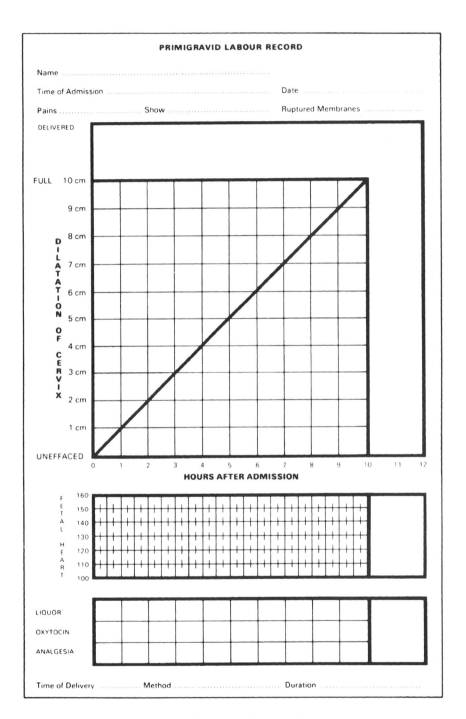

Fig. 25-1. Advancement of cervical dilatation charted on a partogram.

Childbirth Education

Education of mothers is regarded as a key component of the active management of labor. The standardization of treatment during labor permits standardized childbirth classes to be offered. Women are taught in advance how their labor will be managed; they are assured that their labor will almost certainly last less than 12 hours and that they will never be left alone during that time. Also, to be sure that the information taught in childbirth classes is current and accurate, the classes are taught by nurse-midwives who also work on the labor unit.[3]

SAFETY

The debate about the safety of active management of labor was triggered when O'Driscoll and colleagues[5,6] challenged what they believed to be the commonly held belief that the increasing use of cesarean section during the period from 1965 to 1980 had contributed in a major way to the dramatic decrease in perinatal mortality that had occurred over that same period.[7] O'Driscoll and colleagues noted that during that period, cesarean section rates at the National Maternity Hospital remained fairly stable and under 5 percent, while the perinatal mortality rate showed a decline parallel to that occurring in the United States[5] (Fig. 25-2). They asserted that "the same perinatal mortality rates can be achieved with less than one-third the number of cesarean sections."[5] Leveno and colleagues[8] at Parkland Hospital in Dallas, Texas challenged this statement, raising questions about the comparability of perinatal outcomes at the two institutions. Comparing 1983 data from the National Maternity Hospital and Parkland Hospital, they noted a sevenfold higher rate of intrapartum fetal death (1.4 per 1,000 at the National Maternity Hospital versus 0.2 per 1,000 at Parkland Hospital), and a doubling in the risk of neonatal seizures (2.3 per 1,000 at the National Maternity Hospital versus 1.0 per 1,000 at Parkland Hospital) among infants weighing at least 2,500 g. The authors suggest that the lower rates of these adverse outcomes at Parkland Hospital were related to the more liberal use of cesarean section for fetal distress at their institution (0.7 percent at the National Maternity Hospital and 2.1 percent at Parkland Hospital). Examining the cesarean delivery

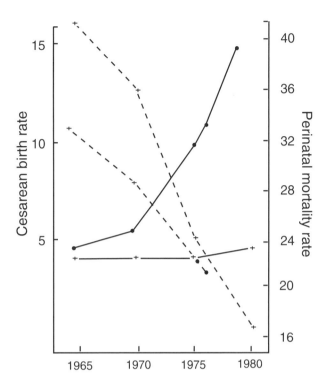

Fig. 25-2. Cesarean birth rates per 100 deliveries are represented by solid lines and perinatal mortality rates per 1,000 deliveries by broken lines. During the years 1965 to 1980, the cesarean section rates at the National Maternity Hospital (represented by crosses) remained fairly stable, while the perinatal mortality rate experienced a decline parallel to that occurring in the United States, (represented by circles).

rates by indication at the two institutions, however, makes it clear that differences in the use of cesarean deliveries for fetal distress were not responsible for most of the disparity in the overall cesarean section rates[8] (Table 25-1). The greatest disparity in the rates of cesarean section was for "labor problems" such as failure to progress.

Three years later, O'Driscoll et al[9] responded to the reported disparity in perinatal outcome by pointing out that the rates of occurrence of rare events such as intrapartum death and seizures in term infants are likely to vary considerably from year to year based on chance alone. O'Driscoll et al therefore compared 3 years of data from the National Maternity Hospital with 2 years of experience at Parkland

Table 25-1. Indications for Primary Cesarean Section, 1983

	National Maternity Hospital (n = 8,068)		Parkland Hospital (n = 10,988)		Difference in Rate (%)
	No.	Rate (%)	No.	Rate (%)	
Labor problems	94	1.2[a]	551	5.0[b]	3.8
Fetal distress	53	0.7	228	2.1	1.4
Malpresentation	54	0.7	205	1.9	1.2
Other	152	1.9	127	1.2	−0.7
Total cesarean sections	353	4.4	1111	10.1	5.7

[a] Includes failure of labor to progress, prolonged labor, failed induction of labor, and cephalopelvic disproportion.
[b] Includes cephalopelvic disproportion, failure of labor to progress, failed forceps delivery, and failed induction of labor.
(Data from Leveno et al.[8])

Hospital. They noted comparable rates of overall perinatal mortality, neonatal seizures in infants weighing 2,500 g or more, and overall intrapartum fetal deaths. Leveno et al[10] countered that while the overall perinatal mortality rates appeared comparable, the comparison was confounded by population differences, and that when stratified according to birth weight ($\leq$2500 g and >2500 g), perinatal mortality at the National Maternity Hospital was higher for infants of both low and normal weight.

The only point of agreement in this trans-Atlantic dispute was that "a note of caution be sounded before comparison is made between perinatal results taken from medical centers located on different continents."[5] It is difficult to compare the perinatal mortality rates and draw conclusions about specific obstetric practice in two different units.[5] To determine

the safety of active management, therefore, one must look at its performance in a variety of settings and in clinical trials. Outside of the National Maternity Hospital, active management of labor has not been found to be associated with an increase in fetal or neonatal death or with other adverse events during labor[11–13] (Table 25-2) or the neonatal period[11–15] (Table 25-3). Specifically, the potential increase in the rates of neonatal seizures and intrapartum fetal death that concerned Leveno et al has not been noted.

Much of the concern about the safety of the active management of labor protocol has arisen from anxiety associated with the use of high-dose oxytocin. It has been postulated that high-dose oxytocin might cause hyperstimulation of the uterus, resulting in decreased uteroplacental blood flow and fetal hy-

Table 25-2. Distribution of Adverse Labor Events in AML and UC

		Frigoletto et al[15a] (%)	López-Zeno et al[14] (%)	Hogston et al[13] (%)	Boylan et al[12] (%)	Akoury et al[11] (%)
Cesarean section for fetal distress	AML	2.2	0.9	0.9	4.3	1.6
	UC	1.2	1.7	1.2	3.9	3.2
Shoulder dystocia	AML	2	1.7	0.4	—	—
	UC	2	1.1	0.5	—	—
Intrapartum meconium	AML	10.0	8.0	—	—	—
	UC	8.2	10.7	—	—	—
Placental abruption	AML	0.3	0	—	—	—
	UC	0	0	—	—	—

Abbreviations: AML, active management of labor; UC, usual care.
[a] Includes women with a singleton pregnancy and spontaneous onset of labor at $\geq$36 weeks' gestation, excluding breech presentation and women with specified medical complications.

Table 25-3. Distribution of Adverse Neonatal Outcomes in AML and UC

		Frigoletto et al[15a] (%)	López-Zeno et al[14] (%)	Hogston et al[13] (%)	Boylan et al[12] (%)	Akoury et al[11] (%)
NICU admission[b]	AML	4	4.0	0.9	—	7.8
	UC	5	3.1	0.7	—	6.2
Neonatal seizures	AML	0.3	0.3	—	0.2	0.2
	UC	0.3	0.3	—	0.4	0
Hyperbilirubinemia	AML	3	—	—	—	3.1
	UC	5	—	—	—	4.3
5-minute Apgar <7	AML	0.4	0.3	0.9	—	1.8
	UC	0.5	0.3	1.4	—	1.7
Birth injuries[c]	AML	1	—	—	—	—
	UC	1.4	—	—	—	—

Abbreviations: AML, active management of labor; UC, usual care; NICU, neonatal intensive care unit.

[a] Includes women with a singleton pregnancy and spontaneous onset of labor at ≥36 weeks' gestation, excluding breech presentation and women with specified medical complications.

[c] Includes nerve injuries and fractures.

[b] Length of NICU admission required varies by study.

poxia.[16,17] Additionally, as water intoxication in the mother[18] and hyperbilirubinemia in the infant[19] have been noted in the literature to be associated with oxytocin use, concerns have been raised about the effect of the higher doses of oxytocin used in active management. Water intoxication is a rare condition. Its occurrence is related to the administration of a large intravenous fluid load in labor, and is increased by the use of electrolyte-free fluids.[20] With current technology, the use of large volumes of fluid is easily avoidable, as oxytocin can be administered by pump.

Several retrospective studies have addressed the safety of high-dose oxytocin by studying outcome within groups of women undergoing labor managed by an active management protocol, and by comparing fetal outcomes for women whose labor was augmented with oxytocin with outcomes for women whose labor is not so augmented. The initial dose of oxytocin in these studies was from 4 to 6 mU/min, which was increased to a maximum of 36 to 40 mU/min. In a study of approximately 700 women, Thorp et al[16] found no significant difference in mean cord blood gas levels between women with oxytocin-augmented and those with non-oxytocin-augmented labor. Additionally, they found no difference in cord blood gas levels in women treated with lower (<14 mU/min) as compared to higher (≥14 mU/min) doses of oxytocin. The largest review of this type

was done by Cahill et al,[21] and covered the 13-year experience of over 30,000 consecutive nulligravid women with term pregnancies, a spontaneous onset of labor, and an infant in a vertex presentation who delivered at the National Maternity Hospital. Overall, the rate of asphyxial death in the oxytocin-augmented and non-augmented groups was comparable. Infants of women in the oxytocin-augmented group had slightly (but not significantly) higher rates of neonatal seizures (2.2 per 1,000 in the augmented and 1.3 per 1,000 in the non-augmented group) and other neurologic abnormalities (1.7 per 1,000 in the augmented and 1.3 per 1,000 in the nonaugmented group).

Two studies of the effects of high-dose oxytocin examined the occurrence of a wide range of adverse outcomes (Table 25-4). Akoury et al,[17] in a study of 1,064 women, found no significant increase in the occurrence of uterine hyperstimulation, fetal distress, low cord pH (<7.20) or neonatal seizures associated with the use of high-dose oxytocin. Satin et al[22] more directly studied the effects on outcome of high- versus low-dose oxytocin in 2,788 women with singleton pregnancies (nulliparous and multiparous) whose fetuses were in a cephalic presentation by implementing routine use of two different oxytocin regimens during two consecutive periods. During the first period, women were treated with an initial dose of 1 mU/min, which was increased to a

Table 25-4. Distribution of Outcomes Associated with Use of High-dose Oxytocin for Augmentation

	Satin et al[22]		Akoury et al[17]	
	High-dose (%)	Low-dose (%)	High-dose (%)	No Oxytocin (%)
Cesarean section for fetal distress	3.6	3.8	2.0	1.4
Shoulder dystocia	1.6	1.2	—	—
Uterine hyperstimulation	51.9	39.0	17.7	14.4
Low umbilical artery blood pH[a]	3.3	4.4	24.1	20.2
NICU admission[b]	6.8	7.0	8.2	9.1
Hyperbilirubinemia	—	—	3.6	1.9
Seizures	0.1	0.1	0.2	0.2
Sepsis	0.3	1.8	—	—

Abbreviation: NICU, neonatal intensive care unit.
[a] Akoury et al: pH <7.2; Satin et al: pH <7.0.
[b] Akoury et al: >24-hr admission; Satin et al: any admission.

maximum of 20 mU/min; during the second period an initial dose of 6 mU/min was employed and increased to a maximum of 42 mU/min. A significantly higher rate of uterine hyperstimulation, defined as contractions of more than 2 minutes duration or more than six contractions within 10 minutes, was noted among women receiving oxytocin augmentation with higher- than among those receiving augmentation with lower-dose oxytocin (52 percent compared with 39 percent). However, the increase was not accompanied by an increase in adverse maternal or fetal outcome. The study found no difference between the groups in the occurrence of infant seizures, an umbilical artery pH below 7.0, or admission to the neonatal intensive care unit (NICU). On the positive side, higher-dose oxytocin was associated with a significantly lower risk of chorioamnionitis in the mother and sepsis in the infant. No cases of uterine rupture or water intoxication were reported in any of the studies.[16,17,21,22]

Overall, the data in the literature are reassuring with regard to the safety of high-dose oxytocin for the augmentation of labor. Examining this issue by comparing women with oxytocin-augmented and those with non-oxytocin-augmented labor is complicated by the inherent difference in the labors of women requiring oxytocin augmentation from those of women who do not require such augmentation. Women who receive oxytocin are those whose labors fail to progress; their labors are longer,[17,18,22] their

infants tend to be larger,[16,22] and they more often require a forceps delivery.[17] Both higher birth weight and long labor have been associated with acidosis even when controlling for oxytocin use.[23] In using sequential populations, the study by Satin et al[22] avoids this difficulty and provides further reassurance about the safety of oxytocin augmentation.

COURSE OF LABOR AND MODE OF DELIVERY
Cesarean Section

Interest in active management of labor in the United States arose from concern about the high rate of cesarean section and the suggestion by O'Driscoll et al[5,6] that its use might serve to reduce the increasing number of cesarean deliveries being performed. O'Driscoll et al[5] specifically noted the large difference between U.S. hospitals and the National Maternity Hospital in the number of cesarean deliveries performed for dystocia. In their setting, only 1.5 percent of nulliparous women required a cesarean delivery for dystocia.[6] This contrasts sharply with the finding in a Texas hospital that the cesarean section rate for dystocia among nulliparous women was 17 percent.[24]

Dystocia was identified by a 1980 U.S. National Institutes of Health (NIH) consensus conference[25] as one of two main contributors to the rapid rise in the cesarean delivery rate in the United States. The conference concluded that the increase in cesarean sections for dystocia was responsible for 30 percent of the overall increase in cesarean births. Data further indicated[27] that cesarean deliveries for dystocia were concentrated among pregnancies yielding infants weighing over 2,500 g, a birth-weight category in which cesarean delivery seemed to offer no survival advantage over vaginal delivery. The second factor identified as a major contributor to the increasing cesarean delivery rate was repeat cesarean section, which was also responsible for 25 to 30 percent of the increase. Dystocia is largely a problem in the labors of nulliparous women. Since women experiencing dystocia during their first labor are those who deliver by repeat cesarean section in subsequent pregnancies, it can be argued that dystocia is primarily responsible for the high cesarean delivery rate in the United States.[5]

Leveno et al,[8] however, contested the assertion by O'Driscoll and colleagues[5,6] that cesarean delivery rates at the National Maternity Hospital could be reproduced in the United States. They maintained that the racial diversity and higher rate of younger and nulliparous patients at their institution (Parkland Hospital) accounted for the higher number of cesarean deliveries performed at that site.[8] O'Driscoll et al,[9] comparing the characteristics of the two populations, concluded that dissimilarities in parity and age distributions could not be responsible for a difference in cesarean section rates of the magnitude observed. They also questioned whether a large change in racial distribution had occurred at Parkland Hospital, noting that such a change would be required to account for the increase in cesarean deliveries that occurred within that institution over time.

A number of studies have been performed to evaluate the effect of active management of labor on the rate of cesarean section. Most of the studies reported are nonrandomized, and compare the labor-and-delivery experience before and after the introduction of active management of labor as the standard of care in a particular hospital. Turner et al[26] reported a 3.4 percent cesarean section rate for the first 1,000 nulliparous women treated under an active management protocol. Overall, the cesarean section rate in nulliparous women in their hospital

dropped from 13.9 percent in the year before to 10.8 percent in the year in which active management was implemented. For those same periods, cesarean sections for dystocia in nulliparas dropped from 4.9 to 1.8 percent. Interestingly, although the protocol was implemented only in nulliparous patients, the rate of cesarean section in multiparous women also decreased after its introduction, suggesting that other changes in labor management may have occurred. Similarly, Akoury[11] compared the rate of cesarean section in 552 actively managed nulliparous women in spontaneous labor with a fetus in the vertex position to a similar number of historical controls. Among women with actively managed labors, the cesarean rate was 4.3 percent, compared with 13 percent in the control group. Forceps were used in 29 percent of the control deliveries but in only 19.4 percent of the actively managed deliveries. Boylan et al[12] reported cesarean section data on 1,843 nulliparous women whose labor was actively managed, and 2,057 historical controls. In their study, active management of labor was employed for nulliparous women if they had a singleton pregnancy with a fetus in a vertex position and no evidence of fetal distress. During the control period, the overall cesarean delivery rate for nulliparous women was 24.3 percent, the cesarean section rate for dystocia was 13.9 percent, and the rate of forceps delivery was 35 percent. After the introduction of active management, the overall cesarean delivery rate fell to 18.8 percent, the cesarean rate for dystocia to 8.8 percent and the rate of forceps deliveries to 30.2 percent.

Hogston and associates[13] examined active management of labor by implementing it in one of two hospital wards while the other continued to provide usual care. Each ward was managed by a different group of physicians. During the study, 448 women delivered on the active management ward and 429 delivered on the control ward. The rate of cesarean section among the women treated with active management was 4.5 percent overall and 2.2 percent for dystocia. For the control ward, the overall cesarean section rate was 5.8 percent with a 3.5 percent rate for dystocia. Forceps use was also somewhat higher in the control ward at 16.3 percent, versus 11.8 percent for the active management group.

Two large randomized studies have addressed the effect of an active management protocol on the need

Table 25-5. Delivery Characteristics in Randomized Trials of AML Compared With NMH

	NMH[a,b] (%)	Frigoletto et al[15c] AML (%)	UC (%)	López-Zeno et al[14] AML (%)	UC (%)
Spontaneous delivery	81	78	74	64	58
Forceps delivery	14	11	14	25	28
Cesarean section	5	11	12	11	14
Labor >12 hr duration	2	9	26	5	19

Abbreviations: AML, active management of labor; UC, usual care; NMH, National Maternity Hospital.

[a] Data from Boylan P, Robson M: Personal communication.

[b] Includes women who are >17 years of age, with a singleton pregnancy, cephalic presentation, and spontaneous onset of labor at ≥36 weeks' gestation.

[c] Includes women with a singleton pregnancy and spontaneous onset of labor at ≥36 weeks' gestation, excluding breech presentation and women with specified medical complications.

for cesarean section (Table 25-5). López-Zeno et al[14] conducted a trial in which they randomized 705 women to be treated under a protocol of active management or traditional management of labor. Only part of the active management protocol was implemented, since the women in the study were randomized after the diagnosis of labor was made and one-to-one nursing was not employed. The authors found a cesarean section rate of 14.1 percent in the control group and 10.5 percent in the active management group. The crude difference was not statistically significant (P, 0.18). After the authors controlled for a large number of variables in a logistic regression analysis, the association became significant. One problem with this study is that the women in both groups were apparently treated by the same providers in the same labor-and-delivery unit, thereby increasing the possibility of bias.

A second randomized trial, conducted by Frigoletto et al,[15] more comprehensively implemented the National Maternity Hospital protocol. In that trial, 1,934 women with low-risk pregnancies were randomized during pregnancy to be treated either with active management of labor or usual care. Women randomized to the active management group received special childbirth classes to teach them the principles of active management of labor. To minimize the influence of implementation of active management on treatment in the usual care group, the active management protocol was implemented in a labor-and-delivery suite remote from the hospital labor-and-delivery unit. Women treated in the active management unit had their labor diag-

nosed and managed by nurse-midwives who worked exclusively for the study, and received one-to-one nursing care. The overall rate of cesarean delivery did not differ between the groups (19.5 percent in the active management group and 19.4 percent in the usual care group).

In the study done by Frigoletto et al, at the Brigham and Women's Hospital in Boston, eligibility for the active management protocol required that a woman reach term without pregnancy complications and have spontaneous onset of labor with the fetus in a vertex position. Because randomization was done during the second trimester of pregnancy, one-third of the women in each group did not meet these criteria at the time of admission to the delivery suite. A secondary analysis of the subgroup of women eligible for the protocol revealed no difference in their cesarean delivery rate (10.9 percent) from that of women who received usual care (11.5 percent).

The two clinical trials examining the active management protocol have yielded conflicting results with regard to the ability of an active management protocol to reduce the cesarean delivery rate for labors that fail to progress. The trial by Frigoletto et al implemented more aspects of the protocol, but its use was associated with no decrease in cesarean deliveries. One explanation for the different findings in the two trials is that the study by Frigoletto et al was better controlled, in that patients in the active management group were treated by dedicated staff in a separate labor unit. The reason for the lower cesarean section rate at the National Maternity Hospital than that achieved by Frigoletto et al is not clear. Interestingly, the difference in the rate of cesarean sections in the study by Frigoletto et al and the study at the National Maternity Hospital was due entirely to an increased number of cesarean sections done during the second stage of labor. The cesarean section rate during the first stage was 5.2 percent while at the National Maternity Hospital the rate was 4.8 percent (Boylan P, Robson M: personal communication). At the National Maternity Hospital, almost no cesarean sections were done during the second stage of labor (in which the cesarean section rate was 0.2 percent) (Boylan P, Robson M: personal communication), while in the active management trial at Brigham and Women's Hospital about one-half of the cesarean deliveries occurred during the second stage (at a rate of 5.8 percent). The forceps delivery rate at the National Maternity Hospital was slightly higher than in the active management group at the Brigham and Women's hospital.

Duration of Labor and Other Outcomes

At the National Maternity Hospital, the duration of labor among nulliparous women is short, with a mean length of 6 hours and 98 percent of women delivering within 12 hours of admission. The duration of labor from admission to delivery has also been consistently reported as being shorter in studies of women treated with the active management protocol.[11-15] In the study by López-Zeno et al,[14] the mean duration of labor in the active management group was 6.5 hours, compared with 8.2 hours in the control group. Similarly, in the study by Frigoletto et al,[15] the median duration of labor in the active management group was 6.2 hours, compared with 8.9 hours in the usual care group.

The results of the study by Frigoletto et al are similar to those of a study by Fraser et al,[27] in which early amniotomy was found to be associated with a shortened labor, but in which its use had no effect on the rate of cesarean delivery. López-Zeno et al also mandated earlier amniotomy in their active management group. In that study, while the active management group had a shorter labor, there was no significant difference in the time from amniotomy to delivery in the study and control groups. This suggests that early amniotomy may be related to the reduced duration of labor associated with active management.

Results of the randomized studies also suggest that other benefits may be associated with the active management of labor. López-Zeno et al[14] found a significantly lower risk of chorioamnionitis (9.9 percent in the active management group versus 4.6 percent in the control group), while Frigoletto et al[15] noted significantly fewer cases of maternal fever in their active management group (6.6 percent) than in the group receiving usual care (10.9 percent). The decrease in febrile outcomes could be related to the shorter duration of labor.

SUMMARY

At the National Maternity Hospital, the active management of labor has been associated with shorter labors and a cesarean section rate lower than that found at most hospitals in the United States, although the cesarean delivery rate at that institution has increased somewhat in recent years, and in 1992 was 8.5 percent. It is uncertain why the best controlled randomized study to date did not show a decrease in cesarean delivery associated with the implementation of active management. Further investigation of differences in labor management at the National Maternity Hospital and hospitals in the United States, particularly during the second stage of labor, may help in understanding differences in cesarean section rates.

REFERENCES

1. O'Driscoll K, Jackson RJA, Gallagher JT: Prevention of prolonged labor. BMJ 2:477, 1969
2. O'Driscoll K, Stronge JM, Minogue M: Active management of labor. BMJ 3:135, 1973
3. O'Driscoll K, Meagher D, Boylan P: Active Management of Labor: The Dublin Experience. Mosby-Year Book, St. Louis, 1993
4. Boylan PC: Active management of labor: results in Dublin, Houston, London, New Brunswick, Singapore and Valparaiso. Birth 16:114, 1989
5. O'Driscoll K, Foley M: Correlation of decrease in perinatal mortality and increase in cesarean section rates. Obstet Gynecol 61:1, 1983
6. O'Driscoll K, Foley M, MacDonald D: Active management of labor as an alternative to cesarean section for dystocia. Obstet Gynecol 63:485, 1984
7. Williams RL, Chen PM: Identifying the sources of the

recent decline in perinatal mortality rates in California. N Engl J Med 306:207, 1982

8. Leveno KJ, Cunningham FG, Pritchard JA: Cesarean section: an answer to the house of horne. Am J Obstet Gynecol 153:838, 1985

9. O'Driscoll K, Foley M, MacDonald D, Stronge J: Cesarean section and perinatal outcome: response from the house of Horne. Am J Obstet Gynecol 158:449, 1988

10. Leveno KJ, Cunningham FG, Pritchard JA: Cesarean section: the house of Horne revisited. Am J Obstet Gynecol 160:78, 1989

11. Akoury HA, Brodie G, Caddick R et al: Active management of labor and operative delivery in nulliparous women. Am J Obstet Gynecol 158:255, 1988

12. Boylan P, Frankowski R, Rountree R et al: Effect of active management of labor on the incidence of cesarean section for dystocia in nulliparas. Am J Perinatol 8:373, 1991

13. Hogston P, Noble W: Active management of labor—the Portsmouth experience. J Obstet Gynecol 13:340, 1993

14. López-Zeno JA, Peaceman AM, Adashek JA, Socot ML: A controlled trial of a program for the active management of labor. N Engl J Med 326:450, 1992

15. Frigoletto FD Jr, Lieberman E, Lang JM et al: Understanding cesarean section rates: a randomized clinical trial of active management of labor. (submitted)

16. Thorp JA, Boylan PC, Parisi VM, Heslin EP: Effects of high-dose oxytocin augmentation on umbilical cord blood gas values in primigravid women. Am J Obstet Gynecol 159:670, 1988

17. Akoury HA, MacDonald FJ, Brodie G et al: Oxytocin augmentation of labor and perinatal outcome in nulliparas. Obstet Gynecol 78:227, 1991

18. Morgan DB, Kirwan NA, Hancock KW et al: Water intoxication and oxytocin infusion. Br J Obstet Gynecol 84:6, 1977

19. Chalmers I, Campbell H, Turnbull AC: Use of oxytocin and incidence of neonatal jaundice. BMJ 2:116, 1975

20. Muller JF, Van Zyl-Smit R: Oxytocin-induced water intoxication. S Afr Med J 68:340, 1985

21. Cahill DJ, Boylan PC, O'Herlihy C: Does oxytocin augmentation increase perinatal risk in primigravid labor? Am J Obstet Gynecol 166:847, 1992

22. Satin AJ, Leveno KJ, Sherman ML et al: High- versus low-dose oxytocin for labor stimulation. Obstet Gynecol 80:111, 1992

23. Yudkin PL, Johnson P, Redman CWG: Obstetric factors associated with cord blood gas values at birth. Eur J Obstet Gynecol Reprod Biol 24:167, 1987

24. Boylan PC, Frankowski R: Dystocia, parity and the cesarean problem, letter. Am J Obstet Gynecol 155:455, 1986

25. National Institutes of Health Consensus Development Conference on Cesarean Childbirth, September 1980. Sponsored by the National Institute of Child Health and Human Development. Publication No. 82-2067. National Institutes of Health, Bethesda, MD, 1981

26. Turner MJ, Brassil M, Gordon H: Active management of labor associated with a decrease in the cesarean section rate in nulliparas. Obstet Gynecol 71:150, 1988

27. Fraser WD, Marcoux S, Moutquin J-M et al: Effect of early amniotomy on the risk of dystocia in nulliparous women. N Engl J Med 328:1145, 1993

Chapter 26

Thrombocytopenia Complicating the Puerperium

Philip Samuels

Affecting approximately 4 percent of pregnancies, thrombocytopenia is the most frequent hematologic complication of pregnancy resulting in consultation. Hospital laboratories vary with regard to their lower limit of a normal platelet count, but it is usually between 135,000 and 150,000/mm^3. Platelet counts generally fall slightly as gestation progresses, because of hemodilution and increased turnover. However, they should not fall below the normal range. In pregnancy, the vast majority of cases of mild to moderate thrombocytopenia are caused by gestational thrombocytopenia, which is discussed below.[1] This form of thrombocytopenia has little chance of causing maternal or neonatal problems.[2] The obstetrician, however, is obliged to rule out other forms of thrombocytopenia that are associated with increased maternal or perinatal morbidity.

With the advent of automated blood cell counters, platelet counts are a routine part of the complete blood count (CBC) obtained at initial prenatal visits and on admission in labor in most settings. Thus, obstetricians identify women with asymptomatic thrombocytopenia when they have no reason to suspect a hematologic problem or even to specifically order a platelet count. Until the late 1980s, it was assumed that all these patients carried a diagnosis of immune thrombocytopenic purpura (ITP), a recognized cause of neonatal thrombocytopenia. Unfortunately, traditional platelet antibody testing cannot distinguish among ITP, thrombocytopenia

---

Common and Rare Causes of Thrombocytopenia Coinciding With Pregnancy

Gestational thrombocytopenia

Severe pre-eclampsia
  HELLP syndrome

Immune thrombocytopenic purpura

Disseminated intravascular coagulation
  Excessive blood loss
  Placental abruption
  Sepsis
  Retained dead fetus
  Amniotic fluid embolus
Systemic lupus erythematosus

Lupus inhibitor/antiphospholipid antibody syndrome

Thrombotic thrombocytopenic purpura

Hemolytic uremic syndrome

Drug-induced thrombocytopenia

Human immunodeficiency virus infection

Type IIb Von Willebrand syndrome

Hematologic malignancies

Congenital thrombocytopenia (May-Hegglin syndrome)

accompanying pre-eclampsia, and gestational thrombocytopenia.[3,4] Yet this distinction is important because each of these diagnoses carries distinct maternal and neonatal implications. This chapter reviews the causes and pathophysiology of thrombocytopenia in pregnancy, and outlines a rational approach to patients with this condition in the third trimester and puerperium.

PATHOGENESIS AND PRESENTATION

Gestational Thrombocytopenia

Patients with gestational thrombocytopenia usually present with mild (platelet count of 100,000 to 149,000/mm^3) to moderate (platelet count of 50,000 to 99,000/mm^3) thrombocytopenia.[5] These patients usually require no therapy, and the fetus appears to be at little if any risk of being born with profound thrombocytopenia (platelet count <50,000/mm^3) or a bleeding diathesis. Gestational thrombocytopenia as a distinct entity was first suggested but not specifically defined in a study published in 1986 by Hart et al.[6] In this study, 28 of 116 pregnant women (24 percent) who were evaluated prospectively during an 8-month period in 1983 had platelet counts below 150,000/mm^3 at least once during pregnancy. In all 17 patients who were followed after delivery, platelet counts returned to normal. Platelet-associated IgG (identified by a positive direct antiglobulin test) was present in 79 percent of these 28 women, and 61 percent had serum antiplatelet IgG (a positive indirect antiglobulin test). None of these women had positive tests for antiplatelet IgG after delivery. Hart and colleagues were actually describing gestational thrombocytopenia before this condition had been recognized as a distinct entity.[6] Samuels et al[3] investigated another 74 women with gestational thrombocytopenia. Forty-six (62 percent) of these patients had circulating antiplatelet IgG in their plasma (a positive indirect test). These 46 women gave birth to two neonates with thrombocytopenia, both having platelet counts above 50,000/mm^3. Burrows and Kelton have further shown, with large series, that there is little risk to the mother or neonate in cases of gestational thrombocytopenia.[5,7,8] In one study they showed that none of a group of 334 women with gestational thrombocytopenia or their infants experienced bleeding complications.[8] In their earlier study of 1,357 healthy, pregnant women, Burrows and Kelton[5] found that 112 (8.3 percent) had platelet counts below 150,000/mm^3). The lowest platelet count was 97,000/mm^3. The incidence of thrombocytopenia (platelet count <150,000/mm^3) in the infants of these 112 women was 4.3 percent, which was not statistically significantly different from that among infants born to healthy pregnant women without thrombocytopenia (1.5 percent). None of these infants had platelet counts below 100,000/mm^3.

The decrease in platelet count in gestational thrombocytopenia is not merely due to dilution of platelets with an increasing blood volume. It appears to be due to an acceleration of the normal increase in platelet destruction that occurs during pregnancy.[1] The increase in platelet-associated IgG seen in these patients may merely reflect immune complexes adhering to the platelet surface, rather than specific antiplatelet antibodies. Patients who have gestational thrombocytopenia do not require any special therapy during the puerperium unless their platelet counts fall below 20,000/mm^3 or they experience clinical bleeding. These complications, however, are rare, and it is difficult to determine whether these patients, with profound thrombocytopenia, have gestational thrombocytopenia or immune thrombocytopenic purpura of new onset. Options for maternal therapy are discussed later in this chapter.

Severe Pre-eclampsia and the HELLP Syndrome

Pre-eclampsia complicates from 5 to 13 percent of pregnancies, usually presenting in the third trimester and most commonly in primigravid patients.[9] Between 5 and 15 percent of patients with pre-eclampsia will develop a platelet count below 100,000/mm^3 during the course of their illness.[10,11] Pre-eclampsia is therefore the second most common cause of thrombocytopenia in pregnancy.

The obstetrician, however, must remember that a pre-eclamptic patient must have a platelet count below 100,000/mm^3 to be classified as thrombocytopenic. Gestational thrombocytopenia and immune thrombocytopenic purpura only require a platelet count of less than 135,000 to 150,000/mm^3 for their diagnosis. When a pre-eclamptic patient develops a platelet count of less than 100,000/mm^3, her disease is reclassified as severe pre-eclampsia regardless of other criteria. Very rarely, thrombocytopenia may be one of the earliest manifestations of pre-eclampsia. The thrombocytopenia associated with pre-eclampsia appears to result from increased platelet destruction rather than decreased platelet production. The relative increases in thromboxane and prostaglandin F$_{2\alpha}$ (PGF$_{2\alpha}$) seen in pre-eclampsia may contribute to platelet activation and destruction, leading to the observed reduction in platelet counts.[12,13] The increased mean platelet volume (MPV) seen in patients with pre-eclampsia, as well as bone marrow specimens that show increased numbers of megakaryocytes, suggest an increase in the presence of circulating immature platelets.[14,15] This implies that increased platelet destruction without the ability to rapidly release platelets into the peripheral circulation is responsible for the low platelet counts observed in some pre-eclamptic patients. Several other mechanisms may also be responsible for the increased platelet destruction seen in this disorder. These potential mechanisms include activation of the coagulation system with increased thrombin production leading to platelet activation and clearance, the adherence of circulating platelets to damaged endothelium, and the clearance of IgG-coated platelets by the reticuloendothelial system. Although it has been shown that antiplatelet antibodies are present in pre-eclampsia, it is uncertain whether these are specific antiplatelet antibodies or merely immune complexes adhering to platelets.[4,16,17] In either situation, the immunoglobulin-coated platelets would be readily removed by the reticuloendothelial system. Redman et al[18] has shown that platelet metabolic abnormalities may actually precede the development of thrombocytopenia or other overt signs of pre-eclampsia. Others have confirmed these findings and have shown they may be present as early as the first trimester.[19–21] These laboratory phenomena, although not clinically useful, have led some investigators to hypothesize that platelet abnormalities may play a central role in the pathogenesis of pre-eclampsia.

The syndrome of hemolysis, elevated liver enzymes, and low platelets (HELLP syndrome) has received much attention because of its unique name, but it really appears to be a variant of severe pre-eclampsia. A platelet count of less than 100,000/mm^3 is a prerequisite for diagnosing HELLP syndrome. Although the syndrome is a variant of severe pre-eclampsia, with similar pathophysiology, some major distinctions make it different from the latter condition. Many of the patients in whom HELLP syndrome is diagnosed are multiparous, the mean maternal age is greater, and the disease often occurs before 36 weeks' gestation.[22,23] Also, although all patients with HELLP syndrome have thrombocytopenia, only 70 to 85 percent have proteinuria, and hypertension is not universal in these patients.[24,25] The mechanism of thrombocytopenia is probably similar to that in severe pre-eclampsia. These clinical differences are delineated here so that this diagnosis is not overlooked if one looks only at the traditional criteria for pre-eclampsia. Some infants born to mothers with severe pre-eclampsia and HELLP syndrome may be thrombocytopenic, but their platelet depressions are generally mild, with counts usually above 100,000/mm^3. There is little or no neonatal hemorrhagic morbidity attributable to thrombocytopenia in these infants. Studies relating to thrombocytopenia in these infants are confusing because many were born prematurely, and prematurity with or without sepsis can be associated with thrombocytopenia, thus confounding the issue.[26,27] Nonetheless, the preponderant evidence indicates that infants born to pre-eclamptic mothers do not need special care because of the risk of being born with thrombocytopenia. They do, however, have other potential problems that may require special care.

Immune Thrombocytopenic Purpura

Although it affects only 1 to 3 per 1,000 pregnancies, ITP has received much attention in the obstetrics literature because of the potential for profound neonatal thrombocytopenia in infants born to mothers with this condition. In general, pregnancy has not been shown to cause maternal ITP or to change the severity of the disease if it already exists. Other studies, however, have shown that in individual patients, exacerbations of ITP often occur during pregnancy and ameliorate after parturition.[3,28,29] Harrington et al[30] were the first to demonstrate that this disorder was humorally mediated. Shulman and associates[31] showed that the mediator of ITP is IgG. These findings were confirmed when Cines and Schreiber[32] de-

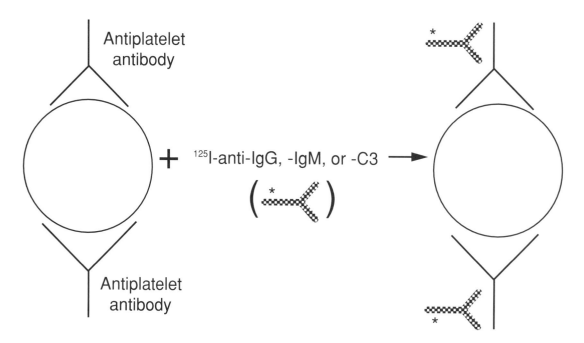

Fig. 26-1. Original direct platelet antibody test as described by Cines and Schreiber[32] in 1979. The test detects immunoglobulins that are bound to platelets (platelet-associated antibodies). In the test, maternal platelets are incubated with radiolabelled anti-IgG, anti-IgM, or anti-C3. Platelets that have antibodies bound to them pick up this radioactive anti-immunoglobulin and can be quantitated by scintillation counting. Many variations of this original test have been developed. Instead of using radioimmunoassay, one can use the principles of enzyme-linked immunosorbent assay (ELISA), immunofluorescence, or flow cytometry to detect platelets with immunoglobulin bound to them.

veloped the first platelet antiglobulin test in 1979. These assays are illustrated in Figures 26-1 and 26-2. After platelets are coated with antibody, they are removed from circulation by binding to the F_c receptors of macrophages in the reticuloendothelial system, especially the spleen. Approximately 90 percent of women with ITP will have platelet-associated IgG.[32] Unfortunately, this is not specific for ITP, as studies have shown that these tests are also positive in women with gestational thrombocytopenia and pre-eclampsia.[3,4] New assays have shown that the autoantibodies responsible for ITP are directed against specific platelet surface glycoproteins, including the IIb/IIIa and Ib/IX complexes.[33] Studies of the binding of antibodies to these and other specific epitopes on platelet surface glycoproteins are ongoing and may eventually yield tests that are useful for distinguishing among the various thrombocytopenic disorders. It will be several years before any results are

forthcoming, and it is doubtful that these tests will be available on an emergent basis, although they will be helpful during the antepartum period. They will not be useful, however, in the patient who presents with thrombocytopenia for the first time during labor.

To make the issue more confusing, the pathogenesis of ITP in children and adults usually differs. Childhood ITP usually follows a viral infection and presents clinically with petechiae and bleeding.[34] This form of ITP is generally self-limited and disappears over time. Adults, conversely, have milder bleeding and easy bruisability, and are often diagnosed after a prolonged period of subtle symptoms. Adult ITP usually runs a chronic course, and long-term therapy is often eventually needed. Many pregnancies occur in women during late adolescence and their early twenties. Among women in these groups who have a history of ITP, it may be difficult to ascer-

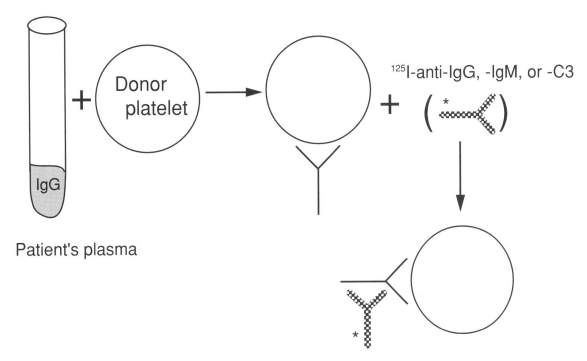

Fig. 26-2. Indirect platelet antibody test as described by Cines and Schreiber.[32] This test detects free, unbound antiplatelet antibodies that are circulating in the patient's plasma. Normal donor platelets are incubated with plasma from a patient with suspected ITP. If circulating antiplatelet antibodies are present, they will bind to the donor platelets. These antibodies are detected by the method described in Fig. 26-1. These unbound, circulating antibodies have been implicated as cause of thrombocytopenia in infants born to mothers with ITP.[3]

tain whether the condition is childhood ITP or early adult ITP. Also, no study has shown whether the risk of neonatal thrombocytopenia is similar for both forms of ITP.

ITP differs from other types of thrombocytopenia in pregnancy because of the risk of profound neonatal thrombocytopenia. Before 1990, this was confounded by the assumption that all patients with unexplained thrombocytopenia during gestation had ITP. Only after 1990 did gestational thrombocytopenia become recognized as a distinct entity.[2,3] This has posed a problem, in that cases of gestational thrombocytopenia have diluted many studies and have made it difficult to determine the true incidence of neonatal thrombocytopenia.

Peterson and Larson,[35] in 1954, were the first to recognize that profound thrombocytopenia (platelet count <50,000/mm^3) may develop in infants born to women with ITP. Territo et al,[36] in 1973, made the first effort to predict which infants were at in-

creased risk of being born with profound thrombocytopenia. They demonstrated, in a small number of patients, that fetuses born to mothers with platelet counts below 100,000/mm^3 were at greatest risk. Many larger studies have since shown that this arbitrary cutoff, while generally valid, is not useful in individual cases. Subsequently, a number of efforts have been made to use noninvasive parameters to assess the risk of severe neonatal thrombocytopenia (including the use of maternal glucocorticoids, whether the mother has undergone a splenectomy, and the presence of antiplatelet antibodies). None of these parameters, however, has had the desired positive or negative predictive values. Table 26-1 lists several studies in which all patients had true ITP, and delineates the rates of profound neonatal thrombocytopenia. Even these carefully performed studies show wide ranges in the rates of such thrombocytopenia.

In 1980, Scott et al[39] were the first to institute di-

Table 26-1. Incidence of Profound Neonatal Thrombocytopenia in Mothers Known to Have ITP

Report	Total Patients With ITP	Infants With Platelet Count <50,000/mm³	95% Confidence Interval (%)
Karapatkin et al[37]	19	6 (31.6%)	20.9–52.5
Burrows and Kelton[8]	60	3 (5%)	0–10.5
Noriega-Guerra et al[38]	21	8 (38.1%)	17.3–58.9
Samuels et al[3]	88	18 (20.5%)	12.0–28.9
Pooled	188	35 (18.6%)	13.0–24.0

rect fetal platelet determination in a series of women with ITP by using fetal scalp sampling. This procedure, however, requires operator skill, an engaged fetal vertex, a dilated cervix, ruptured membranes, and the ability to obtain a pure sample of fetal blood without any contamination by maternal blood or amniotic fluid. The procedure has proven to be technically difficult in the hands of many practicing obstetricians who do not perform fetal scalp sampling on a regular basis. In many cases, amniotic fluid in the vagina contaminates the specimen. Amniotic fluid contains procoagulants that cause fetal platelet clumping and spurious thrombocytopenia. With the development and increased use of ultrasound-guided cordocentesis in the mid-1980s, accurate in utero sampling of fetal platelets has become feasible. Some authors advocate routine use of this technique in mothers with ITP.[40–42] Some maternal-fetal specialists believe that there is minimal risk involved with cordocentesis. Ghidini and colleagues,[43] however, reviewed the complications of cordocentesis at centers that had performed more than 100 such procedures. They found a 1.4 percent risk of perinatal death in low-risk fetuses of more than 28 weeks' gestation who underwent the procedure. The complication rate may be appreciably higher when larger numbers of severely thrombocytopenic neonates have been studied. Bleeding may occur in up to 41 percent of cordocentesis cases, but in most cases stops within 60 seconds. Complication rates will be higher as this procedure becomes increasingly performed by less experienced operators. Furthermore, cordocentesis is expensive when one includes the

cost of the procedure, the physician consultation fee, the ultrasonographic guidance, and the fetal monitoring that must accompany the procedure. Indeed, the risks, associated costs, and low yield in which profoundly thrombocytopenic infants are identified do not justify the routine use of cordocentesis among thrombocytopenic mothers.

The major reason why invasive testing has identified so few thrombocytopenic neonates has been the inclusion of many women with gestational thrombocytopenia in the series in which it has been used. Gestational thrombocytopenia, previously cited as the most common cause of thrombocytopenia in the third trimester, was not recognized until 1986, when it was first alluded to by Hart et al.[6] In 1990, Burrows and Kelton,[8] as well as Samuels et al,[3] firmly established gestational thrombocytopenia as an entity distinct from ITP. In the latter study, Samuels and colleagues showed that roughly 50 percent of women with presumptive ITP who were referred to two major medical centers over a period of 10 years actually had gestational thrombocytopenia.

It is likely that the inclusion of large numbers of women with gestational thrombocytopenia in recent studies of maternal "ITP" has led to the spurious impression that the natural history of ITP has changed.

In a recent meta-analysis, Burrows and Kelton[44] found a 14.6 percent incidence of profound thrombocytopenia in infants born to mothers with ITP. This meta-analysis did not, however, take into account that many of the studies included did not exclude patients with gestational thrombocytopenia. Therefore, the risks of profound thrombocytopenia may well be greater than the incidence reported in this analysis. Moreover, Burrows and Kelton reported a neonatal morbidity rate of only 24 per 1,000, with few serious complications. Both they and Cook,[45] conclude that there is no increased fetal morbidity associated with a platelet count of less than 50,000/mm³. This conclusion is remarkable, considering that there is no pediatric or adult state in which a platelet count of less than 50,000/mm³ is not associated with increased morbidity from bleeding. The reason why the situation for the fetus or neonate with an incompletely developed hemostatic system should be different is not readily apparent. Samuels et al[3] reported a neonatal morbidity rate of

278 per 1,000 in infants born to mothers with true ITP. However, the sample size in their study was too small to determine whether mode of delivery or degree of neonatal thrombocytopenia had an impact on this morbidity. Nonetheless, their study does point out that ITP does not always carry a benign course for the neonate. The neonatal morbidities associated with the condition included intraventricular hemorrhage (IVH), hemopericardium, gastrointestinal bleeding, and extensive cutaneous manifestations of bleeding.[3]

Thrombotic Thrombocytopenic Purpura and the Hemolytic Uremic Syndrome

Thrombotic thrombocytopenic purpura (TTP) and the hemolytic uremic syndrome (HUS) are characterized by microangiopathic hemolytic anemia and severe thrombocytopenia. Pregnancy does not predispose a patient to these conditions, but they should be considered when evaluating the gravid woman with severe thrombocytopenia. TTP is characterized by a pentad of findings.[46,47] The complete pentad occurs in only about 40 percent of patients, but approximately 75 percent present with a triad of microangiopathic hemolytic anemia, thrombocytopenia,

---

Characteristic Findings in Thrombotic Thrombocytopenic Purpura[a]

Microangiopathic hemolytic anemia[b]

Thrombocytopenia[b]

Neurologic abnormalities[b]
  Confusion
  Headache
  Paresis
  Seizures

Fever

Renal dysfunction

[a] The complete pentad of findings is seen in only 40 percent of patients with TTP.

[b] This triad is found in 74 percent of patients with TTP.

---

and neurologic changes.[48] Pathologically, these patients have thrombotic occlusions of arterioles and capillaries. These occur in multiple organs, and there is no specific clinical manifestation of the disease. The clinical picture will reflect the involved organs. The pathophysiology of TTP remains elusive, but diffuse endothelial damage and impaired fibrinolytic activity are among its hallmarks.[49] In many ways, the pathophysiology of TTP mirrors that of severe pre-eclampsia. Weiner[50] has published the most extensive literature review concerning TTP. In this series of 45 patients, 40 developed the disease antepartum, with 58 percent of cases occurring before 24 weeks' gestation. The mean gestational age and onset of symptoms was 23.5 weeks.

This finding may be helpful in attempts to distinguish TTP from other causes of thrombocytopenia and microangiopathic hemolytic anemia occurring during gestation. In Weiner's review, the fetal and maternal mortality rates were 80 percent and 44 percent, respectively.[50] This series included many patients who contracted the disease before plasma infusion/exchange therapy was used for treating TTP. The disorder may be confused with rarely occurring severe pre-eclampsia of early onset. In pre-eclampsia, antithrombin III (AT III) levels are frequently low, however, which is not the case with TTP.[51] The test for AT III may therefore be a useful discriminator between these two disorders.

Although HUS has many features in common with TTP, it usually has its onset in the postpartum period. Patients with HUS display a triad of microangiopathic hemolytic anemia, acute nephropathy, and thrombocytopenia. HUS is rare in adults, and the thrombocytopenia is usually milder than that seen in TTP, with only 50 percent of patients having a platelet count below 100,000/mm^3 at the time of diagnosis. The thrombocytopenia worsens as the disease progresses.[52] A major difference between TTP and HUS is that from 15 to 25 percent of patients with the latter condition develop chronic renal disease.[47] HUS often follows infections with verotoxin-producing enteric bacteria.[53] Cyclosporine therapy, cytotoxic drugs, and oral contraceptives may predispose adults to HUS.[34,55,56] The majority of cases of HUS occurring in pregnancy develop at least 2 days after delivery.[47,49] In fact, in one series, only 9 of 62 (6.9 percent) of cases of pregnancy-associated HUS occurred antepartum.[50] In four of these nine cases symptoms developed on the day of delivery. The mean time from delivery to development of HUS in patients in this series was 26.6 days. Maternal mortality may exceed 50 percent in postpartum HUS.

EVALUATION DURING LATE PREGNANCY AND THE PUERPERIUM

Before deciding on a course to follow in treating the patient with thrombocytopenia during labor and delivery, the obstetrician must evaluate the patient and attempt to ascertain the etiology of her low platelet count. Important management decisions depend on arriving at an accurate diagnosis. A complete medical history, although time consuming, is critically important. It is essential to learn whether the patient has previously had a depressed platelet count or bleeding diathesis. It is also important to know whether these clinical conditions occurred coincidentally with pregnancy. A complete medication history should be elicited, as certain medications, such as heparin, can result in profound maternal thrombocytopenia. The obstetric history should focus on whether there have been any maternal or neonatal bleeding problems in the past. Excessive bleeding from an episiotomy site or cesarean delivery incision site, a need for blood component therapy, easy bruising, or bleeding from intravenous infusion sites during labor should alert the physician to the possibility of thrombocytopenia in a previous pregnancy. The obstetrician should also question whether the infant born of a prior pregnancy had any bleeding diathesis or if there was any problem following a circumcision. Clearly, the obstetrician should also ask questions that will help to ascertain whether the patient is developing severe pre-eclampsia or HELLP syndrome as the cause of her thrombocytopenia. Importantly, all pregnant thrombocytopenic women should be carefully evaluated for the presence of risk factors for human immunodeficiency virus (HIV) infection, since this infection can cause an ITP-like syndrome.

After a thorough history is obtained, a physical examination of the patient should also be performed. Blood pressure should be determined to ascertain whether the patient has impending pre-eclampsia. The physician should also look for ecchymoses or petechiae. If the patient is developing HELLP syndrome, scleral icterus may be present. The eye grounds should be examined for evidence of arteriolar spasm or hemorrhage. An accurate assessment of the gestational age should also be done. This is important, since some of the etiologies of thrombocytopenia in pregnancy, as are discussed later, depend on the gestational age.

It is imperative that a peripheral blood smear be examined by an experienced hematologist or pathologist whenever a case of pregnancy-associated thrombocytopenia is diagnosed. This individual must determine whether microangiopathic hemolysis is present. This will help in establishing a diagnosis. This specialist can also rule out platelet clumping, which will result in a factitious thrombocytopenia. Other laboratory evaluation should be performed as necessary to rule out pre-eclampsia and HELLP syndrome, as well as disseminated intravascular coagulation (DIC). After determining the etiology of thrombocytopenia, the physician can better determine whether imminent delivery is necessary, the thrombocytopenia should be treated before initiating delivery, or the low platelet count should be ignored.

THERAPY DURING LABOR AND DELIVERY

Gestational Thrombocytopenia

Gestational thrombocytopenia, the most common form of thrombocytopenia encountered in the third trimester, requires no special therapy. The most important therapeutic action is to restrain from therapies and testing that may harm the mother or fetus. Patients with mild to moderate gestational thrombocytopenia and no antenatal or antecedent history of thrombocytopenia should be treated as normal pregnant patients. Gestational thrombocytopenia may exist in cases in which the maternal platelet count drops below 75,000/mm^3, but there is not enough published data on such low maternal counts to reach a conclusion whether there are any maternal or fetal risks. These patients should therefore be treated as if they have de novo ITP. Although approximately 4 percent of patients have gestational thrombocytopenia, less than 1 percent have gestational thrombocytopenia with platelet counts below 100,000/mm^3.[8]

Pre-eclampsia and HELLP Syndrome

Unlike other hematologic problems in pregnancy, in which a hematologist may play an important consulting role in treating the patient, the bulk of management of the pre-eclamptic patient falls on the obstetrician. When a pre-eclamptic patient becomes thrombocytopenic with a platelet count of less than 100,000/mm^3, she is classified as having severe pre-eclampsia and the usual mode of therapy is delivery. Most cases of pre-eclampsia occur in late pregnancy, but a significant proportion of cases of severe pre-eclampsia with thrombocytopenia will occur before 34 weeks' gestation. If the patient is stable and has isolated thrombocytopenia without other manifestations of severe pre-eclampsia, one may consider administering betamethasone or dexamethasone and waiting 24 to 48 hours for this therapy to be maximally effective in enhancing fetal pulmonary maturity. Such conservative therapy holds risks for both mother and fetus. There is a high risk of placental abruption or stillbirth. The mother may develop other sequelae of severe pre-eclampsia. Therefore, if this route of management is taken, the patient should be kept in the labor unit and undergo continuous fetal monitoring until delivery. The default therapy is delivery, and only in special circumstances should one consider waiting 24 to 48 hours for enhancement of fetal pulmonary maturity. The thrombocytopenia itself may not warrant therapy. Patients usually do not experience abnormal surgical bleeding unless they have a platelet count below 50,000/mm^3, and spontaneous bleeding rarely occurs if the platelet count is above 20,000/mm^3. As previously mentioned, the thrombocytopenia associated with pre-eclampsia is secondary to rapid destruction of platelets. Consequently, rapid treatment of severe bleeding resulting from thrombocytopenia in these patients requires the administration of platelets. Moreover, because of the ongoing pathophysiology of the disease, the lifespan of transfused platelets is extremely short. Routine platelet transfusion in the absence of bleeding is recommended only if the platelet count is less than 20,000/mm^3, and in these instances the obstetrician should be working toward delivery of the patient.[57] If a cesarean delivery is planned, the platelet count should be at least 50,000/mm^3. Again, because of the short half-life of platelets in pre-eclamptic thrombocytopenia, a platelet transfusion, if elected, should be given immediately before the surgical procedure. Platelet transfusions, however, can be withheld until the patient exhibits excessive bleeding during surgery.

In cases of pre-eclampsia or HELLP syndrome, the platelet count usually continues to fall for an additional 24 to 48 hours. In one study, 90 percent of 61 patients with thrombocytopenia associated with pre-eclampsia had increasing platelet counts by 72 hours after delivery.[11] In another study, all 25 patients with thrombocytopenia had achieved a normal platelet count by 4 days after surgery.[58] In a study of 158 patients with HELLP syndrome, all platelet counts had returned spontaneously to normal within 6 days.[59] In some patients, however, the platelet count remains persistently low, and this is often associated with an increasing lactate dehydrogenase (LDH) level, suggesting ongoing hemolysis and multisystem dysfunction. In a small series, seven patients' thrombocytopenia resolved after plasma exchange therapy.[60] It is debatable, however, whether this therapy helped or whether the patients would have recovered without it. Nonetheless, in the patient who has persistent profound thrombocytopenia and other signs of multisystem dysfunction at 5 to 6 days after delivery, plasma exchange may be considered. This should, however, be reserved only for the extremely ill patient, and should be done only after consultation with a hematologist or hematopathologist.

Immune Thrombocytopenic Purpura

Treatment of the gravid woman with ITP during the late third trimester and puerperium requires attention to both mother and fetus. As in other cases of thrombocytopenia discussed in this chapter, maternal therapy needs to be instituted only if there is evidence of a bleeding diathesis or to prevent a bleeding diathesis if surgery is anticipated. Again, there is usually no spontaneous bleeding unless the platelet count falls below 20,000/mm^3. Surgical bleeding does not usually occur until the platelet count is less than 50,000/mm^3. The conventional means for increasing the platelet count in the patient with ITP include glucocorticoid therapy, intravenous γ-globulin therapy, platelet transfusion, and splenectomy.

If at term the patient has a bleeding diathesis or a platelet count below 20,000/mm^3, there is usually a need to raise the platelet count in a relatively short time. Although oral glucocorticoids can be used for this, intravenous glucocorticoids may work more rapidly. Any steroid that has a glucocorticoid effect can be used. However, hematologists have the greatest experience with methylprednisolone. It can be given intravenously and has very little mineralocorticoid effect. It is important to avoid steroids with strong mineralocorticoid effects because these agents can disturb electrolyte balance, cause fluid retention, and result in hypertension, confounding issues surrounding delivery. The usual dose of methylprednisolone is 1.0 to 1.5 mg/kg *total body weight* intravenously per day in divided doses. It usually takes about 2 days to see a response, but may take 10 days for a maximum response, although this is rare. Even though methylprednisolone does have very little mineralocorticoid effect, some does exist. Because of the large dose that is administered, it is important to follow the patient's electrolytes. There is very little chance of methylprednisolone causing neonatal adrenal suppression because very little crosses the placenta. The drug is metabolized by placental 11β-ol dehydrogenase to an inactive 11-keto metabolite. After the patient has shown an acceptable increase in platelet count with intravenous methylprednisolone, she can be started on oral prednisone in late pregnancy. The usual dose is 60 to 100 mg/day. The oral drug can be given in a single dose, but there is less gastrointestinal upset with divided doses. The physician can rapidly taper the dose to 30 or 40 mg/day, but should taper it slowly thereafter. Since the patient previously had a very low platelet count or would not be undergoing therapy, the physician should titrate the dose to keep the platelet count around 100,000/mm^3. If the physician begins therapy with oral prednisone, the usual initial daily dose is 1 mg/kg total body weight. The response rate to glucocorticoids is about 70 percent. It is important to realize that patients who have been taking glucocorticoids for a period exceeding 2 to 3 weeks may have adrenal suppression and should receive increased doses of steroids during labor and delivery to avoid an adrenal crisis. Tapering should be done slowly thereafter. Also, patients who have been receiving glucocorticoids for some time may experience significant side effects, including fluid retention, hirsutism, acne, striae, poor wound healing, and *Monilia* vaginitis. In very rare circumstances patients receiving long-term steroid therapy during gestation may develop osteoporosis or cataracts. Again, the chance of any fetal or neonatal side effects from the glucocorticoids is remote.

Although glucocorticoids are the mainstays of treatment for maternal thrombocytopenia, these medications will fail in up to 30 percent of cases. In such instances the next medication to use is intravenous immunoglobulin. This agent probably works by binding to the F$_c$ receptors on reticuloendothelial cells and preventing destruction of platelets. They may also adhere to receptors on platelets and prevent antiplatelet antibodies from binding to these sites. Liquid and lyophilized forms of intravenous immunoglobulin are available. The usual dose is 0.4 g/kg/day for 3 to 5 days. However, it may be necessary to use as much as 1 g/kg/day. The response usually begins within 2 to 3 days and usually peaks within 5 days. The duration of the response is variable, and the timing of the dose is extremely important. If a peak platelet count is needed for delivery, the obstetrician should institute therapy about 5 to 8 days before the planned induction or cesarean section. Although intravenous immunoglobulin is a blood product, its method of preparation makes it safe for use. Plasma is thawed and pooled. After the cryoprecipitate is removed, the plasma undergoes Cohn-Oncley cold ethanol fractionation,[62] which inactivates viruses.[63] Furthermore, the liquid form of intravenous immunoglobulin is incubated for 21 days at pH 4.25, which removes and inactivates both enveloped and nonenveloped model viruses.[64,65] These include viruses modeled after HIV, hepatitis C virus, hepatitis B virus, cytomegalovirus virus, Epstein-Barr virus, and Herpes simplex virus. Intravenous immunoglobulin has also been tested against nonenveloped ribonucleic acid (RNA) and deoxyribonucleic acid (DNA) viruses.[66,67] A recent review of the literature could find no cases of viral transmission with the liquid formula of immunoglobulin that had been incubated at pH 4.25. Although intravenous immunoglobulin is very expensive, it should be used before contemplating splenectomy, since some patients with ITP will experience remission after delivery.[68]

Splenectomy can also be used to raise the maternal platelet count, but is usually reserved for cases of midtrimester thrombocytopenia that do not respond to other medications. It is reserved for situations in which the physician cannot keep the platelet count above 20,000/mm^3 with other forms of therapy.[69] It can be used postpartum if the patient does not respond to other forms of therapy. In extremely emergent cases in which there is life-threatening bleeding, or in cases in which other treatment modalities fail to elicit a response, splenectomy can be safely performed at the time of cesarean section after extending a midline incision cephalad.

Platelet transfusions are indicated when there is clinically significant bleeding while the physician is awaiting an effect of other therapies. Platelets can be given immediately preoperatively if the maternal platelet count is less than 50,000/mm^3, before or during a splenectomy, or before or during a cesarean section. They can be used before a vaginal delivery if the mother's platelet count is below 20,000/mm^3. Each "pack" of platelets will increase the platelet count by approximately 10,000/mm^3. The half-life of the transfused platelets is extremely short because the same antibodies and reticuloendothelial cell clearance that affect the mother's endogenous platelets will also affect the transfused platelets. However, platelet transfusion at the time of a skin incision will usually provide enough hemostasis to permit performing the surgical procedure.

Certain surgical precautions should probably be taken for the patient with profound thrombocytopenia who undergoes cesarean delivery. The obstetrician should use electrocautery liberally. The bladder flap should probably be left open in order to avoid hematoma formation. When the parietal peritoneum is closed, subfascial drains are helpful if hemostasis is imperfect. Some physicians choose to employ delayed primary closure of the skin, but this is controversial.

Although the treatment of maternal thrombocytopenia is fairly straightforward, the need for evaluation of the fetal platelet count, and how this information should alter patient management, remain controversial. Although recent papers by Cooke[45] and Burrows and Kelton[44] have attempted to show that there is no risk in delivering a profoundly thrombocytopenic fetus vaginally, these meta-analyses are only generalizations. There is no one series

large enough to permit adequate conclusions about the best mode of delivery for the profoundly thrombocytopenic fetus, nor have any randomized studies been carried out concerning the delivery of these patients. The purpose of this chapter is not to recommend a mode of delivery for the profoundly thrombocytopenic fetus, but to outline which fetuses are at risk of being born with thrombocytopenia and to allow the obstetrician to make decisions about delivery after discussion with the patient. As previously shown, (Table 26-1), anywhere from 5 to 38 percent of fetuses born to mothers with ITP will have platelet counts below 50,000/mm^3. Several studies have tried to determine whether administering glucocorticoids to the mother would increase the fetal platelet count in utero.[37,38,70]

Although the study by Karapatkin[37] gave promising results, other studies have not corroborated its findings. Furthermore, studies have shown that splenectomy has no bearing on neonatal platelet counts. The study by Samuels et al[3] showed that 19.2 percent of ITP patients receiving no therapy for the condition gave birth to profoundly thrombocytopenic infants, as compared with 22.7 percent of those receiving prednisone alone, 23 percent of those who had undergone a splenectomy and received prednisone, and 17.8 percent of those who had undergone only splenectomy. The rate of profound neonatal thrombocytopenia was not significantly different among any of these groups. Even if there is no difference in perinatal morbidity between vaginal and cesarean delivery, there are advantages of knowing whether a fetus is at risk of being born with a platelet count below 50,000/mm^3. The use of scalp electrodes and vacuum extraction are examples of interventions that should probably be avoided in the profoundly thrombocytopenic fetus. A prolonged second stage of labor in the nulliparous patient who is carrying a severely thrombocytopenic fetus might be avoided. Furthermore, because of the potential for neonatal morbidity, it might be safest if the profoundly thrombocytopenic infant were delivered in a tertiary care setting. In the study by Samuels et al[3] there were cases of severe gastrointestinal bleeding, hemopericardium, IVH, and severe cutaneous manifestations of bleeding in infants born to mothers with ITP.[3] Cordocentesis, the only method currently available for accurately determining the fetal platelet count before the onset of labor, is both expensive and invasive. Furthermore, it carries an inherent risk of causing an adverse fetal outcome. Yet, fear of an adverse outcome in the setting of a neonate with an unknown platelet count has led obstetricians to overuse this invasive technique and surgical delivery. Cordocentesis should be reserved for those patients with true ITP and not those with gestational thrombocytopenia. Moreover, because of the risk of complications, cordodentesis should be performed in close proximity to the labor-and-delivery unit. If the fetal platelet count is below $50,000/mm^3$, the obstetrician should discuss potential ramifications of the procedure with the patient. The patient and obstetrician should together decide on an appropriate place and mode of delivery. Figures 26-3 and 26-4 show our recommendations for use of cordocentesis both when platelet antibody testing is available and when it is not. Furthermore, as previously mentioned,

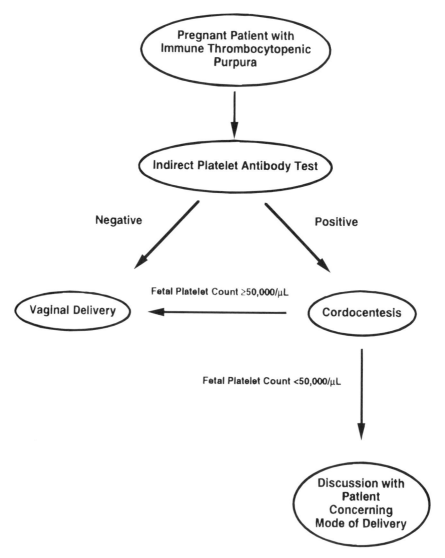

Fig. 26-3. Recommended management of the gravid woman with ITP in the late third trimester and puerperium, when indirect platelet antibodies can be identified by a laboratory that has experience with testing pregnant patients.

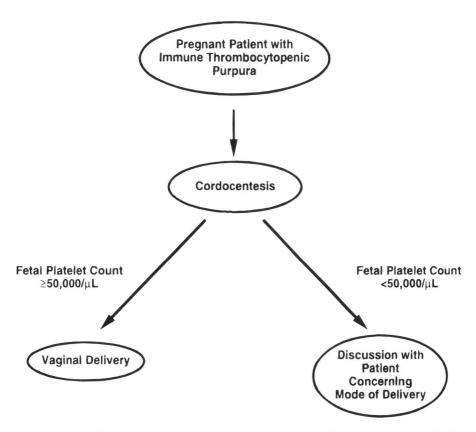

Fig. 26-4. Recommended late pregnancy and puerperal management of the gravid woman with ITP antedating pregnancy when indirect platelet antibody testing is unavailable.

there are no data defining the risks of neonatal thrombocytopenia when the mother with gestational thrombocytopenia has a platelet count below 75,000/mm³. The lower the maternal platelet count, the more likely the mother is to have ITP of new onset.

Thrombotic Thrombocytopenic Purpura and the Hemolytic Uremic Syndrome

Before the use of plasma exchange, maternal and fetal outcomes in pregnancies complicated by TTP were uniformly poor.[50] The first application of plasma exchange for treating TTP during pregnancy was reported in 1984.[71] A later report described a patient in whom chronic TTP had caused previous fetal deaths but experienced a successful pregnancy when treated with aspirin, dipyridamole, and plasma infusion.[72] No large series of patients with TTP in pregnancy have been described. How-

ever, case reports suggest that the prognosis in TTP has improved greatly with plasma infusion and plasma exchange. We recently cured a patient who had had a relapse of TTP 5 years after her initial episode. She was at 23 weeks' gestation and required plasma exchange daily for more than 3 weeks before remission began. Occasionally, patients with TTP who do not respond to other therapy may respond to splenectomy.

HUS has been much more difficult to treat, and only a few case reports of its treatment have appeared. Supportive therapy remains the mainstay of management in HUS.[50,71] Dialysis is often necessary, with close attention given to fluid management. Platelet function inhibitors have also been used in two cases of HUS during pregnancy.[73,77] Plasma infusion and plasma exchange can be tried, but the results have not been as good as in cases of TTP.[75]

Vincristine has been used with some success for HUS in nonpregnant patients, but has not been tried during pregnancy, and prostacyclin infusion, although effective in children, has also not been used during pregnancy.[76,77]

In summary, the treatment of thrombocytopenia during gestation depends on its etiology. The obstetrician need not act on the mother's platelet count unless it is below 20,000/mm^3, or is below 50,000/mm^3 with evidence of clinical bleeding or if surgery is anticipated. In these cases, the treatment will depend on the diagnosis. Furthermore, whether delivery needs to be expedited or can be delayed also depends on the etiology of thrombocytopenia. The fetal/neonatal platelet count need be considered only if the mother carries a true diagnosis of ITP or has presumed gestational thrombocytopenia with a platelet count of less than 75,000/mm^3, since the latter may actually represent de novo ITP. The key to managing these patients is to arrive at an accurate etiology for the thrombocytopenia and to approach the management of the patient and her fetus rationally.

REFERENCES

1. McRae KR, Samuels P, Schreiber AD: Pregnancy-associated thrombocytopenia: pathogenesis and management. Blood 80:2697, 1992
2. Aster RH: Gestational thrombocytopenia. A plea for conservative management. N Engl J Med 323:264, 1990
3. Samuels P, Bussel JB, Braitman LE et al: Estimation of the risk of thrombocytopenia in the offspring of pregnant women with presumed immune thrombocytopenic purpura. N Engl J Med 323:229, 1990
4. Samuels P, Main EK, Tomaski A et al: Abnormalities in platelet antiglobulin tests in preeclamptic mothers and their neonates. Am J Obstet Gynecol 107:109, 1987
5. Burrows RF, Kelton JG: Incidentally detected thrombocytopenia in healthy mothers and their infants. N Engl J Med 319:142, 1988
6. Hart D, Dunetz C, Nardi M, Porges RF et al: An epidemic of maternal thrombocytopenia associated with elevated antiplatelet antibody in 116 consecutive pregnancies: relationship to neonatal platelet count. Am J Obstet Gynecol 154:878, 1986
7. Burrows RF, Kelton JG: Fetal thrombocytopenia and its relation to maternal thrombocytopenia. N Engl J Med 329:1463, 1993
8. Burrows RF, Kelton JG: Low fetal risks in pregnancies associated with idiopathic thrombocytopenic purpura. Am J Obstet Gynecol 163:1147, 1990
9. Lindheimer MD, Katz AI: Hypertension in pregnancy. N Engl J Med 313:675, 1985
10. Gibson B, Hunter D, Neame PB, Kelton JG: Thrombocytopenia in preeclampsia and eclampsia. Semin Thromb Hemost 8:234, 1982
11. Katz VL, Thorp JM, Rozas L, Bowes WA: The natural history of thrombocytopenia associated with preeclampsia. Am J Obstet Gynecol 163:1142, 1990
12. Maklia UM, Viinikka L, Yikorkala O: Evidence that prostacyclin deficiency is a specific feature in preeclampsia. Am J Obstet Gynecol 148:772, 1984
13. Walsh SW, Behr MJ, Allen NH: Placental prostacyclin production in normal and toxemic pregnancies. Am J Obstet Gynecol 151:110, 1985
14. Giles C, Inglis TCM: Thrombocytopenia and macrothrombocytosis in gestational hypertension. Br J Obstet Gynaecol 88:1115, 1981
15. Romero P, Duffy TP: Platelet disorders in pregnancy. Clin Perinatol 7:327, 1980
16. Massobrio M, Benedetto C, Bertini E et al: Immune complexes in preeclampsia and normal pregnancy. Am J Obstet Gynecol 152:578, 1985
17. Schena FP, Manno C, Selvaggi L et al: Behaviour of immune complexes and the complement system in normal pregnancy and preeclampsia. J Clin Lab Immunol 7:21, 1982
18. Redman CWG, Bonnar J, Bellin L: Early platelet consumption in preeclampsia. BMJ 1:467, 1978
19. Zemel MB, Zemel PC, Berry S et al: Altered platelet calcium metabolism as an early predictor of increased peripheral vascular resistance and preeclampsia in urban black women. N Engl J Med 323:434, 1990
20. Haller H, Oeney T, Hauck U et al: Increased intracellular free calcium and sensitivity to angiotensin II in platelets of preeclamptic women. Am J Hypertens 2:238, 1989
21. Kilbey MD, Pipkin FB, Cockbill S et al: A cross sectional study of basal platelet intracellular free calcium concentration in normotensive and hypertensive primigravid pregnancies. Clin Sci 78:75, 1990
22. Sibai BM, Taslimi MM, El-Nazer A et al: Maternal-perinatal outcome associated with the syndrome of hemolysis, elevated liver enzymes, and low platelets in severe preeclampsia-eclampsia. Am J Obstet Gynecol 155:501, 1986
23. Schiff E, Friedman SA, Mercer BM, Sibai BM: Fetal

lung maturity is not accelerated in preeclamptic pregnancies. Am J Obstet Gynecol 169:1096, 1993

24. Weinstein L: Syndrome of hemolysis, elevated liver enzymes, and low platelet count: a severe consequence of hypertension in pregnancy. Am J Obstet Gynecol 142:159, 1982

25. Sibai BM: The HELLP syndrome (hemolysis, elevated liver enzymes, and low platelets): much ado about nothing? Am J Obstet Gynecol 162:311, 1990

26. Kleckner HB, Giles HR, Corrigan JJ: The association of maternal and neonatal thrombocytopenia in high-risk pregnancies. Am J Obstet Gynecol 128:235, 1977

27. Brazy J, Grimm JK, Little VA: Neonatal manifestations of severe maternal hypertension occurring before the thirty-sixth week of pregnancy. J Pediatr 100:265, 1982

28. Cines DB: Idiopathic thrombocytopenic purpura complicating pregnancy. Med Grand Rounds 3:344, 1984

29. Kelton JG, Inwood MJ, Narr RM et al: The prenatal prediction of thrombocytopenia in infants of mothers with clinically diagnosed immune thrombocytopenia. Am J Obstet Gynecol 144:449, 1982

30. Harrington WJ, Minnich V, Arimura G: The autoimmune thrombocytopenias. p. 166. In Toscantins LM (ed): Progress in Hematology. Grune & Stratton, Orlando, FL, 1956

31. Shulman NR, Marder VJ, Weinrach RS: Similarities between known anti-platelet antibodies and the factor responsible for thrombocytopenia in idiopathic purpura. Ann NY Acad Sci 124:499, 1965

32. Cines DB, Schreiber AD: Immune thrombocytopenia. Use of a Coombs antiglobulin test to detect IgG and C3 on platelets. N Engl J Med 300:106, 1979

33. He R, Reid DM, Jones CE, Shulman NR: Spectrum of Ig classes, specificities, and titers of serum antiglycoproteins in chronic idiopathic thrombocytopenic purpura. Blood 83:1024, 1994

34. Yeager AM, Zinkham WH: Varicella-associated thrombocytopenia: clues to the etiology of childhood idiopathic thrombocytopenic purpura. Johns Hopkins Med J 146:270, 1980

35. Peterson OH Jr, Larson P: Thrombocytopenic purpura in pregnancy. Obstet Gynecol 4:454, 1954

36. Territo J, Finkelstein J, Oh W et al: Management of autoimmune thrombocytopenia in pregnancy and in the neonate. Obstet Gynecol 51:590, 1973

37. Karapatkin M, Porges RF, Karapatkin S: Platelet counts in infants of women with autoimmune thrombocytopenia: effects of steroid administration to the mother. N Engl J Med 305:936, 1981

38. Noriega-Guerra L, Aviles-Miranda A, de la Cadena OA et al: Pregnancy in patients with autoimmune thrombocytopenic purpura. Am J Obstet Gynecol 133:439, 1979

39. Scott JR, Cruikshank DR, Kochenour NK et al: Fetal platelet counts in the obstetric management of immunologic thrombocytopenic purpura. Am J Obstet Gynecol 136:495, 1980

40. Moise KJ, Carpenter RJ, Cotton DB et al: Percutaneous umbilical cord blood sampling in the evaluation of fetal platelet counts in pregnant patients with autoimmune thrombocytopenic purpura. Obstet Gynecol 160:427, 1989

41. Kaplan C, Daffos F, Forstier F et al: Fetal platelet counts in thrombocytopenic pregnancy. Lancet 336:979, 1990

42. Sciosia AL, Grannum PA, Copel JA, Hobbins JC: The use of percutaneous umbilical blood sampling in immune thrombocytopenic purpura. Am J Obstet Gynecol 159:1066, 1988

43. Ghidini A, Sepulveda W, Lockwood CJ, Romero R: Complications of blood sampling. Am J Obstet Gynecol 168:1339, 1993

44. Burrows RF, Kelton JG: Pregnancy in patients with idiopathic thrombocytopenic purpura: assessing the risks for the infant at delivery. Obstet Gynecol Surv 458:781, 1993

45. Cook RL, Miller RC, Katz VL, Cefalo RC: Immune thrombocytopenic purpura in pregnancy: a reappraisal of management. Obstet Gynecol 78:578, 1991

46. Moschcowitz E: Hyaline thrombosis of the terminal arterioles and capillaries: a hitherto undescribed disease. Proc NY Pathol Soc 24:21, 1924

47. Miller JM, Pastorek JG: Thrombotic thrombocytopenic purpura and the hemolytic uremic syndrome in pregnancy. Clin Obstet Gynecol 34:64, 1991

48. Ridolfi RL, Bell WR: Thrombotic thrombocytopenia purpura: report of 25 cases and a review of the literature. Medicine 60:413, 1981

49. Kwaan HC: Clinicopathologic features of thrombotic thrombocytopenic purpura. Semin Hematol 24:71, 1987

50. Weiner CP: Thrombotic microangiopathy in pregnancy and the postpartum period. Semin Hematol 24:119, 1987

51. Weiner CP, Kwaan HC, Xu C et al: Antithrombin III activity in women with hypertension during pregnancy. Obstet Gynecol 65:301, 1985

52. Nield GH: Haemolytic uraemic syndrome. Nephron 59:194, 1991

53. Karmali MA, Petrie M, Lim C et al: The association between idiopathic hemolytic uraemic syndrome and infection by verocytotoxin producing *Escherichia coli*. J Infect Dis 151:775, 1985

54. Shulman H, Striker G, Deeg HJ et al: Nephrotoxicity of Cyclosporin A after allogeneic marrow transplantation: glomerular thromboses and tubular injury. N Engl J Med 305:1392, 1981

55. Giroux L, Bettez P: Mitomycin C nephrotoxicity: a clinicopathologic study of 17 cases. Am J Kidney Dis 6:28, 1985

56. Brown CG, Robson AP, Robson JG et al: Haemolytic uraemic syndrome in a woman taking oral contraceptives. Lancet 1:1479, 1973

57. Weinstein L: Preeclampsia/eclampsia with hemolysis, elevated liver enzymes, and thrombocytopenia. Obstet Gynecol 66:657, 1985

58. Neiger R, Contag SA, Coustan DR: The resolution of preeclampsia-related thrombocytopenia. Obstet Gynecol 77:692, 1991

59. Martin JN, Blake PG, Perry KG et al: The natural history of HELLP syndrome: patterns of disease progression and regression. Am J Obstet Gynecol 164:1500, 1991

60. Martin JN, Files JC, Blake PG et al: Plasma exchange for preeclampsia. Am J Obstet Gynecol 162:126, 1990

61. Berchtold P, McMillan R: Therapy of chronic idiopathic thrombocytopenic purpura in adults. Blood 74:2309, 1989

62. Rousell RH: A new intravenous immunoglobulin in adult and childhood idiopathic thrombocytopenic purpura: a review. J Infect, suppl., 15:59, 1987

63. Mitra G, Wong MF, Mozen MM et al: Elimination of infectious retroviruses during preparation of immunoglobulins. Transfusion 26:394, 1986

64. Schwartz RS: Overview of the biochemistry and safety of a new native intravenous gammaglobulin, IGIV, pH 4.25. Am J Med 83:46, 1987

65. Schwartz RS: Biochemistry and safety of native intravenous gammaglobulin (IGIV, pH 4.25). J Clin Apheresis 4:89, 1988

66. Eousell RH, Budinger MD, Pirofsky B, Schiff RI: Prospective study on the hepatitis safety of intravenous immunoglobulin, pH 4.25. Vox Sang 60:65, 1991

67. Rousell RH, Good RA, Pirofsky B, Schill RI: Non-A non-B hepatitis and the safety of intravenous immunoglobulin pH 4.25: a retrospective survey. Vox Sang 54:6, 1988

68. Kelton JG, Inwood MJ, Barr RM et al: The prenatal prediction of thrombocytopenia in infants of mothers with clinically diagnosed immune thrombocytopenia. Am J Obstet Gynecol 144:449, 1982

69. Moise KF Jr: Autoimmune thrombocytopenic purpura in pregnancy. Clin Obstet Gynecol 34:51, 1991

70. Carloss HW, MacMillan R, Crosby WH: Management of pregnancy in women with immune thrombocytopenic purpura. JAMA 244:2756, 1980

71. Lian ECY, Byrnes JJ, Harkness DR: Two successful pregnancies in a woman with chronic thrombotic thrombocytopenic purpura. Int J Obstet Gynecol 29:359, 1989

72. Ezra Y, Mordel N, Sadovsky E et al: Successful pregnancies of two patients with relapsing thrombotic thrombocytopenic purpura. Int J Obstet Gynecol 29:359, 1989

73. Thorsen CA, Rossi EC, Green D, Carone FA: The treatment of the hemolytic-uremic syndrome with inhibitors of platelet function. Am J Med 66:711, 1979

74. Ponticelli C, Rivolta E, Imbasciatti E et al: Hemolytic uremic syndrome in adults. Arch Intern Med 140:353, 1980

75. Olah KS, Gee H: Postpartum haemolytic uraemic syndrome precipitated by antibiotics. Br J Obstet Gynaecol 97:83, 1990

76. Gutterman LA, Levin DM, George BS, Sharma HM: The hemolytic-uremic syndrome: recovery after treatment with vincristine. Ann Intern Med 98:612, 1983

77. Beattie TJ, Murphy AV, Willoughby MLN, Belch JJF: Prostacyclin infusion in haemolytic-uraemic syndrome of children. BMJ 283:470, 1981

Chapter 27

Optimal Route of Delivery for the Very-Low-Birth-Weight Infant

Richard Molteni, Michael Trautman, and Diane Lorant

The era of modern perinatal care was ushered in during the early and middle 1970s. The development of neonatal intensive care had occurred earlier in both Europe and the United States, but was only partially successful in lowering neonatal and perinatal mortality rates on both sides of the Atlantic. A developing interest in maternal-fetal medicine, both in the laboratory and in the clinical arena, ushered in even more dramatic improvements. No longer were the two disparate disciplines of neonatology and obstetrics blaming each other for the unfortunate outcomes of many survivors of these earlier experimental interventions. Now both disciplines joined forces within academic medical centers and national committees to better understand the determinants of healthy survival for both mother and neonate. These cooperative efforts combined in an era of strong federal research funding to produce consistent improvements in obstetric and neonatal outcome. Over the past two decades, technologic advances combined with regionalization of perinatal care have led to substantial improvement in low morbidity survival in the small preterm infant. At each step, newly acquired knowledge and advancing technology pushed the limits of viability constantly lower until healthy survival to 28 gestational weeks has become and "expected" outcome in most neonatal intensive care units (NICUs).

The past half decade has continued that same trend. One recent report, not atypical for many academic perinatal centers, notes that 79 percent of infants born at 25 weeks, 56 percent of infants born at 24 weeks, and 15 percent of infants born at 23 weeks are surviving perinatal care.[1] With such substantial numbers of very-low-birth-weight (VLBW) infants now surviving, obstetricians have continued to adopt more aggressive approaches to prenatal, labor, and delivery care. This extension of time-honored obstetric techniques and management styles to a group of lower birth weight fetuses has proven a successful strategy to this point in time. Yet often we have rushed rapidly forward with poorly conceived or tested interventions, applied them indiscriminately, and only later asked which were truly necessary, efficacious, or cost effective. These questions continue to beg a response in this population of fetuses and neonates. Local "traditions," "religion," strong prejudice, and inaccurate data, often lacking statistical verification, form the basis of many strategies and local standards of care.

Beginning in the early 1980s, despite a lack of valid statistics, routine cesarean sections began to be included in the more active obstetric management of VLBW infants.[2,3] Often, despite small patient numbers and poorly controlled data, delivery by cesarean section has been advocated, and at times elevated to the status of "standard of care," based on a presumption that it is less traumatic for the VLBW infant than delivery by the vaginal route. Malloy et al[3] reported an increase in the cesarean section rate for VLBW infants (500 to 1,499 g) from 24 percent in 1980 to 44 percent in 1984. Coincident with this increased rate of operative delivery is an increase in total hospital costs and rising rates of maternal morbidity.

DELIVERY METHOD

Cesarean Section

A large body of information from the United States and Europe[4–11] would indicate that delivery of the VLBW infant by cesarean section is advantageous, both in terms of short-term advantages (mortality and risk of intracranial hemorrhage) and long-term advantages (incidence of cerebral palsy, permanent neurologic injury, and mental retardation). This has not, however, been a universal finding. A few studies[12–16] have actually defined a definite disadvantage to the routine use of operative delivery for the preterm infant. A higher incidence of respiratory distress in operative deliveries has been has been claimed to contribute to an increase in the incidence of intracranial hemorrhage (ICH). High ventilator pressures, a higher incidence of air leaks, and recurrent episodes of elevated intracranial and arterial pressures (e.g., agitation and endotracheal tube suctioning) represent possibilities offered for this association. The effect of the newer pulmonary surfactant preparations (natural, exogenous, calf lavage, minced cow or pork) on this relationship has not yet been adequately evaluated. While such opinions do stand in direct contrast to most articles dealing with this subject, they suffer from no greater design difficulties than those that conclude a definite advantage to cesarean sections.

A few studies[17,18] have claimed an advantage of operative delivery only when the fetus has been "protected" from the dangers of uterine contractions and such delivery is accomplished before labor has begun. For example, Barrett and colleagues[19] reported that the initiation of labor significantly increased neonatal mortality among infants with birth weights between 501 and 1,000 g. However, in their study, VLBW neonates delivered in the absence of labor were of significantly greater gestational age

(despite lower birth weights) than those born after labor had been initiated. Fetal dysmaturity may well have predisposed this group to intrauterine stress and accelerated lung maturation,[20] thereby secondarily influencing both survival and the risk of ICH. A number of confounding variables are of concern in the interpretation of these studies. When elective cesarean sections are performed at very young gestational ages, severe maternal disease (e.g., pregnancy-induced hypertension [PIH]) is often present. Therefore, most of these mothers and their fetuses have been transferred and managed intensively at high-risk perinatal centers. Worsening maternal disease or early indicators of fetal compromise (ultrasonographic or fetal testing) may have led to higher rates of elective operative delivery in such populations. The potential for greater maturity of these fetuses (e.g., PIH) or their delivery in an environment in which optimal neonatal care is constantly available could also lead to or accentuate observed differences in study findings. These studies consider a different group of fetuses than those whose mothers enter labor with spontaneous preterm rupture of membranes and a high incidence of amniotic and fetal infection. Currently, there are no conclusive data supporting the benefit of delivery of the VLBW infant before the onset of labor.

There are also a number of obstetric and neonatal studies that have claimed an advantage for cesarean delivery in terms of Apgar score at birth,[4,18] fetal heart rate (FHR) patterns during labor,[9] and long-term morbidity[10] in their VLBW subjects. These studies are poorly controlled or completely uncontrolled for race, sex, socioeconomic status, fetal growth status, and resuscitation or nursery course. In studies that have compared the rate of ICH in vaginally or cesarean delivered neonates, the timing of the neonatal ultrasound or computed tomographic (CT) scan has usually also not been standardized, and its chronologic relationship to the actual delivery has therefore not been clearly established. Maternal drug use, both licit and illicit, before and during labor, has often not been considered, and urine samples have not been obtained. The conclusions of these studies must therefore be considered suspect. Mortality, morbidity, the incidence of ICH, and long-term outcome are usually lumped into wide ranges of birth weight or gestational age categories (e.g., the VLBW infant of <1,500 g or the extremely low-birth-weight [ELBW] fetus <1,000 g). Mortality and morbidity change dramatically, often in 100-g increments, and in days rather than weeks, in the lowest birth weight groups. Analyses that fail to more carefully stratify their study patients into narrower categories are thwarted by inherent errors, especially when small numbers of patients are compared.

Prospective studies of operative delivery for VLBW infants have come with great difficulty. The refusal to consider well-designed, randomized prospective outcome studies has been largely justified on ethical grounds. The prospective study Wallace et al, did attempt to compare the outcome of preterm infants born vaginally with that of infants born by cesarean section. This study considered singleton infants of 26 to 33 weeks estimated gestational age, in vertex presentation, without known congenital abnormalities. The authors aborted their study after 40 deliveries because in 63 percent of these cases the actual birth weight was more than 1,500 g, thus subjecting women to cesarean section when there was no (theoretical or assumed) benefit to the fetus. Lacking such prospective information, we have come to depend on numerous retrospective studies in an attempt to determine whether the operative delivery route is inherently safer. The problem encountered with such studies is that almost universally, the infants delivered by cesarean section are larger and gestationally older than their vaginally delivered pairs. This consistent finding probably represents a primary-care physician bias against performing a cesarean section for fetal indications when the possibility of nonviability or severe neurologic injury appears high. It is exactly for this reason that controlled studies are essential. When infants delivered by cesarean section are not matched for gestational age and birth weight with those delivered vaginally, the morbidity and mortality among the two groups can never be directly or accurately compared.

Several studies have attempted to apply more exacting statistical analyses in an attempt to account for these confounding variables (Table 27-1). Kitchen et al,[22,23] assessed the 2-year outcome of 577 infants with birth weights of 500 to 999 g who were born between 1977 and 1987. Severe disability in this study was defined as a mental developmental index

Table 27-1. Cesarean Section Does Not Lower Morbidity or Mortality in Low-Birth-Weight Infants

Author	Weight (g)	Difference in Outcome (Vaginal versus Cesarean Section)
Kitchen et al[23]	500–999	No difference in mental disability or cerebral palsy
Low et al[24]	<2,000	No difference in intrapartum asphyxia
Malloy et al[25]	<1,500	No difference in mortality or intracranial hemorrhage

(MDI) on the Bayley scales of infant development of less than 2 SD below normal, nonambulatory cerebral palsy, or blindness. The mean MDI for children born by cesarean section was 95.1 ($\pm$ 23.1), a mean score that compared favorably to a score of 92.2 ($\pm$ 19) in children born vaginally. Additionally, only 80 percent of children born by cesarean section were free of major handicaps, compared to 87.9 percent of those born vaginally. The authors analyzed their data by logistic regression and concluded that the mode of delivery did not influence disability-free survival to 2 years of age. Kitchen et al also evaluated the rate of neonatal complications during the first week of postnatal life. Among infants delivered by cesarean section, 84.3 percent required intermittent positive pressure ventilation (IPPV) or continuous positive airway pressure (CPAP); by contrast, only 58.5 percent of infants delivered vaginally required similar types of respiratory support. Stepwise regression analysis of the obstetric variables indicated that cesarean section was only marginally associated (but not statistically significantly) with an increase in the use of ventilatory support. Nor were any significant differences observed in the following variables when contrasted by mode of delivery: Apgar scores at 1 and 5 minutes, time of onset of regular respirations, use of sodium bicarbonate in the delivery room, rectal temperature, first arterial pH obtained on admission, duration of assisted ventilation, and supplemental oxygen administration. Low et al[24] also looked for an association between intrapartum asphyxia in infants weighing less than 2000 g and mode of delivery. This study defined intrapartum asphyxia as an umbilical artery buffer base of less than 34 mmol/L. Control patients were utilized and matched for each neonate defined with asphyxia. Low and colleagues discovered no difference in the incidence of cesarean section when asphyxiated and control infants were compared. Since the umbilical artery buffer base in infants delivered by cesarean section was not less than in infants delivered vaginally, the authors concluded that it was unlikely that delivery by cesarean section could be considered less "traumatic" or "hypoxemic" for the VLBW infant than delivery by the vaginal route.

Single-center studies are often criticized for their small numbers of births in the 500- to 750-g range, the range of birth weight (in the gestationally appropriately grown group) in which mortality and morbidity should be highest. A few larger multicenter studies are available for review. Malloy et al[25] reported the mortality and intracranial hemorrhage rates of 1,765 infants with birth weights below 1500 g accumulated from seven centers. They noted that mortality among the 501 to 750-g infants was 53.1 percent when delivery occurred by cesarean section, as compared to 64.3 percent among infants delivered vaginally. Among the 501 to 750-g infants born operatively, the incidence of ICH (grades II to IV) was 37.8 percent, compared to a rate of 50.4 percent in infants delivered vaginally. A cursory review of these statistics would appear to favor VLBW delivery by cesarean section. However, among the 501 to 750-g infants, 84 percent of those born by cesarean section were intubated immediately at delivery, while this same therapy was applied to only 74 percent of infants born vaginally. Additionally, the mean gestational age for the infants delivered by cesarean section was significantly higher (26.2 weeks) than that of the vaginally born (24.5 weeks) infants. To adjust for these confounding variables, the authors used logistic regression models, adjusting for gestational age, pre-eclampsia, fetal presentation, and the presence of labor before cesarean section. The adjusted odds ratios for cesarean section compared to vaginal delivery in the 501- to 750-g birth weight group were 1.05 (95% confidence interval, 0.54 to 2.07) for neonatal death and 0.84 (95% confidence interval, 0.40 to 1.79) for ICH. Logistic regression demonstrated no advantage to cesarean section in any of the weight strata studied. The authors concluded that cesarean delivery was not associated with a lower risk of mortality or ICH.

Forceps Use and Large Episiotomies

A number of other myths have developed over the years when optimal techniques for VLBW delivery are discussed. For example, a much earlier body of literature suggests that delivery of the VLBW infant should include a large episiotomy with forceps assistance to protect the delicate preterm fetal head from the trauma of compression/decompression injury during delivery.[26] More recent studies have failed to substantiate this recommendation. Barrett and colleagues[19] study of 72 singleton infants weighing between 501 and 1,000 g and born vaginally found no difference in the incidence of hyaline membrane disease, patent ductus arteriosus, ICH, or death when the use of a wide episiotomy or forceps was compared to delivery in spontaneous group of equivalently sized infants. In a larger retrospective study, the mortality and morbidity of 394 low-birth-weight (LBW) infants (1,000 to 2,500 g) delivered by low forceps were compared to those of 671 LBW infants who delivered spontaneously.[27] The investigators also found no difference in morbidity or mortality, again arguing against the routine use of prophylactic low forceps delivery. Maltau et al prospectively compared the incidence of retinal hemorrhage in infants 29 to 35 weeks' gestational age born spontaneously with that in infants delivered by gentle forceps extraction.[28] While retinal hemorrhage has never been considered to equate with ICH, this study found no difference in the incidence or severity of retinal hemorrhage by mode of delivery.

PREVENTION OF INTRACRANIAL HEMORRHAGE

For modern obstetrics, the overwhelming question as it relates to route of delivery will continue to center on the incidence of intracranial bleeding in the VLBW group. To parents, regardless of the minimal grade of the bleed, this event represents a major catastrophe in their child's course. Their expectations for the child, as well as the intensity of their own involvement in the child's care, often change after this event. One might assume that recent dramatic advances in perinatal care would have eliminated ICH except in the smallest or sickest neonates at the edges of viability. Unfortunately, even a cursory review of the literature indicates that modern obstetric and neonatal care have only moderately affected the incidence of this complication in the VLBW infant. Easily overlooked, however, is the marked reduction in prevalence and severity of ICH in the older gestational age groups (>1,000 g), comprising neonates compromisingneonates in whom previous incidence figures for ICH were similar to now quoted rates in the ELBW infants currently populating most NICUs. More remarkable, and a true tribute to modern perinatal management, is the negligible increase in the overall incidence and severity of bleeding episodes as the gestational ages of infants selected for obstetric and neonatal intensive care continue to decrease. Unfortunately, the exact management approach (obstetric or neonatal) responsible for the reduced incidence and severity of ICH in these larger birth weight infants has not been determined. Yet even within this birth weight group (1,000 to 2,000 g), some cases of severe bleeding and periventricular leukomalacia can still be expected.

In order to evaluate potential therapies or management techniques for preventing ICH, it is first important to understand the anatomy and physiology of the relevant area of the fetal and neonatal brain, and its unique fragility in the preterm infant. The subependymal germinal matrix is the "birthplace" of all neural cells. The neurons are formed in this highly vascular region of the brain and then migrate radially along their axonal "vines," traveling to their final anatomic resting places. This radiative pattern of migration is essential to the normal development and function of the central nervous system. Once they have taken up their final anatomic position, further interconnection between neurons continues (synaptic formation and interconnection). Later, myelinization is initiated, a process that continues long after birth. An injury during this vulnerable period may lead to a diminished number of neurons (future cerebral atrophy and microcephaly), disorganized migration and radiation (hypsarrhthymia), or aberrant electrical interconnections (seizure disorder). Under normal circumstances the subependymal germinal matrix has involuted and disappeared by 34 postconceptional weeks, making remote the possibility of a serious bleed into the intraventricular space. The initiation of such a subependymal hemorrhage (SEH) in the region of the germinal matrix is thought to follow either a significant increase in cerebral blood flow and blood pressure or a sudden and marked elevation in cerebral venous pressure. The capillaries of the germinal matrix are a single cell in thickness. During hypoxemia, as a protective mechanism similar to the diving reflex in seals, cerebral blood flow (and blood pressure) increases, delivering more blood of lower oxygen content to the brain. In this way the brain's oxygen delivery (the product of oxygen content and blood flow) is maintained and tissue ischemia and cell death are prevented. This same physiologic phenomenon occurs in less intense fashion during hypercarbia. Although this response is a well developed and critical reflex in the term infant, it can lead to a "blowout" lesion in the tissue-paper-thin germinal matrix of the preterm infant. Elevation of cerebral venous pressure, such as after a pneumothorax or cardiac failure, leading to cerebral venous stasis, can also result in ischemia and bleeding into this same region of the brain.

In the premature infant, hypoxemia commonly leads first to subependymal bleeding. Once this event has been initiated, extension can occur medially into the cerebral ventricles or laterally into the white matter of the cerebral hemispheres. Bleeding that is limited to the subependymal area (or the subarachnoid region (or both) is considered a grade I hemorrhage and has little known long-term significance. Whether this lack of association with mental capacity or neurologic function remains true at the most immature gestational ages (23 to 24 weeks) has yet to be proven. A grade II hemorrhage implies extension from the subependymal area into the ventricular cavity without dilatation (hydrocephalus) of the ventricular space. More commonly, little neurologic impairment has been described with this grade of hemorrhage. A grade III hemorrhage implies that ventricular dilatation has followed bleeding within the ventricular space. A small percentage of these infants do progress to hydrocephalus, which requires surgical drainage, and some infants experience a degree of associated motor deficit. Those bleeding episodes that progress laterally into the white matter of the brain (grade IV) carry a very poor prognosis. This is particularly true when they are accompanied by ischemic changes in the neural cells surrounding the ventricular space, the condition known as periventricular leukomalacia (PVL).

PVL is largely due to the immature cerebral vascular pattern in neonates of this degree of immaturity. Blood vessels feeding the areas of brain surrounding the ventricular cavity (periventricular region) are end arteries with poor or absent collateral connections. Any event that reduces the perfusion pressure (high intraventricular pressure, high cerebral venous pressure, or low arterial pressure) in this area of the brain will lead to ischemic damage to these cells. The resulting pathologic changes (leukomalacia) are apparent when cerebral imaging studies (ultrasound, CT scan and magnetic resonance imaging [MRI]) are used. When these changes are associated with intraparenchymal bleeding (grade IV hemorrhage), the worst prognostic indicators are operative.

Prenatally as well as postnatally, any event that leads to prolonged cerebral hypertension, hypoxemia, or hypercarbia can induce such a hemorrhage in the gestationally immature (<34 week) fetus. After delivery, most initial hemorrhages are recognized within the first 12 hours after birth, indicating that labor, delivery, resuscitation, and stabilization have either set the stage for or actually produced the initial hemorrhage in the germinal matrix. These same stimuli, in addition to abnormalities of clotting and platelet function (heparin therapy, indomethacin, infection), contribute to the initiation of postnatal bleeding or to the extension of previous bleeding into other areas of the brain.

For many years it was suggested that an "atraumatic" operative delivery might eliminate this complication. At our present level of knowledge and sophistication we must conclude that intracranial bleeding is, at least to some finite degree, the inevitable byproduct of ELBW, regardless of the method or mode of delivery. This is not to conclude that delivery mode makes no contribution to LBW mortality, morbidity, or ICH. Nor should such a conclusion signal or sanction a new era of passive indifference to the labor management of the parturient with a VLBW infant. Rather, this conclusion recognizes lessons already learned and the need for even more carefully crafted research interventions in this group of high-risk infants. In a similar attempt to diminish its incidence, a wide variety of postnatal interventions have been suggested or attempted for diminishing the risk of systemic and cerebral hypertension and consequent SEH. The introduction of high-dose sedation and paralysis as well as "minimal touch" protocols represent just such nursery attempts. None have been proved statistically valid. Efforts to improve the coagulation status of the neonate with platelet and fresh frozen plasma transfusions have also been attempted, again with unconvincing results.

Despite these disappointing results, ICH continues to plague both the high-risk obstetrician and the neonatologist. Of major import to the obstetrician has been the single question of an optimal delivery route for this group of infants. In the absence of well-controlled and randomized studies, the biases of caregivers and researchers must be acknowledged and clearly recognized when conclusions are drawn from their work. A controlled study, randomized to delivery mode, with sufficient numbers of patients to yield valid conclusions, has yet to be accomplished in the VLBW/ELBW population. The reasons for this failure are myriad. Strong obstetric and neonatal prejudice arguing for one mode of delivery or the other, the ethical dilemma of exposing a mother "unnecessarily" to an operative delivery (a necessary requirement if the study is truly randomized), and an inherent inaccuracy in gestational age estimation (as much as 2 weeks by any modality) that may double the fetal mortality rate at the lower ends of the gestational curve represent but a few of the reasons for this failure. Despite the absence of randomized controls and sufficient study entrants, a number of studies have purported to demonstrate a clear advantage, in terms of incidence or severity of hemorrhage,[4–7,18] of delivery by the operative route. Most studies, however, suffer from one or more of the following design flaws:

1. Inaccurate gestational age dating by (ultrasonography, maternal dates, or postnatal testing). Mortality, morbidity, and ICH attack rates change dramatically with each succeeding day at the lowest gestational age groups.
2. The aggressive or conservative bias of the obstetrician or obstetric group completing the study. Individual philosophy has been repeatedly shown to influence the operative delivery rate

(and survival statistics) at each gestational age to which neonatal intensive care has been extended over the past 20 years. At times, marked variations in individual approaches can be shown to be due to inaccurate mortality or morbidity information within the age groups chosen for study. At other times variation is due to the application of expected rates of bleeding or morbidity calculated from populations delivered and managed 5 or more years ago. It is only as the child approaches school age that accurate follow-up information can be obtained.

3. The inclusion or exclusion of outborn infants in addition to inborn infants when rates or severity of complication are calculated. The inclusion of maternal transfers whose medication and labor management have differed before transfer to a tertiary site also imposes bias.

4. The routine use of "protective" low forceps or "large" episiotomies to prevent mechanical "trauma" to the fetal head.

5. The effect of labor, its length and complications, and medication use (e.g., pitocin, analgesics, sedatives).

6. The nutritional and clotting sufficiency state of the mother (e.g., vitamin K factors, pre-eclampsia with low platelets, steroids, aspirin, antibiotics, heparin).

7. The effect of chorioamnionitis and subsequent fetal infection as a variable or co-variable in the occurrence or severity of bleeding or brain ischemia.

8. The type, number, and duration of use of tocolytics. For example, indomethacin is known to impair fetal renal and platelet function, as well as diminishing cerebral and gastrointestinal blood flow.

9. The neonate's condition at birth, location of birth, need for resuscitation, extent of resuscitation, and effective and efficient stabilization.

10. The effect of intact or ruptured membranes in protecting the fetal head from mechanical trauma throughout labor.

11. The importance of growth status (large, appropriate, or small for gestational age), in addition to birth weight and gestational age, as a risk factor for neurologic complication and poor outcome.

12. The type and depth of anesthesia (regional or general), as well as the types of anesthetic agents used.

13. The very critical issues of why a particular patient experienced preterm labor or premature rupture of her membranes. The etiology of this pregnancy complication may play a crucial role in the origin or extension of any hemorrhage.

14. The effect of a variety of postnatal events that increase cerebral venous pressure (e.g., fluid overload, hypoxic or septic cardiac failure, patent ductus arteriosus with cardiac failure, pneumothorax and other pulmonary air leaks, high-end expiratory and mean airway ventilator pressures) or diminish cerebral arterial flow (e.g., patent ductus arteriosus).

15. The undetected presence of other anomalies in the growth or development of the central nervous system that may have independently contributed to bleeding in or injury to this system.

16. The use of forceps or vacuum extraction and the occurrence of a controlled or precipitous delivery.

17. The type of mechanical ventilation, sedation, paralysis, and analgesia afforded to the neonate, as well as the frequency of a number of "routine" nursery care procedures (e.g., suctioning, needle sticks, intubation) utilized at the perinatal center. Each is capable of increasing systemic arterial or cerebral pressure, leading to a rupture of the fragile germinal matrix.

18. The presence of other complicating nursery factors (infection, DIC, thrombocytopenia, the existence and treatment of a patent ductus arteriosus, frequency and severity of apnea, and other nursery drug therapies).

These events represent only a few of the variables that could significantly alter the outcome, and therefore the conclusions, of small retrospective studies of the optimal delivery route for the VLBW/ELBW infant. Definitive studies will require multicenter cooperation and large clinical trials. Studies that include only small numbers of infants lead only to local conclusions and management styles, often grounded in strong bias. Nevertheless such "conclusions" may rapidly and inappropriately become the local "standard of care" for this group of infants.

A quick look at the available numbers of VLBW/ELBW infants born nationwide is revealing. If the VLBW group of infants represent 0.7 percent (0.3 percent <1,000 g) of annual births in the United States (about 4.0 million), then we should expect only 12,000 infants of less than 1,000 g to be born nationally. In Utah, for example, this amounts to only 105 infants per year. In addition the prenatal, intrapartum, and postnatal management of these patients is no longer confined to our 120 university-associated medical centers, but is now spread among a large and ever growing number of smaller tertiary perinatal centers. The university medical centers (the centers reported in most published studies) are often relegated to managing the sickest group of these neonates and mothers, potentially biasing their published results. By contrast, each of these developing perinatal centers manages but a small percentage of this total VLBW population, and studies at these sites, unless multi-institutional, preclude the accumulation of statistically meaningful data. Large trials, with patients randomly enrolled, will also require careful stratification by birth weight, gestational age, growth status, prenatal risk factors, race, social status, and sex before their results will be capable of widespread clinical application.

At this point in the evolution of perinatal medicine, a few factors *do* seem relevant in determining the appropriate management of the labor and delivery of the VLBW infant. The first concept is historically the most essential. Failure to consider an emergent and/or operative delivery solely because of the presumed fetal gestational age (>24 weeks) or birth weight (>600 g) for the equivalent indications that would lead to such delivery for larger or older fetuses will increase the risk of death, serious morbidity, and significant ICH in this group of infants.[29–33] Since the weight of some infants of higher birth weight and gestational age will be mistakenly underestimated[12] and will therefore lead to the same nonintervention, the rate of morbidity in the higher gestational age/birth weight group will also be adversely affected. Second, it has been repeatedly demonstrated that overall, fetal outcome is enhanced by timely maternal transfer, management, and delivery in a tertiary care center.[32] Third, any event in labor, during resuscitation, or over the first few postnatal days that

suddenly and severely elevates cerebral venous pressure (e.g., pneumothorax, air leaks, interstitial emphysema, and neck compression) or increases cerebral arterial pressure (hypoxemia, hypercarbia, volume infusions, fluid overload, or pressors) can lead to bleeding in the subependymal germinal matrix, with the potential for rupture into the cerebral ventricle or brain parenchyma.[34] At the same time, any event that leads to diminished cerebral perfusion pressure (elevated venous pressure, low arterial blood pressure, or elevated intracranial pressure) can lead to ischemic neuronal injury and cell death.

PRETERM BREECH INFANT

The occurrence of an ICH is usually associated with the effects of hypoxemia on systemic blood pressure, cerebral arterial pressure, and cerebral venous pressure. Resultant elevations, decreases, and fluctuations in these pressures are critical physiologic prodromes. Trauma to the fetal brain usually results in subarachnoid or subdural bleeding, or can lead to cerebral tissue contusion or a parenchymal hematoma. In the VLBW infant delivered vaginally, the breech presentation increases risk by adding the possibility of an entrapped aftercoming head. Although frequently accompanied by cord compression and resultant hypoxemia, this complication could also lead to an increase in cerebral venous pressure, cerebral venous stasis, and a subsequent ICH. When systemic arterial pressure fails to increase (the expected response to hypoxemia), inadequate cerebral perfusion pressure (cerebral arterial pressure minus venous pressure) may result. This can result in venous stasis, diminished oxygen delivery to the arterial side of the circulation, and ischemic injury to the fetal brain.

There is a propensity for breech presentation and an increased risk of head entrapment in the preterm infant. The disparity between head and body (buttocks) size in the VLBW infant is accentuated in ELBW infants, for whom a head to body discrepancy is even greater. This same high risk of central nervous system injury and ICH after breech vaginal delivery has not been recognized (when neonates with anomalies are eliminated) in the term neonate or the larger preterm infant (>32 weeks).[35,36]

In addition to prematurity, a breech presentation is also associated with a number of anomalies, chromosomal defects, syndromes, and congenital abnormalities, many of which involve the central nervous system. Diminished fetal movement and short umbilical cords, often accompanying the neurologically abnormal infant, increasing the likelihood of a breech presentation in these fetuses. These same conditions are also associated with a higher incidence of preterm labor and preterm rupture of membranes.

Unfortunately, these differences or variables are often not stated or reported when comparison of the breech versus the vaginally delivered preterm infant is made in the literature. A number of studies have reported a two- to threefold increase in both the perinatal and neonatal mortality rate in the preterm breech infant when cesarean section is not chosen.[35–44] This mortality has been attributed to ICH, hypoxemia, cord prolapse, and congenital anomaly. These complications are rarely reported separately in these studies. In the older group of preterm infants, above 25 to 28 weeks' gestation, this same increase in mortality rate (particularly from head entrapment) has not been recognized.[45–47]

While the evidence favoring cesarean section for the preterm VLBW breech-presenting infant appears stronger, the evidence accumulating for such a relationship for vertex-delivered infants cannot be considered firm. Once again, large multicentered, randomized studies will be necessary to definitively answer this question.

MULTIPLE GESTATION PRETERM INFANTS

Multiple gestational pregnancies have been demonstrated to have higher neonatal morbidity and mortality rates than singleton pregnancies.[48] Most researchers, however, have attributed this finding to the complications and diseases associated with prematurity rather than to twinning per se. Although cesarean section has been advocated for nonvertex presentations,[49] the data supporting these conclusions are not firm (Table 27-2). McCarthy et al[50] demonstrated in 1981 that although cesarean section did not appreciably reduce the risk of neonatal death for a vertex-presentation twin, it did improve outcome for breech and other presentations. Rydhstrom et al[51–53] demonstrated that during the period between 1973 and 1985, their cesarean section rate increased from 7 to 10 percent to 45 to 50 percent. Although this 12-year interval was associated with a concomitant sharp decrease in the perinatal mortality rate, the rates of cerebral palsy and mental retardation were unchanged. Their analysis failed to reveal any significant impact of abdominal birth on the fetal outcome for LBW twins, even when presentation was considered. Chervenak et al[54] reported 93 vertex-breech and 42 vertex-transverse twin gesta-

Table 27-2. Cesarean Section Does Not Lower Morbidity or Mortality in Twin Gestation Preterm Infants

Author	Difference in Outcome (Vaginal versus Cesarean Section)	
	Vertex	Nonvertex
McCarthy et al[50]	No difference in mortality	Better outcome with cesarean section
Rydhstom et al[51–53]	No difference	No difference
Chervenak et al[54]	No difference in ICH or mortality in infants >1,500 g	No difference in ICH or mortality in infants >1,500 g
Morales et al[55]	No difference in ICH or mortality in infants <1,500 g	No difference in ICH or mortality in infants <1,500 g
Davison et al[56]	No difference	No difference
Adam et al[57]	No difference	No difference in mortality or morbidity in infants >1,000 g
Grieg et al[58]	No difference	No difference

tions in 1982. Seventy-eight percent of the vertex-breech and 53 percent of the vertex-transverse twins were delivered vaginally. Among infants weighing less than 1,500 g there were six neonatal deaths and four cases of documented ICH, while for infants with birth weights greater than 1,500 g there were no documented cases of neonatal death or ICH. Chervenak and colleagues concluded that for infants with birth weights above 1,500 g, routine cesarean section for vertex-breech or vertex-transverse twin gestation may not be necessary. Their data do not prove that vaginal breech delivery of a LBW second twin is necessarily more damaging than delivery by cesarean section. Nevertheless, they suggested that vaginal breech delivery of either a single or twin infant with a birth weight below 1,500 g is not advisable.

Morales et al,[55] in a study of nondiscordant twins weighing under 1,500 g, concluded that second twins were characterized by a higher incidence of respiratory distress syndrome (RDS) and more severe grades of ICH. For vertex-vertex twins, cesarean delivery was not shown to result in an improved outcome. Morales and colleagues did demonstrate, however, that the incidence of RDS was significantly increased in neonates in the group delivered operatively. Among twins with one fetus in a nonvertex presentation, those born via cesarean section demonstrated a lower incidence both of severe grades of ICH and of mortality. However, after multivariate analysis to correct for differences in birth weight between each group, no advantages for cesarean delivery could be demonstrated. Therefore, differences in birth weight, rather than in mode of delivery, accounted for the observed differences in the neonatal outcome of non-vertex-presenting twins. Davison et al[56] studied 54 breech-extracted vaginal second twins weighing between 750 and 2,000 g. They were compared to 43 sets of twins delivered by cesarean section for malpresentation. There were no significant differences in any measure of outcome when vaginal breech-extracted twins were compared with second twins delivered by cesarean section. Adam et al[57] reviewed 578 twins delivered from 1980 to 1987. Their study population included 397 pairs of twins with birth weights above 1000 g without lethal anomalies, and in whom the first twin presented in the vertex position. There were no statistically significant differences in perinatal mortality or morbidity

when the non-vertex-presenting second twin was delivered vaginally or by cesarean section. Adam and colleagues concluded that vaginal delivery, irrespective of the position of the second twin, is acceptable in selected cases when the fetal weight is above 1,500 g and the gestational age is beyond 32 weeks. In a retrospective study of 457 sets of twins delivered between 1985 and 1990, Grieg et al[58] concluded that other than for a lower 1-minute Apgar score, the presentation and mode of delivery of the second twin was not associated with a significant difference in any of their outcome measures. Their data did not support routine cesarean delivery for twins of any birth weight when the second twin was in a nonvertex presentation. Fishman and associates[59] reviewed 781 consecutive twins gestations in which the second twin was delivered vaginally. Of the 390 infants reported, 207 were delivered in the vertex and 183 in the breech position. There were no significant differences between the vaginal breech and vaginal vertex deliveries in any of the neonatal outcome measures studied, even when study infants were stratified by birth weight. Fishman and associates' results suggest that vaginal delivery of the nonvertex second twin is a safe intrapartum management option for the infant weighing over 1500 g. Despite this information, operative delivery of the non-vertex-presenting twin will be the prevailing preference until a larger collaborative study can be performed to examine both VLBW and ELBW infants.

CONCLUSION

In conclusion, although cesarean section has been advocated in the past for the delivery of the VLBW infant in the hope of sparing the infant the "trauma" of a vaginal delivery, there is no evidence to support cesarean section as the optimal route of delivery for the VLBW infant. At present, there exists a body of evidence that would support routine operative delivery for the VLBW infant. However, it is far from clear that this conclusion is based on a statistically valid relationship. The differences in morbidity or mortality between the two groups are usually small and of questionable statistical validity. With small sample sizes, a change of only one or two patients from one group to another is sufficient to remove any statistical power from the conclusion espoused. Perhaps there is a real benefit to cesarean section that has not been demonstrated because of the lack of a well-controlled, prospective, multicenter trial to adequately answer this question. Studies performed to date are plagued by small numbers and confounding variables that favor a better outcome for infants delivered surgically. The literature certainly does not yet indicate an advantage of operative delivery for the lowest birth weight (<1,000 g) or gestationally most immature (<27 weeks) infants. While most authors believe that there will be a demonstrated advantage of such delivery for these infants, few studies[4] defined a clear-cut benefit. The current literature supports an approach to the VLBW infant that is similar to that for older preterm and term infants. Cesarean section should be reserved for those cases in which there is either a maternal or fetal indication for operative delivery, rather than being used as a routine mode of delivery because of extreme prematurity.

REFERENCES

1. Allen MC, Donohue PK, Dusman AE: The limit of viability—neonatal outcome of infants born at 22 to 25 weeks' gestation. N Engl J Med 329:1597, 1993
2. Hack M, Fanaroff AA: Outcomes of extremely-low-birth-weight infants between 1982 and 1988. N Engl J Med 321:1642, 1989
3. Malloy MH, Rhoads GG, Schramm W, Land G: Increasing cesarean section rates in very low-birth weight infants. JAMA 262:1475, 1989
4. Philip AGS, Allan WC: Does cesarean section protect against intraventricular hemorrhage in preterm infant. J Perinatol 9:3, 1991
5. DeCrespigny LC, Robinson HP: Can obstetricians prevent neonatal intraventricular hemorrhage? Aust NZ J Obstet Gynaecol 23:146, 1983
6. Beverly DW, Chance GW, Coates CF: Intraventricular hemorrhage: timing of occurrence and relationship to perinatal events. Br J Obstet Gynaecol 91:1007, 1984
7. Morales WJ, Koerten J: Obstetric management and intraventricular hemorrhage in very low birth weight infants. Obstet Gynecol 68:35, 1986
8. Anderson GD, Bada HS, Sibai BM: The relationship between labor and route of delivery in the preterm infant. Am J Obstet Gynecol 158:1382, 1988
9. Strauss A, Kirz D, Modanlou HD et al: Perinatal events

and intraventricular-sub-ependymal hemorrhage in very low birthweight infants. Am J Obstet Gynecol 151: 1022, 1985
10. Hoffman EL, Bennett FC: Birth weight less than 800 grams: changing outcomes and influences of gender and gestation number. Pediatrics 86:27, 1990
11. Barrett JM, Boehm FH, Vaughn WK: The effect of type of delivery on neonatal outcome in singleton infants of birth weight of 1,000 grams or less. JAMA 250: 625, 1983
12. Paul RH, Koh KS, Monfared AH: Obstetric factors influencing the outcome of infants weighing from 1,001 to 1,500 grams. Am J Obstet Gynecol 133:503, 1979
13. Welch RA, Bottoms SF: Reconsideration of head compression and intraventricular hemorrhage in the vertex very low birth weight fetus. Obstet Gynecol 68: 29, 1986
14. Yu VYH, Bajuk B, Cutting D et al: Effect of mode of delivery on outcome of very low birthweight infants. Br J Obstet Gynaecol 91:633, 1984
15. Kitchen WH, Yu VYH, Orgill AA et al: Collaborative study of very low birthweight infants: correlation of handicap with risk factors. Am J Dis Child 137:555, 1983
16. Ross G, Schechner S, Frayner S: Perinatal and neuro-behavioural predictions of one year outcome in infants <1500 grams. Semin Perinatol 6:317, 1982
17. Hawgood S, Spong J, Yu VYH: Intraventricular hemorrhage: incidence and outcome in a population of very low birthweight infants. Am J Dis Child 138:136, 1984
18. Tejani N, Rebold B, Tuck S et al: Obstetric factors in the causation of early periventricular-intraventricular hemorrhage. Obstet Gynecol 64:1510, 1984
19. Barrett JM, Boehm FH, Vaughn WK: The effect of type of delivery on neonatal outcome in singelton infants of birth weight of 1,000 grams or less. JAMA 250: 625, 1983
20. Gluck L, Kulovich MV: Lecithin/sphingomyelin ratios in amniotic fluid in normal and abnormal pregnancy. Am J Obstet Gynecol 115:539, 1973
21. Wallace RL, Schifrin SB, Paul RH: The delivery route for very-low-birth-weight infants. J Reprod Med 29: 736, 1984
22. Kitchen WH, Permezel MJ, Doyle LW et al: Changing obstetric practice and 2-year outcome of the fetus of birth weight under 1000 g. Obstet Gynecol 79:268, 1992
23. Kitchen W, Ford GW, Doyle LW et al: Cesarean section or vaginal delivery at 24 to 28 weeks' gestation: com-

parison of survival and neonatal and two-year morbidity. Obstet Gynecol 66:149, 1985

24. Low JA, Wood SL, Killen HL et al: Intrapartum asphyxia in the preterm fetus <2000 gm. Am J Obstet Gynecol 162:378, 1990

25. Malloy MH, Onstad L, Wright E: The effect of cesarean delivery on birth outcome in very low birth weight infants. Obstet Gynecol 77:498, 1991

26. Bishop EH, Isreal SL, Briscoe CC: Obstetric influences on the infant's first year of life. Obstet Gynecol 26:628, 1965

27. Schwartz DB, Miodovnik M, Lavin JP: Neonatal outcome among low birth weight infants delivered spontaneously or by low forceps. Obstet Gynecol 62:283, 1983

28. Maltau JM, Egge K, Moe N: Retinal hemorrhages in the preterm neonate. Acta Obstet Gynecol Scand 63:219, 1984

29. Fairweather DVI: Obstetric management and follow-up of the very low birth weight infant. J Reprod Med 26:387, 1981

30. Sachs BP, McCarthy BJ, Rubin G et al: Cesarean section: risk and benefits for mother and fetus. JAMA 250:2157, 1983

31. Smith ML, Spencer SA, Hull D: Mode of delivery and survival in babies weighing less than 2000 grams at birth. BMJ 281:1118, 1980

32. Stewart AL, Turcan DM, Rawlings G et al: Prognosis for infants weighing 1000 grams or less at birth. Arch Dis Child 52:97, 1977

33. Bowes WA, Halgrimson M, Simmons MA: Results of the intensive perinatal mangement of very low birth weight infants (501 to 1500 grams). J Reprod Med 23:245, 1979

34. Perlman JM, Volpe JJ: Intraventricular hemorrhage in extremely small premature infants. Am J Dis Child 140:1122, 1986

35. Croughan-Minihane MS, Petitti DB, Gordis L et al: Morbidity among breech infants according to method of delivery. Obstet Gynecol 75:821, 1990

36. Myers SA, Norbert G: Breech delivery: why the dilemma. Am J Obstet Gynecol 156:6, 1987

37. Kauppila O, Gronroos M, Aro P et al: Management of low birth weight breech delivery: should cesarean section be routine? Obstet Gynecol 57:289, 1981

38. Bowes WA, Taylor ES, O'Brien M et al: Breech delivery: evaluation of the method of delivery on perinatal results and maternal mortality. Am J Obstet Gynecol 135:965, 1979

39. Kiely JL: Mode of delivery and neonatal death in 17,587 infants presenting by the breech. Br J Obstet Gynaecol 98:898, 1991

40. Gravenhorst JB, Schreuder AM, Brand R et al: Breech delivery in very preterm and very low birthweight infants in the Netherlands. Br J Obstet Gynaecol 100:411, 1993

41. Main DM, Main EK, Maurer MM: Cesarean section versus vaginal delivery for the breech fetus weighing less than 1500 grams. Am J Obstet Gynecol 146:580, 1983

42. Lyons ER, Papsin FR: Cesarean section in the management of the breech presentation. Am J Obstet Gynecol 130:558, 1978

43. DeCrespigny LJC, Pepperell RJ: Perinatal mortality and morbidity in breech presentation. Obstet Gynecol 53:141, 1979

44. Duenhoelter JH, Wells CE, Reisch JS et al: A paired controlled study of vaginal and abdominal delivery of the low birth weight breech fetus. Obstet Gynecol 54:310, 1979

45. Bodmer B, Benjamin A, McLean FH et al: Has cesarean section reduced the risks of delivery in the preterm breech presentation. Am J Obstet Gynecol 154:244, 1986

46. Nisell H, Bistoletti P, Palme C: Preterm breech delivery: early and late complications. Acta Obstet Gynecol Scand 60:363, 1981

47. Karp LE, Doney JR, McCarthy T et al: The premature breech: trial of labor or cesarean section? Obstet Gynecol 53:88, 1979

48. Ho SK, Wu P: Perinatal factors and neonatal morbidity in twin pregnancy. Am J Obstet Gynecol 122:979, 1975

49. Cetrulo CL, Ingardia CJ, Sbarra AJ: Management of multiple gestation. Clin Obstet Gynecol 23:533, 1980

50. McCarthy BJ, Sachs BO, Layde PM et al: The epidemiology of neonatal death in twins. Am J Obstet Gynecol 141:252, 1981

51. Rydhstrom H, Ingemarsson I, Ohrlander I: Lack of correlation between a high cesarean section rate and improved prognosis for low-birthweight twins (<2500 g). Br J Obstet Gynaecol 97:229, 1990

52. Rydhstrom H: Prognosis for twins with birth weight <1500 grams: the impact of cesarean section in relation to fetal presentation. Am J Obstet Gynecol 163:528, 1990

53. Rydhstrom H, Ingemarsson I: A case-control study of the effects of birth by cesarean section on intrapartum and neonatal mortality among twins weighing 1500–2499. Br J Obstet Gynaecol 98:249, 1991

54. Chervenak FA, Johnson RE, Berkowitz RL et al: Is routine cesarean section necessary for vertex-breech and vertex-transverse twin gestations? Am J Obstet Gynecol 148:1, 1984

55. Morales WJ, O'Brien WF, Knuppel RA et al: The effect of mode of delivery on the risk of intraventricular hemorrhage in nondiscordant twin gestation under 1500 g. Obstet Gynecol 73:107, 1989

56. Davison L, Easterling TR, Jackson CJ, Benedetti TJ: Breech extraction of low-birth-weight second twins: can cesarean section be justified? Am J Obstet Gynecol 166:497, 1992

57. Adam C, Allen AC, Baskett TF: Twin delivery: influence of the presentation and method of delivery on the second twin. Am J Obstet Gynecol 165:23, 1991

58. Greig P, Veille J-C, Morgan T, Henderson L: The effect of presentation and mode of delivery on neonatal outcome in the second twin. Am J Obstet Gynecol 167:901, 1992

59. Fishman A, Grubb DK, Kovacs BW: Vaginal delivery of the nonvertex second twin. Am J Obstet Gynecol 168:861, 1993

Chapter 28

Obstetric Infections

Sebastian Faro

Infectious complications in the pregnant patient have a variety of etiologies, and many are often very subtle in their presentation. The diseases that result from these infectious processes range from unnoticed to mild and to serious conditions resulting in significant morbidity and mortality for both the mother and the fetus or neonate. The diseases may be caused by bacteria, viruses, fungi, protozoa, and parasites. The pregnant patient is vulnerable to the same infections as the nonpregnant patient, but many of these infections have unique characteristics that are associated with pregnancy. Therefore, these infections not only put the mother at risk, but may also infect the fetus and leave both the mother and infant with long-term sequelae. One additional unique characteristic associated with infection in the pregnant patient is that the disease may not involve the fetus directly but may be responsible for premature rupture of membranes as well as preterm delivery. The preterm infant is also at risk of postbirth infection and neurologic injury, as well as other organ injury or insult. Ironically, the infectious agents are in many instances bacteria that constitute the mother's vaginal flora, and in other instances are organisms introduced from the exogenous environment.

VAGINAL ECOSYSTEM

Infection involving the uterus and its contents should be viewed as a pelvic infection. Conceptually, this differs from gyneologic pelvic infection in that

there is a greater propensity for dissemination and adverse consequences for the fetus. Therefore, there must be a basic understanding of what constitutes a healthy vaginal ecosystem. The ecology of the vagina is complex and consists of an interaction between the host and the endogenous vaginal microflora. The host provides nutrients for the microflora, but also produces a variety of metabolic products, alkaline substances, amino and other acids, carbohydrates, peptides, proteins, and fragmented nucleic acids as well as immunoglobulins, and white blood cells (WBCs) that may attack microbes and hormones. All of these substances have the ability to affect microbes either favorably or unfavorably. Consequently, there exists a delicate equilibrium between all components of the vaginal ecosystem that has the net effect of suppressing more pathogenic resident bacteria and in some instances inhibiting organisms that are foreign to this ecosystem from establishing residence in it. However, this equilibrium is extremely delicate and can easily be disturbed by a variety of factors, including antibiotics, repeated douching, sexual practices and frequency, other disease involving the genital tract as well as distant from the genital tract, and steroids.

The bacteria that constitute the endogenous vaginal flora include gram-positive and gram-negative aerobic, facultative, and obligate anaerobes. These microorganisms exist as saprophytes or commensals. They may behave independently of one another or synergistically or antagonistcally toward one another. This interaction, along with other environmental factors, regulates the growth of all organisms within this ecosystem and therefore helps to determine the endogenous or resident microflora of the vaginal ecosystem at any given time. A healthy vaginal microflora contains a mixed population of bacteria with a density of 10^5 to 10^6/ml of vaginal secretion.[1,2] In a healthy vaginal ecosystem the dominant bacterium is *Lactobacillus acidophilus,* which produces lactic acid and is responsible for maintaining the pH of the system at 3.8 to 4.2. This pH favors the growth of nonpathogenic bacteria and suppresses the growth of pathogens. However, this hydrogen ion concentration does not impair or inhibit the growth of yeast, such as *Candida albicans.* The lactobacilli also produce hydrogen peroxide, which is toxic to anaerobic bacteria because they do not possess catalase,[3] the enzyme responsible for the breakdown of hydrogen peroxide to water and hydrogen.

The equilibrium of the vaginal ecosystem is in a dynamic state of flux that can easily be disturbed by both endogenous and exogenous factors. However, this equilibrium is maintained by the interaction of the bacteria that make up the healthy endogenous flora, of the vagina, and exherts an antagonistic effect on the pathogenic bacteria that commonly inhabit the lower genital tract. This is accomplished by a variety of substances produced by the endogenous bacteria, such as bacteriocins, enzymes, and other inhibiting factors. However, if the pH is increased to more than 4.5, the healthy flora are suppressed and the pathogens dominate. In the case of bacterial vaginosis (BV), *Gardnerella vaginalis* and *Mycoplasma hominis* become dominant early in the transition. As the local oxygen concentration decreases, the anaerobic bacteria assume a dominant role. This results in a further reduction in oxygen concentration until virtually all oxygen is depleted, decreasing the hydrogen ion concentration and increasing the pH to values between 5 and 6. This creates an environment that is virtually hostile to lactobacilli and the other bacteria that are characteristic of a healthy vaginal ecosystem. Both *G. vaginalis* and *M. hominis* can be isolated from the vagina in women with a vaginal pH of 3.8 to 4.2, and no other clinical parameters to suggest BV. This fact reinforces the concept of the

---

Bacterial Make-Up of a Healthy Vaginal Ecosystem

Lactobacillus acidophilus

Nondescript streptococci

Staphylococcus epidermidis

Diphtheroides

Corynebacterium

Escherichia coli

Proteus sp.

Enterobacter sp.

Bacteroides sp.

Bacteroides bivius

Bacteroides melaninogenicus

Fusobacterium sp.

Peptostreptococcus

Eubacterium

Veillonella

---

vaginal ecosystem as a complex system that exists in a dynamic state; the interaction between the bacteria and the other constituents of the ecosystem is a delicate relationship. Whether a healthy state will exist in the lower genital tract depends on many factors, endogenous as well as exogenous. These factors will also determine which bacteria will assume a dominant role and, therefore, the potential for infection. Occasionally, group B streptococci will inhabit and become the dominant bacteria in the vagina. Colonization rates for group B streptococci range from 5 to 25 percent, depending on geographic location.[4–7] These organisms have achieved a position of prime importance to both the physician providing obstetric care and the pediatrician.

Evaluation

All patients who are or are contemplating pregnancy should have an evaluation of the lower genital tract, just as one would routinely obtain specimens from the endocervix for sexually transmitted disease

(STD). The first evaluation that can be performed is easy and inexpensive, and involves determining the pH by using pH test strips that have a pH range from 4.0 to 6.0 in increments of 0.5 units. A vaginal pH of under 4.5 usually indicates that there is no overgrowth of anaerobic bacteria. However, a pH below 4.5 does not necessarily rule out the presence of a disturbed vaginal microflora, since the patient may, for instance lack or have a noticeable reduction in lactobacilli and have a flora dominated by one bacterial morphotype, such as short uniform bacilli, cocci, or yeast forms. Therefore, a microscopic examination of the vaginal should still be performed to determine whether (1) yeasts are present; (2) bacilliary forms are present, which would indicate lactobacilli; (3) if bacillary forms are absent, there is a dominant morphotype; (4) clue cells are present; (5) the squamous cells present are typical or atypical; and (6) yeast forms are present. If in studying the morphotypes of bacteria present, coccal forms predominate one should consider *Streptococcus agalactiae* as being present. This would indicate that a vaginal specimen as well as a urine specimen should be obtained for culture of this organism. The characteristics of the vaginal discharge are listed in Table 28-1.

Another step in the evaluation of vaginal discharge is to obtain a specimen of the discharge from the lateral vaginal wall with a cotton-tipped applicator and to place this in a test tube containing 2 to 3 ml of saline to dilute the discharge. Following this, a drop to two of the diluted discharge is placed on a glass slide and covered with a coverslip. The preparation should be examined with the aid of a microscope under $40\times$ magnification. This will allow the physician to determine whether yeast, BV, or trichomoniasis is present or whether there is an absence of bacillary forms. If there is difficulty in determining whether hyphal of budding yeast forms are present, a drop of discharge can be mixed with 10 percent potassium hydroxide to eliminate nonfungal forms. The fungal cell wall is composed of the polymer chitin, which is resistant to strong alkali. Thus, with two simple and inexpensive procedures, a variety of causes of vaginitis can be diagnosed and the status of the vaginal ecosystem ascertained. This is important because these common conditions of the lower genital tract may play a significant role in determining pregnancy outcome.

YEAST VAGINITIS

The true incidence of vuvlovaginitis caused by a fungal infection, most commonly *C. albicans*, is unknown. Thomason et al[8] found that 23.9 percent of patients with vaginitis seen in an infectious disease ambulatory care clinic had yeast vaginitis. However, every physician providing health care for women is quite familiar with the frequency with which this disease is encountered. Speculation about the factors predisposing to infection caused by this yeast has gone on for a long time. Regardless of the theories and nonmedical treatments that have been proposed, yeast infection is thought to be one of the most common and may be the second most common cause of vaginitis.[9] Pregnancy, a hyperestrogenic

Table 28-1. Characteristic of Vaginal Discharge as Related to the State of the Vaginal Ecosystem

Character	Healthy	BV	GBS	Yeast
Discharge	White to slate gray	Dirty	White to clear	White
Consistency	Thin	Thin, frothy	Thin	Thick, pasty
pH	3.8–4.5	>4.5	3.8–4.5	<4.5
Odor	None	Foul	None	Sweet
KOH	Negative	Negative	Negative	Positive
Whiff test	Negative	Positive	Negative	Negative
Microscopic	Clean[a]	Clue cells[b]	Clean	Hyphae or budding cells

Abbreviations: BV, bacterial vaginosis; GBS, group B streptococcus.
[a] Clean squamous epithelial cells do not have bacteria adherent to the cytoplasmic membrane; the free floating bacteria are dominated by a single morphotype (bacilli).
[b] Clue cells are squamous epithelial cells that are covered with adherent bacteria, and neither the cytoplasmic membrane nor the intracellular organelles could be ascertained.

state, appears to predispose women to yeast infection, and it is estimated that 30 to 40 percent of pregnant women will have asymptomatic colonization by *C. albicans* or other yeast species.[10] A similar situation is seen in women using the oral contraceptive pill. Reinforcing the concept that increased colonization by *Candida* species is associated with a hyperestrogenized state is the notable rarity of this infection in premenarchal and postmenopausal women. There is a noticeable increase in infection among women in the reproductive age group that coincides with higher estrogen levels. Another predisposing factor is diabetes, which is not uncommon in pregnancy. The infection may even serve to indicate that a diabetic screening test should be performed, perhaps earlier in the pregnancy than normal (at 25 weeks' gestation). It should be pointed out that Robinson et al[15] found no difference in glucose tolerance test results when comparing pregnant women with and without vaginal moniliasis.

However, the exact relationship between pregnancy and candidiasis is not understood. In 1934, Cruickshank et al[16] postulated that because there was an increase in glycogen in the vagina during pregnancy, this influenced colonization by yeast. There is little doubt that lactic acid is found in the vagina, but it has not been established that the lactobacilli in the vagina are glycogenolytic bacteria and that this is the mechanism that allows yeasts to have a growth spurt and cause symptomatic vaginitis. Lactobacilli do convert glycogen to lactic acid, which facilitates maintenance of the vaginal pH at a more acidic level, with a hydrogen ion concentration that is preferred by yeasts. In 1937, Bland et al[17] conducted an experiment in 12 pregnant and 12 nonpregnant women, all of whom had their vagina inoculated with *C. albicans*. They found that 10 of the 12 pregnant women developed monilial vaginitis, whereas only 4 of the 12 nonpregnant women became symptomatic. This observation lends support to the hypothesis that pregnancy creates a vaginal ecosystem that is conducive to the growth of yeast.

Although there is definitely an increase in vaginal colonization by yeast during pregnancy, there appears to be a dramatic increase in the third trimester. Coincident with this increase in vaginal colonization is an increase in oral and rectal colonization.[13–15] During the postpartum period there is a decline in vaginal colonization by yeast. Therefore, there is a change in the vaginal ecosystem that is influenced by hormonal change, having a net effect on the consitutents of the vaginal flora.

Many varieties of yeast can potentially cause vuvovaginitis. However, approximately 90 percent of infections are due to *C. albicans* with the remaider caused by *C. glabrata, C. tropicalis, C. pseudotropicalis, C. krusei, C. guilliermondii,* and *C. papapsilopsis.* Yeasts form part of the normal microflora of the human body, and humans are therefore the most important source of candidial infection. The gastrointestinal tract appears to be the main reservoir for yeasts which can be recovered in up to about 40 percent of individuals. Yeasts have been isolated from the lower genital tract in 29 percent of women with a healthy vaginal ecosystem.[16–19] Thus, it is likely that most infections are derived from existing colonization, and the activation of infection is likely to be due to a change in the equilibrium of the vaginal ecosystem.

Diagnosis

The patient with clinical vulvovaginitis usually presents with complaints of vaginal or vulvar itching (or both), and a burning sensation with sexual intercourse. The affected tissue becomes erythematous and there may be excoriations. On occasion, when the symptoms are severe, the labia may become edematous. The discharge is classically described as consisting of patches of thick white exudate, commonly referred to as a "cottage cheese-like discharge." However, the discharge may range from being thick and pasty to white, homogenous liquid. Vaginal candidiasis may also be present in association with other causes of vaginitis, and the discharge may appear atypical.

The diagnosis must be established with accuracy, since an improper diagnosis will result in treatment failure. The external genitalia should be closely inspected for the presence of blisters, ulcerations, and excoriations. A cotton-tipped swab should be used to wipe the external genitalia to retrieve a specimen. The cotton swab should then be immersed in saline to prepare a wet-mount slide for microscopic examination. A separate specimen should be obtained from the vagina and prepared in a similar fashion. If pseudohyphae or budding yeast cells are not observed, a slide with a drop of the specimen should be prepared, one drop of 10 percent KOH should be added, and the preparation should be examined microscopically. If no yeast or fungal forms are detected a specimen should be obtained for culture. Yeast can easily be grown by inoculating the specimen on either Nickerson's or Sabouraud's medium.[20–22] Specialized techniques for establishing a diagnosis of candidiasis are not necessary, since cases not detected by microscopic examination of the vaginal discharge will be determined by culture. There is no need to wait for the culture results to institute treatment once other causes of vaginitis have been ruled out. It would be a rare event to find an individual with symptoms and signs of a yeast infection and not detect yeast morphotypes by microscopic examination or culture of the vaginal discharge.

Recurrent Infection

It is almost impossible to determine the exact route by which a patient has acquired a yeast infection. However, there has been much discussion about two basic routes for such infection: contamination from the rectum and transmission during sexual intercourse. It has been demonstrated that *Candida* can be recovered from the rectum in 100 percent of women with vulvovaginal candidiasis.[23,24]

Since pregnancy favors the growth of yeast, patients with repeated episodes of yeast infection should be considered as having incomplete treatment and not necessarily as having recurrent infection. The usual dosing regimens are those used for the nonpregnant patient, and may well be inadequate for the pregnant patient. The pregnant patient with a yeast infection is more likely to benefit from a maintenance program than from treatments for acute episodes of infection. I would not use ketoconazole or fluconazole in the pregnant patient.

Treatment

A variety of antifungal agents are available for the treatment of yeast vaginitis. Many of these agents have not been tested in pregnant patients. Their use is based on the minimal adverse effects documented in nonpregnant patients. Agents such as amphotericin B, ketoconazole, and fluconazole are contraindicated for use in the pregnant patient.

Antifungal Preparations

Clotrimazoles (Imidazoles)
  Lotrimin
  Mycelex
  Mycelex G
  Gyne-Lotrimin
  Butoconazole (Femstat)
  Terconazole (Terazole)
  Miconazole (Monistat)
  Ketoconazole (Nizoral)
  Fluconazole (Diflucan)
Polyenes
  Amphotericin B (Fungizone)
  Candicidin (Vanobid)
  Nystatin
  Candex (Mycostatin)
  Mycolog II (Nystatin and triamcinolone)

These agents should not be used indiscriminately; rather, the diagnosis should be established by confirming the presence of yeast or hyphal forms by microscopic examination of the vaginal discharge. There is no need to obtain a specimen for the culture of yeast unless the patient has persistent problems of vaginal itching or burning and yeast forms cannot be identified microscopically. The preparations listed in Table 28-2 are all vaginal creams or tablets except for ketoconazole, which is available only for oral use in 200-mg tablets, and fluconazole, which is

Table 28-2. Treatment for *Neisseria gonorrhoeae* and *Chlamydia trachomatis* Infections

Agent	Dosage
Ceftriaxone	250 mg IM one time
Erythromycin	500 mg PO, qid × 10 days
Ceftriaxone	250 mg IM one time
Azithromycin	500 mg PO bid, one time
Ceftriaxone	250 mg IM one time
Clindamycin	300 mg PO tid × 10 days
Amoxicillin/clavulanic acid (Augmentin)	500 mg PO tid × 10 days

available for both intravenous and oral use (neither agent should be used in the pregnant patient).

When using the vaginal imidazoles, the patient should be instructed to insert one applicator-full or vaginal tablet carefully into the vagina, and to avoid traumatizing the cervix which may cause bleeding. The physician should examine the cervix before prescribing the medication to determine that there is no cervical dilatation. This will ensure that the patient will not rupture the amniotic membranes when inserting the applicator containing the medication.

BACTERIAL VAGINOSIS

A description of an unhealthy vaginal ecosystem is provided earlier. However, it is important to remember that BV may be totally asymptomatic and therefore the patient may not indicate that she is experiencing any difficulty with regard to her lower genital tract. Since there is a possible relationship between BV and premature labor, premature rupture of the amniotic membranes, and postpartum endometritis, it is important that the physician examine the vaginal discharge at the initial visit and at other opportune times during the pregnancy. The patient should be questioned about whether she has noted any change in her vaginal discharge (i.e., color change,odor), or vaginal itching or burning or other discomfort since her last visit, and if so, an examination should be performed.

A pH above 4.5 is an indication that the vaginal ecosystem is disturbed and further evaluation is needed (Table 28-1). There is basically one intravaginal treatment for the pregnant patient with BV: clindamycin 2 percent vaginal cream, with one applicator-full given daily for 7 days. However, this has not been shown to be effective in preventing preterm labor or preterm delivery.[29] A recent study in which pregnant women who had delivered a previous preterm infant and were treated with metronidazole for current diagnosis of BV found a reduction in preterm births.[30] Thus, although the data are not strong in establishing a cause-and-effect relationship in BV, there does appear to be a strong relationship. Therefore, if the examination of the pregnant patient at the time of her initial visit reveals BV, treatment should be undertaken. The patient should be re-examined at her next visit, and if there is a persistence

of BV, it should be determined whether sexual intercourse has taken place. If sexual intercourse has occurred, a second course of treatment should be instituted and the patient should either refrain from intercourse or insist that her partner wear a condom or be treated. That she has persistent BV should indicate that this condition can be perpetuated by sexual intercourse. Treatment of the partner can be accomplished with poral netronidazole, 250 mg tid for 7 days.

Although there are no concrete data that establish a cause-and-effect relationship between BV and interruption of pregnancy or postpartum endometritis, the available data do suggest that such a relationship exists.[31-34] Until it is established that a relationship does not exist, it would be in the mother's and fetus's interest to attempt to restore an unhealthy vaginal ecosystem to a healthy state. This approach is neither time consuming nor costly, and from a clinical point of view may therefore turn out to be very cost effective if it can reduce prematurity and postpartum endometritis. In addition, that the patient has BV or repeated episodes of BV does establish that she is sexually active and should encourage the physician to question her about her sexual behavior. This will enable the physician to determine whether the patient is at risk of acquiring an STD.

TRICHOMONIASIS

Vaginal trichomoniasis is a sexually transmissible disease and should be considered as a possible indicator for other STDs. When a diagnosis of trichomoniasis is established, it is important to determine whether the patient or her partner has entered into significant risk behavior. The patient's endocervix should be cultured for both the gonococcus and *Chlamydia*. Consideration should also be given to screening for syphilis and hepatitis B. The patient who is positive for gonorrhea and or *Chlamydia* should definitely be screened for syphilis and hepatitis. If the tests for syphilis or hepatitis B (or both) is positive, the patient should be tested for human immunodeficiency virus (HIV).

Treatment of the patient with trichomoniasis is difficult. Metronidazole is contraindicated in pregnancy, especially in the first trimester, although there are no data to support this position. Patients who have symptomatic infection and are more than 10 weeks pregnant can and probably should be treated with oral metronidazole. A single 2 g dose may be difficult for the patient to tolerate, especially if she is experiencing nausea. Therefore, I prefer 250 mg tid for 7 to 10 days. Intravaginal metronidazole gel should not be used in the treatment of vaginal trichomoniasis because the organism may also be present in the urethra, bladder, and Skene's and Bartholin's glands. Since there is inadequate absorption of metronidazole when it is administered as an intravaginal jel, trichomonads present at extravaginal sites would be unaffected and the patient is likely to experience a repeated episode or persistent infection. In addition, the efficacy of intravaginal metronidazole gel in the treatment of vaginal trichomoniasis has never been demonstrated.

Resistance to oral metronidazole is not a common problem, and patients who fail to respond to oral therapy should initially be evaluated for recurrent infection or noncompliance. In the event that the patient is not being reinfected and is compliant in taking the medication, the presence of a resistant strain of *T. vaginalis* should be considered. Metronidazole sensitivity testing against *T. vaginalis* is not routinely performed in clinical laboratories. Therefore, the patient could be treated with a combination or oral and intravaginal metronidazole as follows: 250 mg tid PO for 10 days and a 500-mg intravaginal suppository once a day for 10 days. The suppository would have to be prepared by the pharmacist, since it is not otherwise available. A specimen of the vaginal discharge should be cultured for isolation, identification, and propagation of the organism. If the organism can be cultured, its sensitivity to metronidazole may be determined.

CERVICITIS

Cervicitis can be caused by a variety of conditions that may or may not be infectious. It is important that the physician eliminate those causes that can be treated, and not become involved in those situations for which treatment does not exist. The treatable bacterial causes of cervicitis are *Nelsseria gonorrhoeae* and *Chlamydia trachomatis*. Other possible bacterial causes of cervicitis, such as the myoplasmas and ureaplasmas, cannot be easily eradicated and there-

fore, no attempt should be made to culture them. The relationship of mycoplasmas and ureaplasmas to significant cervical infection and interruption of pregnancy has not been established. Cervical colonization by *Mycoplasma* and *Ureaplasma* is not very responsive to antibiotic treatment, and their eradication from the lower genital tract is therefore not easily achieved.

Patients found to have gonorrhea or *Chlamydia* should be treated as though they were infected with both organisms. Infection with either or both of these organisms may have significant morbidity, especially if the patient develops disseminated infection, which is known to occur with *N. gonorrhoeae* infection. Although dissemination is less likely to occur with *C. trachomatis*, there is still the possibility of neonatal infection. There are two options for treatment in the pregnant patient, both of which rely on the patient being compliant. Consequently, if there were a single agent to treat both infections, it would reduce the need for intramuscular injection and also reduce cost. Treatment may be instituted before knowing which of the two bacteria or both may be present, and if the gonococcus is present, whether it is β-lactamase producing strain. The possible treatment regimens are listed in Table 28-2. Whichever treatment regimen is used, patients who are culture positive for either or both bacteria must be recultured after they have completed therapy.

It is advisable to encourage the patient with an *N. gonorrhoeae* or *C. trachomatis* infection to refrain from having sexual intercourse, and if this is not possible, the patient should use a condom. Treatment is also prescribed for the patient's partner. After approximately 3 weeks, usually the time of the patient's next prenatal visit, specimens are obtained from the endocervical canal for the isolation of *N. gonorrhoeae* and *C. trachomatis*. If the gonococcus is isolated, it is tested for β-lactamase production, especially if the patient was treated with amoxicillin/clavulanic acid. The penicillins as a class of antibiotics have been shown to be effective in the treatment of chlamydial cervicitis.[35-38]

Although these two organisms have the potential to adversely effect the outcome of the pregnancy, it is important to remember that they may function in a similar manner with regard to the maternal and fetal compartments. That is, *N. gonorrhoeae* will more than likely exhert an immediate effect with regard to the pregnancy, and is more likely to cause disseminated maternal disease, whereas *C. trachomatis* is more likely to cause neonatal disease. The physician must also be vigilant in the detection of STDs to prevent their spread within the community.

The ease with which these organisms are transmitted makes it imperative that the patient be educated about the means of their transmission as well as other STDs, and the significance of this to the community, local and distant. This can create problems between the patient and her partner, but it is important that the patient understand the significance of these infections in relation to her personal health and the well-being of her pregnancy. It is also important that both she and her partner realize that infection with one sexually transmitted organism raises the real possibility of being concomitantly infected with a second sexually transmitted organism that may pose a serious treat to survival, such as hepatitis B or HIV. Thus, the physician has a genuine opportunity to prevent the transmission and acquisition of serious STDs, and can have an important impact on the community in doing so. This can be accomplished by the physician assuming an active role in the diagnosis and management of STDs. It is also important to understand the epidemiology of these diseases if the physician is to have an effect on the STD pool within the community.

STREPTOCOCCUS AGALACTIAE

Streptococcus agalactiae has become a significant organism not only for the obstetrician and neonatologist but also for the gynecologist. This bacterium has become the center of much debate between obstetricians and pediatricians. The latter group favors universal screening of all obstetric patients for *S. agalactiae* infection, whereas, obstetricians favor screening of high-risk patients and patients with prolonged rupture of membranes. The controversy centers around the lack of a sensitive test for the presence of this bacterium in the genitourinary and rectal area in pregnant patients. A second complicating factor is that the organism apparently has the ability to wax and wane. Colonization rates vary from a low of 5 percent to highs of 25 percent or more.[39–41] Therefore, screening only once during a pregnancy may

fail to detect those individuals who subsequently become positive for the organism. A second issue concerns the point in the gestation at which the patient should be screened. A third issue is whether all patients who are group B streptococcus (GBS)-positive should be given antibiotic prophylaxsis during labor. The problems surrounding these issues are (1) the lack of a reliable and rapid test that is inexpensive; (2) the risk of adverse reactions with antibiotic prophylaxis given to all patients who are GBS positive; (3) selection of resistant bacterial strains when antibiotic prophylaxis is administered to a large number of patients; (4) the cost effectiveness of screening and administering prophylactic ampicillin to all known carriers of group B streptococci; and (5) whether infection can really be prevented.

It has been demonstrated that resistant bacterial strains can be selected from the pool of endogenous bacteria that reside in the vaginal ecosystem when patients are subjected to antibiotic prophylaxis. This has been demonstrated when cephalosporins are given prophylactically to patients undergoing cesarean section.[42–45] Prophylactic administration of ampicillin during labor to patients colonized by group B streptococci has been shown to select for resistant strains of *Escherichia coli* and *Klebsiella pneumoniae*.[46]

Thus, the subject of whether all pregnant patients should be screened for group B streptococci can be approached from two viewpoints: a scientific one in which the data are analyzed and conclusions developed from a logical evaluation of the data; and a personal one of putting oneself in the patient's position and letting emotion rule without relying on logical conclusions based on scientific and clinical data.

The first step in trying to develop a management protocol for this problem is to realize that no matter which approach is taken, not all GBS infections are going to be prevented. This is mainly because in some cases, infection of the fetus will have occurred before the patient goes into labor. This may also result in the presence of ruptured amniotic membranes. A second possibility is that the patient may be colonized by such a high inoculum that first exposure to an antibiotic during labor may allow insufficient time for significant erradication of the infecting bacterium. It is important to remember that at any given point in time, the patient is colonized by a population of bacteria, and that all the organisms within that population will not be in the same phase of growth. An antibiotic such as ampicillin will be effective against only those bacteria that are actively growing. Ampicillin, like all penicillins, interferes with synthesis of the bacterial cell wall, and those bacteria that are not actively growing and dividing will therefore not be affected by it. Moreover, since the patient will most likely be receiving intravenous fluids, the antibiotic will be actively excreted by the kidney. Thus, there is a possibility that the concentration of antibiotic in the blood will drop well below the threshold required for eradicating the organism. However, this does not mean that nothing should be done. Rather, the patient should be approached with a plan that is logical.

I recommend that the problem of GBS be discussed with the patient, explaining that there is controversy surrounding this subject and that no approach is available that would guarantee that her baby would be free of the risk of infection. My own opinion, based on clinical experience is that although a great deal of literature is available on the topic of GBS infection during pregnancy, there are no studies available that support any one position. Therefore, I would like to suggest several concepts and recommendations. GBS colonization varies from one location to another, and in many areas, studies have not been done to determine rates of colonization. I would recommend that if a physician is to perform universal screening, it be done at 25 weeks' gestation. This represents a point of potential viability if the fetus is delivered and a level III neonatal intensive care unit (NICU) is available. If the patient should enter labor prematurely, the physician will at least know whether GBS has been documented. If the patient was initially negative, she could be treated as positive if this was desired, or the physician could await the results of rescreening culture. The issue of the organism waxing and waning has always intrigued me, and I wonder if in reality this represents a decrease in the population to such a low point that it is not detected by routine culture methods, and whether, given the right environmental conditions, the organism might increase to detectable numbers. This is why many investigators favor the use of an enrichment step, such as Todd-Hewitt broth and subculturing on blood agar, to maximize the retrieval of group B streptococci.

The next issue concerns the administration of prophylactic antibiotics. The recommended agent is ampicillin, and there appears to be controversy over the appropriate dose. However, many individuals have overlooked the problem of drug distribution and excretion in the pregnant patient. In fact, one must consider the possibility of drug distribution and excretion being different in the laboring as opposed to the nonlaboring patient, and this in turn being different from the situation in the nonpregnant patient. Patients who develop preterm labor should perhaps be considered as infected and possibly requiring a different drug regimen. Since there is synergy between ampicillin and gentamicin against GBS, perhaps this regimen should be used in high-risk situations. Currently, when a GBS-colonized patient is admitted in labor, I administer ampicillin in a dose of 2 g IV every 6 hours during labor with a subsequent dose in the postpartum period. If cesarean section becomes necessary, I change the antibiotic to either ampicillin/sulbactam (Unasyn) or piperacillin/tazobactam (Zosyn). Patients who are admitted with risk factors but whose GBS status in not known are started on piperacillin/tazobactam or ampicillin/unasyn initially.

Another interesting aspect of group B streptococcus is its role in postpartum endometritis. This bacterium has the ability to cause early onset infection, within 12 hours after delivery. This is characterized by high temperatures, tachycardia, and elevated WBC count, and uterine tenderness.[47,48] Patients whose temperatures spike immediately following or within the first 24 hours after delivery should be considered infected, and antibiotics should not be withheld. These patients may become overtly septic and can present a septic shock-like picture.

CHORIOAMNIONITIS

Chorioamnionitis presents an interesting situation that may often be overlooked by the physician. Every physician recognizes chorioamnionitis when the patient is febrile and has tachycardia, uterine tenderness, and an elevated WBC count with a left shift, and when the fetus also has tachycardia. However, chorioamnionitis may often be more subtle and overlooked. The concept of occult infection is especially important when the patient presents in preterm labor with or without premature rupture of membranes. Such patients are likely to be at greater risk of complications because they are likely to receive tocolytic agents as well as steroids. Therefore, it is extremely important that the physician rule out the presence of infection and recognize its most subtle signs.

The evaluation of such patients should begin with a thorough history, to determine whether there have been risk factors associated with the development of premature labor or rupture of the membranes, with a specific quest for exposure to STDs or development of an altered vaginal ecosystem. It should also be determined whether there has been exposure to anyone with an illness. The investigation should begin with a thorough physical examination and a specific search for a focus of infection outside the pelvis. An attempt should be made to detect any signs of a viral illness, respiratory infection, or urinary tract infection before focusing attention on the uterus and its contents.

The uterus should be palpated for the presence of tenderness or pain as well as for contractions. The uterus should then be monitored for contractions and its resting tone should be determined. Infectious processes such as appendicitis, infection or abscess of Meckel's diverticulum, cholecystitis, or infection of any organ that might cause inflammation of the uterine serosa can stimulate the uterus to contract. The fetal heart rate (FHR) should be monitored to determine its baseline, rate, and degree of variability. A pelvic examination should begin with inspection of the vulva, followed by examination of the vagina with a speculum. Care should be taken not to abrade the cervix, prevent bleeding. Specimens should be obtained from the endocervical canal for culture of *N. gonorrhoeae* and *C. trachomatis*. The swab should be checked for the presence of mucous, and if positive the patient should be treated for both *N. gonorrhoeae* and *C. trachomatis*. A specimen should also be obtained from the lateral wall of the lower vagina. This should be sent for gram stain and culture for GBS. If gram-positive cocci are seen on Gram stain, I interpret this as indicating possible GBS infection and institute antibiotic therapy (Unasyn or Zosyn).

A complete blood count (CBC) with WBC differential, serum electrolytes, blood urea nitrogen (BUN),

serum creatinine, and C-reactive protein should also be obtained. Comparison should be made between the patient's WBC count and differential at her first prenatal visit and their current values. A WBC count that has at least doubled from the count obtained at the patient's first prenatal visit should be considered significant (e.g., an original WBC count of 4,500 and current count of 10,000). In addition, a 10 percent or greater increase in band forms is significant. The patient's vital signs should be monitored every hour for the first 6 hours to determine whether there is any significant change in temperature and pulse rate. If the patient is being examined in the morning, her oral temperature should be no higher than 98.6°F. A temperature greater than 99.6°F should be considered a possible clue to impending symptomatic infection. The patient should then be further evaluated.

An amniocentesis should be performed and the fluid should be processed with a Gram stain, assay for glucose concentration, and culture for aerobic, facultative, and obligate anaerobes. A negative Gram stain does not necessarily mean that bacteria are not present but may be at a concentration below 10^3/ml of amniotic fluid. The number of WBCs per high-power field should be determined, and if there are more than 5 WBCs, this finding should be interpreted as an indication of infection. A glucose concentration of less than 15 mg/ml of amniotic fluid suggests that infection may be present and that phagocytosis may have occurred.

Patients in premature labor who have intact membranes and a negative work-up for infection can be given tocolytic therapy. Patients who do not respond to tocolysis should be considered infected until proven otherwise. Whether steroids are administered to such patients depends on the philosophy of the particular labor-and-delivery service. The patient with ruptured membranes presents a more difficult problem, and if the evaluation is negative for infection I would not give steroids in this situation for fear that the patient might be infected but has not manifested any signs or symptoms. A (CBC) and WBC differential should be obtained before instituting therapy. The WBC differential is important because the patient may not manifest a high WBC count initially but may demonstrate an increase in band forms. Again, the patient's WBC count should be compared to the count obtained at the first prenatal visit. A repeat blood count should be obtained within 4 to 6 hours to determine whether there are any significant changes. C-reactive protein can be measured and should initially be obtained on a serial basis to establish any rising trend.

Before instituting antibiotics, tocolysis, or steroids, all laboratory test results should be obtained and specimens collected for the isolation of bacteria. In addition to specimens of amniotic fluid, venous blood should be obtained for the isolation of aerobic, facultative, and obligate anaerobic bacteria. A urine specimen should be collected aseptically and processed for uropathogens. I would also recommend Gram staining of the urine, which can yield almost immediate confirmation of the presence of bacteria and whether they are gram-negative or -positive, as well as whether they are of coccal or bacillary morphotype.

In choosing an antibiotic, one must first consider which bacterium or bacteria are most likely to be involved. The organisms to be considered as prime candidates are *S. agalactiae* and *E. coli*. It is also important to remember that the most likely offending bacteria are derived from the patient's own vaginal ecosystem. Therefore, anaerobic bacteria should also be considered, as must *N. gonorrhoeae* and *C. trachomatis*. Collectively, this requires either the use of a combination of antibiotics or one of the new β-lactam agents such as piperacillin/tazobactam (Zosyn), or ampicillin/sulbactam (Unasyn) or ticarcillin/clavulanate (Timentin). These two agents have a spectrum of activity that includes coverage of aerobic, facultative and obligate anaerobes, and both the gonococcus and *Chlamydia*. Piperacillin/tazobactam, ticarcillin/clavulanic acid, or ampicillin/sulbactam would also seem to be a logical choice because they provide good activity against the Enterobacteriaceae, whereas there is reluctance to use an aminoglycoside in the pregnant patient unless there is serious infection, for fear of inflicting fetal toxicity. However, it should be pointed out that the three combinations are not equal in their antibacterial activity. Antibiotics should be given only if the patient is proven to be infected or there is a strong suspicion of infection. They should not be given to these patients for prophylaxis, since this might enhance the selection of resistant bacteria.

If the patient is in preterm labor and infection is ruled out, then attempts can be undertaken to inhibit uterine contractions. The initial tocolytic agent should be one that has the fewest side effects and does not put the patient at significant risk of pulmonary edema. It is important to remember that when tocolytic agents such as terbutaline or ritodrine are used and the patient is infected, capillary leaks may develop in the pulmonary bed. This can lead to pulmonary edema and even adult respiratory distress syndrome (ARDS). Therefore, it is critical that infection be ruled out before instituting tocolytic therapy. In order to minimize the side effects of tocolysis, an agent such as magnesium sulfate should be the initial therapy. However, if the patient is not actually in labor, but has an irritable uterus that is unresponsive to hydration, a trial of subcutaneously administered terbutaline can be attempted. If the patient is unresponsive but continues to have noticeable contractions, intravenous magnesium sulfate can be administered. Patients who are unresponsive to tocolysis or break through it should be considered infected. Antibiotic therapy should be given to these patients.

If at the time of delivery a cesarean section has been performed, specimens should be obtained for the culture of microorganisms even if the patient has been receiving antibiotics. The patient most likely to develop postpartum endometritis, bacteriemia, or septic shock is one with a substantial infection. If bacteria have made their way into the myometrium to begin the septic process, even though the patient may have received from one to three doses of antibiotic, enough residual bacteria should be present to isolate and identify on culture. The culture will also be beneficial if a resistant organism is present.

It appears that the best specimen for the culture of aerobic, faculatative, and obligate bacteria is a myometrial biopsy specimen obtained at the time of cesarean section. A study performed by Smith et al found that if the tissue specimen was obtained prior to delivery of the infant, bacteriologic examination reflected that bacterial invasion of the myometrium had occurred prior to delivery and that the inoculum size was 100,000 or more colonies per milliliter of homogenized tissue. The infections tended to be unimicrobial, and anaerobes constituted a minority of the organisms present. However, antibiotic therapy is begun prior to knowing the bacteriologic results,

---

Bacteria Commonly Associated With Intrapartum and Postpartum Infection

Streptococcus agalactiae

Escherichia coli

Enterococcus faecalis

Gardnerella vaginalis

Prevatella bivia

Peptostreptococcus

---

and the choice of antibiotic must therefore reflect the possible involvement of a variety of bacteria. The β-lactam antibiotics can simplify antibiotic usage by reducing cost, toxicity and nursing time while offering the physician an opportunity to meet the criteria listed earlier without a difference in the spectrum of activity from that of combinations such as clindamycin and an amnioglycoside.

One bacterium that is not commonly seen today but is still likely to present a challenge is the group A streptococcus (GAS), *Streptococcus pyogenes*. This is the organism that was the cause of childbed fever or puerperal sepsis described by both Semelweiss and Holmes. It is highly virulent and like GBS can cause disease that manifests itself early in the intrapartum or postpartum period. Unlike GBS, GAS is associated with a significant degree of mortality, and can

---

B-Lactam Antibiotics for Treatment of Intra- and Postpartum Infection

Penicillins
  Ampicillin/sulbactam (Unasyn)
  Piperacillin/tazobactam (Zosyn)
  Ticarcillin/clavulanate (Timentin)

Cephalosporins
  Cefotetan
  Cefoxitin
  Ceftizoxime

---

cause a septic shock-like syndrome and mysositis, as well as a necrotizing fasciitis.

That patients with GAS infection are likely to develop an elevated WBC count during labor should initiate a more thorough evaluation by the physician if there is a shift in the WBC differential toward an increase in band forms or an elevated temperature, or both. An elevated temperature should not be considered as transient or as representing dehydration. Patients whose oral temperatures are elevated should have their temperature rechecked every hour to identify whether the elevation is transient. Patients whose temperature does not rapidly return to normal should be considered infected until the opposite is proven. They should be thoroughly evaluated with appropriate tests and cultures. It should be remembered that both GAS and GBS usually cause early onset infection that usually has a virulent course. Both of these bacteria tend to be highly susceptible to the penicillin class of antibiotics, and early recognition of infection, appropriate evaluation and the early institution of appropriate antibiotic therapy should result in immediate resolution of the infection.

LISTERIA MONOCYTOGENES

Listeria monocytogenes is a gram-positive, microaerophilic, motile bacillus that was described in 1926 by Murray et al.[49] Brunn[50,51] isolated *L. monocyctogenes* from neonatal patients and from adults with fatal meningitis. The organism was finally named after Dr. Joseph Lister. It is an interesting bacterium in that it infects animals but may be transmitted on vegetables and dairy products. The infection can be quite serious, with significant mortality. The overall incidence is 0.7 cases per 100,000 population, with an estimated 1,850 cases of bacteremia or meningitis per year in the United States, resulting in 425 deaths.[52]

Transmission of the bacterium may occur through various vectors. Listeriosis is believed to be primarily transmitted by dairy products, such as pasteurized and unpasteurized milk, and biologically fertilized vegetables, cheese, ice cream, and cream, and also by improperly processed poultry, and from one human to another.[53–59]

The pregnant patient who contracts a *Listeria* infection may be asymptomatic or develop "flu-like" symptoms, a mononucleosis-like syndrome, or bacteremia or meningitis.[60] *Listeria* infection may proceed through a long incubation period of several weeks, thus making the distribution of the disease widespread in both time and location. Typically, the pregnant patient with a documented infection is managed by delivery of the fetus. Fleming et al[61] reported a case of maternal listeriosis managed with antibiotics, with successful maintenance of the pregnancy. *L. monocytogenes* was isolated from the patients blood and was eradicated by ampicillin administered in a dose of 2 g IV every 4 hours for 14 days. Faro et al[62] managed a case of *Listeria* bacteremia and intra-amniotic infection by administering ampicillin in a dose of 2 g IV every 4 hours. In this case the patient's bacteremia resolved within 48 to 72 hours of therapy but the intra-amniotic infection could not be resolved. Serial amniocentesis was performed weekly during ampicillin therapy, and after 3 weeks the bacterium could still be isolated from the amniotic fluid. The concentration of ampicillin in the infected amniotic fluid was 41 μg/ml and the MIC_{90} was above 50 μg/ml. However, the MIC_{90} when determined in Mueller-Hinton agar and in sterile amniotic fluid was less than 4 μg/ml. Thus, the antibiotic does not appear to be biologically active in infected amniotic fluid. This latter patient went on to deliver at 30 weeks, and the infant survived without any difficulties and is now 7 years old and doing well.

It cannot be emphasized too strongly that patients who present with preterm labor, whether their membranes are ruptured or not, should be suspected of being infected until proven otherwise. Since many intra-amniotic infections as well as chorioamnionitis or deciduitis may be occult, it is important to perform a thorough evaluation. The clue to occult infection is the presence of preterm labor or preterm rupture of membranes with or without labor. Managing intra-amniotic infection, choriamnionitis, or deciduitis with the use of antibiotics and attempting to maintain a pregnancy in utero requires that the patient understand the risks involved (i.e., sepsis, septic shock, intrauterine death, disseminated intravascular coagulopathy [DIC], and possibly maternal death). It also requires that the physician evaluate the patient several times a day and have the capability to evacuate the uterus rapidly. A proficient and efficient microbiology department as well as a clinical laboratory must be on site to perform all tests that are or may be necessary.

POSTPARTUM ENDOMETRITIS

It is important to remember that most cases of postpartum infection are caused by the patient's own vaginal flora. Therefore, even if the patient is known to be colonized by GBS, one should not exclude the possibility that another bacterium may be responsible for or involved in the infection. This is the reason that a narrow-spectrum antibiotic such as a penicillin should not be used to treat such infection, and why a broad-spectrum agent such as a β-lactam antibiotic or a combination of antibiotics such as ampicillin, clindamycin, and gantamicin should be administered. A specimen for culture should be obtained either at the time of cesarean section, if there is a high index of suspicion, or when a diagnosis of postpartum endometritis is made.

The specimen should be obtained by (1) inserting a sterile speculum into the vagina; (2) removing all lochia and clots; (3) introducing a small sponge on a ring forceps into the uterine cavity to remove clots and assist in drainage of the uterus; and (4) introducing a pipette into the uterus, taking care not to brush against the vaginal or cervical walls, advancing it to the fundus, and taking a biopsy of the uterine lining.[63,64] This is necessary if one wants to attempt to culture the infected tissue and not the uterine lochia. Even this specimen will not be truly representative of the actual site of infection, which is the myometrium, but represents the best possible specimen at this time. The specimen should be put into an anaerobic transport vial and taken to the laboratory for culture, isolation, identification, and bactetial sensitivity testing of aerobic, faculatative, and obligate anaerobes, *Chlamydia*, mycoplasmas, and ureaplasmas.

If a specimen is obtained at the time of cesarean section, the best specimen would be a biopsy specimen of the myometrium at the incision site, obtained before entry into the amniotic cavity or delivery of the infant. This tissue specimen should be placed in an anaerobic transport vial for processing, as described above. If the placenta is to be cultured, it is best to incise a cotlyedon of the placenta and retrieve a piece of the deep tissue to reduce the possibility of contamination. Another possible sampling technique is to separate the amnion from the chorion, swab the opposing surfaces and place the swab into an anaerobic transport vial. The objective of meticulously obtaining a specimen for culture is to reduce the possibility of obtaining contaminating organisms from the lower genital tract.

It is also important to obtain a specimen of urine for culture. It is highly likely that the patient will have asymptomatic bacteriuria. It is also likely that bacteria will traverse the bladder wall and gain entrance to the uterus during labor or delivery. This is especially true for highly virulent organisms. Blood cultures should also be obtained at this time.

Once the specimens have been obtained, antibiotics should be administered. Patients with uncomplicated infection that is detected early will usually begin to show improvement within 48 hours after initially receiving antibiotics. Patients who do not show improvement or whose infection becomes more severe should be re-evaluated to confirm the original diagnosis or establish a new diagnosis. A differential diagnosis should be established to assist in determining the management approach that is to be taken. It is extremely important that the antibiotic initially administered be given ample opportunity to achieve its objective. However, it must be understood that an antibiotic given for prophylaxis may select for a resistant organism. The antibiotic initially chosen for therapy, if it is of the same class as the prophylactic agent (i.e., a cephalosporin) may increase the chance of selection. This selection process may not be initially apparent, but can be seen in patients in whom there appears to be an initial defervescence but a failure of the body temperature to truly reach a nadir of 98.6°F, with a subsequent significant temperature elevation. If a culture of the endometrium is repeated at this time, it is not uncommon to find a pure culture of a bacterium resistant to the antibiotic being administered. Although this is not a common finding, it is my approach to use a cephalosporin such as cefotetan or cefoxitin for prophylaxis, and to treat a subsequent endometritis with ampicillin/sulbactam, piperacillin/tazobactam, or ticarcillin/clavulanic acid.

All patients who develop postpartum endometritis are given antibiotics empirically. However, if endometrial cultures are obtained at the time the initial diagnosis is established, the laboratory can be of as-

---

Differential Diagnosis for Patients Failing Initial Antibiotic Therapy for Postpartum Endometritis

Infection present outside the pelvis

Presence of a resistant bacterium or bacteria

Infected retrovesicle hematoma

Septic pelvic vein thrombosis

Myometrial microabscesses

Necrosis of the myometrium

Pelvic abscess

Bacteremia

Viral infection

Drug fever

---

sistance if the patient does not respond to treatment. It is unrealistic to expect that a patient will respond to an antibiotic within 48 hours after receiving the initial dose. If the patient is not responding, the laboratory should be able to determine whether there is any growth on aerobic culture plates. If there is growth, a Gram stain can be done to determine whether the organism is gram-positive or gram-negative, and whether its morphotype is bacillary or coccal. This will assist in making appropriate alterations in antibiotic therapy.

Patients who fail to respond to a cephalosporin, such as cefoxitin and for whom the laboratory reports the growth of gram-negative rods should have an amnioglycoside added to their regime. The organism in such cases is most likely to be a resistant *E. coli* or *Enterobacter cloacae*. If the organism is a gram-positive coccus, it is most likely *Enterococcus faecalis*, since the cephamycins have activity against group B streptococci and staphylococci. The likelihood of the patient acquiring a methicillin-resistant *Staphylococcus* within the hospital is small. Therefore, the addition of ampicillin to the treatment regimen should be adequate. There is no need to discontinue the cephamycin, since the ampicillin will provide more than adequate coverage against anaerobes. Discontinuing the original antibiotic and substituting clindamycin plus gentamicin will not accomplish anything because the spectrum of these two agents does not provide increased gram-positive coverage (e.g., there is no activity against enterococcus or *Listeria*) if this is also a concern.

Patients receiving an expanded-spectrum penicillin (ampicillin/sulbactam, ticarcillin/clavulanic acid, or piperacillin/tazobactam) who are not responding to it should have an aminoglycoside added to their regimen. However, it is important to understand that the addition of a β-lactamase inhibitor does not increase the activity of the parent agent against enterococcus. Therefore, ticarcillin or ticaricillin/clavulanic acid may well prove ineffective against the enterococcus because the MIC$_{90}$ of ticarcillin for the organism is at best 32 μg/ml. Adding an aminoglycoside will also not provide sufficient synergy against enterococcus. However, both ampicillin and ticarcillin have good activity (ampicillin MIC$_{90}$ 2 μg/ml, piperacillin MIC$_{90}$, 4 μg/ml) and there is excellent synergy when an aminoglycoside is added to either of these agents. If a gram-negative bacterium is isolated, the addition of an amnioglycoside will provide the necessary activity.

If the patient has an enterococcal bacteremia, it is imperative that a combination of a penicillin and an amnioglycoside be used. In this instance either piperacillin/tazobactam or ampicillin/sulbactam can be employed. This is necessary to provide activity against the enterococcus while also maintaining gram-negative faculatative and obligate anaerobic activity. This is important because even though the patient may be bacteremic, the endometritis must also be treated. The latter may be due to a single organism, but may well also be polymicrobial, and the anaerobic culture results will not be known at the same time as the aerobic and blood culture results.

There have been many studies by many investigators demonstrating the effectiveness of agents such as the cephamycins and expanded-spectrum penicillins in treating postpartum endometritis. These agents have also been shown to be as effective as combinations such as clindamycin or metronidazole plus an aminoglycoside.[65–67]

VIRAL INFECTIONS

Viral infections in pregnancy are many and varied, ranging from infections with the common cold virus to infections by specific viruses that may or may not have a detrimental effect on the mother and fetus. It is not the intent of this discussion to be inclusive, but rather to mention those viruses that commonly occur in the pregnant patient. There is a common thread in all viral infections with regard to their presentation, independent of whether the patient is pregnant. All viral infections pass through an incubation phase during which the patient will very likely experience symptoms common to all such infections. These include fever, which may be low grade (i.e., <101°F) or high (i.e., ranging between 101° and 104°F), general malaise, myalgia, and arthralgia. It is during this phase that the viremia usually occurs. Shortly after or during the viremia the patient may develop a rash, which is often characteristic of a particular virus. It is during the viremia and development of the rash that the mother can transmit the infection to her fetus and any other contacts. The transmission of most viral infections, with the exception of the sexually transmitted viral infections, occurs through droplets spread by coughing, sneezing, and kissing.

Since the viral infections are not distinguished by characteristic symptoms or signs at an early stage in their development, it is important that all pregnant patients experiencing a prodrome of infection should notify their obstetrician or other health-care provider about having contracted an illness. It is important that the health-care provider not only conduct a telephone conversation and conclude that the individual has the "flu," but encourage the patient to come to the office and be examined. I prefer to have the patient come toward the end of the day unless there is an obvious reason why she should be seen immediately. I prefer a late afternoon office visit because this is the time that the patient's temperature is more likely to be rising, and when there are likely to be fewer patients in the office who may be inadvertently exposed to her illness.

The patient should be questioned about possible exposure to children or individuals who have recently been ill. It should be remembered that in many viral infections there is a great possibility of the absence of symptoms. Therefore, a patient who is symptomatic provides an opportunity to document an adverse event and a possible explanation should her infant be born with a deficiency. The attitude that viral infections are not treatable and that nothing can be done for them is erroneous and can no longer be tolerated. There is treatment for some viral infections and management options for many of these diseases, but first a diagnosis must be established.

Herpes Simplex

The incidence of herpes simplex infection in a population not exposed to a high frequency of STDs is estimated to be 0.25 to 3.0 percent, while in a population that is sexually promiscuous it ranges from 1.6 to 8 percent.[68] The incidence of herpes in a pregnant population is not different from that in a nonpregnant population ranging from 0.1 to 4 percent.[69,70] One interesting question that has not been satisfactorily resolved is the significance of asymptomatic genital viral shedding in a pregnant patient at term. Studies of the coincidence of asymptomatic viral shedding have shown that approximately 0.1 to 0.4 percent of pregnant women known to have had a herpetic infection will shed virus in the absence of a lesion at delivery, and that 0.01 to 0.04 percent of the neonates born to these women will acquire the infection.[71] Women with acute herpetic lesions at the time of delivery will transmit the disease to their newborns in 40 to 60 percent of cases and the mortality rate can reach as high as 50 percent. Among the survivors, 15 to 25 percent will have significant ocular and or central nervous system damage.[72,73]

There are no well-controlled studies of acyclovir in pregnant patients with herpes, but it would appear that this drug is well suited for use in the pregnant patient with acute herpetic infection. The drug is not activated in cells that are not infected with the virus, and therefore does not pose a threat to the fetus. The drug is used in the treatment of neonates, and should therefore not be withheld from the pregnant patient, especially if at 36 weeks' gestation or longer, who is in labor or near delivery. It would seem that the patient who has acute or recurrent disease near term is a candidate for treatment with acyclovir.

Cytomegalovirus

The cytomegalovirus is a member of the herpesvirus class, but is not sensitive to acyclovir. Infection with the organism is relatively common, affecting from 1 to 2 percent of all newborns. Most pregnant women acquire the infection from children or chronically ill patients. Usually the infection is asymptomatic or the patient may develop what she believes is the "flu," and does not inform her obstetrician that she has been or is ill.

The patient will experience a viremia during the acute phase of the illness. However, in contrast to most other viral infections, there is usually no rash associated with cytomegalovirus infection. The fetus can be infected in utero by hematogenous spread of the virus, or during vaginal birth. Cesarean section does not offer any protection against infection because during operative delivery the fetus is exposed to large volumes of maternal blood and vaginal secretions.

As advised earlier, patients should inform their physician of all illnesses. Neither the patient nor the physician should conclude that the patient has the flu or a cold on the basis of information given over the telephone. The physician should question the patient about possible contacts, her other children, and whether she works in an institution where she is exposed to children or individuals with chronic illness. If there is any suspicion that the patient may have a cytomegalovirus infection, appropriate serum antibody titers should be obtained. The patient may shed virus in bodily fluids yet be totally asymptomatic. This viral shedding may occur over long periods. Cervical secretions can serve as a reservoir for the virus, and among infected women 3 to 4 percent will shed the virus. However, newborns infected through cervical secretions during labor usually do not develop significant infection.[74,75] The virus may also be transmitted via breast milk. Cytomegalovirus has been isolated in 13 percent of lactating women and 58 percent of the infants of these women became viremic.[76]

Infants infected in utero and born with symptomatic infection tend to have petechial hemorrhages, hepatosplenomegaly, jaundice, thrombocytopenia, microcephaly, and chorioretinitis. Some pregnant women experience fetal death in utero. Women who experience fetal death in utero, neonatal death, or the birth of child with the stigma of cytomegalovirus infection are quite apprehensive about subsequent pregnancies. When they become pregnant they want something done to prevent infection, but this cannot be accomplished. Recurrent infection may be due to reactivation of a latent cytomegalovirus infection rather than to a new infection. Infected individuals do develop antibodies, which reduce the virulence of subsequent neonatal infection but do not provide complete immunity.[77]

Varicella-Zoster

Varicella-zoster is a member of the herpesvirus class and is responsive to acyclovir. The varicella component affects approximately 2 percent of women of childbearing age. Among pregnant women, approximately 0.1 to 0.5 percent develop varicella. It is interesting that in one study, from 11 to 33 percent of adults with varicella developed pneumonia, of whom 17 percent died, whereas among pregnant women 41 percent died.[78] In another review 29 percent of 77 patients with acute varicella developed pneumonia and 45 percent died.[79] Thus, varicella in pregnancy is not a disease to be taken lightly, especially since, with the advent of acycylovir, mortality from varicella pneumonia has been reduced to a minimum.

Pulmonary symptoms usually begin 2 days before the onset of the rash. Not all patients who develop pneumonia will develop severe symptoms; approximately one-third of infected individuals will develop a mild, nonproductive cough. Others will develop a rapidly progressive disease with high fever and a constellation of respiratory signs such as dyspnea, tachycapnea, pleural effusion, and in some cases pulmonary edema. Patients who develop a rash should be seen immediately because the respiratory manifestations of varicella infection usually develop 2 days before the onset of the rash, and within 6 days after its development. It is therefore imperative that these patients be examined thoroughly, and if not found to have pulmonary involvement be instructed about the changes in their physical condition that are likely to occur within the next 6 to 10 days.

The most common scenario is for a pregnant patient to call the obstetrician and report that she has been exposed to someone with chickenpox. The patient usually does not recall ever having had chickenpox, and her parents are not helpful. The physician should not administer any therapy at this time. A varicella titer should be obtained and the result must be known within 24 hours because the physician will have a 72-hour window in which to adminis-

ter varicella-zoster immunoglobulin (VZIG) in an attempt to prevent or reduce the severity of acute symptomatic varicella infection.[80,81]

Treatment of acute symptomatic varicella and varicella pneumonia can be accomplished with acyclovir. The patient should be treated as early in the course of developing pneumonia as possible. Delay often results in an advanced pneumonic process and secondary bacterial infection. The usual dose is 10 mg/kg body weight given intravenously in three divided doses every 8 hours.[82–84] Patients who have acute varicella but do not have pneumonic involvement could be considered for treatment with oral acyclovir, but, there are no data to support the use of oral acyclovir in the treatment of varicella.

Varicella infection acquired by the mother within a few weeks of delivery may create a bad prognosis for the newborn. The incubation period after exposure to the virus ranges from 10 to 17 days, maternal viremia occurs within 12 to 48 hours before the development of the rash, and maternal antibodies do not appear in the maternal blood for 4 to 5 days after onset of the rash. Therefore, infants born before the development of maternal IgG antibody are at risk of serious varicella infection. The mortality rate for newborn infants who develop varicella between 5 and 10 days of life is 31 percent.[85]

Mothers exposed to varicella but who deliver within 2 weeks of exposure usually do not put their newborns at risk because viremia has not occurred before delivery. Infants who develop the disease after 10 days of life usually experience a mild case of varicella. Mothers exposed to the virus and who are antibody-negative should receive VZIG for maternal indications only, since the VZIG will have no beneficial effect on the fetus. Approximately 50 percent of infants born to mothers with varicella of recent onset will develop acute disease.[86]

Women who develop their disease near term and appear to be on the verge of beginning labor should have their delivery delayed for approximately 5 days. This will allow enough time for the development of maternal antibodies and their transfer across the placenta, which will result in passive immunization and offer protection to the fetus and newborn. Obviously, one must weigh the risk of inhibiting labor against the risk of delivery. Infants born during the maternal incubation period, although at no significant risk of developing varicella, also lack the passively acquired antibody to it. They should therefore be kept isolated from the mother and should not be breast feed until the rash has been present for at least 5 days, since infants can acquire the virus as well as maternal antibodies to it through breast milk.

The fetus is at significant risk from varicella infection at two periods during its development: before the completion of organogenesis and if born before the development of maternal antibodies. Congenital sequelae of varicella include intrauterine growth retardation (IUGR), limb aplasia, scarring, neurologic deficits, and ophthalmaologic defects. Infection at any other time during pregnancy may result in deficits, but these may not be noticeable at the time of birth. The defects may become apparent as the child grows older and shows ophthalmogic abnormalities or psychomotor deficits, or develops seizures.[87–90]

Parvovirus B19

Parvovirus B19 infection is commonly referred to as "fifth disease" or "slapped cheek disease" and is due to a single stranded deoxyribonucleic acid (DNA) virus. Infection with parvovirus B19 was first recorded in 1975.[91] However, it was not until 1985 that the virus was found to cause serious infection, producing aplastic anemia in a patient with sickle cell anemia.[92]

Infection with parvovirus B19 is responsible for a variety of diseases, including erythema infectiosum (EI), also known as fifth disease; transient aplastic anemia (TAC) in patients with chronic hemolytic anemia; intrauterine fetal death; spontaneous abortions; arthralgias; arthritis; nonimmune fetal hydrops; and chronic anemia in immunodeficent patients.[93–106]

It is important to know the characteristics of the disease as it presents in children, because the disease tends to be asymptomatic in adults. It is most likely acquired through respiratory secretions, and passes easily among individuals in the same household, gatherings within limited spaces such as school rooms, and in any other situations in which the pregnant patient may be exposed to children. The characteristic disease in children is erythema infectiosum (fifth disease or slapped cheek disease). Affected children are very likely to develop a facial rash that

manifests itself as "rosy-cheeks," hence the alternative name of "slapped cheek disease." The rash can and often does appear distributed over other parts of the body as well. It is reticulated or lace-like on the trunk and extremities.[107] The virus has an incubation period of up to 20 days. Approximately 20 to 50 percent of adults tend to be asymptomatic. Symptomatic adults may develop a typical flu-like syndrome, arthralgias, arthritis, a reticulated rash, pruritis or rubella-like exanthems.[107]

Following exposure to an individual with active disease, serum and respiratory secretions become positive within 5 to 10 days.[109,110] The rash usually appears within 17 to 18 days. Viremia is usually present only during the initial 5 days, and infection is therefore transmitted through serum or respiratory secretions.[107] Exposure to the virus results in acquisition of the disease in 50 to 90 percent of persons within a household, whereas exposure in a school setting will result in a 10 to 60 percent frequency of infection among students and 20 to 30 percent of the staff will contract the disease.[95,106] Vertical transmission from the maternal compartment to the fetal compartment can occur, but its actual risk is unknown.[91,108]

Intrauterine fetal death from parvovirus B19 infection has been reported, and the overall fetal loss rate reported in one study was approximately 17 percent.[108] In the latter study it appeared that infections occurring within in the first and second trimester were more likely to result in fetal loss than those occurring during the third trimester. In this study, 10 percent of all the fetal deaths were attributed to parvovirus B19. Serologic studies performed on liveborn infants delivered from infected women revealed that less than one-third were positive, indicating that vertical transmission is incomplete.[109] In a study of four women exposed to parvovirus B19 and found to have IgM antibodies to the virus, three of the four had fetuses that became hydropic.[99] These same investigators reported a review of 37 cases of infected mothers with 14 infected fetuses, of whom 11 were found to be hydropic. It is not surprising that parvovirus B19 can cause fetal hydrops, since the virus has a predilection for the hematopoietic system. Porter et al[110] reported a review of 50 fetuses with nonimmunologic hydrops and found 8 percent to be positive for B19 DNA.

Diagnosis of parvovirus B19 infection can be made from serum IgM and IgG antibodies. The IgM antibody is detectable 3 days after symptoms of erythema infectiosum appear, and will remain up to about 60 days after infection occurs. The IgG antibody appears approximately 7 days after the onset of the illness and persists for years. Pregnant women tested for parvovirus B19 should always have IgM titers measured, since if acute infection is suspected they will remain for up to 60 days. IgG antibody titers should also be measured if there is suspicion of infection. Individuals known to or who are strongly suspected of being infected should have their fetuses examined by ultrasonography, and this should be done serially. If there is evidence of hydrops, an intrauterine blood transfusion should be performed.[111]

Viral Hepatitis

Hepatitis can result from a variety of insults as well as infection, and may be caused by many different microorganisms, including viruses. However, the most common viral infections of the liver involve the specific viral agents listed in Table 28-3.

Hepatitis A

The hepatitis A virus (HAV) is responsible for what has been referred to as infectious hepatitis. This is because it is commonly transmitted via the fecal–oral route, however, the infection has increased among homosexuals and is now classified as an STD.[112] That hepatitis A can be transmitted from contaminated food and culinary items or sexual activity puts pregnant women also at risk.

Hepatitis A, like other types of viral hepatitis, presents as a gastroenteritis with fever, nausea, vomiting, fatigue, and tenderness and pain in the right epigastrium. The patient may or may not develop jaundice. The disease does not progress to a chronic carrier state and is therefore self limiting. Although most cases are mild, serious infection may occur, with liver disease resulting in hepatic failure and death. In the United States, there were approximately 21,000 cases of hepatitis A annually from 1985 to 1990, with 70 fatalities.[113]

Because of the nonspecific clinical symptoms and signs of hepatitis, specific infection is diagnosed by serologic testing for specific antibodies[114] (Table 28-3). Early in the course of the infection or acute disease, the presence of IgM antibody specific to HAV establishes that infection is present.[114] Elevated titers of anti-HAV IgM will remain in the maternal serum for several months and then decline rapidly. Anti-HAV IgG will appear in the maternal serum within 1 to 2 weeks after the titer of IgM begins to rise. Unlike the IgM antibody, anti-HAV IgG will persist for years and will therefore serve as a marker of past infection as well as of patients who received

Table 28-3. Common Causes of Viral Hepatitis

Viral Agent	Diagnostic Test	Effect
Hepatitis A (infectious hepatitis)	Anti-HAV IgM	Indicates acute infection
	Anti-HAV IgG	Past exposure/immunity
Hepatitis B (serum hepatitis)	Hb_sAg	Carrier/infectious
	Hb_eAg	Highly infectious
	Anti-HB_e	Reduced infectibility
	Anti-HB_c	Indicates convalescence
	Anti-HB_s	Indicates recovery
Hepatitis C (non-A, non-B)	Anti-HCV	Indicates exposure/infection
	Elevated ALT, AST	Acute disease
Hepatitis D (delta agent; delta hepatitis)	HDV-Ag	Acute/chronic infection
	Anti-HDV IgM	Acute infection
	Anti-HDV IgG	Exposure/current disease
Hepatitis E	No clinical test available	

Abbreviatons: HAV, hepatitis A virus; HB$_s$Ag, hepatitis B surface antigen; HB$_e$Ag, hepatitis B e antigen; HB$_c$, hepatitis B core, (antigen); HCV, hepatitis C virus; HDV, hepatitis D virus; ALT, alanine aminotransferase; AST, aspartate aminotransferase.

immune serum globulin (ISG) for prophylaxis against hepatitis A. Anti-HAV IgG can also be used to document active infection by obtaining serum samples 2 to 3 weeks apart and noting a fourfold rise in the titer; in patients who have recovered from the acute disease the IgG titer will remain stable.

The pregnant patient who contracts HAV infection usually requires supportive care, since there is no specific treatment for acute disease. Patients who are suffering from nausea and vomiting should be given intravenous fluids and antiemetics. The mainstay of treatment is watchful waiting, with replacement of fluids and nutrients as needed.

Prevention is the key to the management of HAV infection as well as other types of viral hepatitis. The pregnant patient as well as anyone exposed to HAV should be given 0.02 ml/kg body weight of ISG within 2 weeks of the exposure.[115] There have been no reported cases of transmission of HAV infection in utero, and therefore no teratogenic or congenital effects of infection during pregnancy.

Hepatitis B

Unlike hepatitis A, which has a short incubation period, hepatitis B has a rather long incubation period of up to 2 months. It also has been referred to as serum hepatitis because its transmission is primarily via infected blood or blood products or other body fluids. Today, most cases of hepatitis B are transmitted through contaminated syringe needles among drug abusers, or through sexual contact in homosexuals, bisexuals, and the sexual partners of individuals who are at risk.[116] The Centers for Disease Control reports that there are approximately 600 to 700 deaths annually as a direct result of hepatitis B,[117] and estimates that approximately 4,000 to 5,000 deaths each year are secondary to acute and chronic liver disease as a result of hepatitis B virus (HBV) infection.[118]

The clinical presentation of HBV infection is not unlike that with HAV. Ninety percent of patients who contract HBV infection will undergo spontaneous resolution of the disease within 6 months of the onset of illness. Less than 1 percent will develop acute fulminating liver disease and liver failure with death. However, 10 percent of patients will progress to chronic infection. The patient may develop chronic active disease, as determined by an elevated titer of

hepatitis B surface antigen (HB$_s$Ag) that persists for longer than 6 months. Individuals who evolve to a chronic carrier state have normal liver enzymes but an elevated HB$_s$Ag titer. Patients with chronic active disease are differentiated from those with acute infection by the presence of elevated liver enzymes for more than 6 months.[119] Patients with chronic active and persistent HBV infection are of particular concern because they are at risk of cirrhosis or hepatocellular carcinoma.[120]

The pregnant patient who contracts HBV infection is no different, nor requires any different management, than the nonpregnant patient who becomes infected. However, the fetus is also vulnerable to infection, which may occur transplacentally in utero or during delivery. Infection in utero is not associated with teratogenic effects.[121] In contrast to infection in the adult population, fetal or neonatal infection is associated with a 90 percent risk of the development of chronic HB$_s$Ag carriage and, ultimately, liver disease.[120] There are opportunities for infection in utero throughout pregnancy, when fetal-maternal and maternal-fetal hemorrhages occur. If a maternal-fetal blood exchange should occur during the time the mother is experiencing HBV viremia, the infant is at risk of becoming infected.[122] Infants born to HBV-positive mothers, whether exposed to the virus in utero or at the time of delivery if the mother has the hepatitis B antigen (HB$_e$Ag), have up to a 90 percent chance of becoming infected. Prevention of neonatal infection is crucial to preventing progressive disease in the offspring and in preventing spread of the disease. A large number of infections are transmitted laterally and not vertically.[123,124]

The diagnosis of HBV infection, like that of other viral forms of hepatitis, is established serologically. HB$_s$Ag is the first marker to be detected and appears before the onset of clinical symptoms. Patients who recover from infection develop antibody to the surface antigen of the virus (anti-HB$_s$) and their serology for HB$_s$Ag becomes negative. A patient whose HB$_s$Ag test remains positive for more than 6 months is considered to be a chronic carrier. Patients who exhibit HB$_e$Ag are considered highly infectious, whereas those who develop antibody to the e antigen, anti-HB$_e$, are not very likely to pass the infection. The presence of IgM or IgG antibody (or both) to core antigen (HB$_c$Ag) indicates that the patient is manifesting an immunologic response to the infection. Anti-HB$_c$ is also found in patients with chronic infection.[125]

Patients with HBV infection should be monitored during the course of the acute illness by testing for the presence of anti-HB$_s$ and anti-HB$_e$, as well as liver function, as reflected by aspartate aminotransferase (AST) and alanine aminotransferase (ALT). The patient should receive fluids intravenously if there is nausea and vomiting. If the patient is suspected of exposure, hepatitis B immunoglobulin should be administered (0.06 ml/kg body weight IM). The patient should also receive HBV vaccine, for which pregnancy is not a contraindication. The vaccine most frequently used is a yeast recombinant preparation given in a series of three intramuscular injections; the initial injection is followed by the second at 1 month and by the third 6 months later.[126,127]

All pregnant patients should be screened for HB$_s$Ag. It would seem logical, toward preventing HBV infection and the transmission of the infection, that all patients who test negative for anti-HB$_s$ be given the vaccine. In fact, all sexual partners of pregnant patients should also be vaccinated. It is only through vaccination of all individuals who have not been exposed to the virus that spread of this infection can be curtailed. Currently, the recommendation is to vaccinate all those at risk and the newborn. This recommendation does not inhibit the spread of the disease, but only protects those likely to be exposed. Therefore, it would seem rational to vaccinate all individuals who have not been exposed to the disease and thereby prevent its spread, which may be associated with significant morbidity and mortality.

Hepatitis C

Hepatitis C (formerly called non-A, non-B hepatitis) occurring during pregnancy is not associated with an adverse outcome.[128] Although teratogenicity has not been associated with this infection, there is approximately a 50 percent transmission rate in utero in 85 percent of pregnant women with chronic hepatitis C virus (HCV) infection.[129,130] Since there is no vaccine or other effective therapy for HCV infection, it is reasonable to expect that children born to HCV-infected women are also likely to become chronic carriers.

HCV was thought to be primarily contracted from infected blood at the time of transfusion.[131] Recent studies have shown that HCV is commonly found in the same population that harbors HBV and HIV. This finding strongly links the spread of HCV to sexual contact and nonmedical parenteral means (i.e., intravenous drug abuse).[131,132]

Approximately 2 to 3 percent of all pregnant women carry antibodies to HCV. This low carriage rate precludes screening of all pregnant women for the virus, but those women in high-risk groups should be screened. Screening at risk populations is indicated because HCV infection is in most cases asymptomatic. HCV is believed to be the major cause of liver disease in the United States.[130] Since the severity of the initial illness is not related to subsequent morbidity, and a fairly large number of patients tend to be asymptomatic, there is no way to predict who will or will not experience chronic hepatitis, which is why screening is indicated.

The diagnosis of HCV infection has only recently become available, and the tests used for this are still plagued by a significant degree of false positivity. An additional problem with testing for HCV is that in many cases antibody to the virus may take up to 1 year to develop.[129] Testing is currently performed to detect the poresence of an HCV polypeptide, C100-3, and antibody to a core antigen of HCV.[133–135]

Management of the pregnant patient exposed to a known carrier of HCV or suspected of being exposed (e.g., through an accidental needle stick or neonatal exposure) consists of giving ISG. Although there is

---

Women At Risk of Hepatitis C

Transfusion received before 1990

Positive for HB$_{Ag}$

Positive for HIV

Known parenteral drug user

History of repeated STD

no strong evidence that this will be beneficial, it is a reasonable course of action.[136,137]

Hepatitis D

Hepatitis D virus (HDV) was originally referred to as the "delta agent" and was associated with an unusual presentation in patients known to have hepatitis B.[138] It was found that the hepatitis D agent could not function by itself, but required the presence of the HBV.[139] Thus, a patient who contracts hepatitis D must be infected with HBV, for it is this symbiosis that is required for HDV to replicate. When the two agents are present there is increased morbidity and mortality. Mortality among patients with acute hepatitis involving both the D and B viruses can reach 10 percent, whereas with HBV alone it is 1 percent. Individuals infected with HBV alone stand a 5 to 10 percent chance of becoming chronic carriers, whereas when HDV is present this chance increases to 75 percent. Persons with HDV and HBV who develop chronic hepatitis have up to an 80 percent chance of developing cirrhosis and portal hypertension.[138]

Patients who have severe or repeated relapses of hepatitis B should be tested for hepatitis D. This should consist of serologic testing for IgM and IgG antibodies to the virus. Interestingly, infected individuals will have high levels of IgM during the acute phase of disease, but low levels of IgM will persist for years in patients with chronic disease. The presence of IgG should be taken to mean that the disease is resolving.

Infection in pregnancy can result in vertical transmission.[140] There is no specific treatment, and exposed patients should receive ISG. Vaccination against HBV should be instituted as protection against this virus, and will result in protection against HDV infection.

Hepatitis E

Hepatitis E was originally thought to be non-A, non-B hepatitis that was transmitted enterically. However, it is now thought to be a specific viral infection that is transmitted enterically, and is a major form of hepatitis in developing countries. It has also been found to be a significant form of hepatitis in individuals returning to the United States from these endemic areas.[141]

The infection is similar to that caused by HAV. The incubation period is similarly short, ranging from 5 to 9 weeks, and also presents with gastrointestinal symptoms followed by hepatitis. The disease may be severe and fatal, but a carrier state has not been detected. The mortality associated with hepatitis E may be secondary to the nutritional state of the patient. In the United States there has not been significant mortality associated with hepatitis E virus (HEV) infection.

Because of the recency of the discovery of HEV, its significance in pregnancy has not been established. However, if non-A, non-B hepatitis can serve as a model, HEV can be expected to cause severe disease in the pregnant patient. It can be speculated that severe HEV infection may result in a mortality rate of 20 percent.[142] It is doubtful that such a mortality would occur in the United States in the absence of significant underlying disease.

Hepatitis E should be suspected in individuals with hepatitis who test negatively for HAV, HBV, and HCV. Routine clinical testing is not available for establishing a diagnosis of HEV infection. The Centers for Disease Control and Prevention should be contacted, and the Hepatitis Branch may request further testing in cases that test negatively for HAV, HBV, HCV, and non-A, non-B hepatitis.

Management of patients with hepatitis E consists of supportive therapy. Again, there is no specific therapy for patients with the disease. The use of ISG obtained from patients in the United States will probably be of little value. This is because HEV is uncommon in the United States, and the ISG pool will probably contain little or no anti-HEV.

REFERENCES

1. Levison ME, Trestmen I, Quach R et al: Quantitative bacteriology of the vaginal flora in vaginitis. Am J Obstet Gynecol 133:139, 1979
2. Hill GB, Eschenbach DA, Holmes KK: Bacteriology of the vagina. Scand J Urol Nephrol, suppl., 86:23, 1984
3. Eschenbach DA et al: Prevalence of hydrogen peroxide-producing *Lactobacillus* species in normal women and women with bacterial vaginosis. J Clin Microbiol 27:251, 1989
4. Greenspoon JS, Wilcox JG, Kirschbaum TH: Group B streptococcus: the effectiveness of screening and

chemoprophylaxis. Obstet Gynecol Surv 46:499, 1991

5. Hoogkamp-Korstanjte JAA, Gerards LJ, Cats BNP: Maternal carriage and neonatal acquisition of group B streptococci. J Infect Dis 145:800, 1982

6. Dillon HC Jr, Gray E, Pass MA, Gray BM: Anorectal and vaginal carriage of group B streptococci during pregnancy. J Infect Dis 145:794, 1982

7. Regan JA, Klebanoff MA, Nugent RP: The epidemiology of group B streptococcal colonization in pregnancy. Obstet Gynecol 77:604, 1991

8. Thomason JL, Gelbart SM, Broekhuizen FF: Office and clinical laboratory diagnosis of vulvovaginal infections: an overview. p. 93. In Horowitz BJ, Mardh P-A (eds): Vaginitis and Vaginosis. Wiley-Liss, New York, 1991

9. Centers for Disease Control: Nonreported sexually transmitted diseases. MMWR 28:61, 1979

10. Oriel JD, Partridge BM, Denn MJ et al: Genital yeast infections. BMJ 4:761, 1972

11. Anyon CP, Desmond FB, Eastcott DF: A study of *Candida* in one thousand and seven women. NZ Med J 73:9, 1971

12. Davis BA: Vaginal moniliasis in private practice. Obstet Gynecol 34:40, 1969

13. Hilton AL, Warnock DW: Vaginal candidiasis and the role of the digestive tract as a source of infection. Br J Obstet Gynaecol 82:922, 1975

14. Wied GL, Davis ME, Frank R et al: Statistical evaluation of the effect of hormonal contraceptives on the cytologic smear pattern. Obstet Gynecol 27:327, 1966

15. Robinson SC, Nicholas WC, Lee DT et al: The relationship of pregnancy, vaginal candidiasis and glucose metabolism. Can Med Assoc J 96:583, 1967

16. Cruickshank R, Sharman A: Conversion of glycogen of the vagina into lactic acid. J Pathol Bacteriol 39: 213, 1934

17. Bland PB, Rakoff AE, Pincus IJ: Experimental vaginal and cutaneous moniliasis: clinical and laboratory study of certain monilias associated with vaginal, oral and cutaneous thrush. Arch Dermatol Syphilol 36: 760, 1937

18. Pedersen GT: Yeast isolated from the throat, rectum and vagina in 60 women examined during pregnancy and $\frac{1}{2}$ to 1 year after labour. Acta Obstet Gynecol Scand, suppl. 6, 42:47, 1964

19. Pedersen GT: Yeast flora in mother and child. A mycological-clinical study of women followed up during pregnancy, the puerperium and 5–12 months after delivery, and their children on the 7th day of life,

and at the age of 5–12 months. Nord Med 81:207, 1969

20. Carroll CJ, Hurley R, Stanley VC: Criteria for diagnosis of *Candida* vulvovaginitis in pregnant women. J Obstet Gynaecol Br Commonw 80:258, 1973

21. McLennan MT, Smith JM, McLennan CE: Diagnosis of vaginal mycosis and trichomoniasis. Reliability of cytologic smear, wet smear and culture. Obstet Gynecol 40:231, 1972

22. O'Brien JR: Nickerson's medium in the diagnosis of vaginal moniliasis. Can Med Assoc J 90:1073, 1964

23. DeSousa HM, VanUden N: The mode of infection in yeast vulvovaginitis. Am J Obstet Gynecol 80:1096, 1986

24. Miles MR, Olsen L, Rogers A: Recurrent vaginal candidiasis: importance of an intestinal reservoir. JAMA 238:1836, 1977

25. Hillier SL, Martius J, Krohn MA et al: Case control study of chorioamnionic infection and chorioamnionitis in prematurity. N Engl J Med 319:972, 1988

26. Watts DH, Krohn MA, Hillier SL, Eschenbach DA: Bacterial vaginosis as a risk factor for postcesarean endometritis. Obstet Gynecol 75:52, 1990

27. Gravett MG, Hummel D, Eschenbach DA, Holmes KK: Preterm labor associated with subclinical amniotic fluid infection and with bacterial vaginosis. Obstet Gynecol 67:229, 1986

28. Newton ER, Prihoda TJ, Gibbs RS: A clinical and microbiologic analysis of risk factors for puerperal endometritis. Obstet Gynecol 75:402, 1990

29. McGregor JA, Dinsmoor MJ, Gibbs RS: Adjunctive clindamycin therapy for preterm labor: results of a double blind placebo controlled trial. Am J Obstet Gynecol 165:867, 1991

30. Morales WJ, Schorr S, Albritton J: Effect of metronidazole in patients with preterm birth in the preceding pregnancy and bacterial vaginosis: a placebo controlled double blind study. Am J Obstet Gynecol 171: 345, 1994

31. Gibbs RS, Romero R, Hillier SL et al: A review of preterm birth and subclinical infection. Am J Obstet Gynecol 166:1515, 1992

32. Kurk IT, Sivonen O, Savia E, Ylikorkala O: Bacterial vaginosis and pregnancy outcome. Obstet Gynecol 80:173, 1992

33. McGregor JA, French JI, Richter R et al: Antenatal microbiologic and maternal risk factors associated with prematurity. Am J Obstet Gynecol 163:1465, 1990

34. Martius J, Krohm MA, Hillier SL et al: Relationship of bacterial vaginal *Lactobacillus* species, cervical *Chla-*

mydia trachomatis and bacterial vaginosis to preterm birth. Obstet Gynecol 71:89, 1988

35. Csango PA, Gundersen T, Martinsen IM: Effect of amoxicillin on simultaneous *Chlamydia trachomatis* in men with gonococcal urethritis: comparison of three dosage regimens. Sex Transm Dis 121:93, 1985

36. Mann MS, Faro S, Maccato ML, Kaufman RH: Treatment of cervical chlamydial infection with amoxicillin/clavulanate postassium. Infect Dis Obstet Gynecol 1:104, 1993

37. Martin DH, Pastorek JG, Faro S: In vitro and in vivo activity of parenterally administered beta-lactam antibiotics against *Chlamydia trachomatis*. Sex Transm Dis 13:81, 1981

38. Martens MG, Faro S, Maccato M et al: In vitro susceptibility testing of clinical isolates of *Chlamydia trachomatis*. Infect Dis Obstet Gynecol 1:40, 1993

39. Lewin EB, Amstey MS: Natural history of group B streptococcus colonization and its therapy during pregnancy. Am J Obstet Gynecol 139:512, 1981

40. Baker CJ: Summary of the workshop on perinatal infection due to group B streptococcus. J Infect Dis 136:137, 1977

41. Baker CJ, Barrett FF: Transmission of group B streptococci among parturient women and the neonates. J Pediatr 83:919, 1973

42. Faro S, Phillips LE, Martens MG: Perspectives on the bacteriology of postoperative obstetric-gynecologic infections. Am J Obstet Gynecol 158:694, 1988

43. Faro S, Martens MG, Hammill HA et al: Antibiotic prophylaxis: is there a difference? Am J Obstet Gynecol 162:900, 1990

44. Faro S, Cox SM, Phillips LE et al: Influence of antibiotic prophylaxis on vaginal flora. J Obstet Gynecol, suppl. 1, 6:4, 1986

45. Phillips LE, Faro S, Martens MG et al: The microbiology of postpartum endometritis in high risk patients delivered by cesarean section. Curr Ther Res 42:1157, 1987

46. McDuffie RS Jr, McGregor JA, Gibbs RS: Adverse perinatal outcome and resistant *Enterobacteriaceae* after antibiotic usage for premature rupture of membranes and group B streptococcus carriage. Obstet Gynecol 82:487, 1993

47. Faro S: Group B streptococcus and puerperal sepsis. Am J Obstet 138:1219, 1980

48. Faro S: Group B hemolytic streptococci and puerperal infections. Am J Obstet Gynecol 139:686, 1981

49. Murray EGD, Webb RE, Swann MBR: A disease of rabbits characterized by large mononuclear leukocytosis caused by a hitherto undescribed bacillus *Bacter-*

ium monocytogenes (n.sp) J Pathol Bacteriol 29:407, 1926

50. Burn CG: Characteristics of a new species of the genus *Listerella* obtained from human sources. J Bacteriol 30:373, 1935

51. Burn CG: Clinical and pathological features of an infection caused by a new pathogen of the genus *Listerella.* Am J Pathol 12:341, 1936

52. Broome CV: Listeriosis: can we prevent it? ASM News 59:444, 1993

53. Seeliger HPR: Listeriosis. Hafner Publishing, New York, 1961

54. Schlech WF, Lavigne PM, Bortolussi RA et al: Epidemic listeriosis-evidence for transmission by food. N Engl J Med 308:203, 1983

55. Fleming DW, Cochi SL, MacDonald KL et al: Pasteurized milk as a vehicle of infection in an outbreak of listeriosis. N Engl J Med 312:404, 1985

56. Ho JL, Shands KN, Friedland G et al: An outbreak of type 4b *Listeria monocytogenes* infection involving patients from eight Boston hospitals. Arch Intern Med 146:520, 1986

57. Toaff R, Krocluk N, Rabinovitz M: Genital listeriosis in the male. Lancet 2:482, 1962

58. Larssen S, Ciderberg A, Invarsson S: *Listeria monocytogenes* causing hospital acquired enterocolitis and meningitis in newborn infants. BMJ 2:473, 1978

59. Hudson WR, Mead GC: *Listeria* contamination at a poultry plant. Lett Appl Microbiol 9:211, 1989

60. Monif GRG: Infectious Diseases in Obstetrics and Gynecology. P. 96. Harper & Row, Hagerstown, MD, 1974

61. Fleming AD, Ehrlich DW, Miller NA, Monif NA, Monif GRG: Successful treatment of maternal septicemia due to *Listeria monocytogenes* at 26 weeks gestation. Obstet Gynecol 66:52S, 1985

62. Faro S, Maccato M, Phillips LE, Riddle G: *Listeria monocytogenes*: maternal bacteremia and intra-amniotic infection treated successfully. J Infect Dis Obstet Gynecol (submitted)

63. Martens MG, Faro S, Hammill H et al: Comparison of two sampling devices: cotton-tipped swab and double lumen catheter with a brush. J Reprod Med 34:875, 1989

64. Martens MG, Faro S, Hammill HA et al: Transcervical uterine cultures with a new endometrial suction curette. A comparison of three sampling methods in postpartum endometritis. Obstet Gynecol 74:273, 1989

65. Maccato M, Riddle G, Faro S: Cefotetan susceptibility testing against anaerobic bacteria from obstetrical

and gynecologic sources: comparison of five different methods. Infect Dis Obstet Gynecol 1:23, 1993

66. Faro S, Martens MG, Hammill HA et al: Ticarcillin/clavulanic acid versus clindamycin and gentamicin in the treatment of post-cesarean endometritis following antibiotic prophylaxis. Obstet Gynecol 73:808, 1989

67. Martens MG, Faro S, Hammill HA et al: Sulbactam/ampicillin versus metronidazole/gentamicin in the treatment of post-cesarean endometritis. Diagn Microbiol Infect Dis 12:189s, 1989

68. Jeansson S, Molin L: On the occurrence of genital herpes simplex virus infections. Acta Dermatol Venereal 54:479, 1974

69. Tejani N, Klein SW, Kaplan M: Subclinical herpes simplex genitalis infections in the perinatal period. Am J Obstet Gynecol 135:547, 1979

70. Scher J, Bottone E, Desmond E, Simons W: The incidence and outcome of asymptomatic herpes simplex genitalis in an obstetric population. Am J Obstet Gynecol 144:906, 1982

71. Prober CG, Hensleigh PA, Bauchel FD et al: Use of routine viral cultures at delivery to delivery to identify neonates exposed to herpes simplex virus. N Engl J Med 318:882, 1988

72. Brown ZA, Vontver LA, Benedetti J et al: Genital herpes in pregnancy: risk factors associated with recurrence and asymptomatic viral shedding. Am J Obstet Gynecol 153:24, 1985

73. Nahmias AJ, Josey WE, Naib Z et al: Perinatal risk associated with maternal genital herpes infection. Am J Obstet Gynecol 110:825, 1971

74. Amstey MS, Monif GRC: Genital HSV infection in pregnancy. Obstet Gynecol 44:394, 1974

75. Stagno S, Pass RF, Divorsky ME, Alford CA: Maternal cytomegalovirus infection and perinatal transmission. Clin Obstet Gynecol 25:563, 1982

76. Gehrz RC, Marher SC, Knon SO et al: Specific cell-mediated immune defect in active cytomegalovirus infection of young children and their mothers. Lancet 2:844, 1977

77. Stagno S, Reynolds DW, Pass RF, Alfour CA: Breast milk and the risk of cytomegalovirus infection. N Engl J Med 302:1073, 1980

78. Huang E-S, Alford CA, Pass RF et al: Molecular epidemiology of cytomegalovirus infection. Women and their infants. N Engl J Med 313:1270, 1985

79. Harris RE, Rhoades ER: Varicella pneumonia complicating pregnancy: report of a case and review of the literature. Obstet Gynecol 25:734, 1965

80. Young NA, Greshon AA: Chicken pox, measles and mumps. P. 375. In Remington JS, Klein JO (eds):

Infectious Disease of the Fetus and Newborn. WB Saunders, Philadelphia, 1983

81. Brunell PA, Roxx A, Meller L, Kuo B: Prevention of varicella by zoster immune globulin. N Engl J Med 280:1191, 1969

82. Ross ASH: Modification of chicken pox in family contacts by administration of gamma globulin. N Engl J Med 267:369, 1962

83. Lansberger EJ, Hager WD, Grossman JH: Successful management of varicella pneumonia complicating pregnancy. J Reprod Med 31:411, 1986

84. Eder SE, Apuzzio JJ, Weiss G: Varicella pneumonia during pregnancy. Treatment of two cases with acyclovir. Am J Perinatol 5:16, 1988

85. Hankins GD, Gilstrap LC, Patterson AR: Acyclovir treatment of varicella pneumonia in pregnancy. Crit Care Med 5:336, 1987

86. Meyers JD: Congenital varicella in term infants: risks considered. J Infect Dis 129:215, 1974

87. Grandien M, Granstrom G: Effect of zoster immunoglobulin for varicella prophylaxis in the newborn. Scand J Infect Dis 17:343, 1985

88. Brunell PA: Varicella-zoster infection. p. 131. In Amstey MS (ed): Virus Infections in Pregnancy. Grune & Stratton, Orlando FL, 1984

89. Alexander I: Congenital varicella. BMJ 2:1074, 1979

90. Dodion-Fransen S, DeKegel D, Thirty L: Congenital varicella-zoster infection related to maternal disease in early pregnancy. Scand J Infect Dis 5:149, 1973

91. Cossart YE, Field AM, Cant B, Widdows D: Parovovirus-like particles in human sera. Lancet 1:72, 1975

92. Pattison JR, Jones SE, Hodgson J et al: Parvovirus infections and hypoplastic crisis in sickle-cell anemia. Lancet 1:664, 1981

93. Anderson MJ, Jones SE, Fisher-Hoch SP et al: Human parvovirus, the cause of erythema infectiosum (fifth disease). Lancet 1:1378, 1983

94. Anderson MJ, Lewis E, Kidd IM et al: An outbreak of erythema infectiosum associated with human parvovirus infection. J Hyg (Lond) 93:85, 1984

95. Plummer FA, Hammond GW, Forward K et al: An erythema infectiosum-like illness caused by human parvovirus infection. N Engl J Med 313:74, 1985

96. Serjeant GR, Goldstein AR: B19 virus infection and aplstic crisis. p. 85. In Pattison JR (ed): Parvovirus and Human Disease. CRC Press, Boca Raton, FL, 1988

97. Knott PD, Welply GAC, Anderson MJ: Serologically proved intrauterine infection with parvovirus. BMJ 289:1660, 1984

98. Brown T, Anand A, Ritchie LD et al: Intrauterine

parvovirus infection associated with hydrops fetalis. Lancet 2:133, 1984

99. Rodis JF, Hovick TJ Jr, Quinn DL et al: Human parvovirus infection in pregnancy. Obstet Gynecol 72: 733, 1988

100. White DG, Woolf AD, Mortimer PP et al: Human parvovirus arthropathy. Lancet 1:419, 1985

101. Reid DM, Reid TMS, Brown T et al: Human parvovirus-associated arthritis: a clinical laboratory description. Lancet 1:422, 1985

102. Kurtzman GJ, Ozawa K, Cohen B et al: Chronic bone marrow failure due to persistent B19 parvovirus infection. N Engl J Med 317:287, 1987

103. Smith MA, Shah NR, Lobel JS et al: Severe anemia caused by human parvovirus in a leukemia patient on maintenance chemotherapy. Clin Pediatr 27:383, 1988

104. Kurtzman GJ, Cohen B, Meyers P et al: Persistent B19 parvovirus infection as a cause of severe chronic anemia in children with acute lymphocytic leukemia. Lancet 2:1159, 1988

105. Anderson LJ: Role of parvovirus B19 in human disease. Pediatr Infect Dis J 6:711, 1987

106. Chorba T, Coccia P, Holman RC et al: The role of parvovirus B19 in aplastic crisis and erythema infectiosum (fifth disease). J Infect Dis 154:383, 1986

107. Anderson MJ, Higgins PG, Davis LR et al: Experimental parvovirus infection in humans. J Infect Dis 152:257, 1985

108. MMWR: 38:81, 1989

109. Public Health Laboratory Service Working Party on Fifth Disease: Study of human parvovirus (B19) infection in pregnancy. Commun Dis Rep 87 20:3, 1987

110. Porter JH, Khong TY, Evans MF et al: Parvovirus as a cause of hydrops fetalis: detection by in situ DNA hybridisation. J Clin Pathol 41:381, 1988

111. Schwarz TF, Roggendorf M, Hottentrager B et al: Human parvovirus B19 infection in pregnancy. Lancet 2:522, 1986

112. Centers for Disease Control: Hepatitis A among homosexual men—United States, Canada and Australia. MMWR 41:155, 1992

113. Centers for Disease Control: Summary of notifiable diseases, United States. MMWR 40:63, 1991

114. Snydman DR, Dienstag JL, Brink EW et al: Use of IgM hepatitis A antibody testing, investigating a common source, food-borne outbreak. JAMA 245:827, 1981

115. Centers for Disease Control: Update on adult immunizations, recommendations of the Immunization Practices Advisory Committee. MMWR 40 (RR-12): 86, 1991

116. Centers for Disease Control: Protection against viral hepatitis: recommendations of the Immunization Practices Advisory Committee. MMWR 39(RR-2):13, 1990

117. Centers for Disease Control: Summary of notifiable diseases—United States. MMWR 40:63, 1991

118. Centers for Disease Control: Hepatitis B virus a comprehensive strategy for eliminating transmission in the United States through universal childhood vaccination: recommendation of the Immunization Practices Advisory Committee. MMWR 40(RR-13):1, 1991

119. Robinson WS. Hepatitis B virus and hepatitis delta virus. p. 1204. In Mandell GL, Douglas RG, Bennett JE (eds): Principles and Practices of Infectious Diseases. 3rd Ed. Churchill Livingstone, New York, 1990

120. Beasley RP, Hwqang L-Y: Epidemiology of hepatocellular carcinoma. p. 209. In Vyas GN, Dienstag JL, Hoofnagle JH (eds): Viral Hepatitis and Liver Disease. Grune & Stratton, Orlando, FL, 1984

121. Pastorek JG, Miller JM, Summers PR: The effect of hepatitis B antigenemia on pregnancy outcome. Am J Obstet Gynecol 158:486, 1988

122. Ohto H, Lin H-H, Kawana T et al: Intrauterine transmission of hepatitis B virus closely related to placental leakage. J Med Virol 21:1, 1987

123. Stevens CE, Neurath RA, Beasley RP, Szmuness W: Hb$_e$Ag and ant-HB$_e$ detection by radioimmunoassay: correlation with vertical transmission of hepatitis B virus in Taiwan. J Med Virol 3:237, 1979

124. Franks AL, Beig CJ, Kane MA et al: Hepatitis B virus infection among children born in the United States to Southeast Asian refugees. N Engl J Med 321:1301, 1989

125. Hoofnagle JH, DiBisceglie AM: Serologic diagnosis of acute and chronic hepatitis. Semin Liver Dis 11: 73, 1991

126. Kelen GD, Green GB, Purcell RH et al: Hepatitis B and hepatitis C in emergency department patients. N Engl J Med 326:1399, 1992

127. Lynch-Salamon DI, Combs CA: Hepatitis C in obstetrics and gynecology. Obstet Gynecol 79:621, 1002

128. Thaler MM, Park C-K, Landers DV et al: Vertical transmission of hepatitis C. Lancet 338:17, 1991

129. Alter HJ, Purcell RH, Shih JW et al: Detection of antibodies to hepatitis C virus in prospectively followed transfusion recipients with acute and chronic non-A, non-B hepatitis. N Engl J Med 321:1494, 1989

130. Alter MJ, Margolis HS, Krawczynski K et al: The natu-

ral history of community acquired hepatitis C in the United States. N Engl J Med 327:1899, 1992

131. Bohman VR, Stettler RW, Little BB et al: Seroprevalence and risk factors for hepatitis C virus antibody in pregnant women. Obstet Cynecol 80:609, 1992

132. Donahue JG, Munoz A, Ness PM et al: The declining risk of post transfusion hepatitis C virus infection. N Engl J Med 327:369, 1992

133. Kuo G, Choo Q-L, Alter HJ et al: An assay for circulating antibodies to a major etiologic virus of human non-A, non-B hepatitis. Science 244:362, 1989

134. Aach RD, Stevens CE, Hollinger FB et al: Hepatitis C virus infection in post-transfusion hepatitis. An analysis with first and second-generation assays. N Engl J Med 325:1325, 1991

135. van der Poel CI, Cuypers HTM, Reesink HW et al: Confirmation of hepatitis C virus infection by new four-antigen recombinant immunoblot assay. Lancet 337:317, 1991

136. Snydman DR: Hepatitis in pregnancy. N Engl J Med 313:1398, 1985

137. Centers for Disease Control: 1989 Sexually transmitted diseases treatment guidelines. MMWR 38:37, 1989

138. Rizzetto M, Canese MG, Arico S et al: Immunofluorescence detection of new antigen-antibody system (delta/anti-delta) associated hepatitis B virus in liver and serum of HBsAG carriers. Gut 198:997, 1977

139. Rizzetto M: The delta agent. Hepatology 3:729, 1984

140. Hepatitis in Pregnancy. ACOG Technical Bulletin American College of Obstetricians and Gynecologists, Washington DC, 1992

141. Bradley DW, Maynard JE: Etiology and natural history of post-transfusion and enterically-transmitted non-A, non-B hepatitits. Semin Liver Dis 6:56, 1986

142. Centers for Disease Control: Hepatitis E among U.S. travelers, 1989–1992. MMWR 42:1, 1993

Episiotomy

John M. Thorp, Jr.

Episiotomy is described by *Williams' Obstetrics* as the most common operation in obstetrics, after clamping and cutting of the umbilical cord.[1] Episiotomy is surgical enlargement of the vaginal orifice just before delivery. Strictly defined, episiotomy refers to incision of the pudenda or external genitalia. Perineotomy refers to incising the perineum (skin and underlying muscles located between the vagina and anus), and would be a more accurate term.[2] Nevertheless, episiotomy is the more commonly used term and will be used throughout this chapter.

HISTORY

Episiotomy is a modern technique. Ould was the first to record its use as an aid in difficult vaginal deliveries in 1742. Broomal advocated its routine use in 1878, claiming that it could prevent "perineal ruptures."[2]

During the 19th century there was much interest in the prevention of perineal trauma during delivery. In 1855, von Ritgen described 4,875 deliveries with only 190 perineal tears. Within this cohort only one patient had a laceration involving the anal sphincter. This remarkable record was accomplished by a procedure called "scarification" (a series of superficial, circumferential vaginal incisions). At the time, scarification was used in 7 percent of all deliveries. Ritgen[3] admonished the physician to strive for "complete protection of the perineum," and warned

against dismissing his findings as "much ado about a perineal tear."

The routine use of episiotomy began after 1920 with papers presented and published by DeLee[4] and Pomeroy.[5] This coincided with the move of deliveries from home to the hospital, a change in attendants from midwives to physicians, diminishing family sizes, and an increase in abdominal deliveries.[6] Routine episiotomy was not hailed as an advance by all. J. Whitridge Williams remarked, after DeLee's presentation in 1920, that he disagreed with everything DeLee said.[7] Unfortunately, decades would elapse before this debate initiated serious scientific inquiry.

PREVALENCE

The prevalence of episiotomy is highly variable by both country and delivery site. Thacker and Banta,[2] in their landmark review article, had U.S. hospital discharge data analyzed and found that in 1979, episiotomy was performed in 62.5 percent of all vaginal deliveries.[2] Unfortunately, that was the last year for which an estimate of the prevalence of the procedure in the United States is available.

Other countries have lower episiotomy rates. The lowest reported prevalence rate (0.3%) comes from a Jamaican series.[8] Rates in Canada and Europe vary from 8 to 30 percent.[9] In most areas reported to date, nulliparous women have a greater likelihood of receiving an episiotomy.[10,11] Other factors associated with the use of episiotomy include regional anesthesia,[12] operative delivery,[13] delivery by a physician rather than a nurse-midwife,[14] and persistent occiput-posterior presentation.[13]

TECHNIQUE

There are two commonly accepted techniques for episiotomy: midline and mediolateral. Midline or median episiotomy is accomplished by making a midline incision directed toward the rectum. Mediolateral episiotomy is begun in the midline and then directed laterally away from the rectum. Both techniques have their own set of advantages and disadvantages (Table 29-1).

The increased prevalence of rectal injury with midline episiotomy[2] has resulted in the adaptation of mediolateral incision as the technique of choice worldwide except in the United States. American accoucheurs have embraced the midline approach, accepting the increased risk of rectal injury in return for less postpartum pain, ease of repair, and better anatomic results. To date, the two techniques have not been compared in prospective controlled studies.

Since Ritgen's 19th-century report,[3] alternative techniques have been described. For instance, May[15] recently wrote about a T-shaped incision made before delivery. He claims that this provides the advantages of midline episiotomy and avoids rectal injury. Unfortunately, there exist no data from which to evaluate alternative techniques.

Precision about the proper timing and depth of episiotomy is not possible. DeLee[4] and Pomeroy[5] originally advocated "early" episiotomy, before distension of the perineum, with incision of the levator muscles. DeLee[4] went as far as to suggest that every

gravid woman should have a "prophylactic" colporrhaphy. Modern advocates have reiterated his suggestions.[16] In my experience, most contemporary episiotomies are not performed early and do not usually include the levator bundles. Thus, the timing and depth of the procedure must be chosen empirically, depending on the beliefs of the operator. Those who flee into the arms of DeLee and Pomeroy to defend routine use of the procedure should be prepared to incise early and deep.

Likewise, operative vaginal delivery with forceps was considered an essential component with episiotomy in protection of the pelvic floor.[4,5,17,18] The concept beneath this was that shortening of the second stage of labor with early episiotomy and prophylactic forceps would diminish pelvic floor distension and improve ultimate function. Both Helwig et al[19] and Coombs et al[20] have shown that midline episiotomy during operative vaginal birth increases the risk of rectal injury (similar to the increase in risk when midline episiotomy is performed in spontaneous births).

REPAIR

General Principles

Many techniques are described for the repair of episiotomy wounds and spontaneous lacerations of the perineum. The repair should be closed in layers.[16] Hemostasis and anatomic restoration without excessive suturing are cardinal principals for success.[1] Full-thickness suturing should be avoided. One should remember that tissue edges need only be approximated; the edges will oppose automatically when the legs are brought together.

Before planning the repair, it is important to accurately assess the extent of damage. Table 29-2 pre-

Table 29-1. Midline Versus Mediolateral Episiotomy

	Midline Episiotomy	Mediolateral Episiotomy
Ease of repair	More	Less
Anatomic results	Good	Variable
Pain postpartum	Less	More
Blood loss	Less	More
Rectal injury	More	Less

Table 29-2. Classification of Lacerations

Laceration	Tissues Involved
First degree	Fourchette, perineal skin, vaginal mucosa
Second degree	Above, fascial/muscles of urogenital diaphragm
Third degree	Above, external anal sphincter
Fourth degree	Above, rectal mucosa

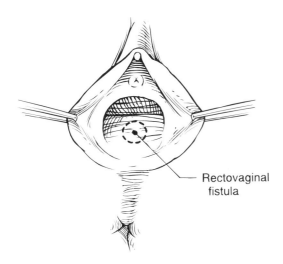

Fig. 29-1. Location of buttonhole injury that could result in rectovaginal fistula.

sents a classification system that is in common use. The repair of spontaneous trauma is almost identical to episiotomy repair. It has been assumed that a midline episiotomy is equivalent to a second-degree laceration.[21] I always try to perform a rectal examination before repair to exclude injury. On occasion the rectum can be entered in a "buttonhole" fashion above the urogenital diaphragm (Fig. 29-1).

Specifics

As stated above, episiotomies, either midline or mediolateral, should be repaired in layers. One should approximate the vaginal mucosa first. I do this with a continuing locked suture, beginning 1 cm above the incision apex to ensure hemostasis. I continue downward to the hymenal ring. Each bite should include vaginal mucosa and endopelvic fascia so as to not compromise pelvic support.

The deep muscles, including the levator bundles if excised, are approximated with three to four interrupted sutures. Care should be taken to not "bunch" the muscle bundles, which may result in dyspareunia. The next layer approximates the urogenital diaphragm and superficial transverse perineal muscles. The bulbocavernosus muscles are then approximated in the midline to reconstruct the introitus. Bunching of tissue with these bites can diminish introital caliber and preclude satisfactory intercourse.

Finally, the skin is reapproximated with a subcuticular suture (Fig. 29-2).

With rectal injuries the rectal mucosa should be reapproximated, again from the apex of the incision or laceration. The bites should be 0.5 cm apart; continuous or interrupted suturing is acceptable. This layer should then be covered with a second that includes endopelvic fascia. The ends of the external anal sphincter are then isolated and approximated with interrupted sutures (Fig. 29-3). Isolation of the severed sphincters can be enhanced by pulling on the presumed muscle bundle with an Allis clamp while palpating sphincter tone with a finger in the rectum. The remainder of the repair is completed as described for episiotomy. Adequate visualization is essential and depends on appropriate traction. This can be ensured either by using a self-retaining retractor or calling for an experienced assistant.

Suture Materials

Chromic catgut has been the traditional suture of choice for the repair of episiotomies and lacerations.[1] A recent review found that derivatives of polyglycolic acid (marketed as Dexon and Vicryl) appear to be better sutures for episiotomy repair.[22] Compared with catgut, their use is associated with 40 percent less pain and need for analgesics. Dexon and Vicryl have one major drawback: the need for suture removal in up to 40 percent of patients.[23,24] The removal of these braided sutures is prompted by their slow hydrolyzation and subsequent irritation. There is a definite need for a synthetic, monofilament, rapidly absorbable suture in the repair of obstetric trauma.

Continuous subcuticular stitching is superior to interrupted, transcutaneous techniques,[22] producing less perineal pain. Histoacryl-tissue adhesive (monomeric n-butyl-2-cyanoacryl) has also been shown to reduce postepisiotomy discomfort.[25]

POSTOPERATIVE CARE

The postpartum perineum has been subjected to a plethora of unproven therapies in an attempt to diminish pain and improve function.[26] Clearly, childbirth is associated with perineal pain,[27] and this is exacerbated by episiotomy.[28] This explains the fre-

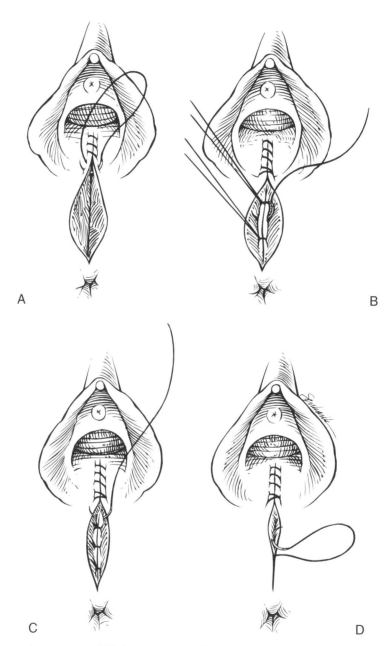

Fig. 29-2. Repair of episiotomy. **(A)** Approximation of vaginal mucosa. **(B)** Approximation of muscles. **(C)** Approximation of superficial muscles. **(D)** Approximation of perineal skin.

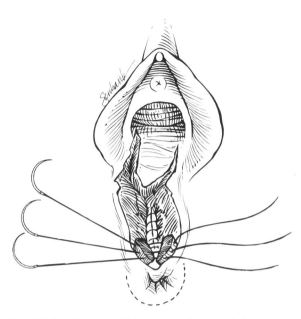

Fig. 29-3. Plication of the severed ends of the external anal sphincter.

quent recruitment of postepisiotomy patients in controlled trials of analgesics.[2]

Most patients with episiotomies will require oral analgesia. Both opiates and nonsteroidal anti-inflammatory drugs (NSAIDs) are effective. The latter have the advantage of not altering mentation. Persistant, severe pain is a warning sign of either urogenital hematoma or cellulitus. Patients with such pain should be examined carefully to exclude these morbid conditions.

COMPLICATIONS

Acute

Bleeding

Episiotomy is reported to increase blood loss.[29,30] In one study 10 percent more gravid women had estimated blood losses exceeding 300 ml with episiotomy than with spontaneous delivery.[31] Severe hemorrhage and large hematomas associated with episiotomy have been reported.[32] Mediolateral episiotomy[1] and "early" incision[16] are thought to result in greater blood loss.

Infection

As with any surgical procedure, infections can occur at the site of the episiotomy. These range in severity from cellulitis[33] to abcess formation.[32] To date there have been no controlled studies of whether spontaneous delivery diminishes or increases this risk.

Necrotizing fasciitis is a catastrophic polymicrobial infection that can complicate episiotomy. There are case reports of maternal deaths from this condition.[34,35] Again, I must re-emphasize that excessive perineal pain in the puerperium should be thoroughly evaluated.

Dehiscence

Up to 10 percent of patients will experience wound disruption after the primary repair of an episiotomy. This is even more likely to occur after third- or fourth-degree lacerations. These disruptions result in a variety of defects, up to two-thirds of which will require surgical repair.[36]

Conventional obstetric doctrine has held that "should repair at the time of delivery fail, a second attempt at repair should be deferred for a minimum of 3 to 4 months."[37] The delay was thought necessary to allow revitalization of tissue. This delay was troublesome to patients who suffered incontinence of feces and flatus and loss of coital function in the interim.

In 1986, Hauth et al[38] reported on eight cases of "early" repair of episiotomy, of which seven were successful. Table 29-3 presents subsequent reports of the results of early repair. To achieve these results the investigators recommend that all patients receive broad-spectrum antibiotics perioperatively. Debridement should be done regularly before surgery, and consists of the removal of visible suture material

Table 29-3. Early Repair of Dehiscence of Episiotomy

Reference	No. Patients	Success[a]
38	8	7/8 (87.5%)
39	20	20/20 (100%)
40	33	31/33 (93.9%)
41	34	32/34 (94.0%)
Total	95	90/95 (94.7%)

[a] Success is defined as intact perineum with hospital discharge.

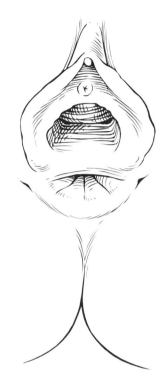

Fig. 29-4. Complete perineal breakdown.

and sharp resection of devitalized tissue. Mechanical bowel preparations before surgery are helpful. Repairs must not be attempted until the wound edges are clean and healthy.

Chronic

Unsatisfactory Anatomic Results

Unsatisfactory anatomic results of episiotomy range in severity from cosmetic problems such as skin tags or asymmetry to debilitating problems such as rectovaginal fistula or complete perineal breakdown. Beisher found that up to 50 percent of women will have a cosmetic defect after mediolateral episiotomy.[42] Fistula and perineal breakdown complicate up to 1 percent of lacerations that involve the rectum[36] (Fig. 29-4). The reader is referred to current reviews regarding the surgical management of fistula and perineal breakdown.[43,44]

Inclusions

Endometriosis[45,46] and metastatic adenocarcinomas[47] and squamous cell carcinomas[48] have been found in episiotomy scars. The first of these two neo-

plasms commonly presents with cyclic pain and the latter with palpable masses. It is assumed that neoplastic cells are implanted at the time of vaginal delivery rather than by hematogenous or lymphatic spread. The exact mechanism of their implantation is unknown. Interestingly, Snyder et al[49] found that perineal condylomata were associated with poor healing of episiotomy repairs.

ARGUMENTS FOR AND AGAINST ROUTINE EPISIOTOMY

Given the high prevalence of episiotomy within the United States noted above, one could describe it as a "routine procedure." Two perceived benefits are often cited to support this practice: prevention of severe damage to the pelvic floor, and prophylaxis against possible future dysfunction of the pelvic floor.[3] Each reputed advantage is assessed in the following sections.

Prevention of Severe Damage

In the literature, the only commonly reported markers of severe trauma to the pelvic floor are third- and fourth-degree lacerations. Lesions of the upper vagina and anterior introitus are consistently underreported.[6]

Tables 29-4 and 29-5 illustrate the incidence over

Table 29-4. Third- and Fourth-degree Lacerations After Midline Episiotomy[a]

Study	No. Patients	Third- and Fourth-degree Lacerations (%)
Giles (1930)	500	3.2
Nuggent (1935)	20	10.0
Chang (1943)	635	0.5
Kaltreider (1948)	15,167	4.5
Ingraham (1949)	9,170	5.0
Smith (1951)	1,500	1.9
McNulty (1953)	6,577	0.9
Jacobs (1960)	5,358	3.0
Dodek (1963)	890	0.4
Harris (1970)	7,477	13.0
Beynon (1974)	1,938	13.5
Coats (1980)	163	23.9
Total	49,395	6.5

[a] Complete bibliography available on request.
(Adapted from Thacker and Banta,[2] with permission.)

Table 29-5. Third- and Fourth-degree Lacerations Without Episiotomy[a]

Study	No. Patients	Third- and Fourth-degree Lacerations (%)
Ritgen[2] (1855)	4,875	0.0
Child (1919)	58	5.2
Nugent (1935)	72	6.4
Brendel (1979)	29	0.0
Gaskin (1980)	801	0.5
Malcki (1980)	379	1.0
Schmint (1980)	102	0.0
Cranch (1981)	799	3.6
Arauso (1982)	2,447	0.0
Buekens et al (1985)	15,237	0.9
Blownal (1985)	13,500	0.4
Sleep and Grant[16] (1986)	457	0.0
Gass et al[7] (1986)	205	0.0
Total	38,961	1.4

[a] Complete bibliography available on request.

the past 140 years of rectal injury with and without antecedant midline episiotomy. From these cumulative data it appears that midline episiotomy is not associated with a decrease in third- and fourth-degree lacerations. Equivalent tables for mediolateral

episiotomy are likewise not convincing that the procedure diminishes the risk of rectal injury.[2]

Table 29-6 outlines retrospective studies and Table 29-7 prospective studies, including randomized controlled trials, that have analyzed the effects of episiotomy on third- and fourth-degree lacerations. Table 29-6 clearly demonstrates that midline episiotomy is associated with an increase in third- and fourth-degree lacerations (range of adjusted odds ratios, 4.2 to 22.5). Mediolateral episiotomy does not appear to protect the rectum from injury except perhaps in nulliparous women.[52]

Prospective studies have been accomplished by allocating subjects to one of two procedures: liberal or restricted episiotomy. The decision to actually perform an episiotomy is made at the discretion of the delivering physician or midwife. These studies are presented in Table 29-7. I analyze the prospective studies as follows. First, women in the limited group showed a trend toward less perineal trauma. These women were more likely to deliver with an intact perineum. Second, midline episiotomy was strongly associated with third- and fourth-degree lacerations, confirming the findings of the retrospective work. Third, mediolateral episiotomy did not prevent rectal injury, as has been claimed. Finally, episiotomy rates of 8 to 40 percent (figures much lower than the

Table 29-6. Retrospective Studies: Effect of Episiotomy on Third- and Fourth-degree Lacerations

Reference	No. Patients	Study Type	Episiotomy Type	Findings
50	41,000	Cohort	Mediolateral	Odds ratio of 28.6 (1.6–5.1) for fourth-degree laceration
51	21,278	Cohort	Mediolateral	Odds ratio of 0.94 (0.6–1.4) for fourth-degree laceration
52	24,114	Cohort	Midline and mediolateral	Mediolateral, odds ratio of 0.4 (0.2–0.9) in nulliparous women; 2.4 (0.9–6.1) in parous women Midline, odds ratio of 4.2 (1.8–10.0) in nulliparous women, 12.8 (5.4–30.3) in parous women
53	241	Cohort	Midline	Odds ratio of 22.5 (7.8–64.6) for fourth-degree laceration
54	2,188	Cohort	Mediolateral	Odds ratio of 2.3 (1.2–4.6) for fourth-degree laceration
55	1,262	Cohort	Midline	Odds ratio 4.3 (1.6–11.7) for fourth-degree laceration
56	2,706	Cohort	Midline	Odds ratio of 8.9 (6.1–13.0) for fourth-degree lacerations
57	9,493	Cohort	Midline	Odds ratio of 4.2 (2.9–5.8) for fourth degree lacerations

Table 29-7. Prospective Studies: Effect of Episiotomy on Third- and Fourth-degree Lacerations

Reference	No. Patients	Group Assignment Method	Episiotomy Type	Liberal	Restricted	Effect on Third- and Fourth-degree Lacerations
57	379	Semirandom	Midline	More third- and fourth degree lacerations	More first degree lacerations and intact perinea	No third- or fourth-degree lacerations without episiotomy
58	189	Random	Mediolateral	More second-degree lacerations	More first-degree lacerations and intact perinea	No third- or fourth-degree lacerations in either group
59	289	Random	Mediolateral	More second-degree lacerations	More first-degree lacerations and intact perinea	No third- or fourth-degree lacerations in either group
60	703	Random	Midline	More second-degree lacerations in multiparous women	More intact perinea in multiparous groups	52/53 third- and fourth-degree lacerations preceeded by episiotomy
61	2,606	Random	Mediolateral	More second-degree lacerations	More first-degree lacerations and intact perinea	No difference in third- and fourth-degree lacerations

actual practice figures in the United States) in the restricted group did not result in excess perineal trauma. Thus, the Argentine Episiotomy Trial Collaborative Group asserted that "routine episiotomy should be abandoned and episiotomy rates above 30 percent cannot be justified."[61]

Trauma to the upper vagina and anterior introitus (clitoris and urethra) must be evaluated. Three prospective studies[57,60,61] have all shown that periclitoral, periurethral, and anterior labial tears are more common is the restrictive groups. Relative risk estimates for such trauma are only modestly elevated, ranging from 1.18 to 1.52. None of the prospective studies (Table 29-7) reports on any injuries to the upper third of the vagina.

Thus, there is no evidence to support the argument that episiotomy limits perineal trauma. There are substantial data from both retrospective and prospective studies indicating that midline episiotomy increases the risk of severe perineal trauma and that mediolateral episiotomy is not protective.

Prophylaxis Against Pelvic Relaxation

The 17th edition of *Williams' Obstetrics*, in defense of episiotomy, states that "It can be said with certainty, that since the era of in-hospital deliveries with episiotomy, there has been an appreciable decrease in the number of women hospitalized for the treatment of symptomatic cystocoele, rectocoele, uterine prolapse, and stress urinary incontinence." Although the two phenomena are associated, there are few data on which to base a claim that episiotomy has caused less pelvic relaxation. Most proponents of this argument cite the 1935 study of Aldridge and Watson[17] and the 1955 study of Gainey.[18]

Both studies compared women delivering in different epochs. In the earlier epochs, patients were less likely to undergo episiotomy. Patients were then followed up (Aldridge and Watson, 6-week follow up; Gainey, 2- to 10-year follow up) and postpartum and pelvic floor damage was assessed. Both studies conclude that the pelvic floor is less likely to be injured after episiotomy.

These studies are open to criticism. First, there is the confounding variable of forceps, which was used with episiotomy. Second, observers were not blinded to the modes of delivery, thereby injecting biases into the assessment. Third, women were compared who delivered within different decades, introducing confounding variables. Finally, episiotomy rates were less than 40 percent and abdominal delivery rates less than 5 percent. Thus, it is difficult to extrapolate these outcomes to current practice.

Two of the randomized trials[59,60] followed their patients postpartum and attempted to assess pelvic floor damage. A 3-year follow-up by postal survey of subjects in the West Berkshire perineal management trial failed to demonstrate diminuition of urinary incontinence by mediolateral episiotomy.[64] The Canadian midline episiotomy trial[60] assessed patients with questionnaires and electromyographic (EMG) perineometry 3 months after delivery. There were no differences between groups in EMG activity or frequency of incontinence.

Multiple observational cohort studies using different modalities, including endorectal ultrasonography,[65] anorectal manometry,[66] pudendal nerve latencies,[67] vaginal manometry,[68] vaginal electromyography with plug electrodes,[69] and vaginal cones,[70] have demonstrated that while vaginal delivery impairs pelvic floor function at least transiently, episiotomy does not mitigate this damage. Manometry[71,72] and questionnaire studies[73] have shown that third- and fourth-degree lacerations, the risk of which is increased by midline episiotomy, are associated with subsequent incontinence of feces and flatus.

CONCLUSION

Episiotomy, much like other medical innovations of the 20th century, was put into widespread use before any scientific testing of its effect. The arguments for its widespread use, while believed by many, do not withstand objective scrutiny. If patients were fully informed of its lack of efficacy and the serious complications it can create, few would consent to having a routine episiotomy. We now have the objective data that will permit our patients to make such a choice. Failure to allow them to do so violates patient autonomy.

REFERENCES

1. Cunningham FG, MacDonald PC, Gant NF et al (eds): Williams' Obstetrics. 19th Ed. Appleton & Lange, E. Norwalk, CT, 1993
2. Thacker SB, Banta HD: Benefits and risks of episiotomy: an interpretative review of the English language literature, 1860–1980. Obstet Gynecol Surv 38:322, 1983
3. Ritgen G: XXIII. Concerning his method for protection of the perineum. Monatschrift fur Geburtskunde 6:21, 1855
4. DeLee JB: The prophylactic forceps operation. Am J Obstet Gynecol 1:34, 1920
5. Pomeroy RH: Shall we cut and reconstruct the perineum for every primipara? Am J Obstet Dis Women Child 78:211, 1918
6. Thorp JM Jr, Bowes WA Jr: Episiotomy: can its routine use be defended? Am J Obstet Gynecol 160:1027, 1989
7. Taylor ES: Comment on episiotomy and third degree tears. Obstet Gynecol Surv 41:229, 1985
8. Doherty PJ, Cohen I: Spontaneous vaginal deliveries and perineal trauma in Lucea, Jamaica. J La State Med Soc 145:531, 1993
9. Vandenbussche P, Wollast E, Buekens P: Some characteristics of antenatal care in 13 European countries. Br J Obstet Gynaecol 92:1297, 1985
10. Thorp JM Jr, Bowes WA Jr, Brame RG, Cefalo R: Selected use of midline episiotomy: effect on perineal trauma. Obstet Gynecol 70:260, 1987
11. Henriksen TB, Bek KM, Hedegaard M, Secher NJ: Episiotomy and perineal lesions in spontaneous vaginal deliveries. Br J Obstet Gynaecol 99:950, 1992
12. Walker MP, Farine D, Rolbin SH, Ritchie JW: Epidural anesthesia, episiotomy, and obstetric laceration. Obstet Gynecol 77:668, 1991
13. Combs CA, Robertson PA, Laros RK Jr: Risk factors for third-degree and fourth-degree perineal lacerations in forceps and vacuum deliveries. 163:100, 1990
14. Wilcox LS, Strobino DM, Baruffi G, Dellinger WS Jr: Episiotomy and its role in the incidence of perineal lacerations in a maternity center and tertiary hospital obstetric service. Am J Obstet Gynecol 160:1047, 1989
15. May JL: Modified median episiotomy minimizes the risk of third-degree tears. Obstet Gynecol 83:156, 1994
16. Paciornik M: Commentary: arguments against episiotomy and in favor of squatting for birth. Birth 17:104, 1990
17. Aldridge AH, Watson P: Analysis of end-results of labor in primiparas after spontaneous versus prophylactic methods of delivery. Am J Obstet Gynecol 30:554, 1935
18. Gainey HL: Postpartum observation of pelvic tissue damage: further studies. Am J Obstet Gynecol 800, 1955
19. Helwig JT, Thorp JM Jr, Bowes WA Jr: Does midline episiotomy increase the risk of third- and fourth-degree lacerations in operative vaginal deliveries? Obstet Gynecol 82:276, 1993
20. Combs CA, Robertson PA, Laros RK Jr: Risk factors for third-degree and fourth-degree perineal lacerations in forceps and vacuum deliveries. Am J Obstet Gynecol 163:100, 1990

21. Cass MS, Dunn C, Stys SJ: Effect of episiotomy on vaginal outlet laceration. J Reprod Med 31:240, 1986

22. Grant A: The choice of suture materials and techniques for repair of perineal trauma: an overview of the evidence from controlled trials. Br J Obstet Gynaecol 96:1281, 1989

23. Mahomed K, Grant A, Ashurst H, James D: The Southmead perineal suture study. A randomized comparison of suture materials and suturing techniques for repair of perineal trauma. Br J Obstet Gynaecol 96:1272, 1989

24. Ketcham KR, Pastorek JG II, Letellier RL: Episiotomy repair: chronic versus polyglycolic acid suture. South Med J 87:514, 1994

25. Adoni A, Anteby E: The use of Histocryl for episiotomy repair. Br J Obstet Gynaecol 98:476, 1991

26. Rhode MA, Barger MK: Perineal care. Then and now. J Nurse Midwifery 35:220, 1990

27. Abraham S, Child A, Ferry J, Vizzard J, Mira M: Recovery after childbirth: a preliminary prospective study. Med J Aust 152:9, 1990

28. Larsson PG, Platz-Christensen JJ, Bergman B, Wallstersson G: Advantage or disadvantage of episiotomy compared with spontaneous perineal laceration. Gynecol Obstet Invest 31:213, 1991

29. Miller RL: A method for reducing episiotomy blood loss. Obstet Gynecol 25:553, 1965

30. Odell LD, Seski A: Episiotomy blood loss. Am J Obstet Gynecol 54:51, 1947

31. Conn LC, Vant JR, Cantor MM: A critical analysis of blood loss in 2000 obstetric cases. Am J Obstet Gynecol 42:768, 1941

32. Proudfit CH, Hunt AB: Episiotomy. Proc Mayo Clin 18:429, 1943

33. Giglio FA, Germany WW, Roberts P: The infested episiotomy. Obstet Gynecol 25:502, 1965

34. Shy KK, Eschenbach DA: Fatal perineal cellulitis from an episiotomy site. Obstet Gynecol 54:292, 1979

35. Ewing TL, Smale LE, Elliott FA: Maternal deaths associated with postpartum vulvar edema. Am J Obstet Gynecol 134:173, 1979

36. Karamijit SK, Yamashita HJ, Wise WE Jr, et al: Delayed repair of obstetric injuries of the anorectum and vagina. A stratified surgical approach. Dis Colon Rectum 37:344, 1994

37. Mattingly RF, Thompson JD (eds): Anal incontinence and recto-vaginal fistulas. p. 669. In: Telinde's Operative Gynecology. 6th Ed. JB Lippincott, Philadelphia, 1985

38. Hauth JC, Gilstrap LC, Ward SC, Hankius GDV: Early repair of an external sphincter anal muscle and rectal mucosa dehiscence. Obstet Gynecol 67:806, 1986

39. Monberg J, Hammen S: Ruptured episiotomia resutured primarily. Acta Obstet Gynecol Scand 66:163, 1987

40. Hankins GDV, Hauth JC, Gilstrap LC III et al: Early repair of episiotomy dehiscence. Obstet Gynecol 75:48, 1990

41. Ramin SM, Ramus RM, Little BB, Gilstrap LC III: Early repair of episiotomy dehiscence associated with infection. Am J Obstet Gynecol 167(4 Part 1):1104, 1992

42. Beischer NA: The anatomical and functional results of mediolateral episiotomy. Med J Aust 2:189, 1967

43. Tancer ML, Lasser D, Rosenblum N: Rectovaginal fistula or perineal and anal sphincter disruption, or both, after vaginal delivery. Surgery 171:43, 1990

44. Given FT Jr, Browning G: Repair of old complete perineal lacerations. Am J Obstet Gynecol 159:779, 1988

45. Wittich AC: Endometriosis in an episiotomy scar: review of the literature and report of a case. J Am Osteopath Assoc 82:22, 1982

46. Sayfan J, Benosh L, Segal M, Orda R: Endometriosis in episiotomy scar with anal sphincter involvement. Report of a case. Dis Colon Rectum 34:713, 1991

47. Van Dam PA, Irvine L, Lowe DG et al: Carcinoma in episiotomy scars. Gynecol Oncol 44:96, 1992

48. Gordon AN, Jensen R, Jones HW III: Squamous carcinoma of the cervix complicating pregnancy: Recurrence in episiotomy after vaginal delivery. Obstet Gynecol 73:850, 1989

49. Snyder RR, Hammond TL, Hankins GD: Human papillomavirus associated with poor healing of episiotomy repairs. Obstet Gynecol 76:664, 1990

50. Bek KM, Laurberg S: Risks of anal incontinence from subsequent vaginal delivery after a complete obstetrical anal sphincter tear. Br J Obstet Gynaecol 99:724, 1992

51. Buekens P, Lagasse R, Dramaix M, Wollast E: Episiotomy and third-degree tears. Br J Obstet Gynaecol 92:820, 1985

52. Shiono P, Klebanoff MA, Carey JC: Midline episiotomies: more harm than good? Obstet Gynecol 75:765, 1990

53. Borgatta L, Piening SL, Cohen WR: Association of episiotomy and delivery position with deep perineal laceration during spontaneous delivery in nulliparous women. Am J Obstet Gynecol 160:294, 1989

54. Henriksen TB, Bek KM, Hedegaard M, Secher NJ: Episiotomy and perineal lesions in spontaneous vaginal deliveries. Br J Obstet Gynaecol 99:950, 1992

55. Wilcox LS, Strobino DM, Baruffi G, Dellinger WS: Episiotomy and its role in the incidence of perineal lacera-

tions in a maternity center and a tertiary hospital obstetric service. Am J Obstet Gynecol 160:1047, 1989

56. Green JR, Soohoo SL: Factors associated with rectal injury in spontaneous deliveries. Obstet Gynecol 73: 732, 1989

57. Thorp JM Jr, Bowes WA Jr, Brame RG, Cefalo R: Selected use of midline episiotomy: effect on perineal trauma. Obstet Gynecol 70:260, 1987

58. Harrison RF, Brennan M, North PM et al: Is routine episiotomy necessary? BMJ 288:1971, 1984

59. Sleep J, Grant A, Garcia J et al: West Berkshire perineal management trial. BMJ 289:587, 1984

60. Klein MC, Gauthier RJ, Jorgensen SH et al: Does episiotomy prevent perineal trauma and pelvic floor relaxation? Online J Curr Clin Trials Doc. No 10, 1992

61. Argentine Episiotomy Trial Collaborative Group: Routine vs selective episiotomy: a randomized controlled trial. Lancet 342:1517, 1993

62. Sleep J, Grant A: West Berkshire perineal management trial: three year follow up. BMJ 295:749, 1987

63. Sultan AH, Kamm MA, Hudson CN et al: Anal-sphincter disruption during vaginal delivery. N Engl J Med 329:1905, 1993

64. Haadem K, Dahlstrom, Lingman G: Anal sphincter function after delivery: a prospective study in women with sphincter rupture and controls. Eur J Obstet Gynecol 35:7, 1990

65. Allen RE, Hosker GL, Smith ARB, Warrell DW: Pelvic floor damage and childbirth: a neurophysiological study. Br J Obstet Gynaecol 97:770, 1990

66. Gordon H, Logue M: Perineal muscle function after childbirth. Lancet, July, 123, 1985

67. Thorp JM Jr, Jones LG, Bowes WA Jr, Droegemueller W: Electromyography with acrylic plug surface electrodes after delivery. Am J Perinatol 1995 (in press)

68. Rockner G, Jonasson A, Olund A: The effect of mediolateral episiotomy at delivery on pelvic floor muscle strength evaluated with vaginal cones. Acta Obstet Gynecol Scand 70:51, 1991

69. Haadem K, Dahlstrom JA, Ling L, Ohrlander S: Anal sphincter function after delivery rupture. Obstet Gynecol 70:53, 1987

70. Sorensen SM, Bondesen H, Istre O, Vilmann P: Perineal rupture following vaginal delivery: long-term consequences. Acta Obstet Gynecol Scand 67:315, 1988

71. Crawford LA, Quint EH, Pearl ML, DeLancey JO: Incontinence following rupture of the anal sphincter during delivery. Obstet Gynecol 82(4 Part 1):527, 1993

Labor-and-Delivery Unit as a Health Screening Center

Terry I. Feng

The health-care system is currently undergoing many changes brought on by concerns about cost, efficiency, access to care, universal coverage, portability of coverage, and coverage for innovative treatments (such as fetal surgery). In addition, the assessment of an individual's health should include an evaluation of all aspects of that person's life and lifestyle. Areas such as nutrition, exercise, smoking, substance abuse, child abuse, and domestic violence need to be addressed when caring for patients. At every occasion on which the patient encounters the health-care system, an opportunity exists to screen for risk-entailing behavior and to reinforce healthy behaviors.

Obstetricians and gynecologists function as the primary health-care providers for most women. Pregnancy is an optimal time to evaluate overall health behavior as well as to modify unhealthy behaviors. During prenatal visits, areas such as exercise, nutrition, substance abuse, domestic violence, and human immunodeficiency virus (HIV) infection should be addressed. Unfortunately, many women do not participate in prenatal care. For some, arrival at the labor-and-delivery area is their first contact with the health-care system. Alternatively, these women may have presented late for prenatal care, had only minimal prenatal care, or received extremely episodic care. Regardless of the pattern of their prenatal care, most women will reliably appear at a labor-and-delivery area for delivery of their infant. Since women will reliably present themselves for care at the time of labor, it is important to consider additional uses of the labor-and-delivery area. One such use would be to screen for specific health risks.

SUBSTANCE ABUSE

Alcohol

It has been more than 20 years since Jones et al[1] coined the phrase "fetal alcohol syndrome" and described the adverse affects of alcohol on the growing fetus. Numerous articles have confirmed the problems of alcohol consumption during pregnancy, which include mental retardation, growth deficiency, and congenital malformations.[2–5] The American College of Obstetricians and Gynecologists (ACOG) has developed several patient education pamphlets that address alcohol and pregnancy.[6,7] The incidence of problem drinking is estimated to be approximately 1 to 2 percent in pregnancy. However, little effort has gone into screening pregnant women for alcohol use.[8,9] Most methods of screening for alcohol consumption have been developed for use in men. The early screening methods involved detailed questionnaires that were given to men in alcohol rehabilitation programs. Later, the questionnaires were significantly shortened and applied pro-

---

Ideal Screening Tool

The ideal "screening tool" should have the following characteristics:

Applicable to the entire population of interest

Low cost

Minimally invasive

Highly specific

Identify a subpopulation at high risk of adverse outcome that would require further evaluation

---

spectively. The questions can be self-administered or asked directly. Two commonly used short screening questionnaires are the Michigan Alcoholism Screening Test (MAST) and the CAGE,[10,11] which consists of four questions.

The CAGE Test

C Have you ever felt you had to *cut* down on your drinking?

A Have people *annoyed* you by criticizing your drinking?

G Have you ever felt *guilty* about your drinking?

E Have you ever felt the need for an *eye opener*?

However, few of these questionnaires have been validated for use among women, and even less so for pregnant women. Sokol et al[12,13] have published extensively on the use of a screening questionnaire in pregnant women, employing the T-ACE questionnaire. Like the CAGE questionnaire, this also involves four questions. The "T" in T-ACE replaces the "G" in the CAGE questionnaire, and is a test for tolerance to alcohol that involves asking "How many drinks does it take to feel high?" An answer of

more than two drinks indicates tolerance. The T-ACE questionnaire could be easily administered to all patients on admission to the labor-and-delivery area. Two or more "Yes" responses on the questionnaire would alert health-care providers to a potential problem that should be further investigated.

Illicit Drug Use

The 1991 National Household Survey on Drug Abuse estimated that 11.1 percent of all women had used an illicit drug within the prior year.[14] Among women aged 18 to 34 years (the primary reproductive years), an estimated 7.8 million had used an illicit drug within the prior year.[14] The use of illicit drugs by pregnant women parallels their use by nonpregnant women. Numerous studies have done anonymous drug screening on patients admitted to labor-and-delivery areas.[15-27] The prevalence of positive urine drug screens ranges from approximately 8 to 15 percent. Several studies have examined the meconium of newborns and reported illicit drugs in as many as 40 percent of cases.[28,29] All of these studies have documented illicit drug use in urban and rural settings, in various geographic locations in the United States, and among patients of both high and low socioeconomic status.[15-27]

Urine screening for substance abuse on admission to the labor-and-delivery unit involves many medicolegal issues that are too complex to address here. However, the medical and public health issues are well defined. Substance-abusing pregnant women have worse perinatal outcomes. They tend to have more premature deliveries, fetal distress, placental abruptions, congenital anomalies, fetal death, and premature rupture of membranes, and less prenatal care.[30,31] These women are also at higher risk of sexually transmitted diseases (STDs), hepatitis, and HIV infection.[32] In addition, substance abuse also causes disruption in parenting, nutrition, family dynamics, and social interactions. Some drug-using women may be involved in illegal activities. The scope of the problem is detailed in a report by the General Accounting Office (GAO) for the U.S. Senate.[30] It identified several areas of concern. Among them are that

> Many drug-exposed infants who might need help are not identified

Drug-exposed infants have more health problems and are more costly to care for

The impact of drug abuse during pregnancy on social welfare and educational systems could be profound

Lack of treatment and prenatal care for women using drugs is contributing to the number of drug-exposed infants

The U.S. Public Health Service expert panel on the content of prenatal care has put a high priority on research involving alcohol and illicit drug use by pregnant women.[31]

It is clear that illicit drug use occurs among pregnant women and that the results are costly. It is also clear that urine drug screening (although imperfect) can identify recent users. Unfortunately, neither medical science nor society has settled on the solution to the problem. Medical science is evaluating such issues as inpatient versus outpatient treatment for drug abuse, drug replacement therapy (methadone), and comprehensive pregnancy and addiction programs. Society is dealing with issues such as incarcerating pregnant addicts, fetus abuse, mandatory drug testing of pregnant women, and confidentiality in matters relating to drug abuse. Although the medical and legal issues are unsettled, the first step in solving the problem will be to identify it.

HUMAN IMMUNODEFICIENCY VIRUS

HIV infection continues to be a growing problem among women of childbearing age. Data from the U.S. Centers for Disease Control and Prevention (CDC) indicate that the prevalence of HIV infection has leveled off in most populations, but continues to rise among women.[33–35] According to the CDC, in 1994, 18 percent of cases of acquired immunodeficiency syndrome (AIDS) occurred among women, representing more than a threefold increase in the proportion reported in 1985. HIV infection is disproportionately represented in disadvantaged minority populations. Three-fourths of the cases of AIDS among women occurred among black and Hispanic women, and the rate among black women was 16 times higher than that for white women. The larg-

est percentage of AIDS cases were reported in women in the Northeast and South (44 percent and 36 percent, respectively). In 1994, many women with AIDS had risk behaviors, including hypodermic drug use or heterosexual contact with a partner at risk or known to have HIV infection. However, 19 percent had no specific HIV exposure reported. Approximately 7,000 HIV-infected women delivered infants in the United States during 1993. If a perinatal transmission rate of 15 to 30 percent is used, this means that approximately 1,000 to 2,000 infants were perinatally infected with HIV during 1993. From 1989 to 1993, HIV infection among pregnant women remained relatively stable at 1.6 to 1.7 per 1,000, although its prevalence varied regionally. Most data on HIV seroprevalence obtained at counseling and testing sites reflect the serologic status of self-motivated volunteers who perceive themselves to be at high risk of exposure to HIV. However, from 50 to 70 percent of infected women may be unaware of any risk factors for HIV infection.[36–39] In a study by Lindsay et al[36] 70 percent of HIV-infected women identified from a routine voluntary prenatal survey did not acknowledge risk factors. Patients who do not seek prenatal care are also at increased risk of HIV infection and other adverse perinatal outcomes. One study has reported an HIV seroprevalence rate of 11 per 1,000 over a 4-year period in nonclinic pregnant patients, which was sevenfold greater than the 1.6 per 1,000 rate of seroprevalence reported in statewide heel-stick blood sampling data.[38]

As new treatment strategies for HIV infection as well as treatments to decrease its perinatal transmission become known, it is of even greater importance to identify HIV-positive women.[40,41] Studies have shown that screening questionnaires for HIV risk-related behavior are not as effective as the routine, voluntary serologic screening of pregnant women.[36,37] A recent study has demonstrated the efficacy of azidothymidine (AZT) in decreasing the risk of perinatal transmission of the virus.[40] Although screening at the time of admission to the labor-and-delivery unit will not allow treatment in the antepartum period, this should not prevent the use of screening. Further studies will indicate whether treatment of the infant in the postpartum period alone will help decrease the incidence of perinatally transmitted HIV infection. In addition, it allows for referral of the mother to specialized HIV clinics. Although the merits of mandatory testing of all pregnant women are beyond the scope of this discussion, the CDC has recently advocated routine voluntary testing of all pregnant women.

DOMESTIC VIOLENCE

During the past decade, domestic violence has been identified as a major cause of emergency department visits by women (Ballard T, personal communication). Different studies have shown that from 20 to 30 percent of women who are seen by emergency department physicians exhibit at least one or more symptoms of physical abuse, and that one-half of all injuries presented by women are the results of a partner's aggression.[42–44] Ten percent of the victims were pregnant at the time of abuse, 10 percent reported that their children had also been abused by the batterer, 86 percent of the victims had suffered at least one previous incident of abuse, and about 40 percent had previously required medical care for the abuse.[43] Approximately 16 percent of American couples experienced an assault during the year in which they were asked about it, and about 40 percent of these assaults involved severely violent acts, such as kicking, biting, punching, chocking, and attacks with weapons.[45] Data on the prevalence of abuse during pregnancy are limited, but several clinic-based studies of pregnant women and two population-based studies have addressed the issue. Prevalence data from clinic-based studies indicate that among all pregnant women, the frequency of abuse ranged from 10 to 26 percent in the prior year.[46–50] The frequency of abuse during the immediate pregnancy ranged from 0.9 to 17 percent.[51,52] Of pregnant women who had been physically abused at some point in their lives, approximately 31 to 71 percent reported abuse during the immediate pregnancy.[47–49,51,52] The population-based survey of abuse during pregnancy employed the pregnancy risk assessment monitoring system (PRAMS).[53] It assessed violence against women over a 12-month period in Alaska, Maine, Oklahoma, and West Virginia. The rates ranged from 3.8 to 6.9 percent. The Second National Family Violence survey compared rates of violence against pregnant women and nonpregnant women of all ages.[54] The overall rate suggested that violence was more common among pregnant than nonpregnant women. However, when the subjects were stratified by age group, there was no significant difference between pregnant and nonpregnant women. Physical abuse is reported four times more often when women are asked directly about it in interviews than when they respond to questionnaires.[55–57]

The ACOG has developed a patient education pamphlet titled "The Abused Woman."[58] It contains useful information for patients and all health-care professionals, and offers a strategy for assessing women about an abusive relationship.

Is Your Current Relationship "Safe"?

Disagreements and arguments, even heated ones, are often a part of a normal relationship; physical violence or other abusive behavior is not. Everyone has a right to get angry, but no one has the right to express anger violently, to hurt you. Does your partner ever

Frighten you with threats of violence or by throwing things when he is angry?

Say it's your fault if he hits you?

Promise it won't happen again, but it does?

A "Yes" answer indicates that you may be involved in an unhealthy relationship. Remember: no woman deserves to be abused. There are alternatives to living in a violent relationship. There are people who can help you sort things out and decide what you would like to change about your life.

Women who respond with a "Yes" answer should be referred to local shelters or to the 24-hour hotline of the National Coalition Against Domestic Violence (1-800-333-SAFE).

Domestic violence is a serious problem in America. The simple screening questionnaire presented here could be used on admission to the labor-and-delivery suite to identify women at risk of physical abuse.

CONCLUSION

Efforts to reduce costs, increase efficiency, and satisfy patient's wishes have led to changes in the labor-and-delivery areas in many hospitals. The traditional labor-and-delivery area has already evolved into labor, delivery, and recovery rooms (LDRs). Some hospitals have also included the postpartum stay in the same rooms (LDRPs).

Unfortunately, some women do not obtain prenatal care, and admission to a labor-and-delivery unit may be their first encounter with the health-care system. It is especially important to screen these women for health problems or risk-entailing behaviors. As the health-care system continues to evolve, it is important to use every patient encounter to its maximum potential. This may involve rethinking the standard uses of various sites of health-care delivery. Admission to the labor-and-delivery area is an opportunity to screen for health problems and to initiate programs to prevent them. This chapter has focused on a few specific problems that can be assessed in the labor-and-delivery suite.

REFERENCES

1. Jones KL, Smith DW, Ulleland CN et al: Pattern of malformation in offspring of chronic alcoholic mothers. Lancet 1:1267, 1973
2. Abel EL, Sokol RJ: Incidence of fetal alcohol syndrome and economic impact of FAS-related mental retardation. Drug Alcohol Depend 19:51, 1987
3. Sokol RJ: The effects of alcohol on pregnancy outcome. p. 69. In Fifth Special Report to the U.S. Congress on Alcohol and Health from the Secretary of Health and Human Services. December 1983
4. Rosett HL, Weiner L, Edelin KC: Treatment experience with pregnancy problem drinkers. JAMA 249:2029, 1983
5. Halmesmaki E: Alcohol counseling of 85 pregnant problem drinkers: effect on drinking and fetal outcome. Br J Obstet Gynaecol 95:243, 1988
6. Alcohol and Women. Women's Health patient pamphlet. American College of Obstetricians and Gynecologists, Washington, DC, September, 1986
7. Drugs and Pregnancy: Alcohol, Tobacco, and Other Drugs. Women's Health patient pamphlet. American College of Obstetricians and Gynecologists, Washington, DC, March, 1994
8. Halliday A, Bush B, Cleary P et al: Alcohol abuse in women seeking gynecologic care. Obstet Gynecol 68:322, 1986
9. Russell M, Bigler L: Screening for alcohol-related problems in an outpatient obstetric gynecologic clinic. Am J Obstet Gynecol 134:4, 1979
10. Selzer ML: The Michigan Alcoholism Screening Test: the quest for a new diagnostic instrument. Am J Psychiatry 127:1653, 1971
11. Ewing JA: Detecting alcoholism: The CAGE questionnaire. JAMA 252:1905, 1984
12. Sokol RJ, Miller SI: Identifying the alcohol-abusing obstetric/gynecologic patient: a practical approach. Alcohol Health Res World 4:36, 1980
13. Sokol RJ, Martier SS, Ager JW: The T-ACE questions: Practical prenatal detection of risk-drinking. Am J Obstet Gynecol 160:863, 1989
14. National Household Survey on Drug Abuse: Population Estimates 1991. National Institute on Drug Abuse, Public Health Service, U.S. Department of Health and Human Services. Washington, DC, 1991
15. Schutzman DL, Frankenfield-Chernicoff MA, Clatterbaugh HE, Singer MD: Incidence of intrauterine cocaine exposure in a suburban setting. Pediatrics 88:825, 1991
16. Chasnoff IJ, Burns WJ, Schnoll SH et al: Cocaine use in pregnancy. N Engl J Med 313:666, 1985
17. Oro AS, Dixon SD: Perinatal cocaine and methamphetamine exposure: maternal and neonatal correlates. J Pediatr 111:571, 1987
18. Frank DA, Zuckerman BS, Amaro H et al: Cocaine use during pregnancy: prevalence and correlates. Pediatrics 82:888, 1988
19. Zuckerman B, Amaro H, Cabral H: Validity of self-reporting of marijuana and cocaine use among pregnancy adolescents. J Pediatr 115:821, 1989
20. Chasnoff IJ, Landress HJ, Barrett ME: The prevalence of illicit drug or alcohol use during pregnancy and discrepancies in mandatory reporting in Pinellas County Florida. N Engl J Med 322:1202, 1990
21. Hollinshead WH, Griffin JF, Scott HD et al: Statewide prevalence of illicit drug use by pregnant women—Rhode Island. MMWR 39:225, 1990
22. Colmorgen GHC, Johnson C, Zazzarino MA, Durinzi K: Routine urine drug screening at the first prenatal visit. Am J Obstet Gynecol 166:588, 1992
23. MacGregor SN, Keith LG, Chasnoff IJ et al: Cocaine use during pregnancy: adverse perinatal outcome. Am J Obstet Gynecol 157:686, 1987
24. Little BB, Snell LM, Klein VR, Gilstrap LC: Cocaine abuse during pregnancy: maternal and fetal implications. Obstet Gynecol 73:157, 1989
25. George SK, Price J, Hauth JC et al: Drug abuse screening of childbearing-age women in Alabama public health clinics. Am J Obstet Gynecol 165:924, 1991
26. Neerhof MG, MacGregor SN, Retzky SS, Sullivan TP: Cocaine abuse during pregnancy: peripartum prevalence and perinatal outcome. Am J Obstet Gynecol 161:633, 1989
27. Zuckerman B, Frank DA, Hingson SCD et al: Effects

of maternal marijuana and cocaine use on fetal growth. N Engl J Med 320:762, 1989

28. Ostrea EM, Brady M, Gause S et al: High prevalence of drug abuse in an obstetric population as detected by analysis of infant's stools (meconium) for drugs. Pediatr Res 27:251A, 1990

29. Ostrea EM Jr, Brady M, Gause S et al: Drug screening of newborns by meconium analysis: a large-scale, prospective, epidemiologic study. Pediatrics 89:107, 1992

30. General Accounting Office: Drug-Exposed Infants: A Generation at Risk. June 1990. U.S. General Accounting Office, U.S. Senate, Washington, DC.

31. Caring for Our Future: The Content of Prenatal Care. A Report of the Public Health Service on the Content of Prenatal Care. U.S. Department of Health and Human Services, Washington, DC, 1989

32. Edlin BR, Irwin KL, Fratique S et al: Intersecting epidemics: crack cocaine use and HIV infection among inner-city young adults. N Engl J Med 331:1422, 1994

33. Update: AIDS Among Women—United States, 1994. MMWR 44:81, 1995

34. Gwinn M, Pappeioanou M, George JR et al: Prevalence of HIV infection in childbearing women in the United States. JAMA 265:1704, 1991

35. Center for Disease Control and Prevention: Heterosexually acquired AIDS-United States, 1993. MMWR 43:155, 1994

36. Lindsay MK, Peterson HB, Feng TI et al: Routine antepartum human immunodeficiency virus infection screening in an inner-city population. Obstet Gynecol 74:289, 1989

37. Barbacci M, Repke JT, Chiasson RE: Routine prenatal screening for HIV infection. Lancet 337:709, 1991

38. Lindsay MK, Feng TI, Peterson HB et al: Routine human immunodeficiency virus infection screening in unregistered and registered inner-city parturients. Obstet Gynecol 77:599, 1991

39. Barbacci M, Chaisson R, Anderson J, Horn J: Knowledge of HIV serostatus and pregnancy decisions, abstract ed. Fifth International Conference on AIDS

40. Conner EM, Sperling RS, Gelber R et al: Reduction of maternal-infant transmission of human immunodeficiency virus type 1 with zidovudine treatment. N Engl J Med 331:1173, 1994

41. Centers for Disease Control and Prevention: Recommendations of the U.S. Public Health Service Task Force on the Use of Zidovudine to Reduce Perinatal Transmission of Human Immunodeficiency Virus. MMWR 43(no. RR-11), 1994

42. Henry SL, Roth M, Gleis LH: Domestic violence—the medical community's legal duty. J Ky Med Assoc 90: 162, 1992

43. Stark E, Flitcraft A, Zuckerman D et al: Wife Abuse in the Medical Setting: An Introduction for Health Personnel. Monograph No. 7. Office of Domestic Violence, Washington, DC, 1981.

44. Berrios DC, Grady D: Domestic violence. Risk factors and outcomes. West J Med. 155:133, 1991

45. Straus MA, Smith C: Family patterns and primary prevention of family violence. Trends Health Care, Law Ethics 8:17, 1993

46. Stewart DE, Cecutti A: Physical abuse in pregnancy. Can Med Assoc J 149:1257, 1993

47. Helton SW, McFarlane J, Anderson ET: Battered and pregnant: a prevalence study. Am J Public Health 77: 1337, 1987

48. Hillard PJA: Physical abuse in pregnancy. Obstet Gynecol 66:185, 1985

49. Campbell JC, Poland ML, Waller JB, Ager J: Correlates of battering during pregnancy. Res Nurs Health 15:219, 1992

50. Berenson A, Stiglich N, Wilkison G, Anderson G: Drug abuse and other risk factors for physical abuse in pregnancy among white non-Hispanic, black and Hispanic women. Am J Obstet Gynecol 164:1491, 1991

51. McFarlene J, Parker B, Soeken K, Bullock L: Assessing for abuse during pregnancy: severity and frequency of injuries and associated entry into prenatal care. JAMA 267:3176, 1992

52. Amaro H, Fried L, Cabral H, Zuckerman B: Violence during pregnancy and substance abuse. Am J Public Health 80:575, 1990

53. Centers for Disease Control and Prevention: Physical violence during the 12 months preceding childbirth—Alaska, Maine, Oklahoma, West Virginia, 1990–1991. MMWR 43:132, 1994

54. How violent are American families? Estimates from the National Family Violence Resurvey and other studies. p. 95. In Straus MA, Gelles RJ (eds): Physical Violence in American Families: Risk Factors and Adaptations to Violence in 8,145 Families. Transaction Publishers, New Brunswick, NJ, 1990

55. McFarlane J, Christoffel K. Bateman L et al: Assessing for abuse: self-report versus nurse interview. Public Health Nurs 8:245, 1991

56. Gelles RJ: Violence and pregnancy: are pregnant women at greater risk of abuse? J Marriage Fam 50: 841, 1988

57. O'Leary KD, Vivian D, Malone J: Assessment of physical aggression against women in marriage: the need for multimodal assessment. Behav Assess 14:5, 1992

58. The Abused Woman. Women's Health patient pamphlet. American College of Obstetricians and Gynecologists, Washington, DC, January, 1989

Chapter 31

Medicolegal Issues

Jeffrey P. Phelan

Medical malpractice claims against obstetricians have risen dramatically during the past two decades. Although obstetricians account for only 5 percent of all physicians, they are named in 12 to 13 percent of all medical malpractice claims filed in the United States today.[1] Of those claims filed, approximately 60 percent are birth-related and often involve an alleged failure to perform or to timely deliver a patient by cesarean section.[2]

As medical malpractice claims have risen, jury awards in excess of 1-million dollars have risen more than 232-fold since 1975.[3,4] Recent information obtained from physician-owned insurance carriers indicates that the average awards in the United States for an infant with central nervous system (CNS) impairment or an Erb's palsy are $650,000 and $350,000, respectively.[5]

Since intrapartum care is frequently associated with the potential for liability, the purpose of this chapter is to familiarize the reader with the concept of foreseeability of harm and its potential application to selected areas of labor-and-delivery care. Unless otherwise stated, the obstetric care discussed is directed at term pregnancies or pregnancies that have achieved at least 37 weeks' gestation. Moreover, the scope of the obstetric issues covers those related to selected aspects of the modified hospital admission test (HAT), such as fetal heart rate (FHR) assessment, fetal presentation, and the estimated fetal weight (EFW). Finally, this chapter is one of many in the field of obstetrics, and does not necessarily represent the standard of care applied by myself or any other practitioner. It merely reflects the transmission of ideas that it is hoped will result in an improvement in perinatal outcome for pregnant women and their unborn children.

FORESEEABILITY

In the case of *MacPherson v. Buick Motor Co.*, Justice Benjamin Cardozo developed the concept of "foreseeability of harm," which is taught to every lawyer in America. In that case, Cardozo wrote that "because the danger is foreseen, there is a duty to avoid the injury . . . if he is negligent where a danger is to be foreseen, a liability will follow."[6]

At first, the application of the concept of foreseeability seems simple. Why, for example, are "Stop" signs placed at intersections? Obviously, they are placed at intersections because it is foreseeable that an accident could occur if two cars enter an intersection simultaneously. Thus, automobile drivers have an obligation to stop before entering the intersection. If a driver fails to stop, enters the intersection, and causes an accident, the driver could be held liable for any resultant injuries.

As demonstrated by the situations in Table 31-1, the medical and the legal professional regard a bra-

Table 31-1. Difference in Perspective Between Obstetricians and Attorneys Regarding FHR Bradycardia

Perspective	Event	Action
Obstetrician	FHR bradycardia	Prompt delivery
Lawyer	FHR bradycardia	Foreseeable? Avoidable?

Abbreviation: FHR, fetal heart rate.

Modified Hospital Admission Test[a]

FHR assessment

Fetal presentation

EFW

[a]Or intrapartum fetal risk assessment on a patient admitted to labor and delivery.

---

dycardic FHR differently. While the typical obstetrician responds reflexively to such an FHR by promptly delivering the patient, the attorney asks whether the obstetrician should have anticipated the bradycardia and delivered the patient before it occurred.

The application of the concept of foreseeability to obstetric care is illustrated in Table 31-2. As demonstrated in the examples given, the risk-management strategies begin with the identification of a problem such as a single footling breech presentation. Once the problem is identified, the foreseeable risk of umbilical cord prolapse can, theoretically, be avoided by taking an active management approach.

HOSPITAL ADMISSION TEST

Whenever a pregnant woman is admitted to the hospital, the admission clinical examination is, in reality, an effort to assess the likelihood of vaginal birth and to foresee the potential for maternal and perinatal morbidity and mortality during labor. In essence, the modified HAT is designed to assess the risks that inure to FHR assessment, fetal presentation, and the

EFW. Using the HAT results, intrapartum risk assessment and clinical management can be determined. For example, the HAT provides an immediate evaluation of current fetal condition, allowing the reallocation of patients to a high- or low-risk status depending on the FHR test results for each fetus at admission.[7] Thus, patients previously considered to be at high risk on admission to the labor-and-delivery unit can be reassigned to the low-risk category according to the results of their HAT. Conversely, fetuses considered to be at low risk on admission to the hospital could be reallocated to the high-risk category. Once the foreseeable risk has passed, the patient would revert to a low-risk status. For example, the conversion of a single footling breech presentation to a vertex presentation reduces the potential for umbilical cord prolapse. Assuming that a funic presentation does not exist, the patient would be considered at low risk of cord prolapse.

With respect to FHR assessment, fetal distress in labor is a common occurrence and a cause of concern for both the patient and her obstetrician. As a result,

---

Table 31-2. Two Obstetric Examples of Foreseeable Risks and Some of the Available Risk-avoidance Strategies

Obstetric Issue	Risk	Risk-avoidance Strategies
Non-frank breech presentation	Cord prolapse	External cephalic version Elective cesarean section Selected vaginal delivery(?)
Macrosomic fetus (EFW >4,500 g)	Shoulder dystocia Erb's palsy	Elective cesarean section Avoid midforceps/vacuum delivery Normal labor curve No fundal pressure

Abbreviation: EFW, estimated fetal weight.

most, if not all, patients who present for labor and delivery are connected to an electronic fetal monitor (EFM) to assess fetal status within a short period after their arrival at the hospital. The basis for FHR assessment soon after admission is to determine the presence or absence of FHR accelerations.[7–10] For example, a reactive nonstress test (NST) within 7 days of delivery is associated with a lower incidence of meconium-stained amniotic fluid, intrapartum fetal distress, perinatal death, and oligohydramnios.[11–15] Moreover, a reactive NST is associated with a low probability of intrauterine fetal death,[13] and represents a sign of fetal well-being.[11–16] A reactive FHR pattern obtained intrapartum is a sign of normal fetal acid-base status and the absence of fetal asphyxia.[17–20] In fact, a fetal pH of 7.20 or higher is significantly more likely to occur in a fetus with a reactive FHR pattern, whether spontaneous[19] or induced[17,18,20] than in one with a nonreactive FHR pattern (Fig. 31-1).

Thus, a reactive FHR pattern found on admission to the labor-and-delivery unit should signify a lower likelihood of fetal distress during labor than that for an outpatient reactive NST. In fact, the presence of fetal distress is about 50 percent lower in patients with a reactive FHR admission test.[8,12,15,21]

In studies involving more than 2,800 patients,[8,12,18,22,23] when a reactive FHR pattern was

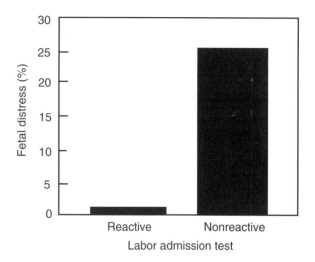

Fig. 31-2. Relationship between fetal heart rate admission test results and incidence of intrapartum fetal distress. (Data from references 8, 15, 18, 22, and 23.)

obtained on admission to the labor-and-delivery unit the likelihood of intrapartum fetal distress was low (Fig. 31-2). Moreover, the type of fetal distress that developed in the reactive group was usually acute.[21] Based on the work of Phelan and Ahn[24] with neurologically impaired infants, the FHR patterns giving rise to intrapartum neurologic impairment were

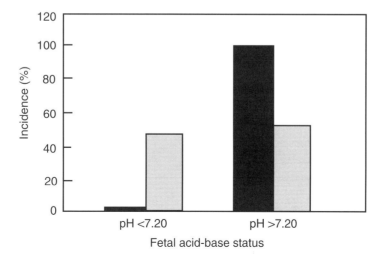

Fig. 31-1. Relationships between a reactive fetal heart rate pattern during labor and fetal acid-base status. Solid bars, reactive; hatched bars, nonreactive.

those that were consistent with Hon's theory of intrapartum asphyxia, comprising a prolonged FHR tachycardia with nonreactivity, FHR decelerations, and absent FHR variability, or a prolonged FHR deceleration lasting many minutes.

Conversely, the absence of FHR accelerations (Fig. 31-2) or a nonreactive FHR test on admission was associated with a greater probability of an adverse fetal outcome.[7,21–23,25] This inverse relationship between the number of FHR accelerations and fetal outcome has also been shown to exist for oligohydramnios[15,25] and FHR decelerations.[15,26] For example, the lower the amniotic fluid volume, the higher the incidence of fetal nonreactivity and FHR decelerations.[15]

Fetal nonreactivity during labor is also associated with higher rates of intrapartum fetal distress.[8,22,23] Specifically, the duration of fetal nonreactivity may be a reflection of the fetal condition.[22–25] Thus, for example, higher rates of operative intervention, perinatal mortality, and neurologic impairment were found for cases in which fetal nonreactivity was present for more than 120 minutes.[22–25] The fetal nonreactivity observed in the cases of 48 neurologically impaired neonates was believed to be the manifestation of a preadmission fetal CNS injury.[24]

Heart rate decelerations are not an uncommon occurrence during an FHR admission test. The work of Phelan and Lewis[26] and of Rutherford[15] indicates that the etiology of FHR decelerations is typically a nuchal cord or diminished amniotic fluid volume. For example, higher frequency of nuchal cords have been described for cases in which a W FHR pattern is observed.[27] By contrast, a V FHR pattern is commonly associated with a reduced amniotic fluid volume.[15,26,28]

If one or more FHR decelerations are observed in association with a reactive FHR pattern on admission to the hospital, a search for the underlying cause of the deceleratory pattern or continuous EFM for a longer period would appear reasonable. However, the likelihood of acute fetal distress during labor in such cases would remain low. If fetal distress did develop, it would usually be manifested as a FHR deceleration lasting for many minutes near the end of labor.[24]

Assuming that a patient satisfies a hospital's criteria for a reactive admission test and has an engaged vertex presentation, she should be considered at low risk of the development of intrapartum fetal distress. This is true regardless of her risk status before labor. As such, she would not necessarily require continuous EFM during labor. Under these circumstances, intermittent FHR auscultation at intervals consistent with a low risk of distress would appear reasonable. In the absence of a number of obstetric or medical conditions, such as oxytocin use, a prior cesarean delivery, infection, or prolonged rupture of membranes, it is my opinion that no fetal monitoring would be obstetrically necessary during labor.

When one or more FHR decelerations are observed during a reactive test on admission for labor, intrapartum fetal distress is more likely to develop than in a similar population without FHR decelerations.[8,9,13,15,26] In such cases, continuous EFM would appear to be reasonable in selected circumstances, depending on the duration of the FHR deceleration. Moreover, the type of fetal distress that would develop, if any, would be similar to that observed in the reactive group, and would generally occur, if at all, near the end of labor. Therefore, continuous EFM or intermittent auscultation would appear to be reasonable options.

The patient with a nonreactive FHR pattern on admission should not be sent home, but should be kept on continuous EFM until the fetal status has been clarified. The duration of nonreactivity before fetal assessment with scalp or acoustic stimulation, a biophysical profile, or a contraction stress test will depend on the circumstances, and will be influenced by a number of factors beyond the scope of this chapter. However, as previously noted, persistent nonreactivity lasting in excess of 90 to 120 minutes in a term fetus should prompt other tests to establish fetal status. To remove any ambiguity, practitioners should consider the establishment of a protocol to address the nonreactive FHR admission test result in their hospitals.

FETAL PRESENTATION

Umbilical cord prolapse remains one of the true emergencies in modern obstetrics.[29,30] Its incidence ranges from 0.09 to 0.8 percent[31–33] and it has been associated with a perinatal mortality rate as high as 50 percent and an unknown incidence of permanent

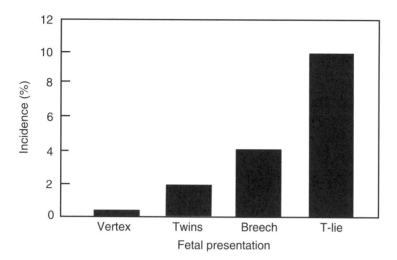

Fig. 31-3. Incidence of umbilical cord prolapse by fetal presentation. T-Lie, transverse lie. (Data from Strong and Phelan,[29] Berkus,[30] and Pathak.[36])

CNS injury.[34] As a result, umbilical cord prolapse continues to be a common source of medical malpractice litigation.[35]

To improve the quality of care and reduce the likelihood of litigation related to umbilical cord prolapse, the second step of the HAT, if not already done before placement of the fetal monitor, is to determine fetal presentation and station. As illustrated in Figure 31-3, the incidence of umbilical cord prolapse is primarily related to fetal presentation and secondarily to the station of the presenting part.[29,30,36] In other words, the common denominator for umbilical cord prolapse is incomplete filling of the maternal pelvis at the time of membrane rupture.[29] As illustrated in Figure 31-4, the more the presenting part fills the maternal pelvis, as with a frank breech presentation, the less likely it is that umbilical cord prolapse will occur.

If, for example, a noncephalic lie or an unengaged vertex presentation is identified on admission, umbilical cord prolapse may be a foreseeable risk. However, the realization of this risk depends on the cervical dilatation, the application of the presenting part to the cervix, and the intrauterine location of the umbilical cord at the time of membrane rupture. In these circumstances, the risk of umbilical cord prolapse may also be suspected from the presence of variable FHR decelerations.[30]

In the term pregnant patient at risk of umbilical

cord prolapse, the clinician should consider the steps outlined below.

Avoidance of membrane rupture

Ultrasonographic evaluation

Continuous EFM

First, the clinician should avoid rupturing the membranes until such time as the clinical circumstances permit it. Before attempting to rupture the membranes, the clinician should consider an ultrasound evaluation using a vaginal probe with color flow Doppler ultrasonography, if available, to search for a funic presentation. If a funic presentation is identified, the patient should be placed in the Trendelenburg position. Then, depending on the fetal presentation and the circumstances, an external cephalic version or a cesarean section can be performed.

As previously suggested in Table 31-2, external cephalic version is an effective means for converting a noncephalic lie to a vertex presentation.[37–44] Doing this can theoretically reduce the risk of cord prolapse. If the version is unsuccessful or the patient prefers a cesarean section, the latter should be performed as soon as is technically feasible. Since mem-

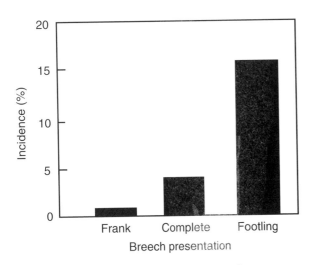

Fig. 31-4. Incidence of umbilical cord prolapse among the different types of breech presentation. (Data from Strong and Phelan,[29] Berkus,[30] and Pathak.[36])

Approach to Patients With Overt Umbilical Cord Prolapse

Knee-chest or Trendelenburg's position

Elevate the presenting part

Fill bladder with normal saline

Administer a uterine relaxant

Apply fetal scalp electrode

Perform cesarean section

---

brane rupture may occur during attempted conduction anesthesia, general anesthesia would appear to be the anesthesia of choice. Before the induction of anesthesia, the patient should be kept supine or in the Trendelenburg position to avoid the potential for cord prolapse.

In the patient at low risk of umbilical cord prolapse and with intact membranes, a careful pelvic examination may warn of the potential for a funic presentation. If during the cervical examination no variable decelerations are observed or the umbilical cord is not palpated, amniotomy can be safely performed. During and immediately after amniotomy, continuous EFM should be used to monitor fetal status.

In cases of overt umbilical cord prolapse,[29,30] timely delivery remains the cornerstone of clinical management. Because few cord prolapses occur at a point in labor at which vaginal delivery can be safely performed, the mainstay of intervention is cesarean delivery. All other management techniques are temporizing measures until a cesarean section can be safely and expeditiously performed.[29]

The first step, if possible, in enhancing umbilical cord blood flow is to elevate the presenting part. This may be accomplished directly with digital pressure, indirectly by placing the patient in the knee-chest or Trendelenburg's position, or by filling the bladder with normal saline. However, this last procedure can be difficult to perform in the anxious atmosphere that frequently accompanies this obstetric emergency.

Rapid abolition of uterine activity with the use of tocolytic agents, such as terbutaline 0.25 mg SC, may be of benefit in the setting of cord prolapse.[45] With uterine relaxation, the presenting part can be more easily elevated and cord compression can be reduced. The net effect is that the fetus can be resuscitated in utero, thus permitting cesarean delivery to be accomplished in an organized, rather than precipitous, manner.[29,30]

Finally, traditional measures such as maternal oxygen administration, the discontinuation of oxytocin infusions, and intravenous fluids should also be considered.

ESTIMATED FETAL WEIGHT

Shoulder dystocia with a resultant Erb's palsy is a common source of malpractice litigation. The central theme in these claims is whether the shoulder dystocia was foreseeable and thus avoidable, and whether, if the shoulder dystocia was not foreseeable, there was a failure to appropriately manage the dystocia when it occurred.

For a shoulder dystocia to be foreseeable, if at all, all three elements listed in the box must be present.[46] If this is not the case, the dystocia cannot be anticipated and is thus not foreseeable; none of the factors listed, in and of themselves, is sufficient to foretell a shoulder dystocia.

The anticipation of a shoulder dystocia begins

```
┌─────────────────────────────────────┐
│    Clinical Findings Indicating Probable     │
│              Shoulder Dystocia               │
│                                              │
│  Fetal macrosomia (EFW >4,500 g)            │
│  Prolonged second stage (>2 hours)          │
│  Midpelvic operative procedure              │
└─────────────────────────────────────┘
```

with an effort to identify fetal macrosomia before or early in labor. According to the American College of Obstetricians and Gynecologists (ACOG), fetal macrosomia is defined as an estimated fetal weight in excess of 4,500 g.[47] This means that an estimation of fetal weight as being average in the case of an infant who subsequently turns out to be macrosomic merely reflects the difficulties in estimating fetal weight. The failure to recognize fetal macrosomia is not based on birth weight, but on whether the clinician made an estimate in good faith of how big the fetus reasonably seemed to be before delivery.

Thus, when the patient presents to the labor-and-delivery unit in labor, a clinical estimate of the fetal weight should be considered part of the patient's admitting evaluation. Once the EFW has been determined it should be documented in the medical records. When the EFW is inconsistent with macrosomia, the factors that suggest fetal macrosomia,[47] even if present, will be less of an issue

in any subsequent litigation. Moreover, the legal focus will shift to the management of the shoulder dystocia and not whether the shoulder dystocia was foreseeable. Moreover, if the EFW is not consistent with fetal macrosomia, an ultrasonographic estimate of fetal weight is, in my opinion, not obstetrically necessary. This is true even when the weight estimate turns out to be incorrect.

In the case in which the clinical EFW suggests macrosomia, and depending on the clinical circumstances, an ultrasonographic estimate of the fetal weight is helpful and can provide additional information to present to the pregnant woman. Assuming that fetal macrosomia is supported by the ultrasound evaluation, the potential risk of shoulder dystocia and its sequelae might also be included in the discussion with the patient.

In these discussions, one has to remember that there is no intrauterine scale. As such, there is no accurate method to weigh the fetus in utero. For example, ultrasound EFWs alone carry a 10 to 15 percent margin of error.[48] This means that the ultrasonographically derived weight estimate could be higher or lower than the estimated weight. An ultrasound EFW of 4,000 g for example, carries a margin of error of ± 1.5 lb.

Given that shoulder dystocia is associated with a prolonged second stage of labor and midpelvic operative procedures, a midpelvic procedure with vacuum or forceps (or both) should be limited to se-

```
┌─────────────────────────────────────┐
│   Clinical Conditions Associated With Fetal   │
│   Macrosomia But Not Necessarily Shoulder     │
│                  Dystocia                     │
│                                               │
│  Pregnancy of 42 weeks or longer             │
│  Maternal weight gain exceeding 44 lb        │
│  Maternal weight exceeding 198 lb            │
│  Delivery of a prior infant weighing more    │
│  than 4 kg                                    │
│  Maternal diabetes mellitus                   │
│                                               │
│  (From ACOG Techical Bulletin,[47] with      │
│  permission.)                                 │
└─────────────────────────────────────┘
```

```
┌─────────────────────────────────────┐
│   Six-step Assessment of Patient with Second  │
│   Stage Labor Longer Than 2 Hours in Whom     │
│     a Midpelvic Operative Procedure Is        │
│                Contemplated                   │
│                                               │
│  1. Is there fetal macrosomia?               │
│  2. Is there an indication?                  │
│  3. Is the maternal pelvis adequate?         │
│  4. What is the position of the fetal head?  │
│  5. Is there evidence of molding, and if so, │
│     how much?                                 │
│  6. Has there been a normal labor curve to   │
│     this point?                               │
│                                               │
│  (From Phelan,[48] with permission.)         │
└─────────────────────────────────────┘
```

Some of the Maneuvers Available to Relieve an Entrapped Shoulder

McRoberts maneuver

Wood's maneuver

Delivery of posterior arm

Rubin maneuver

Zavanelli procedure

(Data from refs. 49 to 54.)

---

lected clinical circumstances and used after a six-step clinical evaluation is conducted to determine its appropriateness.[48] Depending on the results of this evaluation, a midpelvic operative procedure may be a reasonable consideration. Nevertheless, the possibility of shoulder dystocia remains a concern.

Shoulder dystocia is a serious complication of childbirth that occurs in 0.15 to 0.6 percent of all deliveries, usually without warning.[49] When a shoulder dystocia does occur, a number of maneuvers are available to the practitioner. One or more of these methods in combination with suprapubic pressure may be necessary to relieve an entrapped shoulder.[49–54] Fundal pressure should never be used.[47] The subsequent finding of an Erb's palsy in the infant is in most instances unrelated to the maneuver selected,[55] and the condition was probably present before any maneuver was attempted.[56]

SUMMARY

Foreseeability of harm is an important adjunct to intrapartum care. With the modified HAT, the pregnant woman's prospects for vaginal birth or intrapartum complications (or both) can be assessed at the time of her admission for labor and delivery. With this approach, the clinician and nursing personnel are in a better position to determine each patient's risk status and to focus their attention on those patients who are truly at high risk. This approach benefits all patients and should help improve perinatal outcome.

REFERENCES

1. Professional liability survey highlights, claims, experience, merits, duration. American College of Obstetrics and Gynecologists (ACOG) Newsletter: 36:1, 1992
2. Dowden M: Malpractice jury verdicts 1991–1995. OBG Manage 9:6, 1991
3. Harrison TF: The top ten jury awards of 1990. Lawyers Alert 11:4, 1991
4. Ream D: Top ten jury awards of 1991. Plaintiffs' Strategy, Defense Research Institute, May 1992
5. Physicians Owned Insurance Associations of America. May 8, 1993
6. *MacPherson v. Buick Motor Co.*, 217 N.Y. 382, 111 N.E. 1050 (1916)
7. Phelan JP: Labor admission test. Clin Perinatol 21: 879, 1994
8. Ingemarsson I, Arulkumaran S, Paul RH et al: A screening test for fetal distress in labor. Obstet Gynecol 68:800, 1986
9. Ingemarsson I, Arulkumaran S, Paul RH et al: Fetal acoustic stimulation in early labor in patients screened with the admission test. Am J Obstet Gynecol 158:70, 1988
10. Sarno AP, Phelan JP, Ahn MO: Relationship of early intrapartum fetal heart rate patterns to subsequent patterns and fetal outcome. J Reprod Med 35:239, 1990
11. Lee CY, DiLoreto PC, Logrand B: Fetal activity acceleration determination for the evaluation of fetal reserve. Obstet Gynecol 48:19, 1976
12. Phelan JP: The non-stress test: a review of 3000 tests. Am J Obstet Gynecol 139:7, 1981
13. Phelan JP, Cromartie AP, Smith CV: The nonstress test: the false negative test. Am J Obstet Gynecol 142: 293, 1982
14. Smith CV, Phelan JP: Antepartum fetal assessment: the nonstress test. p. 61. In Hill A, Volpe J (eds): Fetal Neurology. Raven Press, New York, 1989
15. Rutherford SE, Phelan JP, Smith CV et al: The four quadrant assessment of amniotic fluid volume: an adjunct to antepartum fetal heart rate testing. Obstet Gynecol 70:353, 1987
16. Lee CY, DiLoreto RC, O'Lane JM: A study of fetal heart rate acceleration patterns. Obstet Gynecol 45: 142, 1975
17. Clark SL, Gimovsky ML, Miller FC: Fetal heart rate response to scalp blood sampling. Am J Obstet Gynecol 144:706, 1982
18. Clark SL, Gimovsky ML, Miller FC: The scalp stimulation test: a clinical alternative to fetal scalp blood sampling. Am J Obstet Gynecol 148:274, 1984
19. Shaw K, Clark SL: Reliability of intrapartum fetal heart

rate monitoring in the postterm fetus with meconium passage. Obstet Gynecol 72:886, 1988

20. Smith CV, Nguyen HM, Phelan JP et al: Intrapartum assessment of fetal well-being: a comparison of fetal acoustic stimulation with acid-base determination. Am J Obstet Gynecol 155:726, 1986

21. Krebs HB, Petres RE, Dunn LJ et al: Intrapartum fetal heart rate monitoring. VI. Prognostic significance of accelerations. Am J Obstet Gynecol 142:297, 1982

22. Brown R, Patrick J: The nonstress test: how long is enough? Am J Obstet Gynecol 141:646, 1981

23. Devoe LD, McKenzie J, Searle NS et al: Clinical sequelae of the extended nonstress test. Am J Obstet Gynecol 151:1074, 1985

24. Phelan JP, Ahn MO: Perinatal Observations in forty eight neurologically impaired term infants. Am J Obstet Gynecol 171:424, 1994

25. Leveno KJ, Williams ML, DePalma RT et al: Perinatal outcome in the absence of antepartum fetal heart rate acceleration. Obstet Gynecol 61:347, 1983

26. Phelan JP, Lewis PE: Fetal heart rate decelerations during a nonstress test. Obstet Gynecol 57:228, 1981

27. Welt SI: The fetal heart rate w-sign. Obstet Gynecol 63:405, 1984

28. Phelan JP: Antepartum fetal assessment: newer techniques. Semin Perinatol 12:57, 1988

29. Strong TH, Phelan JP: Umbilical Cord Prolapse. Fem Patient 16:19, 1991

30. Berkus, M: Coping successfully with cord prolapse. Contemp Obstet Gynecol 22:199, 1983

31. DuToit PFM: Prolapse of the umbilical cord. S Afr Med J 30:1181, 1956

32. Savage EW, Kohl SG, Wynn RM: Prolapse of the umbilical cord. Obstet Gynecol 36:502, 1970

33. Doerr LE: Prolapse of the umbilical cord. J Mich State Med Soc 46:1277, 1947

34. Rhodes P: Prolapse of the umbilical cord. Proc Ry Soc Med 49:937, 1956

35. Rubsamen DS: A greater burden for the obstetrician in managing breech deliveries? Prof Liab News 13:1, 1982

36. Pathak UN: Presentation and prolapse of the umbilical cord. An analysis of 71 cases. Am J Obstet Gynecol 101:401, 1968

37. Ranney B: The gentle art of external cephalic version. Am J Obstet Gynecol 116:239, 1973

38. Van Dorsten JP, Schifrin BS, Wallace FL: Randomized control trial of external cephalic version with tocolysis in late pregnancy. Am J Obstet Gynecol 141:417, 1981

39. Phelan JP, Stine LE, Mueller E et al: Observations of fetal heart rate characteristics related to external cephalic version and tocolysis. Am J Obstet Gynecol 149:658, 1984

40. Stine LE, Phelan JP, Wallace RH et al: Update on external cephalic continuing experience at LAC/USC Medical Center. Obstet Gynecol 65:642, 1985

41. Phelan JP, Stine LE, Edwards NE et al: The role of external version in the intrapartum management of the transverse lie presentation. Am J Obstet Gynecol 151:724, 1985

42. Phelan JP, Boucher M, Mueller E et al: The nonlaboring transverse lie: a management dilemma. J Reprod Med 31:184, 1986

43. Dyson DC, Ferguson JE II, Hensleigh P: Antepartum external cephalic version under tocolysis. Obstet Gynecol 67:63, 1986

44. Morrison JC, Myatt RE, Martin JN et al: External cephalic version of the breech presentation under tocolysis. Am J Obstet Gynecol 154:900, 1986

45. Katz Z, Lancet M, Borenstein R: Management of labor with umbilical cord prolapse. Am J Obstet Gynecol 142:239, 1982

46. Benedetti TJ, Gabbe SG: Shoulder dystocia: a complication of fetal macrosomia and prolonged second stage labor with midpelvic delivery. Obstet Gynecol 52:526, 1978

47. Fetal Macrosomia. ACOG Technical Bulletin No. 159. American College of Obstetricians and Gynecologists, Washington, DC, September, 1991

48. Phelan JP: Medical-legal considerations in the clinical management of the fetus with a growth disorder. p. 365. In Divon MY (ed): Abnormal Fetal Growth. Elsevier Science, New York, 1991

49. Strong TH, Phelan JP: Shoulder dystocia. Fem Patient 13:73, 1988

50. Gonik B, Stringer CA, Held B: An alternative maneuver for management of shoulder dystocia. Am J Obstet Gynecol 145:882, 1983

51. Rubin A: Management of shoulder dystocia. JAMA 189:835, 1964

52. Sandberg EC: The Zavanelli maneuver. A potentially revolutionary method for the resolution of should dystocia. Am J Obstet Gynecol 152:479, 1985

53. Woods CE: A principle of physics as applied to shoulder dystocia. Am J Obstet Gynecol 45:796, 1943

54. O'Leary JA: Cephalic replacement for shoulder dystocia: present status and future role of the zavanelli maneuver. Obstet Gynecol 82:847, 1993

55. Nocon JJ, McKenzie DK, Thomas LJ et al: Shoulder dystocia: an analysis of risks and obstetric maneuvers. Am J Obstet Gynecol 168: 1732, 1993

56. Jennett RJ, Tarby TJ, Kreinick CJ: Brachial plexus palsy: an old problem revisited. Am J Obstet Gynecol 166:1673, 1992

Chapter 32

Self-Preservation and Autonomy: When Maternal and Fetal Well-Being Conflict

Kenneth J. Ryan

When patients and physicians disagree, as they occasionally do over the obstetric management indicated to benefit the fetus, the impasse is designated maternal-fetal conflict by the bioethical pundits. Many articles have been written about the subject. This is, however, a misleading label, because the pregnant women who reject medical advice for various, sometimes seemingly inexplicable reasons, do not necessarily see themselves in conflict with their fetuses or have the desire to harm them. Moreover, the patient's decision may also put her own life or health in jeopardy. The conflict is really about a mix of controlling the application of medical technology, the enforcement of social norms, and clashes of dissonant cultures. Realization of this complexity may be a key to understanding the problem and working toward satisfactory resolutions of it. Fortunately, most pregnant women want to do everything possible to ensure the health and safety of the fetus they carry, and bend over backward to accept the obstetrician's advice. When the patient refuses to do so, in what may at times seem an irrational or irresponsible position, the alternatives have been to have the patient seek a new caretaker if there is time, or to carefully and patiently work through the issues with the patient, using the assistance of family, consultants, and an ethics committee if necessary, or, very rarely one would hope, to forcibly pursue the recommended treatment or call on the courts to enforce

the medical treatment on the recalcitrant patient. Examples in which patients' refusal to follow medical recommendations have occasioned court actions include the rejection of a prohibition against alcohol or drugs during pregnancy, refusal of intrauterine transfusion for a high-zone Rh incompatibility, and failure to adhere to a regimen for the proper management of diabetes during prenatal care. In the labor-and-delivery suite, the major arguments, when they occur, have been over various medical interventions, including early delivery or cesarean birth for fetal indications alone or with maternal problems such as toxemia or placenta previa. Another source of conflict has been the refusal of Jehovah's Witness patients to accept a blood transfusion whether its need is based on a fetal indication. These conflicts create an ethical dilemma in which the physician is torn between two conflicting obligations: the duty to respect the autonomous decisions of the pregnant patient and the duty to medically safeguard the patient and her fetus.

EVOLUTION OF OBSTETRIC CARE AND SOCIAL ATTITUDES TOWARD CHILDBEARING

Two forces have been at work in the last half of the 20th century to modify obstetric care in the United States. The medical and public health professions made a concerted effort to reduce the high levels of first maternal and then fetal morbidity and mortality, largely with advances in technology and emphasis on hospital births. With each improvement in pregnancy outcome, and at cross purposes with organized medicine, the "natural childbirth" movement has tried to demedicalize pregnancy, reduce reliance on technology, and foster alternatives to hospital births, such as birthing centers and home deliveries. The argument for this was that at times, medicine was as much the problem as the solution to improving care. Fortunately, both of these movements, when their excesses were refined, made important positive contributions to obstetric care.

Since the 1930s, maternal mortality has been just about halved in each decade, from roughly 500 deaths per 100,000 live births in 1935 to eight deaths per 100,000 in 1985. The major problems in pregnancy were hemorrhage, infection, and hypertensive disorders. They were successfully attacked by improvements in transfusion and blood products, antibiotics, and life-support technology such as anesthesia, respirators, and fluid and electrolyte treatment, as well as improved surgical technology. Maternal mortality was remarkably reduced for placenta previa in the 1920s with blood replacement and cesarean section, and for toxemia with preventative prenatal care and hospitalization at the earliest signs of pre-eclampsia. In the 1950s Du Vigneaud received the Nobel prize for determining the structure of oxytocin, which could thereafter be synthesized and used clinically. Tocolytics and prostaglandins also became available to aid in obstetric management. It is likely that a considerable improvement in obstetric outcome was also due to a general improvement in public health and nutrition, as well as medical interventions.[1]

With these gains well in hand, medicine turned its attention to improving the outcome for the infant, when perinatal mortality plateaued while maternal outcome continued to improve. The special care or intensive care nursery was introduced, with pediatricians specializing in newborn care. New specialties of perinatology or maternal-fetal medicine were created. Access to the fetus became almost facile, with amniotic fluid sampling and analysis, sonography, fetal surgical techniques, and direct umbilical blood sampling and transfusion. Study of fetal lung development and the predictive tests for fetal lung maturity, starting with the lecithin/sphingomyelin (L/S) ratio and progressing through prenatal glucocorticoid treatment and use of surfactant in the newborn, contributed significantly to a reduced perinatal mortality and morbidity. By the close of the 20th century, it was possible to look at the fetus as a patient separate from the mother. In the past, improvements in outcome for the fetus and infant were achieved through improvements in the pregnant patient's overall condition. It was now possible to address fetal problems more directly, but one thing had not changed: all access to the fetus still involved some breaching of the mother's bodily integrity with x-rays, sonography, needle, or scalpel, and manipulation of the mother's behavior. For the most part, women accepted and applauded these technologic advances, but the ground was at least prepared for some conflicts between maternal and fetal interests and a backlash against the high-technology environment of labor and delivery. Cesarean sections, initially performed largely to save the pregnant patient's life, were increasingly used for fetal indications. The cesarean section rate soared between 1960 and 1990 by almost fivefold, from 5 percent to 25 percent.[2] Contributing to this increase was the fetal distress indication and "failure" to progress in labor. There was concern that this high section rate did not make sense. Electronic fetal monitoring (EFM) added to the cesarean section rate but is now a substantially discredited technology. When finally tested long after it had become a standard of care, EFM proved no more valuable or discriminating for the well-being of the fetus than a nurse listening with a fetoscope.[1] Other evidence was accumulating that the good results in perinatal survival had less to do with the increased cesarean section rate and other obstetric interventions than previously believed. When the backlash did occur it was against the high cesarean section rates, and the high reliance on EFM, and oxytocin and other drugs, as well as the "sterile" ambiance of high-technology medicine.

If the British obstetrician Grantly Dick-Read did not start the natural childbirth movement, he gave great impetus to it with his popular book, *Childbirth Without Fear*, written in the 1930s but reissued in 1959. The thesis was that with proper faith, relaxation, and absence of fear, the birth process could be pain free. This was initially quite popular but never successfully adapted into mainstream obstetrics. The next movement on the scene was psychoprophylaxis, begun in Russia after World War II and picked up by the French physician Ferdinand Lamaze, who championed childbirth classes to teach the deep-breathing techniques that allow women to control their responses to whatever pain and discomforts childbirth had to offer. In the 1960s and 1970s there was a popular revolt against oversedation during labor and the use of general anesthesia in delivery, against isolation of the patient from her family and the restriction of her movements during the birth process. Patients wanted to be awake and aware, some wanted no part of EFM; perineal shaving, episiotomy, and the use of forceps was anathema to many.[3] Gradually this trend was accepted and championed by physicians as well as patients, with the development of combined labor-and-delivery rooms in the hospital that looked like a home bedroom or a hotel room, and featured low-technology deliveries to combat the enthusiasm for out-of-hospital birthing centers and home births. All of this became possible within the framework of advances in obstetrics, newborn pediatrics, and improved general health and nutrition, which made the overall process of childbirth much safer no matter where it occurred. A recent report on outcomes for birthing centers reported reassuringly good results. My own philosophy has been supportive of natural childbirth, with the use only of that technology that is needed and effective. By contrast, prudence dictates that labor and childbirth ought to take place in a location where emergency care for the pregnant patient, fetus, or newborn is readily available should the unforeseen occur.

It should be apparent that a discussion of patient-physician disagreements or maternal-fetal conflict can now be more thoroughly understood from the reference to where we have been over the past 50 or more years in terms of medical advances and social changes in the childbirth process. We should add that the promise of a "perfect" outcome in the 1970s came to be expected for every childbirth as medicine progressed. Failing that, there was a rapid increase in the number and size of malpractice suits and awards for infants who had handicaps or retardation, whether or not the obstetrician could have done anything about it.[2] Over 70 percent of obstetricians could expect to be sued at least once, and in some cases malpractice premiums rose to over $100,000/yr in localities such as Miami and New York City. Patient and physician disagreements could in fact occur both before and after childbirth, and at times could be very costly.

ADVENT OF BIOETHICS AND A CHANGE IN MEDICAL PRACTICE

The backlash against medical technology, especially in childbirth, took place against a background of many social changes during the 1960s and 1970s that centered on assertions of individual rights, a general mistrust of authority in government and the professions, an insistence on civil rights and gender equality, and a pervasive dissatisfaction with the generally unpopular Viet Nam war. The new field of bioethics arose, which was congenial to the popular mood. Although there is some uncertainty about the specific event or technology that triggered this vigorous preoccupation with ethics, there are many candidates. Revelations in the 1970s about federally funded clinical research that was hazardous to the participants and done without their knowledge or consent prompted the Government to form a commission to address the ethical questions that arose. The new technologies of outpatient renal dialysis, respiratory support, and transplantation of the heart and other major organs created ethical dilemmas about triage for scarce resources, as well as about indications for using or foregoing therapy that did not exist before these new modes of therapy were introduced.[4] Concerns about abortion also fueled the interest in ethics. Ethical and legal conflicts between patients or their relatives and medical institutions about starting or stopping life-support systems were ultimately taken to court and became benchmark cases in an evolving public consensus about what should be done in such situations. Case law also developed around the duty of physicians to inform the patient and gain the patient's consent for all medical procedures. Hospital ethics committees became commonplace, and ethics is now formally taught in essentially all medical schools. Relatively late in this process of the development of bioethics, the subject of maternal-fetal conflict arose in case law, in the ethics opinions of professional societies, and in a series of articles analyzing the relevant issues.

Bioethics is an applied ethics that is concerned with action as much as with theory, and a new frame of reference had to be developed to cope with the practical matter of guiding medical practice. The National Commission referred to earlier, responded to its Congressional mandate by fashioning a set of ethical principles in a document called the Belmont Report.[5] These principles were deemed useful for guiding and justifying ethical practices in both clinical research and medicine.

The principles have been rough guides for analyzing and acting on ethical problems, but many other ethical theories have been advanced from the traditions of moral philosophy. These include outcome- and rule-based theories such as utilitarianism or Kantian deontology, and moralities based on rights and on virtues.[6] Most individuals do not make ethical judgements based solely on ethical theories, principles, or means and ends so much as on some combination of them. Analogy and metaphor are widely employed in dealing with ethical dilemmas, often unconsciously. As a consequence, discussing and teaching ethics through the review of specific cases has been quite popular. Such case review is useful and effective as long as it is combined with some strategy for being consistent and systematic in the analysis of events and decisions and application of the conclusions to new cases as they arise. With this background in the evolution of obstetric care, social attitudes toward childbearing, and the development of bioethics, we turn to the cases and writings that are a component of the intrapartum maternal-fetal conflict literature that is the subject of our concern.

INTRAPARTUM MATERNAL-FETAL CONFLICT

It is difficult to imagine much discussion about maternal-fetal or patient-physician conflict before the 1950s, when standards for obtaining informed consent did not exist, when women were given heavy sedation and amnesics during labor, and when the family was kept outside the labor-and-delivery suite. There were the occasional court orders for transfusion to a nonconsenting pregnant patient who was a member of the Jehovah's Witnesses for the benefit of either the fetus or patient, or both. The numerous

Ethical Principles of the Belmont Report

1. *Respect for persons*—recognizing patients as autonomous agents—incorporates two requirements: respecting the wishes of autonomous individuals and protecting those with diminished autonomy. This respect is shown by obtaining informed consent for all research or medical procedures, and by abiding by the decisions of the patient. For patients with diminished autonomy, respect is shown by obtaining substituted or best-interest judgments, occasionally using the courts for this purpose. *Respect for a patient's autonomy* is a modern concept that replaces the paternalism and authoritarian rule that existed from the beginning of medicine until recent times. The trend in society in general toward emphasizing respect for individual rights is consonant with this.

2. *Beneficence*—benefiting patients and avoiding harm—is about securing the well-being of patients and medically safeguarding them. This principle has roots in the traditions of medicine dating back to Hippocratic times. In practice, beneficence is accomplished through risk/benefit evaluations of all preventive, diagnostic, and therapeutic interventions, sometimes including the avoidance of any or all of them. In most cases, however, what constitutes the patient's best interests must ultimately be decided by the patient in accordance with the principle of respect for the autonomous patient, as noted above. At one time, the physician's primary duty was to pursue the patient's best medical interests. In the provision of care, the duty of beneficence must now share primacy with what the patient most desires.

3. *Justice*—fairness in access to and provision of medical care—is a new concept to medicine that, in keeping with the goals of liberal societies, calls for dealing fairly with patients in all aspects of access to and provision of care. This is especially important in view of the power differential between the average patient and the physician, and the tendency for medical institutions to have the state intervene when they disagree with the patient.

conflicts we now see reported are certainly an outgrowth of the changes in obstetric management and social attitudes toward childbearing described earlier, as well as of the advent of a bioethical and legal sensitivity in medical personnel and institutions, and the public. Physicians were previously motivated largely by beneficence toward the medical welfare of the mother and the fetus without being encumbered by the requirement to describe what they wanted to do and to receive prior permission to do it. However, an ethical and legal awareness developed among the health-care professionals, hospital administrators, and patients and their families through the 1970s and 1980s and by the middle of the 1980s a significant number of case reports and articles dealt with maternal-fetal conflict.

It is difficult to obtain an overall perspective on the subject of maternal-fetal conflict, since very few surveys have been done of physician and patient attitudes and practices, and many of the court judgments in cases of such conflict are not precedent-setting. Reliance on the high-profile cases reported in the newspapers may not be typical and could be misleading. Suffice it to say that the subject is an evolving one.

An often referenced article by Kolder et al[7] in the *New England Journal of Medicine* reported the findings of a survey of directors of fellowship programs in maternal-fetal medicine in 1987. Of those who responded, 21 described instances of requests for court orders to enforce medical recommendations made by the medical establishment, and in 86 percent of these cases a court order was obtained. Attempts to override patient wishes by court orders were made in 26 states, while in six instances such orders were denied. In 88 percent of the cases the court order was delivered within 6 hours. In 11 instances in 11 different states, a court order to perform a cesarean section was obtained for indications, including fetal distress, prior cesarean section, and placenta previa. Almost one-half of the fellowship directors polled favored court orders to override patient objections to recommended therapy. What was most telling about the report was that the patients involved were largely black, Asian, or Hispanic (88 percent minority); many were unmarried (44 percent); and 25 percent did not use English as a primary language. This distribution could be interpreted as an unfair selective use of the courts or as evidence of a cultural dissonance between physicians and this segment of the childbearing public, or more likely some combination of both.

REVIEW OF HIGH-VISIBILITY CASES AND RESULTS

It is useful to review some of the referenced and high-visibility cases to identify the range of responses to such conflict and the outcomes (Table 32-1). Field,[8] in her article titled "Controlling Women to Protect the Fetus," cites the case of Ayesha Maydun, a 19-year-old who was in labor for 2 days at home without progress, and after an additional 18 hours of labor in the hospital was deemed to need a cesarean section. Since the patient refused consent, a court order was obtained and an operative delivery was successfully performed. This occurred in 1987 and was provided as a typical case in which court orders are sought and obtained and medical management is orchestrated over the patient's objections. What is not known is how often such forced therapy is really necessary or desirable, and what impact the coercion has on the patient. Insights into these questions will require further study and a look at other cases.

In the 1981 case of Jessie Jefferson in Georgia, it was determined that the patient had a placenta pre-

Table 32-1. Court Cases on Ordering Cesarean Sections

Case	Result
Obstructed labor at term	Operative delivery ordered and accomplished
Placenta previa at term	Normal delivery before court order was executed
Terminal cancer at 25 weeks; attempt to rescue fetus	Ordered cesarean delivery; mother and infant died; court reversed on review
Fetal growth retardation at 37 weeks	Courts up to and including the U.S. Supreme Court refused to intervene

via and needed a cesarean section, which she refused on religious grounds. The medical testimony to the court in support of the doctor's position was that there was a 99-percent chance that a live birth could not be obtained vaginally and a 50-percent chance that the patient would lose her life in such an attempt. The court ordered the recommended medical care, the U.S. Department of Human Resources was awarded custody of the fetus as a "deprived child," and the parents' appeal to the Georgia supreme court was rejected. Mrs. Jefferson thereupon delivered a healthy child vaginally without incident, and in the words of Field,[8] was "more battered by litigation than childbirth." A newspaper article on the event was titled "Supreme Court Orders Cesarean Section—Mother Nature Reverses on Appeal."[7] In another, similar case involving placenta previa, a Michigan court ordered patient compliance but the patient fled and went into hiding until the birth of her infant, which was also by vaginal delivery with a healthy outcome for the newborn. Despite cases of this type, placenta previa at term represents the paradigm circumstance used by Chervenak to ethically justify coerced emergency cesarean delivery if there is "certainty" that a cesarean section would prevent significant harm to the newborn, there is no time for a court order, and the patient does not physically resist the procedure.[9] (This is discussed in more detail in the section, *Ethical Issues.*)

In Colorado, a court order was obtained for a cesarean delivery on an uncooperative patient, on the basis of ominous fetal tracings. A cesarean delivery produced a healthy infant showing no signs of the predicted hypoxia, underscoring the fallibility of some medical predictions even when used as a basis for enforcing patient compliance.[10] Raleigh Fitkin is a case often referred to in relation to court orders for a blood transfusion to a pregnant woman who is a Jehovah's Witness on behalf of the fetus she is carrying. Although the trial court upheld the woman's refusal, the New Jersey Supreme Court in 1964 determined that blood could be administered to save her life or that of the child over her objections. The transfusion never occurred.[10] As George Annas, an expert in health law and ethics noted, this was more than a decade before the New Jersey Supreme Court acted on the Karen Ann Quinlan case and presumably might have a different outcome today. Although many court orders have been obtained and are still being obtained for forced transfusions for the benefit of pregnant patients and their fetuses over the patients' objections, the social awareness of ethical issues is finally catching up with the courts. The courts are now seldom ordering transfusions over the refusal of competent adults, and one can no longer be certain that they will order a transfusion for a pregnant woman for the benefit of her fetus when physicians request this.

The case of A.C. may be a precedent setting case, although it is still the subject of some dispute, since it was quite different from the cases described previously.[8] The patient was a 27-year-old married woman who was pregnant with her first child. She had a history of bone cancer from the age of 13, with numerous hospitalizations and treatments, including a leg amputation, but at the time of her pregnancy the disease had been in remission for 3 years. At a checkup in her 25th week of pregnancy, metastases to the lung were discovered and she was soon hospitalized in a terminal condition. The pregnancy was 26.5 weeks along when the patient's condition deteriorated. The hospital administrators, over the objection of the patient's family and physicians, asked for an emergency court hearing so as to gain permission to deliver the fetus by emergency cesarean section whether or not the patient or her family agreed. The judge, who held the hearing in the hospital, was not clear about what the patient desired, but nevertheless authorized the procedure to save the fetus. The testimony was that the patient might die at any time but that the fetus, if delivered, had a 50 to 60 percent chance of survival. Although there was some confusion about the patient's wishes, her last indication, when the judge was not present, was that she did not want to undergo the surgery. This indication was discounted by the physician who witnessed it because he believed that the environment in which it occurred was not conducive to informed consent. A request for a stay of order was sought but denied by the state court of appeals. The cesarean section was performed but the baby died within 2.5 hours and the mother died within 2 days. It was believed that the operation was a contributing factor in hastening her death. Later, the court of appeals vacated the earlier judgment and decided to hear the case before the entire bench. Beginning in 1988, testimony was heard with surprisingly strong interest despite the death of both the patient and her infant because the case received wide discussion in the lay press and medical, ethical, and legal literature. The final opinion was released in 1990, with the entire bench supporting the majority opinion and only one judge dissenting in part. The court's opinion was that in virtually every case the question of what is to be done is to be decided by the patient on behalf of herself and her fetus. If the patient is incompetent, a substituted judgment should be made. The court considered a cesarean section to be major surgery, and the circumstances for it would have to be extraordinary to justify overriding the patient's wishes.[11]

The opinions in this case were considered limited because of the extreme condition of the patient, the marginal viability of the fetus, and the fact that the case did not cover situations such as placenta previa in which both the mother and the fetus might be in jeopardy. The findings also did not cover more minor treatments such as transfusions in the Jehovah's Witness cases, or cases in which the fetus is at term. It remains to be seen how widely the statement "in virtually all cases" will be interpreted. Both Strong[12] and Curran[11] believe that this case will influence future decisions even in some of these other instances because of the direction it took and the tone it set in making the wishes of a competent pregnant woman paramount. The family of the deceased patient went on to file a civil suit for medical malpractice and civil rights violations against the medical center. In an out-of-court settlement, the hospital agreed to implement a new policy that ensured that ethically difficult decisions would in the future be made by the patient, the family, and the physicians, and not by a routine appeal to the courts. The medical center stated that "respect for patient autonomy compels us to accede to the treatment decisions of a pregnant patient whenever possible." It further stated that "When a fully informed competent pregnant patient persists in a decision which may disserve her own or fetal welfare, this hospital's policy is to accede to the pregnant patient's preference whenever possible." If the treating doctors cannot abide the patient's wishes, they are to seek advice from the hospital ethics committee, or in rare cases in which a substitute is available, the doctor may withdraw from the case.[13]

The most recent case of conflict between a physician and a pregnant patient went all the way to the United States Supreme Court. The patient was a 22-year-old Pentecostal Christian who wanted her trust in God to vouchsafe her decision to have a delivery of a healthy baby by natural means. Her obstetrician believed the baby was not thriving in utero and would either die or be born retarded if an emergency delivery, presumably by cesarean section, was not performed at 37 weeks. When the hospital presented the case to them, the Cook County State's Attorney and public guardian asked the courts to intervene and balance the mother's right to practice her religion and make choices about her obstetric care against the state's interest in protecting the life of her fully developed fetus. The lower court, the Illinois Supreme Court, and the United States Supreme Court, all without comment, refused to intervene. The baby was born vaginally at term on December 30, 1993, weighing only 4 pounds and 12 ounces but otherwise doing well.[14] It is obviously too early to tell whether the child will be normal from a neurologic and intellectual perspective, and it will probably never be known whether an earlier delivery would have made any difference.

LEGAL AND ETHICAL CONSIDERATIONS

The law and morality are distinct but overlapping institutions governing human behavior. Although most laws are morally grounded, this does not guarantee a fair legal system, and some laws are simply wrong from a moral perspective. By contrast, not all moral rules are enforced by law, and some should not be, as in many personal and domestic matters. At the time of our Puritan forebears, church law, civil law, and morality were essentially one, and governed the land. It is clear from a modern perspective that in that era not all laws were moral, since they did not recognize much privacy and gave too much authority to the patriarch, treating women and children as chattel. Today we generally discourage enactment of laws that intrude into the private moral domains that fall within the areas of sex, marriage, childbearing, and raising children, except in the current climate of excessive domestic violence and abuse. Abuse has long been overlooked in our society, at least partly because domestic matters were considered outside the law. Just as our notions of what the law should cover have changed, concepts of morality have changed markedly in the area of medical ethics, as noted above, and both the law and morality are evolving on the subject of maternal-fetal conflict.

Legal Issues

The rulings used to justify court-ordered treatment of pregnant patients have included those set forth in Roe v. Wade and in civil and criminal child neglect statutes, since few other laws are potentially applicable to this area. Roe v. Wade allows for a state interest in the fetus after its viability that can even ban late abortions, but not if the pregnant woman's health or life is at stake. Many argue that once the woman foregoes an abortion before fetal viability, she has a strong obligation to the fetus as it approaches term, and that the state may enforce this. However, in the Court of Appeals review of A.C. described above, the judge argued that Roe v. Wade never gave the fetus primary status or even equal status with the woman when her life or health might be involved, even in the third trimester, and in that decision, a forced cesarean section was considered to be major surgery and a risk to a woman's health.[11] When it comes to applying child neglect laws, the distinction between the free-living child already born and the fetus inside the woman's body is either overlooked or considered irrelevant. Some states have, however, purposely added the fetus to their child abuse statutes to cover maternal-fetal conflicts.[10,15–17]

Judges were at one time more likely than not to support physicians' requests to override patients wishes in general, let alone in the case of a fetus at risk of harm from a nonconsenting and seemingly irrational pregnant woman. There were in fact few precedent-setting decisions that could be referenced for these cases, and both medicine and the law have historically had a paternalistic mindset. However, this is changing, and the courts are today much less willing to force competent adult patients into any medical treatment, even at the risk of their death if they refuse therapy. Physicians sometimes did not inform patients of some serious or fatal risks inherent in a procedure on the grounds it might scare them from agreeing to the procedure when it seemed critical. This sort of paternalistic withhold-

ing of the truth is unimpressive to judges. Failure to obtain adequate informed consent can now be used more effectively against physicians, especially if there is an adverse outcome to a treatment and the patient was not warned of all the relevant risks. In the state of Massachusetts, courts will no longer consider requests for forcing blood transfusions on competent adult patients as long as they are not leaving an orphaned minor child for which no guardian can be found. Whether transfusions would be ordered for the benefit of the fetus in the case of an uncooperative pregnant patient depends more on the judge than the existing law. I participated in a conference for appellate judges from the northern New England states on the subject of maternal-fetal conflict, sponsored by the Women Judges' Fund for Justice. When the participating judges were informally polled about whether they would order a blood transfusion for the benefit of a fetus of a nonconsenting Jehovah's Witness, the response appeared to be equally split between those who would and those who would not. The sex and moral views of the judge seemed to influence the response. There were not many women judges in the group, but they seemed less likely to force treatment on a pregnant woman.

Just as the law is relatively sparse on the subject of forcing therapy, so is it silent on any requirement for physicians to seek court orders in cases of maternal-fetal conflict,[16] although the institution in the case of A.C. seemed concerned about liability if it did not go to court. By contrast, some physicians have been sued by patients, and in the case of A.C. the institution was sued, for violating the patients' rights by taking the patient to court. Although going to court can always be reserved as a last-resort possibility, most commentators now suggest moral persuasion and the use of hospital ethics committees to resolve disputes without relying on the courts, which in any case are becoming less predictable. Clearly, there are also moral arguments about whether one should go to court in a particular instance. We discuss this further in the following section on ethics.

Ethical Issues

There have been many reviews of the ethical issues involved in maternal-fetal conflict, and all essentially agree that the pregnant woman's choices for obstetric care in labor and delivery should be controlling for decisions that do not involve risks to either herself or her fetus (e.g., pain relief, type of monitoring, labor coaching, presence of family members, delivery procedures and methods). The reviews also largely agree that physicians should respect patient preferences or refer the patient to another physician or institution that will. This is based on a widely accepted obligation of respect for patients and their autonomous choices, and a growing public intolerance for management based more on physician or institutional convenience or preference than on patient choice. In other words, if a patient desires a form of "natural childbirth," the use of technology should not be forced on her simply because it makes a physician more comfortable: nor should the value of the technology be oversold to pressure the patient into compliance.

When the patient's choice of intrapartum obstetric management poses a major risk to her life or health (refusal of an urgently needed blood transfusion or a surgical delivery for life-threatening bleeding or toxemia), it usually poses a risk to her fetus as well. Even when a choice poses only a risk to the fetus (fetal distress), all ethical commentators have still wanted to make respect for the pregnant woman's autonomy a serious concern, although some believed that under such circumstances her autonomy should not be absolute.[6] In the latter case there is a desire to balance respect for the patient's autonomy against the beneficence, nonmaleficence, or prudence-based obligations to the patient herself, her fetus, or the medical care team that might be required against strongly held ethical beliefs to provide a form of care that is against all standards of acceptable practice.[6,9] In some cases appeal is made to two or to all three of these bases for challenging the patient's refusal to accept medical advice. These are the cases that have been the basis for seeking court authority or forcing care on the patient in an emergency. Most reviews of the ethical balancing process or court decisions, such as in A.C., have simply used the opinions that the woman should be controlling in "virtually all cases," or that one should almost never go to court, or have held out the appropriateness of going to court in some cases but never specifying the conditions for such action. Chervenak and colleagues, by contrast, have cited as a paradigm situation the existence of "certain" placenta previa

at term with a normal fetus that in the absence of surgery creates a life-threatening risk to both the woman and the fetus and does significant harm to the moral integrity of a health-care team if they cannot provide the cesarean section that is indicated in this setting.[6,9] Chervenak et al believe that patient refusal of recommended care is justification for going to court if there is time for this, or forcing care in an emergency if the patient does not physically resist it. The remainder of this chapter is devoted to reviewing the reasons given for taking this position.

One should begin this review by at least recognizing the importance of anticipating ethical problem cases and practicing what McCullough and Chervenak[6] call "preventing conflict and crisis in clinical practice." This involves a timely and thorough informed-consent process that to my mind should begin when prenatal care is begun and not when a clinical problem occurs. Patients should be informed of the common problems that might arise in any pregnancy and the therapies that are normally used in treating them. The patient should know how her obstetrician ordinarily treats third-trimester bleeding or pre-eclampsia and risks to the fetus, as well as the normal standards of care for transfusion, surgery, and cesarean section so that she can indicate whether she has strongly held or religious beliefs on these matters before they arise. This leaves time for mutual education, development of trust, compromise, counseling, and even selecting another physician if time and circumstances allow. One should be aware that trying to discharge a patient to the care of someone else at the time of a medical crisis and conflict is difficult and hard to justify if one has strong convictions about an obligation to the fetus and going to court to force compliance. Unfortunately, subspecialty referral centers often receive for care patients who they have not previously counseled. Alternatively, the practitioner may be in a crisis environment in which time and the opportunity for discussion and the development of trust are limited, and referral to another physician or institution is simply not medically feasible. In such circumstances it is helpful to have an established institutional plan for dealing with problem cases.

A practical problem with regard to maternal-fetal conflict is its uniqueness. There is no exact analogy in either the law or ethics from which to deal with one "human" entity (the fetus) within the body of another (the pregnant woman), or the obligation of the latter to help or rescue rather than harm the former. Attempts at such analogy are usually strained. One situation sometimes suggested as comparable is the failure of society to legally enforce the breaching of one person's bodily integrity for the benefit of another, as in the forced donation of bone marrow or transplantation of an organ from a parent to a child. Certainly a cesarean section is as formidable as a bone marrow transplant, and a living child is as worthy of consideration as a fetus. This has been an argument given by some judges for refusing to issue a court order forcing therapy on a pregnant woman for the benefit of her fetus.[7] There are no examples of forced therapy involving a breach in the bodily integrity of male or female adults to benefit another person in any situation other than pregnancy. Most agree that a parent should have a moral obligation to do something like this for a child, just as most agree that a pregnant woman should have a moral obligation for the welfare of the fetus she carries. No satisfactory reason has been given for why the state should force therapy in one situation and not the other. This has in turn suggested societal gender bias and an insidious biologic and social determinism in the treatment of pregnant women. Pregnancy is "different," but the question before us is whether it should be.

In the cases of donation of tissue from fetuses, infants, or minor children, there is always the cover of proxy consent that limits charges of coercion. Chervenak and colleagues have rejected the nonexistence of forced adult donation of marrow or of an organ to a child as a suitable analogy for what in my judgment are rather weak reasons. They offer their own analogy of one child standing on the shoulders of another in the deep end of a swimming pool, thereby essentially drowning a smaller child. The lifeguard (obstetrician) would be justified (obligated) in forcibly removing the offending child (pregnant woman) from the shoulders of the smaller child (fetus) to save it. However, I do not find this to be of much help in deciding whether to force therapy on a pregnant woman for the sake of her fetus.[9] All of us choose analogies to both comfort and challenge our intuitions, and one test of their worth has to be how convincing they appear to others.

The justifications for abiding by a patient's decision to refuse therapy for herself or her fetus, using counseling and persuasion rather than coercion for implementing such therapy, or not seeking a court order to implement it include (1) the duty to respect the patient's autonomy and the need to maintain her trust in her medical caretakers; (2) the fallibility of medical judgments; (3) the tendency for patients to shun care and be driven out of the system if it is known that their wishes are not respected; and (4) the unpredictability of courts in responding to medical requests. In any case, most commentators advise that patient choice should especially be honored at the margins of viability, in cases of severe fetal anomaly, with experimental drugs or therapies, or when the risk of harm to the pregnant woman places her life or health at substantial risk that can otherwise be avoided. Going to court is not a benign experience for patients. It has been looked on as an abridgement of patient confidentiality and patient rights. Coercion or forced therapy is an assault on the patient, and although a good outcome for the patient and infant may be given as a post hoc mitigating factor for such a practice, any adverse outcome is an invitation for punitive damages, as in the case of A.C. The failure of some patients to complain after such therapy and to not bring charges against physicians does not justify the means used for effecting therapy. Finally, a state that has no statutes about a duty to rescue, that makes no similar claims on other adults, that provides no universal health coverage, and that offers limited economic and social justice in family matters should not force its will on the pregnant woman, either for her fetus or herself. The idea that therapy can be coerced if the woman does not physically resist sounds suspiciously like the argument that rape does not occur if a woman says no but does not fight back. In any case, there is always the "slippery slope" argument if one does not respect the patient's autonomy on this issue and what is next?

The justifications offered by Chervenak and others[6,9] for seeking court orders or coercing therapy in rare emergency situations include the following:

1. Patient autonomy is not absolute and should be balanced against unreasoned refusal of therapy that will harm the viable, normal fetus

2. The pregnant woman has an obligation to the fetus and the child it will become that should be enforced by the courts if the risk to the mother is slight or at least reasonable by customary standards, and the benefit to the fetus is great and certain. If one can save the woman's life or safeguard her from harms while helping the fetus, so much the better

3. One does not need to make a special plea for consideration of the fetus as a person to invoke an obligation on the part of the pregnant woman and the medical team to have a duty of beneficence to it

4. The fetus has a right to be born free of harm if harm can be reasonably avoided

5. The medical care team should not be restricted by rules or standards for obstetric management that exceed reasonable standards of medical care or are against their moral convictions.

McCullough and Chervenak[6] put forward only one clear-cut case that in their view justifies going to court. This is the situation of a patient with a placenta previa at term who refuses a cesarean section that will almost certainly benefit her and her fetus. The justifications for going to court are the danger to the woman and fetus, the certainty of the situation, and the likelihood of benefit. McCullough and Chervenak[6] also believe that the woman has a duty to the fetus and child it will become and that the state should enforce this obligation. These constitute a powerful series of arguments. By contrast, courts have allowed adults to refuse therapy that would save them, through ethical and legal respect for their autonomy, and the question thereby returns to whether one should treat a pregnant woman differently than other patients on the basis of the presence of a mature fetus. The argument about state-enforced obligations is answered by the charge that the state enforces no similar obligation on anyone but pregnant women because of the uniqueness of the "patient within a patient" that occurs only in pregnancy. The claim that going to court or coercing treatment in such cases is not a form of paternalism is disingenuous. Making someone do what "they're supposed to do" is what paternalism is all about, whether it is for their benefit or not. Finally, attempting to enforce a procedure because the failure to do so upsets the

practice of medicine has not been a sufficiently strong argument to dissuade the legal system from overruling it and allowing patients to refuse blood transfusions, surgery, and food and fluid in a right of self-determination. This position has been difficult for some, but in general physicians have been able to cope with it.

One could go on with point and counterpoint in such a discussion, and each side has telling points[18] that make reasonable arguments, *depending* on whether one wants to live in a community that champions individual rights or one that values a sense of community responsibility.

CONCLUSIONS

Obstetric practice and societal views of childbearing have changed dramatically in the last part of the 20th century. Obstetrics and perinatology have gone from major reductions in maternal and perinatal morbidity and mortality brought by advances in modern biotechnology to an emphasis on birthing centers and low-technology births unless intervention is necessary. The two seem related. The depersonalization and alienation caused by machines in high-technology care, including EFM and soaring cesarean section rates, fostered a move back to nature. The creation of a field of bioethics set the stage for sweeping changes in the patient's relationship to the physician and the health-care system. There is an emphasis in bioethics and now in the law to respect the autonomy of the patient by allowing refusal of all forms of therapy, even those that may save the patient's life. Even a stupid or irrational position on the part of the patient does not in itself prove that the patient is not competent to make medical decisions in the eyes of the law.

The problem of maternal-fetal conflict is a special situation, since there has always been some societal interest in the fetus and a tradition for courts to enforce medical treatment on pregnant women. The results have been mixed, since the courts have occasionally enforced medical treatments that proved clearly wrong and unnecessary. The trend in court rulings seems to be changing, and requests for enforced therapy are being denied more often.

The obstetrician is best served by reviewing possible problems and treatment options with patients early in pregnancy, and anticipating patient non-compliance. This leaves time for discussion, negotiation, and referral if all else fails. In a crisis situation, exhortation of the patient and help from relatives, consultations, and the hospital ethics committee are preferable to seeking a court order. The strongest justification offered for going to court is that both the woman and the fetus would benefit from treatment, as in the case of threatened third-trimester bleeding. When the obstetrician is caught in an emergency without time to seek a court order, most commentators have recommended abiding by the patient's wishes. One opinion has been that one may be "forceful" but may not use force. Fortunately, most women are cooperative and do everything possible for the well-being of their fetus. In the meantime, the ethical and legal analysis of issues involving maternal-fetal and physician-patient conflict will continue to evolve and guide future practice.

REFERENCES

1. Cunningham FG, MacDonald PC, Gant NF et al (eds): Williams' Obstetrics. 19th Ed. Appleton & Lange, E. Norwalk, CT, 1993
2. Ryan KJ: Giving birth in America, 1988. Fam Plan Perspect 20:298, 1988
3. Wertz RW, Wertz DC: Lying-in: A History of Childbirth in America. Free Press, New York, 1977
4. Jonsen AR: The birth of bioethics. Hastings Cent Rep 23:S1 1993
5. The Belmont Report: DHEW Publication No. (OS) 78-0012. U.S. Government Printing Office, Washington DC, 1978
6. McCullough LB, Chervenak FA: Ethics in Obstetrics and Gynecology. Oxford University Press, New York, 1994
7. Kolder VEB, Gallagher J, Parsons MT: Court ordered obstetrical interventions. N Engl J Med 316:1192, 1987
8. Field MA: Controlling the woman to protect the fetus. Law Med Health Care 17:114, 1989
9. Chervenak FA, McCullough LB, Skupski DW: An ethical justification for emergency coerced cesarean delivery. Obstet Gynecol 82:1029, 1993
10. Annas GJ: Forced cesareans: the most unkindest cut of all. Hastings Cent Rep 12:16, 1982
11. Curran WJ: Court-ordered cesarean sections receive judicial defeat. N Engl J Med 323:489, 1990
12. Strong C: Court-ordered treatment in obstetrics. Obstet Gynecol 76:861, 1991
13. Greenhouse L: Hospital sets policy on pregnant patient's rights. New York Times, p. B14. November 29, 1990
14. Terry D: A child is born in court case over cesarean. p. A12. New York Times December 31, 1993
15. Nelson LJ, Milliken N: Compelled medical treatment of pregnant women. JAMA 259:1060, 1988
16. Nelson LJ: Legal dimensions of matenal-fetal conflict. Clinical Obstetrics and Gynecology 35:738, 1992
17. Rhoden NK: Cesareans and Samaritans. Law Med Health Care 15:118, 1987
18. Mathieu D: Preventing Prenatal Harm. Kluwer, Dordrecht, The Netherlands, 1991

Chapter 33

Perinatal Loss

Jaque R. Repke

Despite advances in technology and practice, both nurses and physicians involved in the intrapartum setting will continue to deal with the unwanted outcomes of fetal and infant death. Over the past two decades, the nursing and medical literature have provided improved insight into the best approaches for assisting patients and families with the grieving process. The management of perinatal loss must be dealt with in a collaborative, sensitive, and individualized manner to best serve patients and families dealing with this extremely difficult life crisis. The following sections review the current understanding of the perinatal bereavement process and the rationale for approaches to the management of bereavement, along with clinical-practice guidelines for nurses and physicians practicing in the intrapartum setting (see Appendix 33-1). Perinatal loss in the intrapartum setting can encompass miscarriage, stillbirth, and neonatal death. Approximately 40,000 neonatal deaths occur annually in the United States, and of every 100 pregnancies, from 10 to 20 end in miscarriage before 20 weeks' gestation, while two end in stillbirth after 20 weeks' gestation.[1] The management of perinatal loss has evidenced significant revision and improvement over the past two decades. Research on parental grief responses and therapeutic interventions, as well as the emergence of grief, mourning, and attachment theories, has contributed to more humane and sensitive practices

in these situations. We have come a long way from such protective interventions as sedating the mother throughout labor and delivery, prohibiting contact with the infant after delivery, and giving such inappropriate reassurances as "You can have another baby," and "It's God's will" to women whose infants have died or cannot be saved. It is now well recognized that it is important to involve the patient and her family in all aspects of decision-making. This includes involvement not only in the labor, delivery, and postpartum course, but also in their preferences with regard to spending time with the infant after delivery, planning for the disposition of its remains, and creating tangible memories of the infant.

ATTACHMENT AND LOSS THEORY

The work of Bowlby[2] in attachment and loss theory, together with that of Klaus and Kennel,[3] Kubler-Ross,[4] and others[5,6] provides the framework for perinatal bereavement and mourning. It is now well accepted that attachment to the unborn child occurs for both mothers and fathers. Tangible evidence of the infant's existence, including movement, the sound of the heartbeat, and ultrasound imaging, now available earlier in gestation through vaginal probe ultrasonography, contributes to this attachment. The feeling of loss created when a child dies is predicated on this developed attachment. Prospective parents build hopes and dreams for their unborn child as early as the time that conception is definitively diagnosed. New concepts of self are also created, such as the future role of mother and father. The hopes and dreams for the child's future and new concepts of self, such as that of parent, are also losses that are sustained and must be considered. Perinatal loss is therefore a prospective grief for lost hopes as compared to retrospective grief for one who was known.

ATTACHMENT AND GRIEF RESPONSES

Mothers Versus Fathers

Klaus and Kennel contend that the attachment process commences when the pregnancy is planned and follows progressive milestones. After the pregnancy is confirmed, the couple must come to terms with the life-style changes it creates, overcome this ambivalence, and reach a point of acceptance of the pregnancy. In the next phase of the attachment process, maternal recognition of fetal movement, the baby takes on the dimension of an individual for the mother. From this point until birth, the mother develops a picture of what her ideal baby will look like.

In comparison, the father's initial attachment is described as more intellectual than emotional until the point of fetal movement. With current technologies such as Doppler and vaginal probe ultrasound, hearing the heartbeat or seeing the fetus more than likely facilitates both parents' view of their infant as an individual at earlier points in gestation.[7]

The final phases of attachment, usually shared by both parents, are the birth experience itself; seeing, touching and holding; and finally, caring for the infant.[3]

The initial delay in the father's emotional attachment to the infant, in combination with the obvious physical nature of maternal attachment, results in a different bond between the father and the infant and the mother and the infant. This disparity is the basis on which the grief and mourning process may be asynchronous in couples.

This initial lag in paternal investment may be offset by such things as participation in labor and birth, earlier contact with the infant, witnessing delivery and resuscitation, and being the recipient of initial information if the mother is recovering. Expression of grief for fathers can be difficult if they are influenced by stereotypic expectations of males as strong and unemotional.[8] Feelings of responsibility conflict with those of helplessness or dependency, and fathers can be caught between their own grief and the needs of their wives.[9]

Mothers may perceive their husbands' outwardly stoic behavior as noncaring and nonsupportive. In efforts to spare their wives from their feelings, some husbands may not verbalize their grief reactions. This, as well as the differing maternal and paternal timetable for experiencing grief, can lead to isolation, misunderstandings, stress in the marital relationship, and sometimes divorce.[3] In interviews of 51 fathers, Page-Lieberman and Hughes found that 69 percent acknowledged a difference between spouses in the chronology of grief, and most fathers stated that their intense period of grieving was shorter than that of their wives. Slightly more than half reported that they eventually grew closer to their wives as a result of their loss.[9] These findings have implications for practice in terms of preparing parents for the possibilities of encountering different styles and levels of grieving in their spouses, and encouraging communication both in the hospital as well as when they go home.

Early Versus Late Pregnancy

Research conflicts on findings relative to grief intensity and gestational age. While it would seem logical to assume that the intensity of grief is directly related to the degree of attachment, Peppers and Knapp[10] demonstrated no quantifiable difference in maternal grief response to miscarriage, stillbirth, or infant death. Kirkley-Best,[11] however, described losses later in pregnancy as being associated with greater grief intensity than those in early pregnancy. Similarly, Toedter et al[12] also found a significant correlation between gestational age and grief response. Theut and colleagues[13] empirically examined differences between grief reactions following losses in early versus late pregnancy, and found significantly greater grief in the late loss group. The retrospective nature of these studies, as well as other variations in methodology, make overall conclusions difficult, and further research is warranted in this area to clarify their implications for practice.

Other Considerations

Grief responses will also vary with such factors as previous losses, coping styles, whether the perinatal loss was unexpected as opposed to anticipated, cultural and religious influences, and individual and family strengths.[14] Clinicians must also be careful not to assume that pregnancy loss inevitably and only involves mourning the death of one's baby. Other losses that may be felt include the loss of the role of parent, as well as loss of self-esteem or the revisiting of prior emotional conflicts. Because grief responses may show wide variation, clinicians must be able to evaluate each patient and family within their unique circumstances, attempt to understand what the loss of their infant means to them, and individualize care accordingly.[15]

STAGES OF GRIEF AND MOURNING AND IMPLICATIONS FOR PRACTICE

Grief is defined as the emotions one feels after suffering a loss, such as sadness, anger, guilt, shame, and anxiety. Mourning is the process used to resolve the emotions of grief. Bowlby and Parkes characterize four phases of grief and mourning by the specific behaviors exhibited in each (Table 33-1). It should

be pointed out that these phases should not be construed as separate, progressive entities, since they will overlap and may play out again on the anniversary of the birth or death, as well as on holidays.

Nurses and physicians in the intrapartum setting should guide their care according to an understanding of the first two phases in particular, given that these are the phases and associated behaviors usually encountered during the hospital stay. Discharge planning should include anticipatory guidance for parents, identifying the types of feelings and emotions they may experience on going home, as well as in the latter two phases of grief, which occur outside of the hospital setting. (see Appendix 33-1 for clinical practice guidelines for management of patients experiencing perinatal loss in the intrapartum setting.)

During Labor

The initial phase of shock and numbness is usually the one that will be evidenced in the labor-and-delivery setting. The duration of this phase can vary from a few hours to 4 months after the death, and is characterized by a wide range of behaviors. Parents may be especially unresponsive to stimuli in the midst of labor, and hear only portions of what is said or

Table 33-1. Mourning Process

Phase of Grief	Time Frame	Behavioral Expression
Shock and numbness	Several hours–4 mo	Resistance to stimuli Difficulty in making judgments Altered functioning Emotional outbursts Periods of clarity
Searching and yearning	4–6 mo	Urge to recover the dead infant Sensitivity to stimuli Anger/irritability Guilt Restlessness Questioning
Disorganization and disorientation	6–9 mo	Apathy Despair Impeded functioning Acute awareness of reality
Reorganization	1–2 yr	Sense of weight being lifted Return of energy and judgment-making ability Stable eating and sleeping habits

(Adapted from Bowlby and Parkes,[5] and Davidson,[6] with permission.)

explained to them. Difficulty in decision-making and impaired judgment are also evidenced, along with a feeling of being stunned and, sometimes, emotional outbursts inconsistent with the situation. On the other hand, there will also be periods of clear thinking and understanding. Clinicians must be able to identify these lucid points so that information and explanations can be given as requested, and choices about the immediate time after delivery can be offered. Anticipatory grieving is often found when a death or a condition incompatible with life has been diagnosed before labor, as well as in situations of extreme prematurity and premature labor or miscarriage. At this point, behaviors identified in the *searching and yearning* phase of grief may also be evidenced. In this phase, parents may express guilt for things they may or may not have done during the pregnancy that they feel contributed to their baby's death. They may be searching for answers and may ask many questions, along with exhibiting anger at the unfairness of their situation. This anger may sometimes be directed at clinicians, and if so, should be managed by providing explanations rather than being personalized. Clinicians should direct their actions during labor toward supportive, presencing care, with interventions responsive to the patient's or couple's lead. This approach, as well as several of the behaviors identified above, is illustrated in the following nursing clinical narrative (O'Toole R, New England Medical Center):

She was a married, 29-year-old woman experiencing her first pregnancy after 3 years of infertility. The pregnancy remained uncomplicated until this day, when a routine ultrasound detected that the baby had died. She was in early labor with an epidural anesthetic. She was grieving appropriately with occasional episodes of anger, followed by periods of sadness.

My first impression on entering her room was that it reflected an atmosphere of grief and loss. The most apparent loss being the absence of the clip-clop sound a baby's heart makes when recorded on a fetal monitor. In its place was a profound silence that echoed the devastation this couple was experiencing.

Following my introduction, I decided to express my sorrow for their unfortunate circumstances. My

apologies were met with sad and vacant looks from both Mr. and Mrs. O. Feeling inadequate to provide comfort, solace, or words of encouragement, I decided to sit in silence with them and wait for their cue.

A half an hour passed before Mrs. O. began to vent angry feelings about losing her baby. As she continued to talk, I began to feel more helpful by listening and giving reassuring nods. This helped to establish a sense of trust, which enabled me to explore the needs of this couple.

Both agreed on baptism, but were undecided about holding the baby right away. I assured them that these feelings were normal and apt to change many times before the birth.

In a few short hours, Mrs. O. was completely dilated and ready to push with contractions. As the birth of the baby approached, she began to weep and express her fears concerning the delivery. Her foremost fear was that after the baby's birth she would no longer be considered a mother. As long as the baby remained inside, she was safe from dealing with the full impact of her loss. I intervened at this time because Mrs. O was losing focus on the situation. Her husband stood helplessly by, unable to find the right words to console her. I decided to encourage Mrs. O to take her time and not push until she felt better prepared for the birth.

With the pressure off, and the added benefit of a great epidural, she began to calm down. Dimming the room lights, I left Mr. and Mrs. O alone for the first time that evening. When I returned, Mrs. O said she was ready to deliver the baby. Surprised, I asked her if she was sure. With confidence, she replied, "Thank you for allowing me the extra time to hold onto him. I know he is not mine to keep."

After Delivery

Acknowledging the Infant and Validating the Loss

Because parents want to know their child, it can be important to offer them the opportunity to hold the child after delivery. Although it is not a prescriptive measure, parents should be offered the choice of holding, touching and naming their infant, and planning a memorial service congruent with their cultural and religious background. These actions serve to acknowledge the infant and validate the loss for the parents. In cases in which the infant is severely premature or has a condition that will not be amenable to resuscitative efforts, parents should be offered the opportunity to hold their baby as he or she dies. Taking the infant away to die in a neonatal intensive care unit (NICU) or nursery should not be done unless the parents specifically request it. Knowing that they were with their infant when the baby died is very meaningful to parents. In cases in which there are anomalies or maceration, a sensitive explanation of the baby's appearance can be helpful to prepare parents for viewing their infant. This is important in such situations, since what parents imagine is usually worse than the reality.

Mementos such as photographs, a stockinette cap, bracelets, hand and footprints, and a lock of hair are examples of keepsakes that parents find meaningful in remembering their baby and should be suggested, while also taking cultural and religious preferences into consideration. Baptism and a certificate of birth may, for example, be offered to Christian parents.

Some parents may initially indicate that they do not prefer to see the infant after delivery or do not want mementos. These preferences need to be honored in the management, keeping in mind that some parents will subsequently request that they be able to see or hold their infant. Mementos are typically kept for parents indefinitely, based on experiences of parents calling and requesting these keepsakes at some later point.

Additional Measures

Clinicians should continue to direct their care toward listening to, understanding, and responding sensitively to parents as individuals at this time, recognizing the diversity of grief reactions and facilitating the expression of grief. Extending visiting policies and involving other family members in the grieving process can be offered to the parents. If the parents have chosen a name for the infant, it is important to use the name when referring to the infant with the parents and family.

The timing and manner of requests for decisions about burial, disposition, or autopsy are crucial. Parents should not be rushed through the painful process of digesting the reality of the death of their infant and having to make decisions about autopsy and the disposition of remains, especially when the death was not anticipated or was only recently determined.

Postpartum

In deciding on the site for postpartum care, the mother should be given a choice of location. Some mothers may feel that the postpartum unit acknowledges them as mothers, while others may prefer not to be exposed to other new mothers and infants. Gynecology or antepartum units may be alternatives in these cases. All units caring for these mothers should ensure by some mechanism that all hospital personnel are aware of the loss.

Postpartum care should be guided by assessment and intervention strategies identified in the clinical practice guidelines for perinatal loss. Final decisions about the infant must be made before discharge. Whether or not autopsy has been chosen, it is important to ensure that parents have the opportunity to have their questions answered in simple terms regarding the cause of their infant's death. Covington and Theut[16] in 1993 reported on results of the National Maternal and Infant Health Survey (NMIHS) conducted in 1988 by the National Center for Health Statistics. A qualitative analysis of the 413 responses identified such themes as the need for further information and unresolved questions about the cause of death. Twenty-one percent of respondents who had experienced perinatal loss indicated a lack of understanding about the cause of their infant's death as well as dissatisfaction with the explanations they had received.[16]

If an autopsy is to be done, a plan for communicating its results should be identified and followed through. Information communicated verbally may be difficult to retain and understand. Therefore, written information on the cause of or conditions implicated in the death, as well as their impact on future pregnancies, should be given if possible.

CONSULTATION

In some facilities, the social work department may provide consultative services for parents experiencing perinatal loss. Most social workers have training in grief counseling, and may also be able to identify financial or other resources for parents who may be unable to afford costs for burial.

Although grief responses vary, psychiatric consultation should be sought if the nurse and physician are concerned about abnormal manifestations of parental grief, and in particular if either parent expresses suicidal ideation or exhibits total absence of a grief reaction.

PROVIDING ANTICIPATORY GUIDANCE

Parents should be provided with both verbal and written information about the normality of grief, its stages and length, the kinds and intensities of emotions it entails, and how others will react to it. Literature written specifically for this purpose is available, and should be provided. *When Hello Means Goodbye*[17] is a guide for parents to take home that includes information about perinatal loss, as well as expressions of the feelings and thoughts of parents who have experienced perinatal loss.

The Pregnancy and Infant Loss Center in Wayzata, Minnesota, and Resolve Through Sharing (RTS) Bereavement Services in La Crosse, Wisconsin, are two national organizations that publish resources for parents on such topics as self-care and fathers', siblings', and grandparents' grief, and both can make referrals to support groups nationwide.

Parents should be advised that the most intense grief will be experienced in the first 2 to 4 months after the death of their infant,[18] and will become progressively less symptomatic over time. Explanations about gender differences in grieving are also helpful. Maternal grief reactions may include sleep and appetite disturbances along with guilt, anger and hostility, depression, and uncontrolled crying. Mothers usually desire social support in discussing the death of an infant.[19] Fathers may exhibit social withdrawal and inability to work, in addition to excessive guilt, anger, and hostility. They may exhibit complete denial of death and some may use alcohol as an escape.

Parents should be encouraged to not only support each other, but to reach out beyond the nuclear family for professional help if they so wish. Typically, a support system is present for the initial 4 to 6 weeks and is then withdrawn. At this point, support groups and professional counseling services may become important.[8] Parents should also be advised that anniversaries of the infant's death will evoke initial feelings of grief and loss.

The manner in which others react to them should also be reviewed. While some persons may be supportive and empathetic, others will be uncomfortable and may avoid the parents through a sense of helplessness in knowing what to say or do.[8] Well-intended comments such as "You'll have another baby" may be hurtful, since parents need to have their lost child acknowledged rather than replaced.

Suggesting that a close friend or relative call the couple's circle of friends to inform them of the death may help to prevent painful inquiries about the baby or the pregnancy.

FOLLOW-UP

Patients report that follow-up phone calls by the primary nurse and physician at designated points, such as at 1 and 6 weeks after the loss, are helpful. The intent is to communicate to the parents that they are not alone, and have a resource person available if they need one. In addition, the follow-up provides an opportunity for parents to ask questions they feel are still unanswered.

The physician should address the issue of future pregnancies at some point in the follow-up. While each couple's circumstances must be taken into consideration, pregnancy immediately following a loss is usually discouraged until the loss becomes less all-consuming. A period of 6 months after the loss is a general guideline. Parents must understand that love for their lost infant will always remain. Grief behaviors and the attachment to the lost infant need to subside enough so that attachment may occur with a new infant.[20]

OTHER CONSIDERATIONS

Explanations to Children

Factors influencing a child's response to perinatal loss include their cognitive and developmental level; knowledge about, attachment to and expectations for the infant; and feelings of ambivalence.[8]

If parents experiencing perinatal loss have other children, additional literature developed for this circumstance should be provided.

Strategies for Helping Children Experiencing Perinatal Loss of a Sibling

1. Present facts to children in language they can understand; give details/show pictures if they ask
2. Repetition may be necessary, as also for adults
3. Provide explanations that are honest; give details if they ask
4. Avoid such figurative statements as "the baby has gone to sleep forever," which may cause children to fear going to sleep themselves
5. Encourage children to share their feelings
6. Let the children know they did not cause the death
7. Allow the children to participate in the death ritual if possible

---

Death Coinciding With Birth of a Multiple

Multiple conceptions are on the rise as a result of reproductive technology. The risks of medical complications, premature birth, stillbirth, congenital problems, and sudden infant death syndrome increase with multiple gestations.[21]

Parents face an unusually difficult experience when a loss occurs in a multiple gestation with a sibling survivor from the same pregnancy. Dealing with joy and grief simultaneously poses a complex situation for the patient, her family, and the care providers involved. Knowledge of the perinatal grieving process and awareness of factors unique to this situation are important to guide clinical practice in such cases.

Although some assume that parents grieving for an infant lost in a multiple gestation would experience less of a grief response than those who lose a singleton or all infants in a multiple birth, these parents may actually experience more acute feelings of loss.[22] Conflict results from the dilemma of simultaneously grieving for a lost infant while developing attachment for the surviving sibling(s). Furthermore, Western society has assigned a special status to multiple gestations, resulting in a lost sense of prestige and lost expectations about life as a family

with multiples. Mothers of multiples have reported guilt for having difficulty in forming an attachment to their living infant(s) while grieving for the dead child, as well as feelings of inadequacy, believing that they have either failed in pregnancy or are unable to raise more than the surviving sibling(s). Guilt may also stem from the wish for a child of a certain sex as opposed to another. If the survivor(s) is critically ill, some parents may fear that it will not survive either, and may become so concerned that they lack time and energy to perform the necessary grief work for a lost infant.

Bryan reported that mothers of lost infants in a multiple gestation continue to think of the surviving sibling(s) as member of a twin, triplet, or other set, and refer to them as such. Parents have also reported feeling that the surviving child is aware of the lost sibling and appears lonelier than other children.[23] The grieving process for parents of a lost infant in a multiple gestation may take longer than the grief period experienced by parents mourning a lost infant from a singleton pregnancy. Birthdays, holidays, and anniversaries evoke conflicting emotions. Working through the grief process in these situations can be more difficult, and is therefore important, especially for the surviving sibling.[22,41]

Clinical Practice Implications

Both the primary nurse and the physician need to direct efforts toward acknowledging the loss of an infant in a multiple gestation. The same principles as in a singleton loss should be employed to facilitate early grief work. Opportunities to see, hold, and touch the dead or dying infant should be offered to make the loss real and to verify which infant lived and which infant died. Facilitating this process is important because it offers parents the only opportunity to care for this baby. As with other losses, providing mementos and keepsakes, speaking of the infant by name, and describing or comparing physical characteristics with those of the surviving sibling(s) are acknowledgements of the infant's existence and importance.

Encouraging communication between the parents is of extreme importance. Joint decisions about such issues as memorial services, and concerns over the surviving (and perhaps ill) sibling, are difficult because of the range of emotions involved. Working through feelings of guilt is a task that can be assisted by the primary nurse and physician through their repeated provision of information and reassurance about the normality of guilt feelings.

Following delivery, assistance for parents with the surviving infant(s) in a multiple gestation will differ, depending on the circumstances of the survivor(s). If the surviving sibling is in the NICU, the parents' response may range from severe anxiety to detached disinterest. The mother and father may also be at differing stages of emotional involvement. Continued, repeated information about the status of the surviving infant is important, and the mother should be taken for frequent visits with it while she is still hospitalized.

When the surviving infant is well, staff personnel may also see a wide range of parental interest in learning to care for it and attachment behaviors related to the infant. Acknowledging the normality of these behaviors and reactions on the part of the parents is important. Taking over care-giving tasks for the infant should be done according to the parent's need, acknowledging to them that it is sometimes difficult to form an attachment to a surviving infant.[22]

Anticipatory Guidance

In addition to giving guidance to parents who lose a singleton infant, care givers should prepare the parents to experience the following potential feelings or situations.

Anticipatory Guidance for Parents who Experience Loss in a Multiple Gestation

1. Normal nature of disappointment over the loss of excitement and prestige of having twins, triplets, or greater sets of offspring
2. Difficulty in telling friends and family about the loss—it can be helpful to ask a friend or family member to spread the word; parents may initially want to take someone with them who can provide explanations of their experience

(Continues)

---

3. Feelings of devaluation as a woman, as well as feelings of being punished for earlier ambivalence about the multiple pregnancy or the preference for a child of one sex over another
4. Friends and family may give excessive attention to the surviving infant; let them know of your need to grieve for lost infant also
5. Guilt about enjoying the surviving infant; consider a memorial service for the lost infant either before or at the same time as the surviving infant has a welcoming event
6. Ambivalence and guilt about not being able to care for your surviving infant; it is appropriate to ask for help in caring for your infant until you feel you can do this yourself
7. Birthdays and holidays will always be a reminder of your loss; discuss your feelings with your spouse on these occasions

---

Support groups and literature are available for this specific situation. The Center for Loss in Multiple Birth, Inc. (CLIMB) exists for parents who have experienced the death of one, both, or all of their children during a twin or higher multiple pregnancy, at birth or in infancy. Literature and other resources on such loss, including a quarterly newsletter, are available c/o Jean Kollantai, P.O. Box 1064, Palmer AK 99645.

IMPORTANCE OF EMOTIONAL CARE

Patients and their families who experience perinatal loss require care givers who will take their individual circumstances into consideration and guide their emotional as well as physical care accordingly. Although the interventions identified here have been helpful to many patients, it is of utmost importance to remember that not all families will benefit from a prescribed protocol for the loss of an infant. Listening to patients and taking direction from their cues will allow the necessary individualization to occur. Both nurses and physicians need to acknowledge that, although this aspect of obstetric practice is difficult, the emotional care provided in the labor-and-delivery area is crucial in assisting the patient and her family in the initial stages of the grief process.

REFERENCES

1. Woods J, Esposito J: Pregnancy Loss: Medical Therapeutics and Practical Considerations. Williams & Wilkins, Baltimore, 1987
2. Bowlby J: Attachment and Loss. Vol. 2. Basic Books, New York, 1980
3. Klaus M, Kennell J: Parent-Infant Bonding. 2nd Ed. CV Mosby, St. Louis, 1982
4. Kubler-Ross E: Questions and Answers on Death and Dying. Macmillan, New York, 1974
5. Bowlby J, Parkes CM: Separation and loss within the family. In Anthony EJ, Koupernik C (eds): The Child and His Family. John Wiley & Sons, New York, 1974
6. Davidson GW: Understanding Death of a Wished-for Child. OGR Service Corp, Springfield, IL, 1979
7. Raskin VD: Influence of ultrasound on parents' reaction to perinatal loss. Am J Psychiatry 146:1646, 1989
8. Gardner SL, Merenstein GB: Helping families deal with perinatal loss. Neonat Netw 5:17, 1986
9. Page-Lieberman J, Hughes CB: How fathers perceive perinatal death. MCN Am J Matern Child Nurs 15:320, 1990
10. Peppers LG, Knapp RJ: Maternal reactions to involuntary fetal/infant death. Psychiatry 43:155, 1980
11. Kirkley-Best E: Grief in response to perinatal loss: an argument for the earliest maternal attachment. Dissert Abstr Int 42:2560, 1981
12. Toedter LJ, Lasker JN, Alhadeff JM: The perinatal grief scale: development and initial validation. Am J Orthopsychiatry 58:435, 1988
13. Theut SK, Pedersen FA, Zaslow MA et al: Perinatal loss and perinatal bereavement. Am J Psychiatry 146:635, 1989
14. Gardner SL, Merenstein GB: Grief and perinatal loss. In Merenstein GB, Gardner SL (eds): Handbook of Neonatal Intensive Care. CV Mosby, St. Louis, 1985
15. Leon IG: Perinatal loss: a critique of current hospital practices. Clin Pediatr 31:366, 1992
16. Covington SN, Theut SK: Reactions to perinatal loss: a qualitative analysis of the national maternal and infant health survey. Am J Orthopsychiatry 63:215, 1993
17. Schwiebert P, Kirk P: When Hello Means Goodbye: A Guide for Parents Whose Child Dies at Birth or Shortly After. Perinatal Loss, Portland, OR, 1985
18. Zeanah CH: Adaptation following perinatal loss: a critical review. J Am Acad Child Adolesc Psychiatry 28:467, 1989
19. Wilson AL, Witzke D, Fenton LJ, Soule D et al: Parental response to perinatal death: mother-father differences. Am J Dis Child 139:1235, 1985
20. Kowalski K: No happy ending: pregnancy loss and bereavement: Nurse's Association of the American College of Obstetricians and Gynecologists Clinical Issues 2:368, 1991
21. Hendel J: The death of a twin. Bereavement Magazine July/August, p. 34, 1989
22. Johannsen L: As birth and death coincide. MCN Am J Maternal Child Nurs. 14:89, p. 34, 1989
23. Bryan EM: The death of a newborn twin: how can support for parents be improved? Acta Gen Med Gemellol (Rome) 35:115, 1986
24. Swanson-Kaufman K: There should have been two: nursing care of parents experiencing the perinatal death of a twin. J Perinat Neonatal Nurs 2:78, 1988

SUGGESTED READINGS

Harrigan, R, Naber MM, Jensen KA et al: Perinatal grief: response to the loss of an infant. Neonatal Netw 12:25, 1993

Menke JA, McClead RE: Perinatal grief and mourning: Adv Pediatr 37:261, 1990

Ryan PF, Cote-Arsenault D, Sugarman CC: Facilitating care after perinatal loss: a comprehensive checklist. J Obstet Gynecol Neonat Nurs 20:385, 1991

Szgalsky JB: Perinatal death, the family and the role of the health professional. Neonatal Netw 8:15, 1989

Appendix 33-1

Clinical Practice Guidelines: Collaborative Management of Patients Experiencing Perinatal Loss in the LDR(P) Setting

PURPOSE AND INTENT

These guidelines serve to describe general interventions and principles to be implemented by both primary nurses and physicians who care for patients and their families who experience a perinatal loss, recognizing that it requires willingness on the part of the care giver to be open to each patient's individual distress and to continue to learn about the wide range of responses to loss. It is intended to encourage a situation-specific approach.

SUPPORTIVE DATA

Perinatal bereavement occurs in all pregnancy loss, whether early or late in gestation, or involving the death of a neonate. Loss evokes personal and individual grief responses in patients. Perinatal loss may encompass not only that of the child but also of self-concept or self-esteem of mother, father, sister, brother, or grandparent. Research findings vary on grief intensity and exhibited behaviors for such variables as length of gestation and gender. In addition, usefulness of any given intervention generally found helpful in these situations, may be perceived differently based on culture, religion, previous losses, and coping patterns. Therefore regardless of when the loss occurs, all interventions should be guided by

> Individually attending to the needs of the particular family
>
> Careful consideration of what the loss means to each patient and family in this specific clinical context
>
> A supportive versus prescriptive approach in terms of choices offered by the care giver and acknowledgment of the range of grief responses exhibited by the patient and her family

GOALS AND EXPECTED OUTCOMES
During Hospitalization

> The patient and her family will be provided with a supportive environment throughout labor, delivery, and the postpartum period in order to assist them in working through initial grief stages
>
> The patient and her family will be provided with interventions based on their unique circumstance and personal choices in order to reestablish a sense of control and acknowledge their infant's existence
>
> The patient and her family will be provided with ongoing information, as they request it or are able to understand it, about the cause of death and their resulting feelings

At Discharge

> The patient and her family will be provided with information about how the grief process may progress for them and how others may react
>
> The patient and her family will be told of any follow-up information to be expected related to their infant's death
>
> The patient and her family will be given options for ongoing support

LABOR AND DELIVERY
Assessment

Identify factors that may contribute to individual grief reactions:

> Previous losses: type, timing, coping styles
>
> Prenatal attachment: investment, planning
>
> Nature of the current loss: unexpected versus anticipated, multiple gestation, multiple aspect of loss
>
> Cultural/religious influences
>
> Individual and family strengths

Interventions—General

Provide immediate, honest information if the baby is in distress or when death is known

Provide caring, supportive environment:
  Provide repeated explanations as requested, assure patients they are not at fault
  Acknowledge that guilt feelings are normal
  Express your own sorrow for their situation

Provide comfort measures to meet physical needs of mother and father

Avoid sedation

Principles and Key Points

Use simple explanations and terminology appropriate to mothers's/family's educational level. Involve both parents when any information is given.

Consider epidural analgesia if desired by patient and safe clinically

Sedation may alter grief work if the mother cannot remember labor and delivery. Also alters decision making and ability to choose whether to see or hold the infant after delivery

Presencing

Primary nurse and physician:
  Remain with parents and take parent's lead in wanting presence
  Remain available to answer questions and provide explanations as needed
  Listen to, understand, and respond to patients as individuals
  Encourage expression of feelings and respond in a supportive, nonjudgmental fashion, respecting individual coping styles

Principles and Key Points

Increased dependency may be exhibited, requiring professional presencing; patients may feel isolated if left by themselves

Anticipate diversity in grief reactions and the potential ventilation of a full range of emotions: sadness, anger, despair, humor

Offer Choices

Ask parents if they wish to see, hold, and touch infant after delivery

Allowing the infant who is alive but will die to remain with parents until death occurs

Prepare parents for what they will see, including color, size, bruises, abnormalities, and body temperature

Delay suggestion of an autopsy if parents are in the initial stages of shock and grief

Ask parent to choose postpartum location

Ask parents to consider disposition for fetus'/infants' remains

Extend visitation to other family members and allow them to see the infant, based on the parents' wishes

Ask parents if they wish to have clergy present at any time

Principles and Key Points

For some, making choices provides a sense of control over the situation

Respect the decision to not see, touch, or hold the infant; let parents know they may have the chance again if they reconsider

Recognize that persons experiencing initial grief exhibit both difficulty in decision-making and lucid periods; try to identify lucid periods for decision-making, and involve both mother and father in ongoing decisions

Respect the individuality of parents' unique situations, as well as cultural and religious influences on parental choices

Remain with the parents unless they ask for time alone

If one option is a non-maternity floor, nursing personnel on that floor should be knowledgeable and competent in dealing with perinatal loss

Acknowledge the Infant

Offer option of baptism

Identify characteristics of the infant that are either familial or unique

Speak of the infant by name if the parents have chosen one

Create memories, considering cultural, religious, and personal preferences and permission

> Provide photograph of the baby
>
> Provide remembrances such as footprints, baby bracelets, cap, a lock of hair

Offer opportunity to consider a memorial service for the baby, giving them time to make a decision

Express your sorrow

Principles and Key Points

Any Christian may perform this rite for the parents

If parents decline personal effects of the infant but are not opposed to them, tell them you will maintain and keep them indefinitely in the event they reconsider

---

POSTPARTUM AND DISCHARGE PREPARATION

Assessment

Identify grief behaviors exhibited by both parents

Identify parents ability to communicate with each other

Identify need for consultation: psychiatry, social work

Principles and Key Points

Somatic signs of grief may include shortness of breath, lethargy, sleep and appetite changes, feeling of "empty arms," anxiety, tachycardia

Understand the meaning of behaviors no matter how pathologic, and consider whether they promote or interfere with the grieving process

---

Interventions

Provide physical care to mother

Advise mother that lactation will occur

and assist her in choosing a suppression method

Do not isolate or avoid parents and family

Continue to acknowledge as mother, father, or parents

Call infant by given name when discussing plans for burial, disposition, and autopsy

Communicate situation to all staff and identify room with symbol or sign to alert other hospital personnel

---

Principles and Key Points

Providing consistent care givers is important

Prior to Discharge

Determine parents' wishes regarding autopsy and disposition of infant's remains

Provide parents with assistance as needed in making burial arrangements

Continue to give clear, factual explanations; repeat often

Provide consultation as appropriate

> Offer social work services as needed
>
> Consider psychiatric consultation if either parent expresses suicidal ideation

Provide anticipatory guidance on how the grief process may progress for parents, and how others may react

> Reactions of friends and family
>
> Examples of somatic manifestations of grief
>
> Examples of differences in partner responses to grief
>
> Indications for seeking help

Provide options for ongoing support:

> Inform of availability of support groups
>
> Provide with literature and references in addition to mementos and remembrances

Inform of plans for follow-up

> Autopsy report
>
> > Time frame for receiving and plans for informing of results
>
> Callback at 1 and 4 weeks after loss

Principles and Key Points

Take time with the patient; sit down in the room when discussing wishes and decisions

Maternal Mortality: An International Perspective

Timothy R. B. Johnson and
E. Y. Kwawukume

Labor and delivery are the critical periods leading to expulsion of the products of conception from the mother. Internationally, they remain a time of great risk to women. For the individual woman, the risk of dying from pregnancy is influenced by the risk associated with that pregnancy and by the number of times she becomes pregnant. Each time a woman becomes pregnant she runs the risk of maternal death, and this adds up over her lifetime.

The World Health Organization (WHO) estimates that there are 500,000 maternal deaths worldwide every year.[1] This is almost one death every minute. The vast majority of these deaths are in developing countries. While 25 percent of women of reproductive age live in developed countries, only 1 percent of maternal deaths take place in those countries.[2,3] The discrepancy between developed and developing countries is much greater for maternal deaths than for most other health problems.[4] In this chapter we use many illustrative examples from Ghana, since we believe the problems and issues they represent are universal.

Maternal mortalities are subdivided into direct and indirect obstetric deaths. Direct obstetric deaths are those resulting from obstetric complications of the pregnant state, prenatally, during labor, and in the puerperium. These can be due to omissions, incorrect treatment, interventions, or a cascade of events resulting from any of these three factors. Indirect obstetric deaths are those resulting from pre-existing diseases or diseases that develop during pregnancy and are aggravated by the physiologic effects of pregnancy. On average, three-quarters of maternal deaths in developing countries are direct obstetric deaths.[1] In Ghana and most other African countries, many direct maternal deaths occur toward term and during the intrapartum period in hospitals.[2] The loss of a woman at delivery is a traumatic event that can have far-reaching consequences for the bereaved family, who are not only confronted with her loss but also with the loss of their faith in modern medical care.

There are various unorthodox institutions competing with hospitals for delivery in Ghana, mainly "spiritual houses," fetish priests' houses, and quack doctors. These institutions manage both normal and complicated deliveries. Consequently, there is the need to implement measures that reduce maternal deaths in hospitals, especially during the last stages of labor, so as to restore faith in hospitals and attract more women for appropriate prenatal care and birth in a modern health-care system, including birth centers or hospitals. The aims of intrapartum care are

1. To achieve delivery of a normal healthy infant with minimal physiologic discomfort and maximal psychological satisfaction for the parents
2. To anticipate, recognize, and treat potentially ab-

normal conditions before significant hazard develops for the mother or the infant
3. To provide the mother and the father with a satisfactory and relaxed atmosphere for delivery of their infant, with competent midwives and obstetricians
4. To provide full technical back-up facilities, such as anesthetic, pediatric, and adequate blood bank facilities

In the attainment of these objectives, it is important to bear in mind that most mothers deliver healthy infants spontaneously with minimal assistance, and that they should be encouraged to regard labor as a natural physiologic function. However, a significant minority fail to achieve this goal, even though they have no apparent problems at the onset of labor. This shows the constant need for supervision and the ready availability of staff and facilities for active intervention when it is required. In fact, the premise that labor is a natural physiologic function that should not be subject to interference has been challenged since time immemorial, based on recognition of the unnecessary loss of maternal and fetal life. Many current policies of intervention, such as the use of oxytocic agents to stimulate uterine activity, and the use of obstetric forceps, had their origins two or more centuries ago for improving the quality of intrapartum care.[5]

Korle-Bu Teaching Hospital, in the southern part of Ghana, has a delivery rate of about 10,000 infants per year. The hospital serves mainly as a referral (tertiary care) center for most high-risk pregnant women referred from other hospitals for labor and delivery. It also cares for most of the normal pregnant women in the capital city of Accra, which has a population of about 1.2 million people.

At Korle-Bu Teaching Hospital, it has been noticed that intrapartum, antenatal, and postpartum care are complementary to one another when maternal health is considered. Good intrapartum care may correlate positively with good antenatal supervision, and laxity in antenatal management has tremendous impact on the intrapartum care seen at the hospital. Some mortalities from sickle cell disease, preeclampsia, and anemia in patients who die during the intrapartum period are due to poor antenatal care. Although the antenatal service coverage continues to improve, expanding from 65 percent in 1988 to 90 percent in 1991, there has been a decrease in the average number of visits paid by each woman during her pregnancy, from 2.9 to 2.6 visits.[6]

The maternal mortality in Ghana is estimated to be 390 per 100,000 population.[6] Higher figures are seen in referral hospitals, as in Korle-Bu Teaching Hospital and the School of Medical Sciences in Kumasi.[7] These figures are higher because of the moribund cases referred late to these hospitals from the various districts. Although maternal mortality is due to multifactorial causes, there are institutional factors responsible for the delays in the management of obstetric emergencies, especially such direct emergencies as hemorrhage, pre-eclampsia/eclampsia, and sickle cell crisis.

Intrapartum maternal mortality accounts for about 34.1 percent of all maternal deaths at Korle-BU Teaching Hospital. These are mainly preventable deaths and are due to (1) inefficient blood supply; (2) organizational structure; (3) ancillary diagnostic support; (4) anesthetic cover; and (5) management of labor.

INEFFICIENT BLOOD SUPPLY

Korle-Bu Teaching Hospital consumes about 10,000 to 13,000 U of blood each year. Eighty percent is consumed by women and children. Statistics from the national blood bank show only 25 to 30 percent of voluntary blood donors.

As seen in Table 34-1, the major cause of maternal mortality in Ghana is hemorrhage, and at Korle-Bu Teaching Hospital, hemorrhage accounts for about 40.2 percent of intrapartum maternal deaths. These are due to lack of adequate quantities of blood for prompt transfusion and inefficient blood bank facilities. Compounding the problems posed by hemorrhage is the poor response of husbands or relatives of patient in donating blood willingly in a crisis. With the advent of human immunodeficiency virus (HIV) and acquired immunodeficiency syndrome (AIDS), few volunteers are willing to donate blood, and as a result there is difficulty in securing blood at the appropriate time. Even in centers in which blood is available, relatives often have to deposit some amount of money before the blood is cross-matched. Invariably, poor patients from the villages cannot

Table 34-1. Causes of Maternal Mortality

| | No. of Cases | | | | |
	1991	1992	1993	Total	%
Sickle cell diseases	17	7	16	40	15.7
Abortion	10	5	18	33	12.9
Ectopic pregnancy	6	4	4	14	5.5
Postpartum hemorrhage	12	7	15	34	13.3
Placental abruption	4	3	6	13	5.1
Antepartum hemorrhage	5	—	1	6	2.3
Sepsis	3	3	5	11	4.3
Pre-eclampsia	8	3	6	17	6.7
Eclampsia	14	3	11	28	11.0
Ruptured uterus	1	2	4	7	2.7
Obstructed labor	1	1	4	6	2.3
Severe anemia	6	2	6	14	5.5
Anesthesia	—	—	1	1	0.4
Others	15	3	13	31	12.2
Maternal deaths	102	43	110	255	100
Maternal mortality	10.6	4.7	9.6	8.4	
Total live births	9,630	9,135	11,496	30,261	

readily afford such amounts and have to wait for long periods before blood transfusion takes place. The process of waiting ends with maternal death. A simple remedy would be to have a blood refrigerator near the delivery units so that blood and blood products could be stored for immediate use.

ORGANIZATIONAL STRUCTURES

There is no legislation banning unsupervised deliveries in Ghana. The institutional delivery rate is low, amounting to about 30 percent.[6] Trained and untrained traditional birth attendants (TBAs) are being used as stopgap personnel, but do not have the scientific skills needed to cope with modern trends in obstetrics. The untrained TBAs are the spiritual leaders, fetish priests, and herbalists. Trained TBAs get some knowledge from programs sponsored by the Ministry of Health. These TBAs deliver over 70 percent of infants, but hardly provide adequate statistics. It was estimated by a Ghana-U.S. Agency for International Development (USAID) pilot project begun in 1970 in the Danfa region of Ghana that there are 730 TBAs per 100,000 population compared to 9 physicians and 91 nurses for every

100,000 people. TBAs interviewed in the Ashanti-Akim district of Ghana claimed that they deliver from two to four newborns per month, sometimes more. A total of 29 TBAs serve 18 villages in the district. In most villages there are at least two TBAs, and as many as six or seven in others.[8] The national figure on TBAs has increased remarkably, In 1990, 1,364 TBAs were trained. This number rose to 5,587 in 1993, an increase of 75.9 percent.[9] The TBAs form an essential group for basic training, with the goals of updating their knowledge so that they can identify at-risk groups for early referral and work in a hygienic environment during delivery.

Ghana now has 60 obstetricians. About 95 percent of them are in the cities, mainly Accra and Kumasi, and none in the rural areas. This is also the trend seen in other West African countries.[10]

In the regions in which there are competent obstetricians and midwives, most of the complicated referral labor cases are handled first by the most junior physicians. These physicians might not have been exposed to a sufficient number of obstetric emergencies, and are therefore not sufficiently confident to handle these challenging cases.

There are also trained doctors in obstetric units who are not interested in midwifery. A safer measure would be to have staffing subdivisions, as seen in some industrialized countries such as the United States, where the hospitals have a separate maternal and fetal unit on which both trained and trainee-obstetricians interested in midwifery work together to improve the quality of care.

ANCILLARY DIAGNOSTIC SUPPORT

Intrapartum untrasonography is an important tool in the management of patients with antepartum hemorrhage (APH) during labor. Ultrasonography is not a routine procedure, and therefore, patients arrive in labor bleeding without a clear-cut diagnosis of the type of their APH. Patients are therefore booked for examination under anesthesia (EUA) to rule out placenta previa, a process that can provoke more bleeding. The introduction of ultrasonography at Korle Bu has saved time as well as anesthetic agents and operating room manpower.

There is a need for intrapartum testing of hemoglobin, sickling, white blood cell (WBC) count, and urine, which are lacking in most hospitals, especially during the night. Tests for coagulation profiles are not readily available, and therefore the reliability in differentiating disseminated intravascular coagulation (DIC) from severe placental abruption, for example, is low. About 5 percent of the maternal mortality in Ghana from 1991 to 1993 was due to placental abruption, and about 2 percent developed renal failure. Facilities for such testing, if available, would enhance the clinical accuracy in the management of intrapartum care.

Lack of potent intravenous antibiotics and antihypertensive drugs increases intrapartum maternal mortality in the developing world. Patients who have ruptured membranes for more than 24 hours with sepsis may not get antibiotic coverage during labor. They therefore go through labor with overwhelming infection, ending with maternal and fetal death. The management of eclamptic patients does not follow any sound protocol apart from that in the medical schools. Even here, treatment with agents such as hypotensive drugs and anticonvulsants may represent a problem. Some patients arrive in our labor wards in good time for treatment to be begun, but have to wait for hours without treatment because of shortages of essential drugs. Some relatives are sent out to commercial pharmacies to purchase these drugs before procedures are performed. As shown in Table 34-2, 19.6 percent of 87 intrapartum deaths, were due to eclampsia/PET from cerebral hemorrhage and renal failure, most of which could have been prevented with good intrapartum management. If labor wards can be sufficiently supplied with these drugs, deaths from sepsis and pre-eclampsia would be markedly reduced.

Table 34-2. Intrapartum Deaths

	1991	1992	1993	Total	%
Sickle cell disease	5	3	4	12	13.8
Postpartum hemorrhage	9	3	10	22	25.3
Placental abruption	4	2	4	10	11.5
Antepartum hemorrhage	2	—	1	3	3.4
Sepsis	1	1	1	3	3.4
Pre-eclampsia	4	—	3	7	8.1
Eclampsia	4	1	5	10	11.5
Ruptured uterus	1	1	2	4	4.6
Obstructed labor	1	—	2	3	3.5
Others	4	1	2	7	8.1
Anemia	2	1	3	6	6.9
Total intrapartum deaths	37	13	37	87	100

ANESTHESIA COVERAGE

Most labor wards in Ghana do not have 24-hour anesthesia coverage. Anesthetists are not readily available in the labor wards for emergency interventions. Cases of ruptured uterus and third-trimester bleeding may have to wait for hours before surgery. Obviously, bleeding can become significant under such circumstances, with worsening of the patient's condition before operations are done.

General anesthesia is used in the developing world in all types of major surgery during labor. This sometimes results in failed intubation, aspiration, and death. In addition, pethidine is the main analgesic employed to relieve pain in labor. This drug diminishes gastric motility and makes vomiting more likely. There is a potential risk of aspiration, especially when the patient has eaten before entering labor. Epidural anesthesia, which is not common in most of the developing world, would be beneficial. Laboring patients who need surgery can easily be shifted to the operating table without wasting time or, with epidural anesthesia, being in danger of aspiration.[11]

MANAGEMENT OF LABOR

With the introduction of the partograph, prolonged labor and its complications are on the decline; yet Ghana had approximately 3.5 percent of intrapartum deaths from obstructed labor between 1991 and 1993. This shows that intrapartum monitoring is inadequate. Certainly a few cases may need more sensitive inputs (e.g., scalp electrodes for pH and blood gas measurement) that are not currently available.

Previously scarred uteruses might benefit more from internal pressure monitors, especially in tertiary care hospitals, to reduce the incidence of both uterine rupture and cesarean section, which have a higher maternal mortality rate than vaginal delivery.[12] However, considering the many basic facilities lacking in our labor wards, it would probably be beneficial to have in-service training for both physicians and the nursing staff in the management of labor with the partograph, rather than advanced facilities such as cardiotocography[13] (Fig. 34-1).

Practice behavior also contributes gravely to the increasing maternal death rate. Some herbalists use preparations containing croton species that have very powerful uterotonic effects. With sustained contractions, uterine rupture has been the sequela, especially in the northern parts of Ghana. The dosages of active agents in these herbal preparations are not standardized. There is a general shortage of nurses in our labor wards, and high-risk patients do not get the attention given in the developed world. In addition, the number of patients presenting in labor

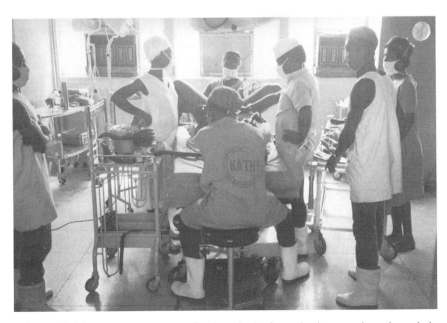

Fig. 34-1. Labor and delivery management suffer from lack of standard protocols and needed equipment.

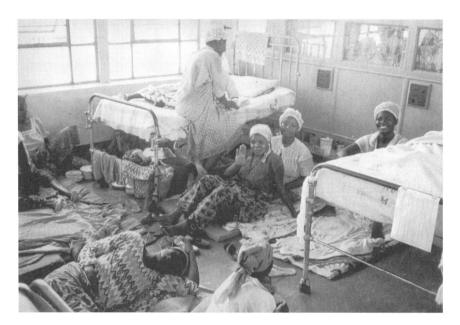

Fig. 34-2. Maternity facilities are overcrowded and understaffed.

is overwhelming, with some laboring on the floor without proper attention and management (Fig. 34-2). Many of the patients that arrive in labor already have serious complications. For one reason or another, some women choose to labor in the home or with relatives until they become exhausted.

SAFE MOTHERHOOD INITIATIVE

The foregoing factors led to the international Safe Motherhood Initiative and specific goals and objectives for the year 2000, with a specific goal of reducing maternal mortality by half. The Safe Motherhood Initiative* focuses on three key areas:

1. Expanding and strengthening maternal health services, including community-based care and backup and support at the first level of referral for women who require skilled obstetric care
2. Increasing access to family planning services
3. Improving women's cultural and legal status and their access to educational and economic opportunities

* For more information about Safe Motherhood, including receipt of regular newsletters, or to received specific information about the partograph, write to The Division of Family Health, World Health Organization, 1211 Geneva 27 Switzerland.

In addition, the WHO has proposed the concept of levels of referral. The introduction of these levels of referral requires more than medical competencies and personnel alone, but also major social and political actions to provide accessibility and transportation for women to these sites of care.

As outlined by the WHO in its documents on level of referral, maternal health services should be designed to provide therapeutic and preventive interventions during pregnancy, skilled care during labor and delivery, and back-up referral services for high-risk patients and complicated cases. The minimal module for maternal health care should include three elements[15]:

1. Community-based services that should reach every pregnant woman
2. Levels of first referral services to provide obstetric care for high-risk patients and to deal with complications
3. Effective linkage between the two levels of care, including two-way communications and referrals

In addition, communication and referral to hospitals (tertiary care) should be available from levels of first referral. As recommended by the WHO, the "essential obstetric functions at the first referral level" should include the following elements:

1. Surgical care, including facilities for performing cesarean sections, surgical treatment of sepsis, repair of ruptured uterus, and management of ectopic pregnancy
2. Anesthesia
3. Medical treatment for complications such as pregnancy-induced hypertension, diabetes, heart disease, and other medical conditions associated with pregnancy
4. Blood replacement in cases of hemorrhage and severe anemia
5. Manual and/or assessment functions for retained placenta and other obstetric complications
6. Family planning functions to provide devices that cannot be fitted at primary health-care clinics
7. Management of women at high risk, comprising patients identified on enrollment at the antenatal clinic or for indications that become evident in the course of pregnancy or labor

REGIONALIZATION IN THE UNITED STATES

The United States has regionalized obstetric and neonatal care into primary, secondary, and tertiary levels that at first glance seem quite different from the WHO levels of referral. The higher technology and availability of maternal transport, and the direction of fetuses to tertiary and even quarternary (heart transplants, fetal surgery, genetic therapy) levels of care have led to the proliferation of neonatal intensive care units (NICUs). These units have been copied in the developing world.

Regionalization of care in the United States was based on tertiary centers, which not only had the facilities to provide complex and sophisticated patient care, but also assumed regional responsibilities for transportation, high-risk patient education, research, and quality control. Similar standards could be introduced at the community, first referral, and consultant levels proposed by WHO. The American College of Obstetricians and Gynecologists (ACOG) and the American Academy of Pediatrics (AAP)[12] have developed recommended guidelines and standards, which are presented as potential models.

NCOG/AAP Guidelines[†]
Medical Staff
Level I

The perinatal care program at a level I hospital should be co-ordinated jointly by the chiefs of the obstetric and pediatric services. In hospitals that do not have separate departments of pediatrics and obstetrics, one physician may be given the responsibility for co-ordinating perinatal care. This administrative approach requires close co-ordination and unified policy statements. Responsibilities of the co-ordinator(s) of perinatal care at a level I hospital include policy development, maintenance of standards of care, collaboration with the nursing department, and consultation with staff at those hospitals providing level II and level III care in the region.

A qualified physician or a certified nurse-midwife (CNM) should attend all deliveries. When CNMs are involved in patient care, their specific role should be delineated by departmental rules and regulations.

Hospitals should ensure the availability of skilled personnel for perinatal emergencies. Anesthesia personnel with credentials for administering obstetric anesthesia should be readily available. At least one person capable of initiating neonatal resuscitation should be present at every delivery. One or two other persons should be available for an emergency resuscitation.

Level II

A board-certified obstetrician with special interest, experience, and in some situations special competency certification in maternal-fetal medicine should be the chief of the obstetric service at a level II hospital. A board-certified pediatrician with special interest, experience, and in some situations subspecialty certification in neonatal medicine should be the chief of the newborn care service. These physicians should co-ordinate the hospital's perinatal care services and, in conjunction with other medical, nursing, and hospital administration staff, develop policies concerning staffing, routine procedures, equipment, and supplies. Small or high-risk neonates should be managed by appropriately qualified

---

[†] From Guidelines for Perinatal Care,[12] with permission.

physicians. The general pediatrician should have the expertise to assume responsibility for the acute, although less critical, care of the infant; understand the need for proper continuity of care and be capable of providing it; and share responsibility with the neonatologist for the development and delivery of effective services for newborns at risk in the hospital and community. Management may be provided by qualified neonatal nurse-practitioners in collaboration with the physician.

The director of obstetric anesthesia services should be board-certified and should have training and experience in obstetric anesthesia. Anesthesia personnel with credentials to administer obstetric anesthesia should be readily available. Policies regarding the provision of obstetric anesthesia, including the necessary qualifications of personnel who are to administer anesthesia and their availability for both routine and emergency deliveries, should be developed. The hospital staff should also include a radiologist and, ideally, a clinical pathologist who are available 24 hours a day. Specialized medical and surgical consultation should be readily available.

Level III

Ideally, the director of the maternal-fetal medicine service at a level III hospital should be a full-time, board-certified obstetrician with special competency certification in maternal-fetal medicine. The director of the regional NICU should be a full-time, board-certified pediatrician with subspecialty certification in neonatal medicine. As co-directors of the perinatal service, these physicians are responsible for the maintenance of standards of care, development of the operating budget, evaluation and purchase of equipment, planning and development of in-hospital and outreach educational programs, coordination of these activities, and evaluation of the effectiveness of perinatal care in the region. They should devote their time to patient-care services, research, and teaching, and they should coordinate the services provided at their hospital with those provided at level I and level II hospitals in the region.

Other maternal-fetal medicine specialists and neonatologists who practice in the level III facility should have qualifications similar to those of the chief of their service. There should be one neonatologist for every 6 to 10 patients in the continuing

care, intermediate care, and intensive care areas. A ration of one physician (including residents or fellows) or one neonatal nurse-practitioner to every four or five patients who require intensive care is ideal for routine daily management. A maternal-fetal medicine specialist and a neonatologist should be readily available for consultation 24 hours a day. Personnel qualified to manage any obstetric or neonatal emergencies should be in house.

Obstetric and neonatal diagnostic imaging, provided by obstetricians or radiologists who have special interest and competence in maternal and neonatal disease and its complications, should be available 24 hours a day. Pediatric subspecialists in cardiology, neurology, hematology, and genetics should be available for consultation. Consultant services in renal function, metabolism, endocrinology, gastroenterology and nutrition, infectious diseases, pulmonary function, immunology, and pharmacology are also needed. In addition, pediatric surgical subspecialists (e.g., neurosurgeons and cardiovascular orthopedic, ophthalmologic, urologic, and otolaryngologic surgeons) should be available for consultation and care. Pathologists with special competency in placental, fetal, and neonatal disease should also be members of the level III hospital staff.

A board-certified anesthesiologist with special training or experience in maternal-fetal anesthesia should be in charge of obstetric anesthesia services at a level III hospital. Personnel with credentials to administer obstetric anesthesia should be available in the hospital. Personnel with credentials to administer neonatal and pediatric anesthesia should be available as required.

Nursing Staff

Delivery of safe and effective perinatal nursing care requires appropriately qualified nurses in adequate numbers to meet the needs of each patient in accordance with the care setting. The number of staff and level of skill required are influenced by the scope of nursing practice and degree of nursing responsibilities within an institution. Nursing responsibilities in individual hospitals vary according to the level of care provided, prescribed practice procedures, number of professional and ancillary staff, and professional nursing activities in continuing education and research. Intrapartum care requires the same labor intensiveness and expertise as on any other intensive care unit, and accordingly should be allocated adequate training and fiscal support.

Changing trends in medical management and technologic advances influence and may increase the nursing workload. Each hospital should determine the scope of nursing practice for each of its nursing units and specialty departments. A multidisciplinary committee composed of representatives from the hospital, medical, and nursing administrations should follow published professional standards and guidelines, consult state nursing practice acts, identify the types and numbers of procedures performed, and identify activities that are performed by non-nursing personnel.

Recommended nurse/patient ratios for perinatal services are shown in Table 34-3. Additional personnel are necessary for indirect patient care activities. Close evaluation of all factors involved in a specific

Table 34-3. Recommended Nurse/Patient Ratios for Perinatal Care Services

Staffing Ratio	Care Provided
1:1–2	Antepartum testing
1:2	Laboring patients
1:1	Patients in second stage of labor
1:1	Ill patients with complications
1:2	Oxytocin induction or augmentation of labor
1:1	Coverage for initiating epidural anesthesia
1:1	Circulation for cesarean delivery
1:6	Antepartum/postpartum patients without complications
1:2	Postoperative recovery
1:3	Patients with complications, but in stable condition
1:4	Recently born infants and those needing close observation
1:6–8	Newborns needing only routine care
1:3–4	Normal mother-newborn couplet care
1:3–4	Newborns requiring continuing care
1:2–3	Newborns requiring intermediate care
1:1–2	Newborns needing intensive care
1:1	Newborns requiring multisystem support
>1:1	Unstable newborns requiring complex critical care

case is essential in establishing an acceptable nurse/patient ratio. Variables such as type of patient, patient turnover, acuity of patients' conditions, patient or parent education needs, bereavement care, mixture of skills of the staff, environment, types of delivery, and use of anesthesia must be taken into account in determining appropriate nurse/patient ratios.

Level I

The perinatal care program at a level I hospital should be under the direction of a registered nurse. Responsibilities include directing perinatal nursing services, guiding the development and implementation of perinatal policies and procedures, collaborating with the medical staff, and consulting with hospitals providing level II and level III care in the region.

Nursing personnel in each perinatal care area, or in combined areas, should be under the direct supervision of a registered nurse. Nursing responsibilities include psychologically and physically preparing the patient and family, applying and monitoring technology, interpreting information and responding appropriately, maintaining an accurate record, and making referrals as necessary. Nursing personnel should be able to identify deviations from normal physiology, especially perinatal emergencies; to institute appropriate actions; and to communicate pathophysiologic processes to primary care providers.

Whenever there are patients in labor in the hospital, the hospital should ensure that a registered nurse is in attendance who has both training and clinical competency in perinatal nursing; can evaluate the condition of the mother, fetus, and neonate; and can assess the degree of risk to which they are subject during labor, delivery, and the neonatal period.

Level II

Each of the obstetric and neonatal patient care areas in a level II hospital should have a head nurse with training and clinical competence in perinatal/neonatal nursing and nursing administration. In addition, specialty certification is highly desirable for all nurse managers, who are responsible for the management of the unit and for supervision of the direct nursing care provided.

In addition to the nursing responsibilities identified in the section on level I hospitals, nursing staff in the labor, delivery, and recovery areas of the level II hospital should be especially able to identify and respond to the obstetric and medical complications of pregnancy, labor, and delivery. Furthermore, the nursing staff of the intermediate care nursery in a level II hospital should be able to monitor and maintain the stability of cardiopulmonary, metabolic, and thermal functions; assist with special procedures, such as lumbar punctures, endotracheal intubation, umbilical vessel catheterization; and exchange transfusion; and perform emergency resuscitation. Nursing staff in this area should be specially trained and able to initiate, modify, or stop treatment when appropriate, even if a physician or neonatal nurse-practicioner is not present according to established protocols. In those units in which neonates receive mechanical ventilation, there is the need for continuous availability of appropriately trained staff who have demonstrated the ability to intubate the trachea, manage mechanical ventilation, and decompress a pneumothorax. These activities may be performed by advanced-practice neonatal nurses. The unit's medical director should supervise the delegated medical acts, processes, and procedures performed by advanced-practice neonatal nurses.

Level III

It is highly desirable for the director/supervisor and head nurses of perinatal nursing services in level III hospitals to not only have training and clinical competence in perinatal/neonatal nursing care, but also specialty certification. The obstetric and neonatal patient care areas should each have a head nurse director responsible for management of the unit and supervision of direct patient care. These nurse managers should have at least a nursing baccalaureate degree.

The nursing staff in each perinatal care area, or in combined areas, should have specialty certification or advanced training and experience in the nursing management of both low-risk and high-risk patients and their families. Nursing staff should also be especially experienced in caring for the obstetric and medical complications of pregnancy or the neonatal period, or both.

The nursing staff in the NICU should have specialty certification or advanced training and experience in the nursing management of the high-risk neonates and their families. Nursing staff should also be experienced in caring for unstable neonates with multisystem problems, and in specialized care technology. A staff comprised entirely of professional registered nurses is preferable. A clinical nurse specialist should be available for consultation and support to the staff for nursing care issues. Additional nurses with special training are required to fulfill regional center responsibilities, such as outreach and transport.

Support Personnel

All Levels

A blood bank technician should always be available for determining blood type, cross-matching blood, and performing Coombs tests. The hospital's infection control personnel should be responsible for surveillance of infections in mothers and neonates, as well as for the development of an appropriate environmental control program. A radiology technician should be readily available 24 hours a day to perform chest radiography. The need for other support personnel depends on the intensity and level of sophistication of the other support services provided. An organized plan of action, including personnel and equipment, for identification and immediate resuscitation should be established.

Levels II and III

The following support personnel should be available in the perinatal care service of level II and level III hospitals[12]:

> At least one full-time medical social worker who has experience with the socioeconomic and psychosocial problems of high-risk mothers and fetuses, sick neonates, and their families (additional medical social workers may be required if the patient load is heavy)
>
> At least one occupational or physical therapist with neonatal expertise
>
> At least one registered dietician/nutritionist who has special training in perinatal nutrition and can plan diets that meet the special needs of high-risk mothers and neonates

Qualified personnel for support services such as laboratory studies, radiologic studies, and ultrasound examinations (these personnel should be readily available 24 hours a day)

Respiratory therapists or nurses with special training who can supervise the assisted ventilation of neonates with cardiopulmonary disease (optimally, one therapist is needed for each four neonates who are receiving assisted ventilation)

The hospital's engineering department should include air-conditioning, electronic, and mechanical engineers as well as biomedical technicians, who are responsible for the safety and reliability of the equipment in all perinatal care areas.

INTERNATIONAL STANDARDS FOR INTRAPARTUM CARE

While the United States and other countries have led the way in regionalization, and similar guidelines and protocols may serve policy makers and planners internationally, there remain many areas of inconsistency in intrapartum care. The introduction of a standardized prenatal record has clearly improved prenatal and intrapartum management in countries of Western Europe, and yet only recently have ACOG prenatal records become available and increasingly accepted in the United States. Clearly, such records permit rapid transfer of information and patients between the various levels of care when problems occur.

The WHO introduced the partogram, or labor curve, as a management tool for prevention of abnormal labor.[14] The partogram has been described and used since the early 1970s in a variety of settings and contents. The excellent WHO partograph is published with a series of user tools, including section I, describing the principle and strategy of the technique: section 2, a user's manual; section 3, consisting of guidelines for operational research; and section 4, a facilitator's guide. It appears that routine use of the WHO partograph could be recommended in all labor-and-delivery centers. The simplified WHO partograph could be introduced by decision makers at the ministry of health as well as to leaders

of the medical and nursing profession in any country and its teaching hospitals (Fig. 34-3). Medical and midwifery schools should be encouraged to teach the principles and use of the partograph in their curriculum. TBAs and other health-care providers should also be involved, since the partograph can be included in the training program provided for them by their local health systems. Access to the partograph, suction bulbs, and hygienic technology can serve to link TBAs with their support system and improve the perception of "technologic medicine" in the community. In countries in which nurse midwives and traditional birth attendants have close relationships, early transfer (e.g., after 12 hours) has been recommended.

The partograph can serve a different purpose or function at different levels of care.[16] At the peripheral site it is used to provide early warning that labor is prolonged and that the woman should be transferred to a hospital. In the hospital setting, movement to the right of the alert line gives a warning and actualizes the critical point at which amniotomy, pitocin, or consultation can be implemented.

We believe the time is right to consider international guidelines and standards for intrapartum care, including

Levels of referral/regionalization

A common record

The partograph

Standard drug lists

Standard instrument and technology lists

Protocols for management

Protocols for blood availability

Lessons can be learned from the community health initiatives in the developing world, as well as from the managed-care/health-care reform initiatives in the United States.

Maternal mortality is an international disgrace.[13] The Safe Motherhood Initiative has identified strategies to reduce this mortality by developing regionalized levels of referral and introducing the partogram. We are approaching an era when rapid information exchange, facsimile communication, computerization, CD-ROM libraries, and other tech-

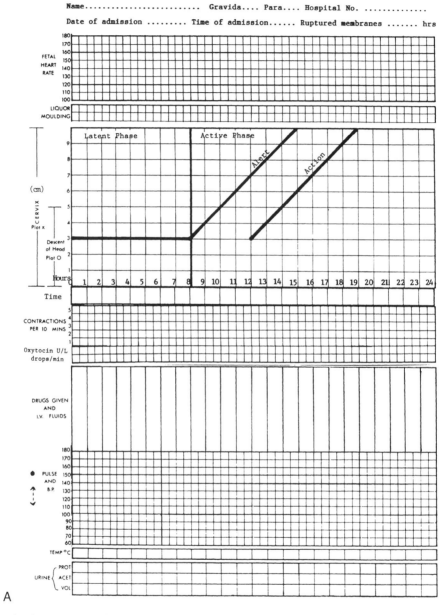

Fig. 34-3. (A & B) Partograph (labor curve) developed by the WHO for introduction and dissemination with extensive supporting educational materials. (From the World Health Organization,[14] with permission.) *(Figure continues.)*

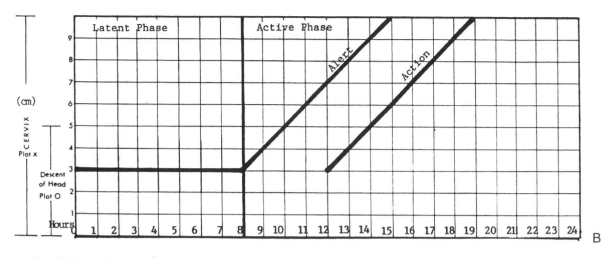

Fig. 34-3. *(Continued).*

nologies will permit us to consider international standards for obstetric services. These might include common records, and management protocols, including the partogram and standard equipment and drug lists. Despite local differences, much can be accomplished by recognizing the similar issues in intrapartum care faced throughout the world, and coming together to develop shared and often common solutions for them.

REFERENCES

1. Prevention of Maternal Mortality: Report of a World Health Organization Interregional Meeting, November 11–15, 1985. (FHE/86.1) World Health Organization, Geneva, 1986
2. Starrs A: Preventing the tragedy of maternal deaths: a report of the International Safe Motherhood Conference, Nairobi, February, 1987. World Bank, Washington, DC, 1987
3. United Nations 1987 World Contraceptive Use. United Nations, Population Division, Department of International Economic and Social Affairs, New York, 1987
4. United Nations Population Chart 1988. United Nations, Population Division, Department of International Economic and Social Affairs, New York, 1988
5. Maine D et al: Prevention of maternal deaths in developing countries: program options and practical considerations. Presented at the International Safe Motherhood Conference, Nairobi, February 10–13, 1987
6. Maternal and Child Health/Family Planning. Annual Report. Ministry of Health, Accra, Ghana, 1991
7. Martey JO, Djan JO, Twum ENL et al: Maternal mortality due to hemorrhage in Ghana. Int J Gynecol Obstet 42:237, 1993
8. Ashanti-Akim District Profile, Ministry of Health, Kumasi, Ghana. January 1980
9. National TBA Training Program, MCH/FP Division. Ministry of Health Statistical Report, Accra, Ghana, January, 1994
10. Omu AE: Traditional midwives in Nigeria. Lancet 1: 620, 1981
11. Okonofua FE, Makinde ON, Ayangade SO: Yearly trends in cesarean section and cesarean mortality at IIe-ife, Nigeria. Trop J Obstet Gynecol (special edition) 1:31, 1988
12. Guidelines for Perinatal Care. 3rd Ed. American Academy of Pediatrics and American College of Obstetricians and Gynecologists, Washington, DC, 1992
13. Lawson JB: The bight of Benin and beyond: reflections on obstetrics in the developing world. Int J Gynecol Obstet 34:101, 1990
14. The Partograph: a managerial tool for the prevention of prolonged labour. World Health Organization Maternal and Child Health Unit, Division of Family Health, Geneva, 1988
15. Fauvaeau V, Stewart K, Khan SA, Chakraborty J: Effect on mortality of community-based maternity-care programme in rural Bangladesh. Lancet 338:1183, 1991
16. Seffah JD, Amaniampong K, Wilson JB: The use of the partograph in monitoring labor in a prior cesarean section, letter. Int J Gynecol Obstet 45:281, 1994

Index

Page numbers followed by *f* indicate figures; those followed by *t* indicate tables.

A

"The Abused Woman," 504

Academy of Pediatrics, *Guidelines for Perinatal Care* of, 8

Accreditation, of nurse-midwifery programs, 46

Acid-base balance, fetal
fetal heart rate correlated with, 372t, 372–373
physiology of, 403–406, 404f, 405t, 406t

Acidemia, fetal. *See* Fetal acidosis.

Acidosis, fetal. *See* Fetal acidosis.

Active management of labor, 419–429
cesarean section and, 426–429, 428t
duration of labor and, 429
outcomes of, 429
principles of, 420–423
childbirth education and, 423
diagnosis and, 420
dystocia and, 421
one-to-one nursing care and, 421
oxytocin administration and, 421
population and, 420
progress during first stage of labor and, 421, 422f
progress during second stage of labor and, 421
rupture of membranes and, 420–421
safety of, 423f, 423–426, 424t–426t

Active phase of labor, disorders of, 93–95
active phase arrest, 94–95
protracted active phase, 93–94, 96–97, 97t

Acute renal failure (ARF), placental abruption causing, 210

Acyclovir
for herpes simplex infections, 476
for varicella-zoster infections, 477

Adenocarcinomas, following episiotomy, 494

Admission criteria
for in-hospital birth units, 58
for obstetric intensive care units, 242

β-Adrenergic agonists
for asthma, 322t, 323
acute, 328–329
chronic, 326
for placental abruption, 210–211

β-Adrenergic blocking agents, for chronic hypertension, 268–269, 269t

α₂-Adrenergic-receptor agonists
for cesarean section, 41–42
for vaginal delivery, 37

β-Adrenergic tocolytic agents, 281–285, 297–304
fetal-neonatal side effects of, 302–304
maternal physiologic effects of, 297–299
maternal side effects of, 284–285, 299–302
for preterm labor, 281–285, 284t
clinical efficacy of, 282–283
clinical use of, 283–285, 284t
mechanisms of action of, 281–282

Advanced practice skills, for nurse-midwives, 61–62

AFLP syndrome, differentiation from HELLP syndrome, 265t

Africa, maternal mortality in. *See* Maternal mortality, in Ghana.

Airway management, during general anesthesia, 42

Albuterol, for asthma, 322t, 323

Alcohol abuse
placental abruption caused by, 208
screening for, 501–502

Alexandria unit, 81

Ambulation, for active phase arrest, 94–95

American Academy of Pediatrics (AAP), standards of, 547

American College of Nurse-Midwives (ACNM), 46

Standards for the Practice of Nurse-Midwifery of, 48–49

American College of Obstetricians and Gynecologists (ACOG)
"The Abused Woman" published by, 504
Guidelines for Perinatal Care of, 8
standards of, 49, 547

American Medical Association, opposition to Sheppard-Towner Maternity and Infant Protection Act, 8

Amino acid solutions, for amniotransfusion, 396

Aminoglycosides, for postpartum endometritis, 474, 475

Aminophylline, for asthma, 322t, 323–324
acute, 329

Amniocentesis
in chorioamnionitis, 470
genetic, in multiple gestations, 125–126
for polyhydramnios, 128
in preterm labor, 279
for pulmonary maturity, in multiple gestations, 130
safety of, in multiple gestations, 125–126

Amniotic fluid
egress of, 389–390
fetal swallowing and, 389
fluid movement across membranes and, 389
maternal hydration and, 389–390
ferning of, 77, 79f
fluxes of, 387–388
modulation of volume of, 390–396
hemodynamic modification for, 390–392
intrapartum amniotransfusion for, 392t, 392–396
production of, 388–389
fetal micturition and, 388–389
pulmonary secretion and, 389
volume during labor, 390